Best Practices

Evidence-Based Nursing Procedures

SECOND EDITION

Best Practices

Evidence-Based Nursing Procedures

SECOND EDITION

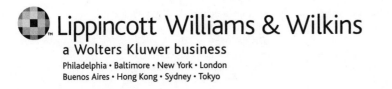

Lippincott Williams & Wilkins
a Wolters Kluwer business

Philadelphia • Baltimore • New York • London
Buenos Aires • Hong Kong • Sydney • Tokyo

STAFF

Executive Publisher
Judith A. Schilling McCann, RN, MSN

Editorial Director
H. Nancy Holmes

Clinical Director
Joan M. Robinson, RN, MSN

Senior Art Director
Arlene Putterman

Editorial Project Manager
Jennifer Kowalak

Clinical Project Manager
Beverly Ann Tscheschlog, RN, BS

Editor
Julie Munden

Clinical Editor
Anita Lockhart, RN, MSN

Copy Editors
Kimberly Bilotta (supervisor), Scotti Cohn,
Heather Ditch, Amy Furman, Dona Perkins,
Dorothy P. Terry, Pamela Wingrod

Designers
Linda J. Franklin (project manager)

Digital Composition Services
Diane Paluba (manager), Joyce Rossi Biletz,
Donna S. Morris

Manufacturing
Beth J. Welsh

Editorial Assistants
Megan L. Aldinger, Karen J. Kirk, Linda K. Ruhf

Design Assistant
Georg W. Purvis IV

Indexer
Barbara Hodgson

**Library of Congress
Cataloging-in-Publication Data**

Best practices : evidence-based nursing procedures. — 2nd ed.
         p. ; cm.
   Includes bibliographical references and index.
   1. Nursing—Quality control. 2. Nursing—Standards.
3. Evidence-based nursing. I. Lippincott Williams & Wilkins.
   [DNLM: 1. Nursing Care—standards—Practice Guideline. 2. Evidence-Based Medicine—methods—Practice Guideline. WY 100 B561 2007]
RT85.5.B475 2007
362.1'730685—dc22
ISBN13: 978-1-58255-532-4
ISBN10: 1-58255-532-X (alk. paper)   2006012245

Contents

Contributors and consultants

Rosemary Ashby, AS, BSN, MS, CGRN, ARNP
Nurse Practitioner
James A. Haley Veterans Hospital
Tampa, Fla.

Judi L. Brendle, RN, MSN
Director of Evidence-Based Practice and
    Nursing Research
Lancaster (Pa.) General Hospital

Kim Cooper, RN, MSN
Nursing Department Program Chair
Ivy Tech Community College
Terre Haute, In.

Nancy DeRosa, BSN, MS, CNA-BC
Manager of the Center for Education and
    Development
Advocate Lutheran General Hospital
Park Ridge, Ill.

Ellie Z. Franges, MSN, CRNP, CNRN, APRN-BC
Nurse Practitioner — Neurosurgery
St. Luke's Hospital & Health Network
Bethlehem, Pa.

Gretchen L. Hunt, RN, MSN, CCRN, CNS
Clinical Education Specialist
Harris Methodist Hospital
Fort Worth, Tex.

Kimiko Cunningham Krutz, RN, MSN, ONC
Clinical Nurse Specialist — Orthopaedic/
    Neurosurgery
Saint Elizabeth Regional Medical Center
Lincoln, Neb.

Christine V. O'Donnell, RN, MSN, BS, CIC
Infection Control Practitioner
James A. Haley Veterans Hospital
Tampa, Fla.

Donna M. Roe, RN, MS, CEN
Clinical Education Manager
St. Joseph Hospital
Nashua, N.H.

Susan Sample, CRNP, MSN
Program Manager of Cardiothoracic Surgery
Lancaster (Pa.) General Hospital

Rita M. Wick, RN, BSN
Education Specialist
Berkshire Health Systems
Pittsfield, Mass.

How to use this book

Throughout *Best Practices: Evidence-Based Nursing Procedures* — after entry titles, after subheads, after paragraphs, bullets, and sentences — you'll find bold initials in the form of icons. These initials identify evidence-based data and their supporting research reports, fundamental principles of science, and the professional associations, health care organizations, and government groups whose standards, protocols, guidelines, and mandates underlie and dictate the very best in clinical health care practice today. Use the list below to identify the organizations represented by the icons.

AABB American Association of Blood Banks

AACN American Association of Critical-Care Nurses

AACT American Academy of Clinical Toxicology

AAD American Academy of Dermatology

AAN American Academy of Neurology

AANN American Association of Neuroscience Nurses

AANS American Association of Neurological Surgeons

AAP American Academy of Pediatrics

AARC American Association for Respiratory Care

ABA American Burn Association

ACC American College of Cardiology

ACG American College of Gastroenterology

ACLS Advanced Cardiac Life Support, American Heart Association

ACIP Advisory Committee on Immunization Practices, a committee of the Centers for Disease Control and Prevention

ACOG American College of Obstetricians and Gynecologists

ACS American Cancer Society

ACSC American College of Surgeons Committee

ADA American Dental Association

ADiaA American Diabetes Association

AF Arthritis Foundation

AGA American Gastroenterologic Association

AHA American Heart Association

AHospA American Hospital Association

AHRQ Agency for Healthcare Research and Quality, formerly Agency for Health Care Policy and Research (AHCPR)

ALA American Lung Association

ANA American Nurses Association

ANNA American Nephrology Nurses' Association

APIC Association for Professionals in Infection Control and Epidemiology

APS American Pain Society

ASGE American Society of Gastrointestinal Endoscopists

ASPEN American Society for Parenteral and Enteral Nutrition

AWHONN Association of Women's Health, Obstetric and Neonatal Nurses

CDC Centers for Disease Control and Prevention

CMS Centers for Medicare & Medicaid Services, formerly Health Care Financing Administration (HCFA)

DNA Dermatology Nurses' Association

EB Evidence-based data

ENA Emergency Nurses Association

FDA Food and Drug Administration

FORUM Child Health Corporation of America's Cooperative Pulse Oximetry FORUM

HIPAA Health Insurance Portability and Accountability Act

HPA Hospice Patient's Alliance

IFFGD International Foundation for Gastrointestinal Disorders

INS Infusion Nurses Society

IOM Institute of Medicine

ISMP Institute for Safe Medication Practices

JCAHO Joint Commission on Accreditation of Healthcare Organizations

JNC Joint National Committee on Prevention, Detection, Evaluation, and Treatment of High Blood Pressure (JNC VI) (a committee of the National Institutes of Health; the National Heart, Lung, and Blood Institute; and the National High Blood Pressure Education Program)

MFR Manufacturer recommendation

NANN National Association of Neonatal Nurses

NAON National Association of Orthopaedic Nurses

NCCMERP National Coordinating Council for Medication Error Reporting and Prevention

NHLBI National Heart, Lung, and Blood Institute

NIA National Institute on Aging

NIH National Institutes of Health

NINDS National Institute for Neurologic Disorders and Stroke

NKF National Kidney Foundation

NOF National Osteoporosis Foundation

NPUAP National Pressure Ulcer Advisory Panel

ONS Oncology Nursing Society

OSHA Occupational Safety and Health Administration

PCP Patient Care Partnership, developed by the American Hospital Association

SCCM Society of Critical Care Medicine

Science Fundamental principles of science

WHS Wound Healing Society

WOCN Wound, Ostomy and Continence Nurses Society

Foreword

Evidence-based practice continues to grow and strengthen in the healthcare world, and nursing is no exception. Indeed, in their 2001 report, "Crossing the Quality Chasm: A New Health System for the 21st Century," the Institute of Medicine encourages health care professionals to provide care using evidence-based practice. Magnet environments integrate research and evidence-based practice into clinical and operational processes. However, although evidence-based practice appears to be in the headlines of journals, conferences, and organizations, many barriers remain in place for the nurse, such as a lack of time and access to the appropriate tools.

Best Practices: Evidence-Based Nursing Procedures, Second Edition, handily allows the nurse to overcome these barriers and more. Thoroughly reviewed and updated, this new edition looks at current research and resources, offering the most up-to-date information in providing nursing care to patients. The book provides quick and easy access to scores of evidence-based nursing procedures — an excellent resource and reference tool for nurses as they become active participants in identifying and developing best practices in nursing practice.

Evidence-based practice takes research utilization to a higher level by encouraging the nurse to use critical thinking skills in individualizing research results to best meet the needs of the patient. *Best Practices: Evidence-Based Nursing Procedures,* Second Edition, has several new key features: each section now provides a new teaching icon, a list of nursing diagnoses to assist the bedside nurse in individualizing and documenting the care plan, including actual problems, risk for problems, and wellness issues. Each entry also includes expected outcomes and complications, allowing the nurse to better prepare for treatment effects.

In addition to these new enhancements, the book retains the same helpful features such as the highlighted icons — *Alert, Controversial issue, Clinical impact,* and *Innovative practice* — as well as invaluable web resources.

As healthcare organizations and associations challenge healthcare professionals to provide evidence-based practice, *Best Practices: Evidence-Based Nursing Procedures,* Second Edition, offers a comprehensive resource to the practicing nurse. The future of healthcare demands excellence, which involves continually updating practice procedures through research and evidence. As the profession of nursing continues to evolve, embedding evidence-based practice as the foundation of nursing care paves the road to excellence.

Judi L. Brendle, RN, MSN
Director of Evidence-Based Practice and Nursing Research
Lancaster (Pa.) General Hospital

What is best practice?

As new procedures and medicines become available, nurses committed to excellence must regularly update and adapt their practices. The approach known as "best practice" is an important tool in helping nurses provide high-quality care to their patients. Best practice refers to the clinical practices, treatments, and interventions that result in the best possible outcome for the patient and the health care facility providing those services.

The concept of best practice comes from the wider health care community. Interest in this concept has grown as a result of increasing requirements that health care providers control costs and show statistical evidence of the effectiveness of a treatment program. Experts began to recognize that treatment of patients with similar diagnoses differed significantly among practitioners and health care systems and that these differences led to inconsistent patient outcomes. They turned their attention to identifying the care that resulted in the best outcomes for patients and encouraging practitioners to provide that kind of care.

Nurses have been part of this effort all along. The Best Practice Network, until recently an affiliation of nursing organizations whose aim was to help nurses implement best practices, defined best practice as a "plan, action, or service that has been improved and implemented to produce superior outcomes." In nursing, determining best practice is a process of identifying high-quality nursing practices, analyzing them, and applying them to local nursing practices. It allows nurses to use information from various sources — not only research and textbooks, but also colleagues and other experts. The best practice approach is generally a team effort, which provides a structure for deciding when and how to use these sources of information.

This process may seem time-consuming and of questionable value to nurses who have clinical experience or who have recently completed educational programs. Yet, even these nurses encounter everyday questions for which there are no ready answers. A best practice approach gives nurses the tools to answer clinical questions intelligently, effectively, and — with a little practice — promptly.

The process of identifying excellent nursing care practices, knowing how to measure them, and putting them to work in clinical practice helps to delineate exactly how nurses contribute to better patient outcomes and gives nurses evidence of the value of their practice. Health care facilities benefit because consistent care based on the most current evidence is efficient and cost-effective. (See *Building best practices,* page 2.)

Identifying best practices

How do we know what a best practice is? The process begins with understanding the common sources of information available to nurses: research data, personal experience, and expert opinion. (See *Research and nursing,* page 2.)

One might be tempted to rely entirely on research-based information. However, such information has several disadvantages. The data are limited in amount and scope. Many studies produce inconclusive results and require further research; others may not address the specific problem the clinician is attempting to solve. Data from research journals can be highly technical and difficult to implement in clinical practice. Finally, the journals that publish such data are expensive and, if obtained, nurses may not have the time to read them.

A nurse's own experience or that of her colleagues is less reliable than research because a single person can be influenced as much by preconceptions as by objective observations. For example, if a nurse believes that a certain medication is the most effective,

1

Building best practices

Identifying and developing best practices is a team effort. Listed here are five basic steps for building best practices in your facility.

● **Limit the size of the team to 8 or fewer members.** Include those who work most closely with the users of the service or the users themselves, and be sure to get a commitment from the members during the initial planning meeting. Hold members accountable to their commitment; eliminate those who don't show up, instead utilize them as consultants.

● **Communicate clearly the reason for creating the team;** clarify the goals, the problem, and the process for improvement to avoid different perceptions of why the team has assembled.

● **Examine the issue,** looking at the positive and negative aspects of the program. Gather information using facts, statistics, experiences, examples, analogies, and expert feedback. Analyze the data for your program and others to identify gaps in care.

● **Determine specific measurable objectives,** indicators to be measured, and timelines.

● **Benchmark,** or compare your results against other services and programs.

Research and nursing

Research is the foundation on which all sciences are based. Its reliance on observations made in a controlled setting limits confusion over which factors actually produce the results. Health care professionals have long recognized the importance of research in the laboratory setting, but recently they have begun to develop ways to make research information more useful in the clinical setting.

Evidence-based nursing is the term used to describe nursing practice based on information obtained from research. For example, a nurse's belief that a certain drug is more effective for pain relief than others may be based on previous experience with that drug. But other factors could be contributing to pain relief, such as the route of administration or the amount of time the nurse spends assessing the patient. Perhaps the drugs produce similar analgesia, but the nurse's approach to care affects the patient's response. Research data help the nurse make evidence-based decisions in choosing one drug over another, and they may provide insight into treatment for a patient who doesn't respond to a medication. Finally, research information tends to be more current than information published in textbooks.

her enthusiasm may affect how patients respond to the medicine. Furthermore, even the most skilled practitioner may not notice that a large percentage of her patients don't respond well. This bias is part of human nature, and it can cloud any practitioner's judgment. Best practice provides other sources of information and a structure for implementing that knowledge in one's practice.

Benchmarking

In addition to an evidence-based approach, benchmarking is one process for identifying sources of best practice information. This collaborative, ongoing process has been used in many fields for centuries; the term originated with the reference marks that craftsmen noted on their workbenches. Today, a benchmark is a measure of performance that serves as a standard for evaluating other results. The concept came to health care in the mid-1990s with the need to increase efficiency without sacrificing quality of care. Health care facilities had to find the most effective management approaches possible. Benchmarking is especially useful for administrative nursing concerns, such as cost and nursing hours required per patient.

Traditionally, benchmarking is done by a team of members from different professions and departments in a hospital or other health care facility. A critical factor in successful benchmarking is careful consideration of the benchmarks that are used and how they were achieved. Without this focus, benchmarks become rules to be followed without understanding the reasons. Thus, successful benchmarking is an ongoing process of planning, data collection, analysis of processes and practices, and implementation for improvement. (See *Benchmarking for best practices*.)

Planning

The first step in benchmarking is for the team to identify clear, concrete, specific goals for patients and the facility. Examples include decreased length of hospital stay, decreased complication rates, and increased patient and family satisfaction.

With goals established, the team next searches for appropriate outcome measures for the identified goals — length of stay statistics, for example. The focus here is external; that is, on measures used at other facilities. Benchmarks aren't always available, especially for nursing-related outcomes, such as pain management and patient and family satisfaction with care. Identifying these gaps is part of delineating nursing's unique contribution to patient care outcomes. If no studies exist for a desired benchmark, the team's study can be the first to set the benchmark.

Collecting data

After deciding on appropriate benchmarks, the team's next step is to find them. Formulating a plan and a timetable for collecting and analyzing the data can help the team avoid becoming bogged down at this stage. Government Web sites, hospital and professional organization Web sites, and benchmarking collaboratives, such as the University Health System Consortium, can all be good sources of data. Research data can be obtained through traditional means, such as going to a medical library or using Internet sources such as PubMed, a database of published health care literature maintained by the National Library of Medicine.

INNOVATIVE PRACTICE

Benchmarking for best practices

Your facility can develop a benchmarking worksheet as a tool to guide the process of benchmarking, keep track of the results, and document accomplishments. When you have identified a goal, complete the following steps on the worksheet and document your findings.

● Find two or three benchmarks that can be used as measures for the stated goal and can be compared across systems. Benchmark categories include cost, clinical outcomes, patient satisfaction, and functional health status.
● Select the resources you'll use to determine best practices. This includes identifying the experts in the field internally and externally, researching and analyzing data internally and externally, looking at national averages or standards and the best outcomes, and examining the published literature (research reports).
● Formulate a data collection plan, including who will collect the data. Establish a timeline for data collection, analysis, and documentation.
● Measure your own performance against benchmarks, comparing your facility's outcomes against national standards or best outcomes.
● Identify practices that produce best results. Studying the differences between those "best" processes and your own could provide innovative strategies to introduce changes.
● Implement new or revised practices. This step could include establishing or updating standardized orders or changing the admission process.
● After implementing a best practice, collect data to determine if outcomes have improved or worsened.

Analyzing processes and practices

The team's next step is to compare the collected data to the information about its own facility to identify gaps between the two. After identifying a difference, the team analyzes the processes that produced the best results and tries to delineate how they differ from local practices. How were shorter patient stays or improved patient satisfaction achieved? Which nursing interventions resulted in fewer complications? How often were they done and when? These kinds of questions are an important part of understanding how to achieve similar results.

Implementing for improvement

Finally, the facility implements changes. Sometimes, repeating exactly what was done at another facility isn't feasible, for example, because the patient populations or staff differ. In such cases, the team must be innovative and adapt the process to the existing environment.

Because the changes are new, the team must regularly evaluate their impact. This means monitoring patient outcomes to find out whether the new procedures improve these outcomes and if the changes created new problems. Inevitably, refinements and adjustments are necessary, which is why benchmarking is an ongoing process.

Evidence-based nursing practice

Nurses can also use benchmarks to compare, measure, and evaluate their own practice outcomes in evidence-based nursing practice. Evidence-based practice is nursing practice built on information obtained from research. For example, perhaps you were taught in nursing school that turning a patient every 2 hours was the way to prevent pressure ulcers. However, in practice you find that this alone doesn't seem to prevent ulcers from developing in your patients. After reading current research on the subject, you know that a patient's nutritional status is also important. This evidence leads you to encourage increased intake of protein as one of your nursing interventions.

Traditionally, nurses haven't regularly used research as a basis for practice. (See *Criticisms of evidence-based practice*.) A survey of staff nurses about how often they used various sources of knowledge for their practice revealed that the most common source was what colleagues or physicians were doing or what they had been taught in nursing school (despite the fact that the surveyed nurses had been out of nursing school for an average of 18 years). Of those who did read about research in journals, about one-third didn't read the research itself but others' reports on it (known as secondary sources).

Of course, it can be daunting for a nurse to consider whether everything she does in her nursing practice is evidence based. However, the idea of evidence-based practice is an ongoing concern, like all aspects of best practice. As questions arise in clinical practice, research is one avenue for answers. With a little practice in finding articles that relate to a question and in making sure that the source is a high-quality one, nurses usually find the straightforward process of implementing evidence-based changes rewarding.

Moving toward evidence-based nursing

The basic steps involved in evidence-based nursing practice resemble those of benchmarking: formulating a clinical question, searching for peer-reviewed articles on that clinical question, critically evaluating and comparing the articles, applying the information from the articles, and evaluating the outcome of the changes made in local practice.

Formulating the clinical question

The clinical question may develop from questions that arise in your practice or from an area in which you want to increase awareness. For example, you may wonder which type of adhesive is most irritating to skin. The manufacturer provides some information, but you know this information isn't entirely objective, so you decide to investigate further.

A good way to begin your research is to start with a specific and concrete question. Having this in mind before searching articles keeps your research focused and saves time. Start by formulating the question in terms of a relationship between a patient (or patient population), an exposure (typically a treatment, a diagnostic test, or a nursing procedure), and the result of the exposure. For example, you may be especially interested in patients whose skin is compromised by long-term steroid use. To focus your research even further, you may look at how adhesives affect the skin, asking yourself if some available adhesive is better than the one you are currently using.

The last step in the research process is to define your outcome. At this point, you decide what questions to ask and what factors to consider. Are you looking for an adhesive that's cost-effective? Safe? Nonirritating?

After carefully considering all factors, it's time to formulate your question: "What type of adhesive is least likely to cause skin irritation in patients with a history of long-term steroid use?" Now the important terms for your search are becoming clear: adhesive, long-term steroid use, and skin irritation. You may have to broaden your scope a bit, but this specific query is a good place to begin.

Searching the literature

Now you're ready to begin looking for articles. The most efficient way to go about finding relevant articles is to use an online index of published articles, such as PubMed, MEDLINE, or CINAHL (Cumulative Index of Nursing and Allied Health Literature). These indexes, also known as databases, list all articles published in a given period by journals in a particular profession (or group of professions). The database tells you what journals it scans for articles to be indexed. Look for a link on the Web site's home page or in the front of a printed index.

Online indexes work the same way as the older print indexes, listing articles and then cross-referencing them by author, journal, and subject. If you're looking for articles on a particular topic, search for them by using a term (keyword) that you think describes the topic. For example, if you want information on pressure sores, you might start with decubitus ulcers. Some online databases help users narrow down the list of results by giving them options, such as listing only articles on the causes or on the treatment of pressure sores. PubMed, a database maintained by the National Library of Medicine, provides these helpful options (or filters, as they're sometimes called).

The database will provide you with a list of articles on the topic you have chosen. Your first search effort may yield a dauntingly long list or a discouragingly short one. This is common, and it just requires some fine-tuning of your request. If the list is too long, try limiting the dates of the search to the past year or two or narrowing your focus to just one aspect of the topic, such as causes, treatments, or specific patient populations. If the list is too short, try broadening your search by being less selective about patients (try all ages, for example). Using online indexes makes this easy to do, and many provide links to click on that tell the database to broaden or narrow your search for you.

Your goal in doing this database search is to find published reports of the results of research projects. If the title of the article leaves you unsure whether the article is a report of a research project, read the abstract carefully. A standard format for research reports contains the following sections: abstract, introduction (occasionally called a review of the literature because it's a brief summary of past related research), methods, results, and a discussion section at the end. An article fitting this format is most likely a report of a research project.

A related type of article, called a literature review, summarizes many individual research reports and is usually written by an expert on that topic. Literature reviews can be valuable sources of summarized information. Most reviews are qualitative; that is, the expert compares the study designs and the researcher's findings and makes judgments as to quality and applicability. Relying on the author to make judgments for you can save time and direct you to additional articles that are more specific to your question. Always check out the references at the end of a literature review for additional articles to read.

A meta-analysis is a quantitative type of literature review. A true meta-analysis converts the results of each individual study to a statistic (called an *effect size*) and then compares studies quantitatively. In health science research, the term meta-analysis is used more loosely to describe a summary that compares studies in a systematic manner (typically a table). Meta-analyses aren't that common, however, so don't limit your search to just this form of review.

In addition to using databases, several journals review and summarize recent research and may provide commentary on the study. Examples of these are *Journal Watch, ACP Journal Club, Evidence-Based Medicine,* and *Evidence-Based Nursing.*

Obtaining the research

When you have identified 8 or 10 articles, obtaining them is the next step. Occasionally, the article is available directly online at no cost or for a fee. Generally, however, you must go to the print journal itself. If you have access to a teaching hospital or university library, most of the articles will be available through them. Your own facility's library may have the article, and if it doesn't, it may be able to obtain a copy for you without charge. Check with your reference librarian.

Abstracts, the condensed summaries that appear at the beginning of many articles, are commonly available online without cost. The question of whether it's acceptable to read only the abstract of an article is difficult. Busy practitioners who have little time to read research and aren't in a position to evaluate the details of a report may decide to read only the abstracts. By not reading the full report you may miss important details about the study population and how data were collected. Another reason for reading full reports is that you'll become more skilled at recognizing reports that lack important information as you become familiar with standard formats and procedures.

Analyzing and comparing data

Evaluating the quality of a research report can be difficult if you haven't had some training in research methodology. In fact, even seasoned researchers debate the quality of studies and how to interpret and apply the results. However, if you follow a few basic rules, you can be sure that the study you read has met a baseline standard of quality.

First and foremost is to use only articles that are published in *peer-reviewed journals.* These journals require outside experts to review articles submitted for publication. Why has this practice evolved? The sciences, including nursing sciences, are based on the idea that it takes many people to observe and agree on what they see to arrive at an objective assessment of what's real. Scientists understand that what people believe can be based on what they want to see rather than what's really there. Even experts can make misjudgments of this nature because the psychological process involved is largely unconscious. Belief in the starting hypothesis, pressure from the organization funding the research, and other factors can color the researcher's interpretation of data. Human nature must be taken into account when doing research, and scientists have developed various tools and guidelines to assure that research reports are based on observable evidence. If other experts in the same field read and review a researcher's report and agree that the research design and the researcher's conclusions are sound, the journal agrees to publish the research report.

If you aren't sure whether a journal is peer reviewed, check the pages that give information on subscription and philosophy of the journal's editors or the pages that give information to authors on how to submit their article for publication. Limiting your reading to articles in peer-reviewed journals increases the likelihood that the research and its report meet basic standards of quality. In addition, more and more journals are including expert commentary on the report within the report itself.

However, even the quality of peer-reviewed research can vary. While this brief introduction can't cover all aspects of how to judge the quality of a research study, two criteria — validity and reliability — are strong indicators of quality.

Validity refers to whether the research project actually measures what it claims to measure. For example, in research on the success of a patient-education program, for example, how do you know whether the researcher is truly measuring a change in patients' behavior (the ultimate goal of patient education) or just their knowledge about what they should be doing? Another aspect of this issue is whether the researchers themselves have unwittingly affected the results of their research. For example, a researcher may wish to know if clothing interferes with an accurate assessment of blood pressure. However, if this researcher is collecting the data (taking the blood pressures), she might read the blood pressure a little differently depending on what she expects to see.

Subjects are also susceptible to this problem. For example, someone who knows whether he's receiving medicine or a placebo might react differently according to his own expectations. To prevent this from happening, research designs keep subjects and researchers from knowing which subjects are in the treatment group. When neither researcher nor subject knows, the study has a *double-blind* design.

Reliability refers to whether the results of the study will be repeatable. Ideally, you shouldn't accept the results of any study as true without finding at least one attempt to repeat it with the same results. In reality, research is rarely repeated exactly. Later studies change the design or the patient population to broaden the knowledge base about the condition and its treatment. So it's rare to find research reports that ask the same question (or test the same hypothesis). But, as the number of studies on the same general topic grows, a picture begins to form that clinicians can use to understand their own patient population.

In considering reliability, it's important to look carefully at the study population. Is the study's population similar to your patient population? Did the researcher use a control group for comparison? A control group is a separate group of study subjects who don't receive the exposure or treatment being studied and who are the basis of comparison for the study group. The control group should be similar in size, age range, gender, socioeconomic status, and baseline health to the study group. Ideally, researchers assign people randomly to either a study or control group. This process, known as *randomizing*, is a hallmark of high-quality research. A final concern is how many subjects were involved in the research project. Research on large numbers of subjects produces more reliable results than smaller studies.

However, not all types of research can use randomization, double-blinding, control groups, and large populations. Understanding the acceptable alternatives requires training and experience.

Comparing the studies you or your team has gathered is the next step, and this can be challenging. You must weigh variables, such as patient population characteristics and quality of the study design. Final decisions usually require discussion and compromise.

Applying best practices

When you have read the literature and discussed it with your colleagues, it's time to consider instituting

---

Strategies for implementation

These 12 strategies can help you implement evidence-based practice.

● Review and assess the extent to which your practice is evidence based.
● Review current literature to find support for your belief that evidence-based practice results in better outcomes.
● Ask questions about your current practice strategies. (For example, is the use of distraction really effective in reducing children's distress during intrusive procedures?)
● Identify colleagues at your facility who have the same interests in the clinical questions you're trying to solve.
● Conduct a collaborative search for studies or systematic reviews in the specific area of your clinical questions.
● Analyze the studies from your search to decide if you have the "best evidence" to guide your practice.
● Develop a practice guideline using the "best evidence."
● Establish measurable outcomes that can be used to determine the effectiveness of your guideline.
● Implement the practice guideline.
● Measure the established outcomes.
● Evaluate the practice guideline to determine if your facility should continue it or change it.
● Develop a system for routinely sharing evidence-based literature and discussing ways to improve practice at your facility such as through evidence-based rounds.

Adapted with permission from Melnyk, B., et al. "Evidence-Based Practice: The Past, the Present, and Recommendations for the Millennium," *Pediatric Nursing* 26(1):77-80, January 2000.

---

new procedures or policies. New care plans and procedure protocols may need to be written and approved to make sure that patients receive consistent care. (See *Strategies for implementation*.) This will also help in the process of evaluating the results of the change in your practice.

Clinical tools

Colleagues and experts from related fields have developed tools for individuals and facilities to use in implementing best practices. The most common clinical tools are procedures, protocols, guidelines, standards of care, critical pathways, and innovative practices.

Procedures

A procedure is a set of steps by which a desired outcome is accomplished. Its purpose is to govern the handling of frequently occurring situations. Procedures are created to provide a safe and consistent course of action for health care workers in specific situations and to provide the best outcome for the patient. Examples of procedures are nasogastric tube insertion and removal and arterial puncture.

Some procedures are similar to protocols (see below) and specify what is to be done; for example, in the case of cardiac arrest in which specific steps are outlined to care for the patient.

A procedure usually includes:
● a description, which identifies the diagnostic criteria that define the problem
● a list of the equipment needed and the necessary preparatory steps
● an outline of the course of action, potential complications, and special considerations
● documentation of what has been done, the results, and the patient's response.

A multidisciplinary team develops procedures. This team may consist of members from every facet of health care (such as medicine, nursing, nutrition, and infection control) and outside of health care (such as lawyers and administrators). Procedures, which are usually based on current research, are frequently revised or updated because health care is constantly changing. They're excellent guidelines for best practices.

Protocols

Protocols are established sets of procedures for action in a given circumstance. Their purpose is to synthesize information into a concise structure that promotes the translation of knowledge into the actions most likely to produce optimal patient outcomes.

Usually, protocols outline the proper sequence of actions that a practitioner should take to establish a diagnosis or begin a treatment regimen. Examples include a pain management protocol that outlines a bedside strategy for managing acute or chronic pain and a wound care protocol. (See *Oral care protocol.*)

Protocols are evidence based and written by nursing or medical experts, commonly with input from other health care providers. They may be approved by legislative bodies such as the boards of nursing or medicine in a given state. Committees or boards of directors may approve other types of protocols specific to their facility.

Use of protocols can facilitate cost-effective, consistent care and provide an educational resource for clinicians to keep abreast of the most current best practices for a specific patient population. Protocols can be flexible, allowing a practitioner to use clinical judgment, or highly directive. Advanced practice nurses commonly use protocols to arrive at a diagnosis or institute treatment regimens.

Guidelines

Guidelines are general outlines for specific courses of action in response to a diagnosis or condition. The Institute of Medicine has defined *clinical practice guidelines* as "systematically developed statements to assist practitioner and patient decisions about appropriate health care for specific clinical circumstances."

Clinical practice guidelines are usually written by expert health care providers who condense a large amount of information into an easily usable format. Guidelines recommend courses of action for a particular diagnosis or condition and therefore reflect value judgments about the relative importance of various health and economic outcomes. They're multidisciplinary and can be used to coordinate care by multiple providers.

Guidelines support the implementation of best practices by integrating individual clinical expertise with the best available clinical evidence. Using them can help the nurse streamline care, control variations in practice patterns, and use health care resources more effectively. Hospital readmission rates frequently decrease after implementation of a guideline such as the Centers for Disease Control and Prevention's *Guidelines for Prevention and Control of Nosocomial Infection.*

Like research-based information, clinical guidelines should be evaluated for the quality of their sources. At least, it's a good idea to read the developers' policy statement about how evidence was selected and what values were applied in making recommendations for care. Guidelines also can be valuable sources of information for evidence-based care. When

Oral care protocol

Assessment	**1.** Determine if the patient is intubated or has a tracheotomy. **2.** Assess lips and oral cavity on admission and at least daily. **3.** Assess for contraindications for oral care every 2 hours, including: – hemodynamically instability – massive oral trauma – practitioner orders that conflict with oral care.
Report to practitioner	**4.** Report abnormal findings from the oropharynx (such as bleeding or ulcerations).
Interventions	**5.** If the patient is intubated or has a tracheotomy, perform every 2 hours: – Replace suction liner, tubing and covered Yankauer every 24 hours – Use suction toothbrush twice a day on even hour and as needed (recommended at 8 a.m. and 8 p.m.) – Brush the teeth using a suction toothbrush with Perox-A-Mint solution. Brush for approximately 1 to 2 minutes, applying suction at completion and as needed during the brushing. Gently brush the surface of the tongue. – Use suction swabs every 2 hours on even hour (with the exception of the twice-a-day brushing times) to clean the teeth and tongue. – Use moisturizing swabs every 2 hours after completion of oral care. Apply mouth moisturizer to mucous membranes, buccal cavity and tongue. **6.** If the patient isn't intubated or doesn't have a tracheotomy, perform every 4 hours at a minimum and as needed. **7.** Every 6 hours or prior to major position changes or extubation, and as needed to assist in controlling secretions, perform deep oropharyngeal suctioning to assist in removing oropharyngeal secretions that have pooled in the hypopharynx, using the disposable hypopharyngeal suction catheter.
Teaching and documentation	**8.** Inform the patient and his family of rationale to decrease the risk for complications. **9.** Report abnormal assessment findings. **10.** Report performed interventions. **11.** Document patient or family teaching or response.

Adapted from Simmons-Trau, D. "Zap Vap With a Back to Basics Approach," *Nursing2006Critical Care*, 1(1):28-36, January 2006, with permission of the publisher.

published, they're considered to define the appropriateness of care by explaining the indications for tests or treatments.

Guidelines and protocols provide an overall framework for delivering a standard of care.

Standards of care

A standard is a statement describing an expected level of care or performance. Standards delineate the role played by a practitioner in a facility and describe a level of care or performance common to advanced specialty practice by which the quality of practice performance can be judged. Professional associations, specific professional groups, and government or regulatory agencies usually develop standards of care. For example, the Board of the American Association of Critical Care Nurses has established standards of care that can be used equally by patients, families, employers, facilities, the public, and regulatory and legislative bodies.

Critical pathways

Critical pathways are care management plans that outline a sequence of events for care of patients with a given diagnosis or condition. (See *Critical pathway: Colon resection without colostomy*, pages 10 to 12.)

(Text continues on page 13.)

Critical pathway: Colon resection without colostomy

At any point in a treatment course, looking at the critical pathway allows you to compare the patient's progress and your performance as a caregiver with standards. This standard critical pathway outlines care for a patient with a colon resection without colostomy.

	Patient visit	**Presurgery day 1**
Assessments	● History and physical with breast, rectal, and pelvic examinations ● Nursing assessment	● Nursing admission assessment
Consultations	● Social service consultation ● Physical therapy consultation	● Notify referring physician of impending admission
Laboratory and diagnostic tests	● Complete blood count (CBC) ● PT/PTT ● Electrocardiogram ● Chest X-ray (CXR) ● Chemistry profile ● CT scan ABD w/wo contrast ● CT scan pelvis ● Urinalysis ● Barium enema and flexible sigmoidoscopy or colonoscopy ● Biopsy report	● Type and screen for patients with Hg level < 10
Interventions	● Many or all of the above laboratory and diagnostic tests will have already been done. ● Check all results and fax them to the surgeon's office.	● Admit by 0800 ● Check for bowel preparation orders ● Bowel preparation* ● Antiembolism stockings ● Incentive spirometry ● Ankle exercises* ● I.V. access* ● Routine VS* ● Pneumatic inflation boots
I.V.s		● I.V. fluids, D_5W ½ NSS
Medication	● Prescribe GoLYTELY or Nulytely 1000-1400 ● Neomycin @ 1400, 1500, and 2200 ● Erythromycin @ 1400, 1500, and 2200	● GoLYTELY or Nulytely 1000-1400 ● Erythromycin @ 1400, 1500, and 2200 ● Neomycin @ 1400, 1500, and 2200
Diet/GI	● Clear liquids presurgery day ● NPO after midnight	● Clear liquids presurgery day ● NPO after midnight
Activity		

KEY:
* = NSG activities
V = Variance
N = No Var.

	1.	2.	3.		1.	2.	3.
	V	V	V		V	V	V
	Ⓝ	N	N		Ⓝ	Ⓝ	Ⓝ

Signatures:

1. _C. Molloy, RN_
2. _____
3. _____

1. _M. Connel, RN_
2. _J. Smith, RN_
3. _P. Joseph, RN_

Critical pathway: Colon resection without colostomy *(continued)*

	Day 0 O.R. day	Postoperative day 1	Postoperative day 2
Assessments	● Nursing admission assessment on TBA patients in holding area ● Postoperative review of systems assessment*	● Review of systems assessment*	● Review of systems assessment*
Consultations			
Laboratory and diagnostic tests	● Type and screen for patients in holding area with Hg level < 10	● CBC	● Electrolyte 7 (EL-7) ● CXR
Interventions	● Shave and prepare in operating room ● NG tube maintenance* ● I/O ● VS per routine* ● Urinary catheter care* ● Incentive spirometry* ● Ankle exercises* ● I.V. site care* ● HOB 30° ● Safety measures* ● Wound care* ● Mouth care*	● NG tube maintenance* ● I/O* ● VS per routine* ● Urinary catheter care* ● Incentive spirometry* ● Ankle exercises* ● I.V. site care* ● HOB 30°* ● Safety measures* ● Wound care* ● Mouth care* ● Antiembolism stockings	● Discontinue NG tube if possible* (per guidelines) ● I/O* ● VS per routine* ● Discontinue urinary catheter* ● Ambulating* ● Incentive spirometry* ● Ankle exercises* ● I.V. site care* ● HOB 30°* ● Safety measures* ● Wound care* ● Mouth care* ● Antiembolism stockings
I.V.s	● I.V. fluids, D_5L	● I.V. fluids, D_5LR	● I.V. fluids D_5 ½ NSS + MVI
Medication	● Preoperative ABX in holding area ● Postoperative ABX X 2 doses ● PCA (basal rate 0.5 mg) ● subQ heparin	● PCA (basal rate 0.5 mg) ● subQ heparin	● PCA (0.5 mg basal rate)
Diet/GI	● NPO/NG tube		● Discontinue NG tube per guidelines: (Clamp tube at 8 a.m. if no N/V and residual < 200 ml, discontinue tube @ 1200)* ● (Check with physician first)
Activity	● 4 hours after surgery ambulate with abdominal binder* ● Discontinue pneumatic inflation boots after patient ambulates	● Ambulate t.i.d. with abdominal binder* ● May shower ● Physical therapy b.i.d.	● Ambulate q.i.d. with abdominal binder* ● May shower ● Physical therapy b.i.d.
Teaching			● Reinforce preoperative teaching* ● Patient and family education p.r.n.* ● Re: family screening
KEY: * = NSG Activities V = Variance N = No Var. **Signatures:**	1. 2. 3. V V V Ⓝ Ⓝ Ⓝ 1. *L. Singer, RN* 2. *J. Smith, RN* 3. *P. Joseph, RN*	1. 2. 3. V V V Ⓝ Ⓝ Ⓝ 1. *L. Singer, RN* 2. *J. Smith, RN* 3. *P. Joseph, RN*	1. 2. 3. V V V Ⓝ Ⓝ Ⓝ 1. *A. McCarthy, RN* 2. *R. Moyer, RN* 3. *L. Walters, RN*

(continued)

Critical pathway: Colon resection without colostomy *(continued)*

	Postoperative day 3	Postoperative day 4	Postoperative day 5
Assessments	● Review of systems assessment*	● Review of systems assessment	● Review of systems assessment*
Consultations	● Dietary consultation		● Oncology consultation if indicated (Dukes B2 or C or high-risk lesion) (or to be done as outpatient)
Laboratory and diagnostic tests	● CBC ● EL-7	● Pathology results on chart	● CBC ● EL-7
Interventions	● I/O* ● VS per routine* ● Incentive spirometry* ● Ankle exercises* ● I.V. site care* ● Safety measures* ● Wound care* ● Antiembolism stockings	● I/O* ● VS per routine* ● Incentive spirometry* ● Ankle exercises* ● I.V. site care* ● Safety measures* ● Wound care* ● Antiembolism stockings	● Consider staple removal ● Replace with Steri-Strips ● Assess that patient has met discharge criteria*
I.V.s	● I.V. convert to saline lock	● Continue saline lock	● Discontinue saline lock
Medication	● Discontinue PCA ● P.O. analgesia ● Resume routine home medications	● P.O. analgesia ● Preoperative medications	● P.O. analgesia ● Preoperative medications
Diet/GI	● Clear liquids if+bm/flatus ● Advance to postoperative diet if tolerating clear liquids (at least one tray of clear liquids)	● House	● House
Activity	● Ambulate at least q.i.d. with abdominal binder* ● May shower ● Physical therapy b.i.d.	● Ambulate at least q.i.d. with abdominal binder* ● May shower ● Physical therapy b.i.d.	
Teaching	● Reinforce preoperative teaching* ● Patient and family education p.r.n.* ● Re: family screening ● Begin discharge teaching	● Reinforce preoperative teaching* ● Patient and family education p.r.n.* ● Discharge teaching re: – reportable s/s – follow-up – wound care*	● Review all discharge instructions and Rx including:* ● Follow-up appointments: – with surgeon within 3 weeks – with oncologist within 1 month if indicated

| **KEY:**
* = NSG Activities
V = Variance
N = No Var.

Signatures: | 1.   2.   3.
V   V   V
Ⓝ   Ⓝ   Ⓝ

1. *A. McCarthy, RN*
2. *R. Moyer, RN*
3. *L. Walters, RN* | 1.   2.   3.
V   V   V
Ⓝ   Ⓝ   Ⓝ

1. *L. Singer, RN*
2. *J. Smith, RN*
3. *P. Joseph, RN* | 1.   2.   3.
V   V   V
Ⓝ   Ⓝ   N

1. *L. Singer, RN*
2. *J. Smith, RN*
3. |

Critical pathways differ from guidelines in that they usually focus on the quality and efficiency of care after treatment decisions have been made. They're also usually multidisciplinary in nature, outlining the duties of all professionals involved with patient care. Finally, critical pathways are designed along specific timelines for indicated actions as well as specifying expected patient outcomes to serve as checkpoints for the performance of the patient and caregiver.

The example on pages 10 to 12 is a plan for treatment and management of a patient admitted for a colon resection without colostomy. The plan specifies assessments, consultations, laboratory and diagnostic tests, interventions, I.V. access, medications, diet, and activity.

Critical pathways are typically generated and used by health care facilities that deliver care for similar conditions to a large number of patients. They're usually developed by multidisciplinary committees made up of clinicians at the particular health care facility. The overall goals are to help establish a standard approach to be used by all providers in the facility, to help various members of the health care team understand their roles, and to provide a framework for collecting data on patient outcomes. Pathways must be based on evidence from reliable sources (benchmarks, research, guidelines); therefore, the committee must gather and use information from peer-reviewed literature and experts outside the facility's professional community.

Innovative practices

These are creative solutions to everyday problems intended to provide small, incremental improvements in nursing care delivery. They're usually limited in scope but not in ingenuity. Examples of award-winning innovative practices include a new documentation system for an admission assessment that triggers other disciplines, such as social services, respiratory care, pastoral care, nutritional care, or enterostomal therapy to perform assessments on the newly admitted patient.

These practices and ideas aren't researched or analyzed by the wider nursing community, and many are therefore less reliable than other sources of information. Even so, they may be extremely important to the growth of knowledge and the advance of practice.

Innovation is a critical part of professional practice because it relies on the expertise and intuition of seasoned clinicians. It stimulates practitioners to question traditional and accepted clinical practice. Clinical innovation is also an impetus for new research and the emergence of best practices.

Evaluating outcomes

Evaluation is the final step in the evidence-based practice process. Evaluating outcomes of best practices allows the nurse to determine the patient's response to the nursing interventions and provides a gauge of the extent to which the initial objectives (or goals) have been achieved.

Outcomes should be documented concisely and objectively. Documentation should show how the outcomes relate to the nursing diagnoses and describe the patient's response to interventions, indicate whether the goals were met, and include additional pertinent data.

As new practices are implemented, the team evaluates and documents the patient's responses. As this happens, you may find that the original care plan needs modification. The nursing practice may shift as problems are resolved and additional information about the patient's state of health is collected.

Supportive references

Angus, J., et al. "Implementing Evidence-Based Nursing Practice: A Tale of Two Intrapartum Nursing Units," *Nursing Inquiry* 10(4):218-28, December 2003.

Clarke, H., et al. "Pressure Ulcers: Implementation of Evidence-Based Nursing Practice," *Journal of Advanced Nursing* 49(6):578-90, March 2005.

Miransky, J. "The Development of a Benchmarking System for a Cancer Patient Population," *Journal of Nursing Care Quality* 18(1):38-42, January-February-March 2003.

Semin-Goossens, A., et al. "A Failed Model-Based Attempt to Implement an Evidence-Based Nursing Guideline for Fall Prevention," *Journal of Nursing Care Quality* 18(3):217-25, July-August-September 2003.

Simpson, R. "Evidence-Based Nursing Offers Certainty in the Uncertain World of Healthcare," *Nursing Management* 35(10):10-12, October 2004.

van Meijel, B., et al. "The Development of Evidence-based Nursing Interventions: Methodological Considerations," *Journal of Advanced Nursing* 48(1): 84-92, October 2004.

Wallin, L., et al. "Sustainability in Changing Clinical Practice Promotes Evidence-Based Nursing Care," *Journal of Advanced Nursing* 41(5):509-18, March 2003.

2

Basic care

According to the American Hospital Association, approximately 37 million people are hospitalized each year. For most people, hospitalization is one of the most difficult times in their life — illness, disrupted routine, loss of privacy, and loss of control over life events. In addition to being the direct caregiver, the nurse may need to provide for the patient and his family, offering teaching, counseling, coordination of services, development of community support systems, and assistance in coping with health-related lifestyle changes. In many facilities, staff nurses, primary nurses, clinical nurse specialists, and advanced practitioners provide some or all of these vital services.

In this chapter, you'll find recommendations of best practice techniques, innovative practices, and controversial issues that can challenge traditional nursing practices. Many are evidence-based **EB**, representing research data, based on fundamental principles of science **Science**, or recommended by product manufacturers **MFR**. Others are endorsed by professional groups, such as the American Nurses' Association **ANA** or the Infusion Nurses Society **INS**. Still others are endorsed by organizations, such as the American Heart Association **AHA**, the American Association for Respiratory Care **AARC**, the American Diabetes Association **ADiabA**, the Wound Ostomy and Continence Nurses Society **WOCN**, the National Pressure Ulcer Advisory Panel **NPUAP**, the American Cancer Society **ACS**, the Joint Commission on Accreditation of Healthcare Organizations **JCAHO**, the Agency for Healthcare Research and Quality **AHRQ**, the Centers for Medicare & Medicaid Services **CMS** (formerly the Health Care Financing Administration), the Joint National Committee on Prevention, Detection, Evaluation, and Treatment of High Blood Pressure **JNC**, and the Centers for Disease Control and Prevention **CDC**. And some are mandated by the American Hospital Association's Patient Care Partnership **PCP**, the Occu-pational Safety and Health Administration **OSHA**, the Hospice Patients Alliance **HPA**, or the Health Insurance Portability & Accountability Act **HIPAA**.

Understanding basic care

First, it's important to review the broader aims of nursing care, such as helping the patient cope with restricted mobility, making his environment comfortable, promoting safety, preventing complications, and helping him return to a normal life.

● *Dealing with impaired mobility.* Whenever a patient's condition restricts or prevents mobility, your nursing goal is to promote independence. You can motivate him by setting goals together to help prevent injury and complications associated with immobility. If the patient faces long-term immobility, it's important for you to help him achieve and maintain a positive self-image.

● *Providing a comfortable environment.* With ongoing assessment of a patient's needs, you can affect a patient's comfort, condition, response to treatment, and overall outcome. You can provide a comfortable environment simply by manipulating physical factors, such as temperature, humidity, and lighting. However, keep in mind that illness is a stressor that may intensify a patient's response.

● *Promoting safety.* Be alert to hazards in the patient's environment, and teach him and his family to recognize them. When caring for a patient with restricted mobility, you must assist him if he's moved, lifted, or transported. By using proper body mechanics, you can prevent injury to the patient and yourself. To help reduce patient and nurse injury, the Occupational Safety and Health Administration has developed guidelines to help prevent musculoskeletal injuries that also include keeping the patient safe at the same time. **JCAHO** **OSHA**

● *Preventing complications.* Immobility poses special hazards for the patient who's confined to bed, such as increased pressure on bony prominences; venous, pulmonary, or urinary stasis; and disuse of muscles and joints. These can lead to such complications as pressure ulcers, thrombi, phlebitis, pneumonia, urinary calculi, or contractures. To prevent complications, be sure to use correct positioning, assistive devices, frequent positioning, and range-of-motion exercises and to provide meticulous skin care.

● *Promoting rehabilitation.* In most cases, the first step toward rehabilitation is walking. Depending on the patient's condition, this may occur gradually. If necessary, use assistive devices, such as canes, crutches, or walkers. Effective rehabilitation may also require you to teach positioning, transfer, and mobilization techniques to the patient and his family. Demonstrating a technique, such as transfer from a bed to a wheelchair during hospitalization, helps the patient and his family to understand it. Practicing it under your supervision gives them the confidence to perform it at home. Encourage the family to provide positive reinforcement to motivate the patient to work toward his goals.

In addition to these nursing care goals, this chapter also covers the basic fundamentals of nursing: admission, transfer, and discharge procedures; patient safety and mobility; and patient transfer techniques and proper body mechanics. In addition to providing a comprehensive review of nursing fundamentals, the chapter also covers procedures, such as arterial puncture, blood pressure and pulse assessment, fecal occult blood testing, venipuncture, urine collection, use of restraints, postoperative and preoperative care, respiratory assessment, care of the dying patient, spiritual care, and postmortem care.

Admission

Admission to the nursing unit prepares the patient for his stay in the health care facility. Every facility follows a different set of policies and procedures for admitting a patient, and a patient's condition determines the extent of the admitting procedure. For instance, a patient who's admitted through the emergency department (ED) may not go through the same interview process as a patient scheduled for admission.

Whether the admission is scheduled or follows emergency treatment, effective admission procedures should accomplish these goals:

● verify the patient's identity using two patient identifiers according to facility policy **JCAHO** and assess his clinical status

● make him as comfortable as possible

● introduce him to roommates and staff members

● orient him to the environment and routine

● provide supplies and special equipment needed for daily care.

Florence Nightingale defined nursing as "the act of utilizing the environment of the patient to assist him in his recovery." Because admission procedures can color the patient's perception of the environment, they have a significant impact on responses to treatment. Nurses should be directly involved in the admission process — assigning a patient to a room, making sure that the necessary diagnostic tests are completed, and providing for continuity of care when the patient is admitted. Admitting personnel (a clerk or secretary) should confer with the nursing staff to make sure that the patient's room assignment is based on the patient's condition, health care needs, and personal preferences. Consideration of these factors during the admission process reduces the patient's anxiety and promotes cooperation, contributing to the patient's recovery.

The initial contact with the patient sets the foundation for your relationship. Be prepared to give the patient and his family, if present, your undivided attention during the admission process. Taking the time to listen to and assess your patient fulfills his physiologic and safety needs and establishes a therapeutic relationship. When orienting the patient and his family to the facility's routine, remember to mention that two or more nurses may care for the patient (depending on shift requirements) during his hospitalization.

The Joint Commission on Accreditation of Healthcare Organizations requires that each patient have an admission assessment performed by a registered nurse. **JCAHO** During this assessment, the nurse must prioritize the patient's needs, and she should always be conscious of the patient's levels of fatigue and comfort. The admission process can be exhausting, especially when the patient is delayed in the admitting office for a room assignment. When the patient is experiencing physical or psychological problems,

INNOVATIVE PRACTICE

Multidisciplinary assessment tool

Health care workers at Baton Rouge General Medical Center in Louisiana have developed an innovative multidisciplinary admission assessment tool. The multidisciplinary team includes health care workers from social services, respiratory therapy, diabetes management, pastoral care, dietary, enterostomal therapy, clinical case management, and physical, speech, and occupational therapy.

During the admission history, the patient is asked a series of questions that "trigger" other health care disciplines to assess the patient. A person from the appropriate department then visits and assesses the patient and provides recommendations for care. The health care team believes that patients benefit from this multidisciplinary approach by receiving necessary assessments earlier in the hospital stay.

the nurse should decide whether any portion of the admission assessment can be postponed.

It's also important to maintain the patient's privacy while obtaining his health history. According to the Patient's Bill of Rights, now referred to as the Patient Care Partnership, the patient has the right to expect this. Examination, consultation, and treatment should be conducted in a way that protects the patient's privacy. **PCP**

Admission routines that are efficient and show appropriate concern for the patient can ease his anxiety and promote cooperation and receptivity to treatment. Conversely, routines that the patient perceives as careless or excessively impersonal can heighten anxiety, reduce cooperation, impair the response to treatment, and perhaps aggravate symptoms.

Equipment

Gown • personal property form • admission form • nursing assessment form • thermometer • emesis basin • bedpan or urinal • bath basin • water pitcher, cup, and tray • urine specimen container, if needed

An admission pack usually contains soap, a comb, a toothbrush, toothpaste, mouthwash, a water pitch-

er, a cup, a tray, lotion, and facial tissues. The pack helps prevent cross-contamination and increases nursing efficiency. Because the patient's pack is included in his bill, he can take it home with him.

Preparation of equipment
• Obtain a gown and an admission pack.
• Position the bed as the patient's condition requires. If the patient is ambulatory, place the bed in the low position; if he's arriving on a stretcher, place the bed in the high position. Fold down the top linens.
• Prepare emergency or special equipment, such as oxygen or suction, as needed.

Implementation
• Adjust the lights, temperature, and ventilation in the patient's room.

Admitting the adult patient
• Greet the patient by name and introduce yourself and other staff present.
• Confirm the patient's identity using two patient identifiers according to facility policy. **JCAHO** Verify the name and its spelling with the patient. Notify the admission office of any corrections.
• Quickly review the admission form and the practitioner's orders. Note the reason for admission, restrictions on activity or diet, and orders for diagnostic tests requiring specimen collection.
• Escort the patient to his room and, if he isn't in great distress, introduce him to his roommate, if he has one. Then wash your hands and help the patient change into a gown or pajamas; if he's sharing a room, provide privacy. Itemize all valuables, clothing, and prostheses on the personal property form or, if your facility doesn't use such a form, in your notes. Encourage the patient to store valuables or money in the safe or, preferably, to send them home along with medications he may have brought. Show the ambulatory patient the bathroom and closets.
• Obtain a complete list of the patient's current medications and dosages and document this information in the patient's medical record. **JCAHO**
• Take and record the patient's vital signs, and collect ordered specimens. Measure his height and weight if possible. If he can't stand, use a chair or bed scale and ask him his height. *Knowing the patient's height and weight is important for planning*

treatment and diet and for calculating medication and anesthetic dosages. **JCAHO**

● Show the patient how to use the equipment in the room. Be sure to include the call system, bed controls, television controls, telephone, and lights.

● Explain the routine at your health care facility. Mention when to expect meals, vital signs checks, and medications. Review visiting hours and restrictions.

● Take a complete patient history. Include all previous hospitalizations, illnesses, and surgeries; current drug therapy; and food or drug allergies. Ask the patient to tell you why he came to the facility. Record the answers (in the patient's own words) as the chief complaint. Follow up with a physical assessment, emphasizing complaints. On the nursing assessment form, record any marks, bruises, or discoloration. (See *Multidisciplinary assessment tool*.) **JCAHO**

● After assessing the patient, inform him of tests that have been ordered and when they're scheduled. Describe what he should expect.

● Before leaving the patient's room, make sure that he's comfortable and safe. Return the bed to the low position, and adjust the pillows and linens. Place the call button and other equipment (such as water pitcher, cup, emesis basin, and facial tissues) within easy reach.

● Post patient care reminders (concerning such topics as allergies or special needs) at the head of the patient's bed *to notify coworkers*. (See *Using patient care reminders*.)

Admitting the pediatric patient

● Your initial goal is to establish a friendly, trusting relationship with the child and his parents *to help relieve fears and anxiety, which can hinder treatment*. Remember that a child younger than age 3 may fear separation from his parents; an older child may worry about what will happen to him.

● Speak directly to the child, and allow him to answer questions before obtaining more information from his parents. **PCP**

● While orienting the parents and child to the unit, describe the layout of the room and bathroom, and tell them the location of the playroom, television room, and snack room, if available.

● Teach the child how to call the nurse. Stress that someone will always be available to take care of his needs such as helping him to the bathroom.

Using patient care reminders

When placed at the head of the patient's bed, care reminders call attention to the patient's special needs and help ensure consistent care by communicating these needs to the facility staff, the patient's family, and other visitors.

You can use a specially designed card or a plain piece of paper to post important information about the patient, such as:

● allergies
● dietary restrictions
● fluid restrictions
● specimen collection
● deafness or impaired hearing (specify which ear)
● foreign-language speaker.

You can also use care reminders to post special instructions, such as:

● complete bed rest
● no blood pressure on right arm
● turn every hour
● nothing by mouth
● infection control or isolation procedures.

Never violate the patient's privacy by posting his diagnosis, details about surgery, or other confidential information he might find revealing or intrusive.

● Explain the facility's rooming-in and visiting policies *so the parents can take every opportunity to be with their child*.

● Inquire about the child's usual routine *so that favorite foods, bedtime rituals, toileting, and adequate rest can be incorporated into the routine*.

● Encourage the parents to bring some of their child's favorite toys, blankets, or other items *to make the child feel more at home in unfamiliar surroundings*.

Special considerations

● If the patient doesn't speak English and isn't accompanied by a bilingual family member, contact the appropriate resource (usually the social services department) to secure an interpreter.

● Keep in mind that the patient admitted to the ED may require special procedures.

● If the patient brings medication from home, take an inventory and record this information on the nursing assessment form. **JCAHO** Instruct the patient not to take any medication unless authorized by the practitioner. Send authorized medication to the pharmacy for identification and relabeling. Send other medication home with a responsible family member or store it in the designated area outside the patient's room until he's discharged. *Use of unauthorized medication may interfere with treatment or cause an overdose.*

● Find out the patient's normal routine, and ask him if he would like adjustments to the facility regimen; for instance, he may prefer to shower at night instead of in the morning. *By accommodating the patient with such adjustments whenever possible, you can ease his anxiety and help him feel more in control of his potentially threatening situation.*

Documentation

After leaving the patient's room, complete the nursing assessment form or your notes, as required. The completed form should include the patient's vital signs, height, weight, allergies, and drug and health history; a list of his belongings and those sent home with family members; the results of your physical assessment; and a record of specimens collected for laboratory tests. Also document any patient teaching you performed.

Supportive references

Bickley, L. *Bates' Guide to Physical Examination and Health History Taking,* 8th ed. Philadelphia: Lippincott Williams & Wilkins, 2003.

Joint Commission on Accreditation of Healthcare Organizations. "Standards: Frequently Asked Questions: Hospital," 2005. *www.jcaho.org/accredited + organizations/standard/faq/hos.html.*

Kozier, B., et al. *Fundamentals of Nursing,* 7th ed. Upper Saddle River, N.J.: Prentice Hall Health, 2003.

Perry, A., and Potter, P. *Clinical Nursing Skills and Techniques,* 6th ed. St. Louis: Mosby–Year Book, Inc., 2005.

Alignment and pressure-reducing devices

Proper body alignment means that the joints, tendons, ligaments, and muscles are in line with the pull of gravity. When the body is aligned — whether the patient is sitting, standing, or lying down — these structures carry no excessive strain. Body balance is achieved when a wide base of support exists, the center of gravity falls within the base of support, and a vertical line can be drawn from the center of gravity through the base of support.

The human body is meant to be mobile, as evidenced by the harmful effects of immobility. The most obvious signs of prolonged immobility commonly occur in the muscles and skin. Common problems resulting from prolonged immobility include:

● disuse osteoporosis — the bones demineralize and become spongy in the absence of weight-bearing exercise and may fracture easily

● disuse atrophy — the muscles decrease in size, losing most of their strength and normal function

● contracture — permanent shortening of the muscle that limits joint mobility; muscle fibers can't shorten and lengthen

● reduced skin turgor — skin atrophy and a shift in body fluids between the compartments of the dermis decrease the skin's elasticity

● skin breakdown — immobility impedes circulation and decreases the supply of nutrients to specific areas.

Positioning to maintain proper body alignment is vital in the prevention of complications, such as joint contractures and deformities. Devices, such as pillows and foam, can reduce pressure on bony prominences by preventing contact between prone areas and support surfaces. **AHRQ** Incorrect positioning or infrequent repositioning of the patient with circulatory problems may result in pressure ulcers, which can develop within 24 hours and require months to heal and thousands of dollars to correct. Frequent repositioning may prevent contractures as well as pressure ulcers. The goal is to maintain the body posture as near as normal to an upright position. The spine should be straight, the head neutral, and all extremities in functional positions.

For patients confined to a bed, special support surfaces and positioning devices can be used to maintain correct body positioning and prevent complications of prolonged bed rest. Specialty beds provide pressure relief, eliminate shearing and friction, and reduce moisture; for example, a kinetic (RotoRest) bed provides continuous passive range of motion (ROM) or oscillation to counteract the patient's immobility. Special support surfaces can include gel or air overlays.

Be sure to follow the manufacturer's instructions before using these products. **MFR**

Positioning devices should be used to maintain the functional position of the wrists, hands, fingers, ankles, and other extremities. The major joints should be placed in extension to prevent hip and knee contractures. Devices include cradle boots to protect the heels and help prevent skin breakdown and footdrop; external hip rotation and abduction pillows to help prevent internal hip rotation after femoral fracture, hip fracture, or surgery; trochanter rolls to help prevent external hip rotation; and hand rolls to help prevent hand contractures. **Science**

Cradle boots, made of sponge rubber with heel cutouts, cushion the ankle and foot without completely enclosing it. Other commercial boots are available, but not all help to prevent external hip rotation. Footboards with antirotation blocks help prevent footdrop and external hip rotation but don't prevent heel pressure. High-topped sneakers may be used to help prevent footdrop, but they don't prevent external hip rotation or heel pressure.

The abduction pillow is a wedge-shaped piece of sponge rubber with lateral indentations for the patient's thighs and straps that wrap around the thighs to maintain correct positioning. Although a properly shaped bed pillow may temporarily substitute for the commercial abduction pillow, it's difficult to apply and doesn't maintain the correct lateral alignment.

The commercial trochanter roll is made of sponge rubber, but one can also be improvised from a rolled blanket or towel. The hand roll, available in hard and soft materials, is held in place by fixed or adjustable straps. It can be improvised from a rolled washcloth secured with roller gauze and adhesive tape.

The primary nursing goal in immobility is to neutralize detrimental effects on the patient and maintain normal function. (See *Preventing pressure ulcers,* page 20.)

Equipment

Cradle boots or substitute • abduction pillow • trochanter rolls • hand rolls (see *Common preventive devices,* page 21)

Preparation of equipment

● If you're using a device that's available in different sizes, select the appropriate size for the patient.

● Always refer to the manufacturer's application guidelines before applying the device. **MFR**

Implementation

● Confirm the patient's identity using two patient identifiers according to facility policy. **JCAHO**
● Explain the purpose and steps of the procedure to the patient and his family.

Applying cradle boots

● Open the slit on the superior surface of the boot. Then place the patient's heel in the circular cutout area. If the patient is positioned laterally, you may apply the boot only to the bottom foot and support the flexed top foot with a pillow.
● If appropriate, apply the second boot to the other foot.
● Position the patient's legs properly *to prevent strain on hip ligaments and pressure on bony prominences.*

Applying an abduction pillow

● Place the pillow between the supine patient's legs. Slide it toward the groin so that it touches the legs all along its length.
● Place both upper legs in the pillow's lateral indentations, and secure the straps *to prevent the pillow from slipping.*

Applying trochanter rolls

● Position one roll along the outside of the thigh, from the iliac crest to midthigh and another roll along the other thigh. Make sure that neither roll extends as far as the knee *to avoid peroneal nerve compression and palsy, which can lead to footdrop.*
● If you've fashioned trochanter rolls from a towel, leave several inches unrolled and tuck this under the patient's thigh *to hold the device in place and maintain the patient's position.*

Applying hand rolls

● Place one roll in the patient's hand *to maintain the neutral position.* Secure the strap, if present, or apply roller gauze and secure with nonallergenic or adhesive tape.
● Place another roll in the other hand if needed.

INNOVATIVE PRACTICE

Preventing pressure ulcers EB

Pressure ulcers have tremendous emotional, physical, and financial consequences to patients and the heath care system. Research shows that complying with the 1992 pressure ulcer prevention guidelines from the Agency for Healthcare Research and Quality reduces the incidence of pressure ulcers. However, a study by the University of Washington, Department of Plastic Surgery, Department of Epidemiology, and the Department of Pediatrics found that despite these guidelines for pressure ulcer prevention, the incidence of pressure ulcers among hospitalized patients hasn't declined.

The authors of the study gathered census data from the National Center for Health Statistics for a period of 14 years from 1987 to 2000. They looked at patients admitted with a primary diagnosis of pressure ulcers as well as those patients admitted for another diagnosis but who developed pressure ulcers while hospitalized. Although no evidence indicated that following the guidelines for pressure ulcer prevention decreased the number of pressure ulcers that developed in hospitalized patients, the study did reveal that pressure ulcers are now being reported in a more thorough manner.

Special considerations

● Remember that the use of assistive devices doesn't replace the need for frequent patient positioning, ROM exercises, and skin care.

TEACHING *Explain the use of the devices to the patient and caregiver. Demonstrate how to use each device, emphasizing proper alignment of extremities, and have the patient or caregiver give a return demonstration so you can check for proper technique. Emphasize measures needed to prevent pressure ulcers.*

Nursing diagnoses

● Impaired physical mobility
● Impaired skin integrity

Expected outcomes

The patient will:
● maintain functional mobility
● exhibit no signs of skin breakdown
● communicate understanding of skin protection measures
● remain free from complications.

Complications

● Contractures and pressure ulcers may occur with the use of a hand roll and possibly with other assistive devices. To avoid these problems, remove a soft hand roll every 4 hours (every 2 hours if the patient

has hand spasticity); remove a hard hand roll every 2 hours.

● All skin surfaces should be assessed every 2 to 4 hours in the nonambulatory patient to assess for potential skin breakdown. **JCAHO** Also, provide vigilance in assessing the nutritional needs of the immobilized patient.

Documentation

Record the use of these devices in the patient's chart and the nursing care plan, include the reason for the device, and indicate assessment for complications. Document any patient teaching performed and the patient's understanding. Reevaluate your patient care goals as needed.

Supportive references

Baranoski, S., and Ayello, E. *Wound Care Essentials Practice and Principles.* Philadelphia: Lippincott Williams & Wilkins, 2004.

Groeneveld, A., et al. "The Prevalence of Pressure Ulcers in a Tertiary Care Pediatric and Adult Hospital," *Journal of Wound, Ostomy & Continence Nursing* 31(3):108-20, May-June 2004.

Jones, J. "Evaluation of Pressure Ulcer Prevention Devices: A Critical Review of the Literature," *Journal of Wound Care* 14(9):422-25, October 2005.

National Pressure Ulcer Advisory Panel: *www.npuap.org/.*

Common preventive devices

Equipment is available to reduce pressure or help maintain positioning, depending on the patient's needs.

Boot

Prevents footdrop, skin breakdown, and external hip rotation

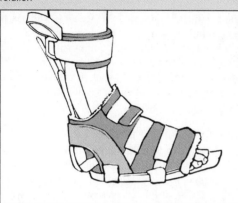

Trochanter roll

Prevents external hip rotation

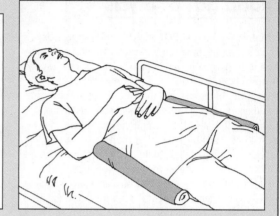

Abduction pillow

Prevents internal hip rotation and hip adduction

Hand roll

Prevents hand contractures

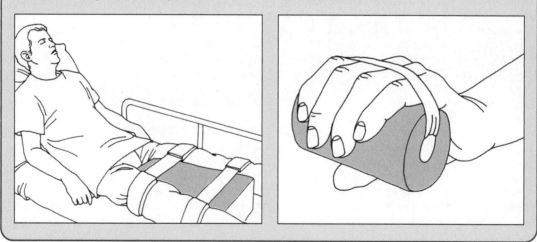

Price, M., et al. "Development of a Risk Assessment Tool for Intraoperative Pressure Ulcers," *Journal of Wound, Ostomy & Continence Nursing* 32(1):19-30, January-February 2005.

Scott, J.R., and Gibran, N.S., et al. "Incidence and Characteristics of Hospitalized Patients with Pressure Ulcers: State of Washington, 1987 to 2000," *Plastic and Reconstructive Surgery* 117(2):630-34, February 2006.
EB

Thompson, P., et al. "Skin Care Protocols for Pressure Ulcers and Incontinence in Long-Term Care: A Quasi-Experimental Study," *Advances in Skin and Wound Care* 18(8):422-29, October 2005.

Arterial puncture for blood gas analysis

Arterial blood gas (ABG) analysis helps assess oxygenation and ventilation and provides vital information to manage a patient's metabolic and respiratory disturbances. ABG analysis evaluates ventilation by measuring blood pH and the partial pressures of arterial oxygen (Pao_2) and partial pressure of arterial carbon dioxide ($Paco_2$). Blood pH measurement reveals the blood's acid-base balance, the Pao_2 indicates the amount of oxygen that the lungs deliver to the blood, and the $Paco_2$ indicates the lungs' capacity to eliminate carbon dioxide. ABG samples also can be analyzed for oxygen content and saturation and for bicarbonate values. Any change in cardiopulmonary status results in changes in ABG values, which reflect changes in the pulmonary and renal systems as they attempt to compensate for imbalances in the body.

Typically, ABG analysis is ordered for patients who have chronic obstructive pulmonary disease, pulmonary edema, acute respiratory distress syndrome, myocardial infarction, or pneumonia. It's also performed during episodes of shock and after coronary artery bypass surgery, resuscitation from cardiac arrest, changes in respiratory therapy or status, and prolonged anesthesia.

A specially trained nurse can draw most ABG samples. When selecting a site for sampling arterial blood, the nurse should keep three key factors in mind. First, superficial arteries are easier to palpate, stabilize, and puncture and puncture of arteries that are surrounded by insensitive body tissues, such as muscle, tendon, and fat, is less painful for the patient. Second, potential complications include vascular spasm, clotting of the vessel, or bleeding that results in a hematoma and vascular compression. Third, if a complication does occur, the artery should have good collateral blood flow. The radial artery best meets these criteria; the brachial artery is usually the best second choice.

Allen's test is a simple clinical maneuver to assess collateral blood flow in the radial artery before an attempt is made to puncture the artery. A positive result indicates that ulnar collateral flow is present, allowing a degree of safety in using the radial artery. (See *Performing Allen's test*.)

If the radial artery is inaccessible or Allen's test is negative, then the brachial artery can be used. However, the brachial artery is one of the most difficult arteries to palpate and stabilize, carries a higher risk of venous puncture because of its location, and can be very painful if the brachial nerve is punctured.

Only nurses who have had additional specialized training should use the femoral artery. This artery is best used in an emergency, such as cardiac arrest or hypovolemic shock, when pulses are difficult to palpate.

Equipment

10-ml glass syringe or plastic luer-lock syringe specially made for drawing blood for ABG analysis • 1-ml ampule of aqueous heparin (1:1,000) • 20G $1^{1}/_{4}$" needle • 22G 1" needle • gloves • alcohol pad • two 2" × 2" gauze pads • rubber cap for syringe hub or rubber stopper for needle • ice-filled plastic bag • label • laboratory request form • adhesive bandage • optional: 1% lidocaine solution

Many health care facilities use a commercial ABG kit that contains all the equipment listed above except the adhesive bandage and ice. If your facility doesn't use such a kit, obtain a sterile syringe specially made for drawing ABG samples, and use a clean emesis basin filled with ice instead of the plastic bag to transport the sample to the laboratory.

Preparation of equipment

● Prepare the collection equipment before entering the patient's room.

● Wash your hands thoroughly, then open the ABG kit and remove the sample label and the plastic bag.

● Record on the label the patient's name and room number, date and collection time, and the practitioner's name. Fill the plastic bag with ice and set it aside.

● If the syringe isn't heparinized, you'll have to do so. Attach the 20G needle to the syringe, and then open the ampule of heparin. Draw all the heparin into the syringe *to prevent the sample from clotting*. Hold the syringe upright, and pull the plunger back slowly to about the 7-ml mark. Rotate the barrel while pulling the plunger back *to allow the heparin to*

Performing Allen's test ⓔⒷ

Rest the patient's arm on the mattress or bedside stand, and support his wrist with a rolled towel. Tell him to clench his fist. Using your index and middle fingers, press on the radial and ulnar arteries. Hold this position for a few seconds.

Without removing your fingers from the patient's arteries, ask him to unclench his fist and hold his hand in a relaxed position. The palm will be blanched because pressure from your fingers has impaired normal blood flow.

Release pressure on the patient's ulnar artery. If the hand becomes flushed, which indicates blood filling the vessels, you can safely proceed with the radial artery puncture. If the hand doesn't flush, perform Allen's test on the other arm.

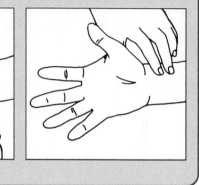

coat the inside surface of the syringe. Then slowly force the heparin toward the hub of the syringe, and expel all but about 0.1 ml of heparin.
● To heparinize the needle, first replace the 20G needle with the 22G needle. Then hold the syringe upright, tilt it slightly, and eject the remaining heparin. *Excess heparin in the syringe alters blood pH and* Pao_2 *values.*

Implementation
● Confirm the patient's identity using two patient identifiers according to facility policy. ⒿⒸⒶⒽⓄ
● Tell the patient that you need to collect an arterial blood sample, and explain the procedure *to help ease anxiety and promote cooperation.* Tell him that the needle insertion will cause some discomfort but that he must remain still during the procedure. ⓅⒸⓅ
● Wash your hands and put on gloves. ⒸⒹⒸ
● Place a rolled towel under the patient's wrist *for support.* Locate the artery and palpate it for a strong pulse.
● Clean the puncture site with an alcohol pad, starting in the center of the site and spiraling outward in a circular motion with friction for 30 seconds or until

the final pad comes away clean. Allow the skin to dry.
● Palpate the artery with the index and middle fingers of one hand while holding the syringe over the puncture site with the other hand. The puncture site should be between your index and middle fingers as they palpate the pulse.
● Puncture the skin and the arterial wall in one motion, following the path of the artery. When puncturing the radial artery, hold the needle bevel up at a 30- to 45-degree angle. When puncturing the brachial artery, hold the needle at a 60-degree angle. (See *Arterial puncture technique,* page 24.)
● Watch for blood backflow in the syringe. Don't pull back on the plunger *because arterial blood should enter the syringe automatically.* Fill the syringe to the 5-ml mark.
● After collecting the sample, press a gauze pad firmly over the puncture site until the bleeding stops — at least 5 minutes. If the patient is receiving anticoagulant therapy or has a blood dyscrasia, apply pressure for 10 to 15 minutes; if necessary, ask a coworker to hold the gauze pad in place while you prepare the sample for transport to the laboratory. Don't ask the patient to hold the pad. *If he fails to apply sufficient*

Arterial puncture technique

The angle of needle penetration in arterial blood gas sampling depends on which artery you're sampling. For a radial artery puncture, which is most commonly used, the needle should enter bevel up at a 30- to 45-degree angle over the radial artery, as shown.

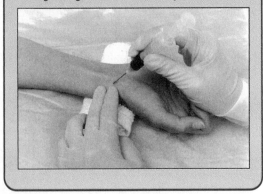

to indicate on the laboratory request slip the amount and type of oxygen therapy the patient is receiving.
● If the patient isn't receiving oxygen, indicate that he's breathing room air. If the patient has received a nebulizer treatment, wait about 20 minutes before collecting the sample.
● If necessary, anesthetize the puncture site with 1% lidocaine solution or normal saline with 0.9% benzyl alcohol. Consider such use of lidocaine carefully *because it delays the procedure, the patient may be allergic to the drug, or the resulting vasoconstriction may prevent successful puncture.*
● When filling out a laboratory request form for ABG analysis, be sure to include the following information *to help the laboratory staff calibrate the equipment and evaluate results correctly:* the patient's current temperature, most recent hemoglobin level, current respiratory rate and, if the patient is on a ventilator, fraction of inspired oxygen and tidal volume. **JCAHO**

Nursing diagnoses
● Deficient knowledge (procedure)
● Risk for infection
● Risk for injury

Expected outcomes
The patient will:
● demonstrate an understanding of the procedure and reason for the test
● remain free from infection
● not develop complications related to the procedure.

Complications
● If you use too much force when attempting to puncture the artery, the needle may touch the periosteum of the bone, causing the patient considerable pain, or you may advance the needle through the opposite wall of the artery. If this happens, slowly pull the needle back a short distance and check to see if you obtain a blood return. If blood still doesn't enter the syringe, withdraw the needle completely and start with a fresh heparinized needle. Don't make more than two attempts to withdraw blood from the same site. *Probing the artery may injure it and the radial nerve. Also, hemolysis will alter test results.*
● If arterial spasm occurs, blood won't flow into the syringe and you won't be able to collect the sample. If this happens, replace the needle with a smaller one

pressure, a large, painful hematoma may form, hindering future arterial punctures at that site.
● Check the syringe for air bubbles. If any appear, remove them by holding the syringe upright and slowly ejecting some of the blood onto a 2″ × 2″ gauze pad.
● Insert the needle into a rubber stopper, or remove the needle and place a rubber cap directly on the needle hub. *This prevents the sample from leaking and keeps air out of the syringe.*
● Put the labeled sample in the ice-filled plastic bag or emesis basin. Attach a properly completed laboratory request form, and send the sample to the laboratory immediately.
● When bleeding stops, apply a small adhesive bandage to the site.
● Monitor the patient's vital signs, and observe for signs of circulatory impairment, such as swelling, discoloration, pain, numbness, or tingling in the arm or leg. Watch for bleeding at the puncture site.

Special considerations
● If the patient is receiving oxygen, make sure that his therapy has been underway for at least 15 minutes before collecting an arterial blood sample.
● Unless ordered, don't turn off existing oxygen therapy before collecting arterial blood samples. Be sure

and try the puncture again. *A smaller-bore needle is less likely to cause arterial spasm.*

Documentation

Record the results of Allen's test, the time the sample was drawn, the patient's temperature, site of the arterial puncture, how long pressure was applied to the site to control bleeding, and the type and amount of oxygen therapy the patient was receiving.

Supportive references

Aaron, S.D., et al. "Topical Tetracaine Prior to Arterial Puncture: A Randomized, Placebo-Controlled Clinical Trial," *Respiratory Medicine* 97(11):1195-99, November 2003.

American Association for Respiratory Care. "AARC Clinical Guideline: Blood Gas Analysis and Hemoximetry. 2001 Revision and Update," *Respiratory Care* 46(5):498-505, May 2001.

Patterson, P., et al. "Comparison of 4 Analgesic Agents for Venipuncture," *AANA Journal* 68(1):43-51, February 2000.

Perry, A.G., and Potter, P.A. *Clinical Nursing Skills and Techniques,* 6th ed. St. Louis: Mosby–Year Book, Inc., 2005. **EB**

Blood pressure assessment

Arterial blood pressure is a measure of the pressure exerted by the blood as it flows through the arteries. Blood moves in waves as the heart contracts and relaxes. *Systolic* pressure occurs during left ventricular contraction at the height of the wave and reflects the integrity of the heart, arteries, and arterioles. *Diastolic* pressure occurs during left ventricular relaxation and directly indicates blood vessel resistance. The difference between systolic and diastolic pressures is called pulse pressure. Blood pressure is measured in millimeters of mercury (mm Hg).

Arterial blood pressure may be measured directly (invasively) or indirectly (noninvasively). The direct method requires electronic monitoring equipment and the insertion of a catheter into an artery. The patient must be in an intensive care unit or setting. Noninvasive measurement requires a blood pressure cuff, a sphygmomanometer, and a stethoscope. The brachial artery is commonly used; however, the radial artery or popliteal artery may also be used.

Cloth or disposable vinyl compression cuffs come in many different sizes. According to the American Heart Association, cuff size should be proportional to the circumference of the patient's limb. (See *Acceptable bladder dimensions for arms of different sizes,* page 26.) Ideally, the width of the cuff should be 40% of the circumference or 20% wider than the diameter of the midpoint of the limb. **AHA JNC** The bladder should encircle at least 80% of the adult upper arm and the entire arm of a child. For an adult, the average bladder is 4³/₄″ to 5¹/₄″ (12 to 13 cm) wide and 8⁵/₈″ to 9¹/₈″ (22 to 23 cm) long. If the bladder is too narrow, the blood pressure reading will be falsely high; if it's too wide, the reading will be falsely low.

Frequent blood pressure measurement is critical after serious injury, surgery, or anesthesia and during an illness or a condition that threatens cardiovascular stability. (Frequent measurement may be done with an automated vital signs monitor.) Regular measurement is indicated for patients with a history of hypertension or hypotension, and yearly screening is recommended for all adults.

Because pressure differences of more than 10 mm Hg exist between the arms of 6% of hypertensive patients, blood pressure should be measured in both arms at the initial assessment and in the arm with the higher pressure for future blood pressure measurements. **EB1**

Blood pressure should be measured using the recommendations set by the Seventh Report of the Joint National Committee on Prevention, Detection, Evaluation, and Treatment of High Blood Pressure (JNC VII). Until recently, patients with hypertension were stratified based on blood pressure readings alone. The JNC VII, however, also considers the patient's individual risk factors so that those with more risk factors are treated more aggressively. (See *Classification of blood pressure,* page 26.) The JNC VII has developed an innovative flowchart to guide the treatment of patients with hypertension. (See *Algorithm for treatment of hypertension,* page 27.)

Equipment

Mercury or aneroid sphygmomanometer • stethoscope • automated vital signs monitor (if available)

Acceptable bladder dimensions for arms of different sizes* `EB2`

Using an improper cuff size can greatly reduce the accuracy of a blood pressure reading. Use the chart below to help you to select the proper cuff size based on the patient's arm circumference.

Cuff	Bladder width (cm)	Bladder length (cm)	Arm circumference range at midpoint (cm)
Neonate	3	6	< 6
Infant	5	15	6 to 15†
Child	8	21	16 to 21†
Small adult	10	24	22 to 26
Adult	13	30	27 to 34
Large adult	16	38	35 to 44
Adult thigh	20	42	45 to 52

* There's some overlapping of the recommended range for arm circumferences to limit the number of cuffs; it's recommended that the larger cuff be used when available.
† To approximate the bladder width:arm circumference ratio of 0.4 more closely in infants and children, additional cuffs are available.

Adapted from Perloff, D., et al. "Human Blood Pressure Determination by Sphygmomanometry," *Circulation* 88(2)2460-467, November 1993, with permission of the publisher.

Classification of blood pressure `JNC` `EB3`

The Seventh Report of the Joint National Committee on Prevention, Detection, Evaluation, and Treatment of High Blood Pressure recommends that a person's risk factors be considered in the treatment of hypertension. The patient with more risk factors should be treated more aggressively.

Category	SBP mm Hg		DBP mm Hg
Normal	< 120	and	< 80
Prehypertension	120 to 139	or	80 to 89
Hypertension, stage 1	140 to 159	or	90 to 99
Hypertension, stage 2	≥ 160	or	≥ 100

Key: SBP = systolic blood pressure; DBP = diastolic blood pressure

Adapted from the Seventh Report of the Joint National Committee on Prevention, Detection, Evaluation, and Treatment of High Blood Pressure. NIH Publication No. 03-5231. Bethesda, Md.: National Institutes of Health; National Heart, Lung, and Blood Institute; National High Blood Pressure Education Program, May 2003.

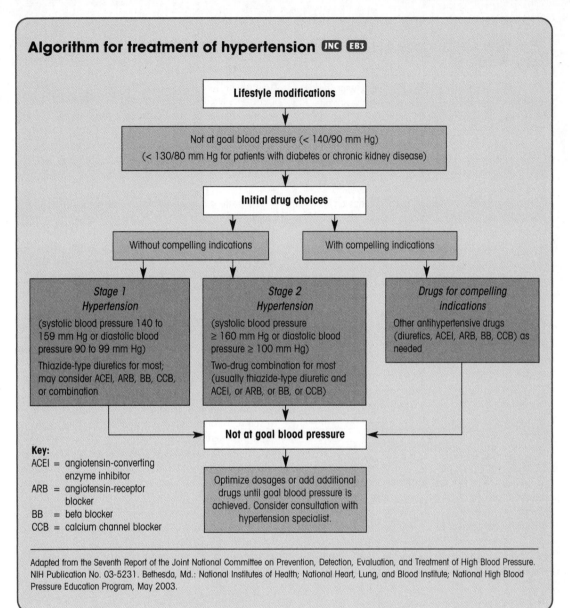

Algorithm for treatment of hypertension JNC EB3

Lifestyle modifications

↓

Not at goal blood pressure (< 140/90 mm Hg)
(< 130/80 mm Hg for patients with diabetes or chronic kidney disease)

↓

Initial drug choices

Without compelling indications | With compelling indications

Stage 1 Hypertension

(systolic blood pressure 140 to 159 mm Hg or diastolic blood pressure 90 to 99 mm Hg)

Thiazide-type diuretics for most; may consider ACEI, ARB, BB, CCB, or combination

Stage 2 Hypertension

(systolic blood pressure ≥ 160 mm Hg or diastolic blood pressure ≥ 100 mm Hg)

Two-drug combination for most (usually thiazide-type diuretic and ACEI, or ARB, or BB, or CCB)

Drugs for compelling indications

Other antihypertensive drugs (diuretics, ACEI, ARB, BB, CCB) as needed

Not at goal blood pressure

Key:
ACEI = angiotensin-converting enzyme inhibitor
ARB = angiotensin-receptor blocker
BB = beta blocker
CCB = calcium channel blocker

Optimize dosages or add additional drugs until goal blood pressure is achieved. Consider consultation with hypertension specialist.

Adapted from the Seventh Report of the Joint National Committee on Prevention, Detection, Evaluation, and Treatment of High Blood Pressure. NIH Publication No. 03-5231. Bethesda, Md.: National Institutes of Health; National Heart, Lung, and Blood Institute; National High Blood Pressure Education Program, May 2003.

The sphygmomanometer consists of an inflatable compression cuff linked to a manual air pump and a mercury manometer or an aneroid gauge. The JNC VII recommends using a mercury sphygmomanometer *because it's more accurate and requires calibration less frequently than the aneroid model.* JNC However, a recently calibrated aneroid manometer may be used. To obtain an accurate reading from a mercury sphygmomanometer, you must rest its gauge on a level surface and view the meniscus at eye level; you can rest an aneroid gauge in any position, but you must view it directly from the front.

Positioning the blood pressure cuff

To properly position a blood pressure cuff, wrap the cuff snugly around the upper arm above the antecubital area (the inner aspect of the elbow). When measuring an adult's blood pressure, place the lower border of the cuff about 1″ (2.5 cm) above the antecubital fossa. The center of the bladder should rest directly over the medial aspect of the arm; most cuffs have an arrow to be positioned over the brachial artery. Next, place the bell of the stethoscope on the brachial artery at the point where you hear the strongest beats.

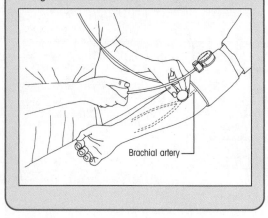

Brachial artery

Cuffs come in sizes ranging from neonate to extra-large adult. Disposable cuffs and thigh cuffs are available. (See *Positioning the blood pressure cuff.*)

The automated vital signs monitor is a noninvasive device that measures the pulse rate, systolic and diastolic pressures, and mean arterial pressure at preset intervals. (See *Using an electronic vital signs monitor.*)

Preparation of equipment
● Carefully choose an appropriate-sized cuff for the patient; the bladder should encircle at least 80% at the upper arm. **JNC** *An excessively narrow cuff may cause a falsely high pressure reading; an excessively wide one, a falsely low reading.* **EB4**
● If you're using an automated vital signs monitor, collect the monitor, dual air hose, and pressure cuff.

Then make sure that the monitor unit is firmly positioned near the patient's bed.

Implementation
● Confirm the patient's identity using two patient identifiers according to facility policy. **JCAHO**
● Tell the patient that you're going to take his blood pressure.
● Have the patient rest for at least 5 minutes before measuring his blood pressure. Make sure that he hasn't had caffeine or smoked for at least 30 minutes. **JNC**
● The patient may lie supine or sit erect during blood pressure measurement. If the patient is sitting erect, make sure that he has both feet flat on the floor *because crossing the legs may elevate blood pressure.* **EB5** His arm should be extended at heart level and be well supported. *If the artery is below heart level, you may get a false-high reading.* Make sure that the patient is relaxed and comfortable when you take his blood pressure *so it stays at its normal level.* **EB4**
● To ensure proper cuff placement on the patient's arm, first palpate the brachial artery. Position the cuff 1″ (2.5 cm) above the site of pulsation, center the bladder above the artery with the cuff fully deflated, and wrap the cuff evenly and snugly around the upper arm. If the arm is very large or misshapen and the conventional cuff won't fit properly, take leg or forearm measurements.
● To obtain a thigh blood pressure, apply the appropriate-sized cuff to the thigh, and auscultate the pulsations over the popliteal artery. To obtain a forearm blood pressure, apply the appropriate-sized cuff to the forearm 5″ (13 cm) below the elbow. Blood pressure sounds can be heard from the popliteal artery.
● If necessary, connect the appropriate tube to the rubber bulb of the air pump and the other tube to the manometer. Then insert the stethoscope earpieces into your ears.
● To determine how high to pump the blood pressure cuff, first estimate the systolic blood pressure by palpation. As you feel the radial artery with the fingers of one hand, inflate the cuff with your other hand until the radial pulse disappears. Read this pressure on the manometer and add 30 mm Hg to it. Use this sum as the target inflation to prevent discomfort from overinflation. Deflate the cuff and wait at least 2 minutes. **EB4**

Using an electronic vital signs monitor

An electronic vital signs monitor allows you to track a patient's vital signs continually, without having to reapply a blood pressure cuff each time. What's more, the patient won't need an invasive arterial line to gather similar data. These steps can be followed with most other monitors.

Some automated vital signs monitors are lightweight and battery operated and can be attached to an I.V. pole for continual monitoring, even during patient transfers. Make sure that you know the capacity of the monitor's battery, and plug the machine in whenever possible to keep it charged. Regularly calibrate the monitor to ensure accurate readings.

Before using a monitor, check its accuracy. Determine the patient's pulse rate and blood pressure manually, using the same arm you'll use for the monitor cuff. Compare your results when you get initial readings from the monitor. If the results differ, call your supply department or the manufacturer's representative.

Check the manufacturer's guidelines because most automated monitoring devices are intended for serial monitoring only and may be inaccurate for a one-time measurement. **MFR**

Preparing the device
● Explain the procedure to the patient. Describe the alarm system *so he won't be frightened if it's triggered.*
● Make sure that the power switch is off. Then plug the monitor into a properly grounded wall outlet. Secure the dual air hose to the front of the monitor.
● Connect the pressure cuff's tubing to the other ends of the dual air hose, and tighten connections *to prevent air leaks.* Keep the air hose away from the patient *to avoid accidental dislodgment.*
● Squeeze all air from the cuff, and wrap it loosely around the patient's arm about 1″ (2.5 cm) above the antecubital fossa. If possible, avoid applying the cuff to a limb that has an I.V. line in place. Position the cuff's "artery" arrow over the palpated brachial artery. Then secure the cuff for a snug fit.

Selecting the parameters
● When you turn on the monitor, it will default to a manual mode. (In this mode, you can obtain vital signs yourself before switching to the automatic mode.) Press the AUTO/MANUAL button to select the automatic mode. The monitor will give you baseline data for the pulse rate, systolic and diastolic pressures, and mean arterial pressure.
● Compare your previous manual results with these baseline data. If they match, you're ready to set the alarm parameters. Press the SELECT button to blank out all displays except systolic pressure.
● Use the HIGH and LOW limit buttons to set the specific parameters for systolic pressure. (These limits range from a high of 240 mm Hg to a low of 0 mm Hg.) Repeat this step three times for mean arterial pressure, pulse rate, and diastolic pressure. After setting the parameters for diastolic pressure, press the SELECT button again to display current data. Even if you forget to do this last step, the monitor will automatically display current data 10 seconds after you set the last parameters.

Collecting the data
● Program the monitor according to the desired frequency of assessments. Press the SET button until you reach the desired time interval in minutes. If you have chosen the automatic mode, the monitor will display a default cycle time of 3 minutes. You can override the default cycle time to set the interval you prefer.
● You can obtain a set of vital signs at any time by pressing the START button. Also, pressing the CANCEL button will stop the interval and deflate the cuff. You can retrieve stored data by pressing the PRIOR DATA button. The monitor will display the last data obtained along with the time elapsed since then. Scrolling backward, you can retrieve data from the previous 99 minutes. Make sure that the patient's vital signs are documented frequently on a vital signs assessment sheet.

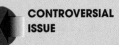

CONTROVERSIAL ISSUE

The diastolic dilemma AHA

The decision of whether to use the fourth or fifth Korotkoff sound as the diastolic blood pressure has long been the subject of controversy. Although the difference in the fourth and fifth sounds is usually less than 5 mm Hg, the sounds may be the same, the fourth sound may 10 mm Hg higher, or sounds may be heard all the way down to zero. The American Heart Association accepts the point at which all sound disappears, the fifth Korotkoff sound, as the diastolic blood pressure. The fifth sound is believed to more closely match the diastolic pressure obtained by direct intra-arterial monitoring and is more easily recognized by health care professionals. The fourth Korotkoff sound is considered the diastolic pressure in infants and children. **EB5**

● When you resume, locate the brachial artery by palpation. Center the bell of the stethoscope over the area of the artery where you detect the strongest beats, and hold it in place with one hand. *The bell of the stethoscope transmits low-pitched arterial blood sounds more effectively than the diaphragm.*

● Using the thumb and index finger of your other hand, turn the thumbscrew on the rubber bulb of the air pump clockwise to close the valve.

● Pump the cuff up to the predetermined level.

● Carefully open the valve of the air pump, and then slowly deflate the cuff — no faster than 2 to 3 mm Hg/second. While releasing air, watch the mercury column or aneroid gauge and auscultate for the sound over the artery. **EB4**

● When you hear the first beat or clear tapping sound, note the pressure on the column or gauge. This is the systolic pressure. (The beat or tapping sound is the first of five Korotkoff sounds. The second sound resembles a murmur or swish; the third sound, crisp tapping; the fourth sound, a soft, muffled tone; and the fifth, the last sound heard.) **EB4**

● Continue to release air gradually while auscultating for the sound over the artery.

● Note the pressure where sound disappears. This is the diastolic pressure — the fifth Korotkoff sound. (See *The diastolic dilemma.*) **EB4**

● After you hear the last Korotkoff sound, deflate the cuff slowly for at least another 10 mm Hg *to ensure that no further sounds are audible.*

● Rapidly deflate the cuff. Record the pressure, wait 2 minutes, and then repeat the procedure. If the average of the readings is greater than 5 mm Hg, take the average of two more readings. After doing so, remove and fold the cuff, and return it to storage. **JNC**

● Document the blood pressure results.

● Explain the importance of follow-up visits based on JNC VII recommendations to your patient. (See *Hypertension: Recommendations for follow-up.*)

Special considerations

● If you can't auscultate blood pressure, you may estimate systolic pressure. To do this, first palpate the brachial or radial pulse. Then inflate the cuff until you no longer detect the pulse. Slowly deflate the cuff and, when you detect the pulse again, record the pressure as the palpated systolic pressure.

● Palpation of systolic blood pressure also may be important *to avoid underestimating blood pressure in patients with an auscultatory gap.* This gap is a loss of sound between the first and second Korotkoff sounds; it may be as great as 40 mm Hg. You may find this in patients with venous congestion or hypotension.

● When measuring blood pressure in the popliteal artery, position the patient on his abdomen, wrap a cuff around the middle of the thigh, and proceed with blood pressure measurement.

● If the patient is anxious or crying, delay blood pressure measurement, if possible, until he becomes calm *to avoid falsely elevated readings.* **EB4**

● Occasionally, blood pressure must be measured in both arms or with the patient in two different positions (such as lying and standing or sitting and standing). In such cases, observe and record significant differences between the two readings, and record the blood pressure and the extremity and position used.

● Measure the blood pressure of patients taking antihypertensive medications while they're in a sitting position *to ensure accurate measurements.*

● Remember that malfunction in an aneroid sphygmomanometer can be identified only by checking it against a mercury manometer of known accuracy. Be sure to check your aneroid manometer this way periodically. Malfunction in a mercury manometer is evident in abnormal behavior of the mercury column. Don't attempt to repair either type yourself; instead, send it to the appropriate service department.

Nursing diagnoses

● Deficient knowledge (disease)
● Health-seeking behaviors (monitoring blood pressure)

Expected outcomes

The patient will:
● state an understanding of the need to monitor his blood pressure
● state an understanding of lifestyle modifications
● express an interest in learning new behaviors to lower his blood pressure
● state his blood pressure range
● maintain blood pressure within the desired limits.

Complications

● *Impaired circulation can affect blood pressure and cause an inaccurate reading.* Therefore, don't measure blood pressure on a patient's affected arm if the:
– shoulder, arm, or hand is injured or diseased.
– arm has a cast or bulky bandage.
– patient has had a mastectomy or removal of lymph nodes on that side.
– patient has an arteriovenous fistula in that limb.
● Don't take blood pressure in the arm on the affected side of a mastectomy *because it may decrease already compromised lymphatic circulation, worsen edema, and damage the arm.*
● Likewise, don't take blood pressure on the same arm of an arteriovenous fistula or hemodialysis shunt *because blood flow through the vascular device may be compromised.* **EB4**

Documentation

In the patient's chart, record blood pressure as systolic over diastolic such as 120/78 mm Hg. Chart an auscultatory gap if present. If required by your facility, chart blood pressures on a graph, using dots or checkmarks. Also, document the limb used and the patient's position. Include patient teaching about lifestyle modifications, drug therapy, and follow-up care. Record the name of any practitioner notified of blood pressure results and any orders given.

Hypertension: Recommendations for follow-up JNC

The Seventh Report of the Joint National Committee on Prevention, Detection, Evaluation, and Treatment of High Blood Pressure recommends the following guidelines.

After antihypertensive drug therapy is initiated, most patients should return for follow-up and adjustment of medications at approximately monthly intervals until the blood pressure goal is reached. More frequent visits will be necessary for patients with stage 2 hypertension or with complicating comorbid conditions. Serum potassium and creatinine levels should be monitored at least one to two times per year. After blood pressure is at goal and stable, follow-up visits can usually occur at 3- to 6-month intervals. Comorbidities, such as heart failure; associated diseases, such as diabetes; and the need for laboratory tests infuence the frequency of visits. Other cardiovascular risk factors should be treated to their respective goals, and tobacco avoidance should be promoted vigorously. Low-dose aspirin therapy should be considered only when blood pressure is controlled because the risk of hemorrhagic stroke is increased in patients with uncontrolled hypertension.

Supportive references

Beevers, G., et al. "ABC of Hypertension. Blood Pressure Measurement. Conventional Sphygmomanometry: Technique of Auscultatory Blood Pressure Measurement," *British Medical Journal* 322(7293):1043-47, April 2001.

Craven, R.F., and Hirnle, C.J. *Fundamentals of Nursing Human Health and Function,* 5th ed. Philadelphia: Lippincott Williams & Wilkins, 2006. **EB4**

Joanna Briggs Institute for Evidence Based Nursing and Midwifery. "Best Practice: Vital Signs," 3(3), 1999. *www.joannabriggs.edu.au/bpmenu.html.*

Keele-Smith, R., and Price-Daniel, C. "Effects of Crossing Legs on Blood Pressure Measurement," *Clinical Nursing Research* 10(2):202-13, May 2001. **EB5**

McAlister, F., and Straus, S. "Evidence-Based Treatment of Hypertension. Measurement of Blood Pressure: An Evidence-Based Review," *British Medical Journal* 322(7291):908-11, April 2001. **EB1**

Perloff, D., et al. "Human Blood Pressure Determination by Sphygmomanometry: Part 1," *Circulation* 88(5): 2460-470, November 1993. **EB2**

Perry, A., and Potter, P.A. *Clinical Nursing Skills and Techniques,* 6th ed. St. Louis: Mosby–Year Book, Inc., 2005.

The Seventh Report of the Joint National Committee on Prevention, Detection, and Treatment of High Blood Pressure. NIH Publication No. 03-5233. Bethesda, Md.: National Institutes of Health; National Heart, Lung, and Blood Institute; National High Blood Pressure Education Program. December 2003. *www.nhlbi.nih. gov/guidelines/hypertension/jcintro.html.* **EB3**

Woods, A. "Improving the Odds Against Hypertension," *Nursing2001* 31(8):36-42, August 2001.

Body mechanics Science

Body mechanics is the term used to describe the efficient, coordinated, and safe use of muscle groups to maintain balance, reduce fatigue, reduce energy requirements, and decrease the risk of injury while moving objects and carrying out activities of daily living. It involves the concepts of *center of gravity, line of gravity,* and *base of support* in relation to body alignment and balance.

The center of gravity is a point in the center of the body at navel level that's the pivot point for forward, back, and lateral balance. The line of gravity is located midline and forms a vertical line from the middle of the forehead to the midpoint between the feet, which form the base of support. When a person moves, the center of gravity moves continuously in the same direction as the body. Balance depends on the interrelationship of the center of gravity, line of gravity, and base of support. During movement, the closer the line of gravity is to the center of the base of support, the more stable the balance. The closer the line of gravity is to the edge of the base of support, the more precarious the balance. If the line of gravity falls outside the base of support, balance is lost.

The broader the base of support and the lower the center of gravity, the greater the stability and balance. Body balance, therefore, can be greatly enhanced by widening the base of support and lowering the center of gravity, bringing it closer to the base of support.

The best practice for body mechanics can be summed up in three principles. First, *keep a low center of gravity* by flexing the hips and knees instead of bending at the waist. This position distributes weight evenly between the upper and lower body, helps maintain balance, and decreases the load on the back muscles by transferring the weight to the stronger leg muscles. Second, *create a wide base of support* by spreading the feet apart. This tactic provides lateral stability and lowers the body's center of gravity. Finally, *maintain proper body alignment* — spine straight, head in neutral position, and all extremities in functional position — and keep the center of gravity directly over the base of support by moving the feet rather than twisting and bending at the waist.

Many patient care activities require the nurse to push, pull, lift, and carry. Application of proper body mechanics enables her to use the appropriate muscle groups when performing nursing care and can prevent musculoskeletal injury and fatigue and reduce the risk of injuring patients.

Implementation

Follow the directions below to push, pull, stoop, lift, and carry correctly.

Pushing and pulling

● Stand close to the object and place one foot slightly ahead of the other, as in a walking position. Tighten the leg muscles and set the pelvis by simultaneously contracting the abdominal and gluteal muscles.
● To push, place your hands on the object and flex your elbows. Lean into the object by shifting weight from the back leg to the front leg, and apply smooth, continuous pressure using leg muscles.
● To pull, grasp the object and flex your elbows. Lean away from the object by shifting weight from the front leg to the back leg. Pull smoothly, avoiding sudden, jerky movements.
● After you've started to move the object, keep it in motion; *stopping and starting uses more energy.*

Stooping

● Stand with your feet 10″ to 12″ (25.5 to 30.5 cm) apart and one foot slightly ahead of the other *to widen the base of support.*
● Lower yourself by flexing your knees, and place more weight on the front foot than on the back foot. Keep the upper body straight by not bending at the waist.
● To stand up again, straighten the knees and keep the back straight.

Lifting and carrying

● Assume the stooping position directly in front of the object *to minimize back flexion and avoid spinal rotation when lifting.*

● Grasp the object, and tighten your abdominal muscles.

● Stand up by straightening the knees, using the leg and hip muscles. Always keep your back straight *to maintain a fixed center of gravity.*

● Carry the object close to your body at waist height — near your center of gravity — *to avoid straining the back muscles.*

Special considerations

● Wear shoes with low heels, flexible nonslip soles, and closed backs *to promote correct body alignment, facilitate proper body mechanics, and prevent accidents.*

● When possible, pull rather than push an object *because the elbow flexors are stronger than the extensors. Pulling an object allows the use of hip and leg muscles and avoids the use of lower back muscles.*

● When doing heavy lifting or moving, remember to use assistive or mechanical devices, if available, or obtain assistance from coworkers. Know your limitations and use sound judgment.

● *Mechanical and other assistive devices have been shown to significantly decrease incidences of low back injury in nursing personnel.* **EB1** **EB2** **EB3**

Supportive references

Collins, J., and Owen, B. "NIOSH Research Initiatives to Prevent Back Injuries to Nursing Assistants, Aides and Orderlies in Nursing Homes," *American Journal of Industrial Medicine* 29(4):421-24, April 1996. **EB1**

Lee, Y., and Chiou, W. "Ergonomic Analysis of Working Posture in Nursing Personnel: Example of Modified Ovako Working Analysis System Application," *Research in Nursing and Health* 18(1):67-75, February 1995. **EB2**

Owen, B. "Preventing Injuries Using an Ergonomic Approach," *AORN Journal* 72(6):1031-36, December 2000. **EB3**

Owen, B., et al. "What Are We Teaching About Lifting and Transferring Patients?" *Research in Nursing and Health* 22(1):3-13, February 1999.

Owen, B., and Fragala, G. "Reducing Perceived Physical Stress While Transferring Residents: An Ergonomic Approach," *AAOHN Journal* 47(7):316-23, July 1999.

Care of the dying patient

Dying is a profound process affecting everyone involved: the dying person, significant others, friends, and caregivers. Beliefs and past experiences will affect how each person deals with the process of dying and death. To be effective in caring for the dying patient, a nurse needs to be knowledgeable about the dying process and comfortable in addressing death.

As a patient approaches death, he needs intensive physical support, and he and his family require emotional comfort. There are two phases, which occur before the actual time of death: the *pre-active phase of dying* and the *active phase of dying*. The pre-active phase may last approximately 2 weeks, while the active phase of dying usually lasts 3 days. Signs and symptoms of the pre-active phase are increased lethargy, withdrawal from social activities, decreased appetite, changes in respiration (periods of apnea) whether awake or asleep, edema in the extremities or the whole body, and an inability to recover from infections or heal from wounds. During this phase, the patient also may report seeing people or loved ones who have already died, and commonly the patient will state that he's dying. **HPA**

Signs and symptoms of impending death (the active phase of dying) include reduced respiratory rate and depth, decreased or absent blood pressure, weak or erratic pulse rate, lowered skin temperature, decreased level of consciousness (LOC), diminished sensorium and neuromuscular control, diaphoresis, pallor, cyanosis, and mottling. Emotional support for the dying patient and his family typically means simple reassurance and the nurse's physical presence to help ease fear and loneliness. More intense emotional support is important at much earlier stages, especially for the patient with a long-term progressive illness, who can work through the stages of dying. (See *Five stages of dying*, page 34.) **HPA**

Patients sometimes request withdrawal of treatment of a chronic illness that causes or prolongs suffering. Health care providers should respect a patient's wishes regarding extraordinary means of life support. The Patient Self-Determination Act of 1991 requires health care agencies serving Medicaid and Medicare patients to provide them with information regarding the various advance directive options, legal documents allowing a patient to decide what medical treatments he'll receive if he becomes unable to make decisions.

Five stages of dying EB1

Elisabeth Kübler-Ross, author of *On Death and Dying*, explained that the dying patient progresses through five psychological stages in preparation for death. Further research has shown that not all patients experience these emotional states in the same order or in the same way. However, knowing about the five stages allows you to more accurately assess the emotional needs of the dying patient.

Denial
The patient refuses to accept the diagnosis. He may experience physical symptoms similar to a stress reaction — shock, fainting, pallor, sweating, tachycardia, nausea, or GI disorders. During this stage, be honest with the patient but not blunt or callous. Maintain communication with him, so he can discuss his feelings when he accepts the reality of death. Don't force the patient to confront this reality.

Anger
When a patient stops denying his impending death, he may show deep resentment toward those who will live on after he dies — you, the facility staff, and his own family. Although you may instinctively draw back from the patient or even resent this behavior, it may help if you understand it as a normal reaction to the loss of control in his life rather than a personal attack. Maintaining a calm manner will help defuse the anger and allow you to help him find different ways to express it.

Bargaining
Although the patient acknowledges his impending death, he attempts to bargain for more time with God or fate for more time. He'll probably strike this bargain secretly. If he does confide in you, don't urge him to keep his promises.

Depression
In the depression stage, the patient may first experience regrets about his past and then grieve about his current condition. He may withdraw from his friends, family, physician, and you. He may suffer from anorexia, increased fatigue, or self-neglect. You may find him sitting alone, crying. Accept the patient's sorrow, and if he talks to you, listen. Provide comfort by touch, as appropriate. Resist the temptation to make optimistic remarks or cheerful small talk.

Acceptance
In acceptance, the last stage, the patient accepts the inevitability and imminence of his death — without emotion. The patient may simply desire the quiet company of a family member or friend. If, for some reason, a family member or friend can't be present, stay with the patient to satisfy his final need. Remember, however, that many patients die before reaching this stage.

CLINICAL IMPACT *The ordinary "Power of Attorney" doesn't give another person the legal right to make decisions about medical care for the patient. Only a "Durable Medical Power of Attorney" authorizes another person to make such decisions for a patient when the patient can't communicate his wishes.*

The patient may have signed a living will. This document, legally binding in most states, declares the patient's desire for a death unimpeded by the artificial support of such equipment as defibrillators, respirators, life-sustaining drugs, or auxiliary hearts. Nurses should know if a living will is legal in their state and their facility's policy regarding a signed living will. If the patient has signed such a document, the nurse must respect his wishes and communicate the physician's "no code" order to all staff members. (See *Evidence-based protocol: Advance directives*.)

An open discussion among the patient, the patient's family, and the health care provider will contribute to rational understanding of the situation so that the patient can make the best decision. Such discussion should distinguish between the desire to avoid suffering and the feeling and fear many patients have of being a burden.

Evidence-based protocol: Advance directives [EB2]

Here's an example of an advance directive protocol.

Assessment criteria
● Determine the patient's age.
● Identify the patient's primary language and any communication barriers.
● Assess the patient's cognitive level and ability to make decisions regarding treatment.
● Find out if the patient already has an advance directive.
● If yes, make a copy and place in the patient's chart.
● If no, provide patient education about advance directives and then ask the patient if he wishes to complete one. If the patient decides he would like to complete an advance directive, refer him to the appropriate resources. If not, document the results of the advance directive assessment in the health care record.

Description of the practice
If a living will has been signed or a health care proxy has been designated, do the following:
● Make sure that the documents can be easily found and accessed in the patient's chart.
● Communicate the document's existence to the practitioner.
● Determine if the designated health care proxy has a copy of the document.

● Review and clarify the document with the practitioner, patient, or proxy so that everyone is clear about the patient's wishes.
If the patient hasn't signed a living will or if a durable Power of Attorney hasn't been executed, do the following:
● Provide the patient (and, if appropriate, his family or significant others) with information about advance directives (brochures, videos, or other materials).
● Ask the patient if he would like to involve family members in discussions about advance directives; be sure to be sensitive to how the patient's beliefs and values may affect the discussion regarding advance directives.
● Be sensitive to the patient's and his family's fears about death in discussions about advance directives.
● Respect the patient's right not to complete advance directives.
● Reassure the patient that by signing an advance directive doesn't mean he'll receive substandard care.
● Know the facility's policy about resolving conflict between the patient and his family and health care providers regarding the patient's treatment.
● Help a patient execute an advance directive, and make suggestions as to whom to give advance directives and where to keep them.
● Make copies of the signed advance directive and place one in the patient's chart and communicate to the staff the patient's wishes.

Adapted from Weiler, K., and Garand, L. "Advance Directives." In Titler, M., series ed. *Series on Evidence-Based Practice for Older Adults.* Iowa City: The University of Iowa College of Nursing Gerontological Nursing Interventions Research Center, Research Dissemination Core, 2001. *www.nursing.uiowa.edu/gnirc,* with permission of the publisher.

Equipment
Clean bed linens ● clean gowns ● gloves ● water-filled basin ● soap ● washcloth ● towels ● lotion ● linen-saver pads ● petroleum jelly ● suction equipment, as necessary ● optional: indwelling urinary catheter

Implementation
● Assemble equipment at the patient's bedside, as needed.

Meeting physical needs
● Take the patient's vital signs often, and observe for pallor, diaphoresis, and decreased LOC.
● Reposition the patient in bed at least every 2 hours *because sensation, reflexes, and mobility diminish first in the legs and gradually in the arms.* Make sure the bed sheets cover him loosely *to reduce discomfort caused by pressure on arms and legs.* [EB3]
● When the patient's vision and hearing start to fail, turn his head toward the light and speak to him from near the head of the bed. Because hearing may be acute despite loss of consciousness, avoid whispering

Understanding organ and tissue donation

A federal regulation enacted in 1998 requires health care facilities to report all deaths to the regional organ procurement organization. This regulation was enacted so that no potential donor is missed and the family of every potential donor understands the option to donate. Although organ donor requirements vary, the typical donor must be between the ages of a neonate and 60, and free from transmissible disease. Tissue donations are less restrictive, and some tissue banks will accept skin from donors up to age 75.

According to the American Medical Association, about 25 types of organs and tissues are being transplanted. Collection of most organs, such as the heart, liver, kidney, or pancreas, requires that the patient be pronounced brain dead and kept physically alive until the organs are harvested. Tissue such as eyes, skin, bone, and heart valves may be taken after death. Contact your regional organ procurement organization for specific organ donation criteria or to identify a potential donor. If you don't know the regional organ procurement organization in your facility's area, call the United Network for Organ Sharing at (804) 330-8500.

or speaking inappropriately about the patient in his presence. **EB3**

● Change the bed linens and the patient's gown as needed. Provide skin care during gown changes, and adjust the room temperature for patient comfort, as necessary.

● Observe for incontinence or anuria, *the result of diminished neuromuscular control or decreased renal function.* If necessary, obtain an order to catheterize the patient, or place linen-saver pads beneath the patient's buttocks. Put on gloves and provide perineal care with soap, a washcloth, and towels *to prevent irritation.*

● Suction the patient's mouth and upper airway *to remove secretions.* Elevate the head of the bed *to decrease respiratory resistance.* As the patient's condition deteriorates, he may breathe mostly through his mouth.

● Offer fluids frequently, and lubricate the patient's lips and mouth with petroleum jelly *to counteract dryness.*

● If the comatose patient's eyes are open, provide appropriate eye care *to prevent corneal ulceration.*

● Provide mouth care for the comatose patient.

● Provide ordered pain medication as needed. Keep in mind that, as circulation diminishes, medications given I.M. will be poorly absorbed. Medications should be given I.V., if possible, *for optimum results.* **EB4**

Meeting emotional needs

● Fully explain all care and treatments to the patient even if he's unconscious *because he may still be able to hear.* Answer questions as candidly as possible, without sounding callous. **EB3**

● Allow the patient and his family to express their feelings, which may range from anger to loneliness. Take time to talk with the patient. Sit near the head of the bed, and avoid looking rushed or unconcerned.

● Notify family members, if they're absent, when the patient wishes to see them. Let the patient and his family discuss death at their own pace.

● Offer to contact a member of the clergy or social services department, if appropriate.

● If a living will and advance directives have been completed, make sure that the documents can be easily located. Notify all relevant care providers of their existence and review them to be sure you understand the patient's wishes. **EB2**

● If no living will has been executed, provide the patient and significant others with information regarding end-of-life issues. Remember to be sensitive, yet straightforward, taking into account cultural, ethnic, and religious issues for the patient and his family. Respect the patient's or his family's right not to complete advance directives if they choose, and inform them that you won't abandon them or provide substandard care because of their choice. **EB3**

Special considerations

● If the patient has signed a living will, the physician will write a "no code" order on his progress notes and order sheets. Know your state's policy regarding living wills. If living wills are legal, transfer the "no code" order to the patient's chart or Kardex and, at the end of your shift, inform the incoming staff of this order.

- If family members remain with the patient, show them the location of bathrooms, lounges, and cafeterias. Explain the patient's needs, treatments, and care plan to them. If appropriate, offer to teach them specific skills so they can take part in nursing care. Emphasize that their efforts are important and effective. As the patient's death approaches, give them emotional support.
- At an appropriate time, ask the patient's family if they have considered organ and tissue donation. Check the patient's records to determine whether he completed an organ donor card. (See *Understanding organ and tissue donation.*)

Nursing diagnoses
- Death anxiety

Expected outcomes
The patient will:
- identify the need to be with others and the need to be alone
- use available support services as needed
- express feelings of peacefulness and comfort.

Documentation
Record changes in the patient's vital signs, intake and output, and LOC. Note the times of cardiac arrest and the end of respiration, and notify the practitioner when these occur.

Supportive references
Harvey, J. "Debunking Myths about Post-Mortem Care," *Nursing2001* 31(7):44-45, July 2001. **EB3**

Jenkins, C., and Bruera, E. "Assessment and Management of Medically Ill Patients Who Refuse Life-Prolonging Treatment: Two Case Reports and Proposed Guidelines," *Journal of Palliative Care* 14(1):18-24, Spring 1998. **EB4**

Kübler-Ross, E. *Questions and Answers on Death and Dying.* New York: Simon & Schuster, 1997. **EB1**

Quill, T., and Byock, I. "Responding to Intractable Terminal Suffering: The Role of Terminal Sedation and Voluntary Refusal of Food and Fluids," *Annals of Internal Medicine* 132(5):408-14, March 2000. Published erratum, *Annals of Internal Medicine* 132(12):1011, June 2000.

University of Iowa Gerontological Nursing Interventions Research Center, 2001. *www.nursing.uiowa.edu/gnirc/.* **EB2**

Discharge

Successful discharge planning is a centralized, coordinated, multidisciplinary process that makes sure that a patient has a plan for continuing care after leaving the health care facility. Sometimes referred to as *continuity of care,* discharge planning seeks to provide services that will enable the patient to become as independent as possible by developing a care plan for ongoing maintenance and improvement of health. (See *Reducing readmissions,* page 38.)

The American Nurses Association describes discharge planning as "the part of the continuity of care process which is designed to prepare the client for the next phase of care and to assist in making any necessary arrangements for that phase of care, whether it be self-care, care by family members, or care by an organized health care provider." **ANA**

The Joint Commission on Accreditation of Healthcare Organizations standards state that discharge planning should be initiated early in the treatment process based on the requirements of the care plan or other written guidelines. Ideally, the admitting nurse who first meets the patient starts the assessment and identifies needs. Staff nurses, social workers, therapists, utilization review, physicians, and others then add to the care plan. The health care facility is responsible for keeping the patient and his family informed of the care process, especially when the facility anticipates some level of care continuing after discharge, while also ensuring compliance with all regulators regarding the patient's confidentiality. **HIPAA JCAHO** This discussion should begin as early as possible and should continue throughout the care process, anticipating and including the time of discharge. Criteria for discharge or terminating treatment are stipulated and may vary with the patient's age, disability, and treatment objectives. Criteria may also vary according to treatment settings, as set forth in the organization's policies and procedures. The standards also state that the information given to the patient and his family at the time of discharge includes:
- conditions that may result in the transfer to another facility or level of care
- alternatives to transfer
- clinical basis for discharge
- anticipated need for continued care after discharge. **JCAHO**

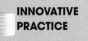

INNOVATIVE PRACTICE

Reducing readmissions EB1

With shorter hospital stays, patients with chronic illness may be discharged before their exacerbation is resolved. Elderly patients, in particular, are prone to readmissions and poor outcomes after early discharge. Researchers at the University of Pennsylvania in Philadelphia found that a special discharge program and home care plan reduced health care costs and readmissions in vulnerable hospitalized elderly patients.

Advanced practice nurses (APNs) with master's degrees and experience in gerontology visited patients and caregivers for discharge planning within 48 hours of patient admission and at least every 48 hours throughout the hospital stay. After discharge, APNs visited patients and caregivers within 48 hours and again 7 to 10 days after discharge. They made additional home visits based on patient needs, were available by telephone 7 days a week, and called patients and caregivers each week.

Care provided by the APNs centered on medications, management of symptoms, nutrition, activity, rest, follow-up care, and psychosocial concerns. APNs monitored the patient's progress and collaborated with the practitioner and other multidisciplinary team members.

At 24 weeks after discharge from the hospital, patients who received comprehensive discharge care by an APN were less likely to be readmitted to the hospital and were hospitalized for fewer days than elderly patients receiving standard discharge planning and intervention.

Reimbursement pressures have resulted in shorter hospital stays for patients. The Omnibus Reconciliation Act of 1986 mandated that all hospitals participating in Medicare have a discharge-planning program. Because of changes with the health care financing system, mainly the prospective payment system (PPS), decreased hospital stays has been the primary goal of many administrators, boards, and medical staff.

When a patient receives Medicare or other insurance payment for hospitalization, the PPS has a set price for each type of discharge diagnosis. Medicare uses diagnosis-related groups (DRGs) to categorize patients into over 400 diagnostic categories, such as fractured hip, heart failure, or urinary tract infection. If the hospitalization costs are less than the prenegotiated rate, the hospital keeps the difference, making a profit. However, if patient care costs more, the hospital loses money on the case because it isn't allowed to bill the patient for charges not covered by DRGs.

Although discharge from the health care facility is considered routine, effective discharge requires careful planning and ongoing assessment of the patient's needs during his hospitalization to ensure the best outcome.

Equipment

Wheelchair, unless the patient leaves by ambulance • patient's chart • patient instruction sheet • discharge summary sheet • prescriptions • plastic bag or patient's suitcase for personal belongings

Implementation

● Confirm the patient's identity using two patient identifiers according to facility policy. JCAHO

● Inform the patient and his family of the time and date of discharge as soon as it's known. If the patient can't arrange transportation, notify the social services department. (Always confirm arranged transportation on the day of discharge.) PCP

● Make a referral to the discharge planning department, if appropriate, in your facility.

● Obtain a written discharge order from the practitioner. If the patient discharges himself against medical advice, obtain the appropriate form. (See *Dealing with a discharge against medical advice*.)

● If the patient requires home medical care, confirm arrangements with the appropriate facility department or community agency.

● On the day of discharge, review the patient's discharge care plan, initiated on admission and modified during his hospitalization, with the patient and his family. List prescribed drugs on the patient instruction sheet along with the dosage, prescribed time schedule, and adverse reactions he should report to the practitioner. Make sure that the drug schedule is consistent with the patient's lifestyle *to prevent im-*

proper administration and to promote patient compliance. Have the patient or family member sign the discharge instruction sheet indicating that they have received and understand the discharge instructions. (See *Discharge teaching goals*.) **EB2**

● Review procedures the patient or his family members will perform at home. If necessary, demonstrate these procedures, provide written instructions, and check performance with a return demonstration. **PCP**

● List dietary and activity instructions, if applicable, on the patient instruction sheet, and review the reasons for them. If the practitioner orders bed rest, make sure that the patient's family can provide daily care and will obtain necessary equipment.

● Check with the practitioner about the patient's next office appointment; if the practitioner hasn't yet done so, inform the patient of the date, time, and location. If scheduling is your responsibility, make an appointment with the practitioner, outpatient clinic, physical therapy, X-ray department, or other health services, as needed. If the patient can't arrange transportation, notify the social services department.

● Retrieve the patient's valuables from the facility's safe and review each item with him. Then obtain the patient's signature *to verify receipt of his valuables.*

● Obtain from the pharmacy any drugs the patient brought with him. Return these to the patient if drug therapy is unchanged. If giving a new prescription, provide an explanation of the dosage, schedule, and adverse effects.

● If appropriate, take and record the patient's vital signs on the discharge summary form. Notify the practitioner if any signs are abnormal such as an elevated temperature. *If necessary, the practitioner may alter the patient's discharge plan.*

● Help the patient get dressed, if necessary.

● Collect the patient's personal belongings from his room, compare them with the admission inventory of belongings, and help place them in his suitcase or a plastic bag.

● After checking the room for misplaced belongings, help the patient into the wheelchair, and escort him to the exit; if the patient is leaving by ambulance, help him onto the litter.

● After the patient has left the area, strip the bed linens and notify the housekeeping staff that the room is ready for terminal cleaning.

● After discharge, follow up with a telephone call to the patient or caregiver. **EB2**

Dealing with a discharge against medical advice

Although a patient can choose to leave a health care facility against medical advice (AMA) at any time, the law requires clear evidence that he's mentally competent to make that choice. In most health care facilities, an AMA form serves as a legal document to protect you, the practitioners, and the facility if problems arise from a patient's unapproved discharge.

The AMA form should clearly document that the patient knows he's leaving against medical advice, that he has been advised of the risks of leaving and understands them, and that he knows he can come back.

If a patient refuses to sign the AMA form, document this refusal on the form and enter it in his chart. Use the patient's own words to describe his refusal.

Provide routine discharge care. Even though your patient is leaving AMA, his rights to discharge planning and care are the same as those for a patient who's signed out with medical advice. So, if the patient agrees, arrange follow-up care, and offer other routine health care measures.

TEACHING

Discharge teaching goals

Your discharge teaching should aim to ensure that the patient:
● understands his illness
● complies with his drug therapy
● carefully follows his diet
● manages his activity level
● understands his treatments
● recognizes his need for rest
● knows about possible complications
● knows when to seek follow-up care.

Remember that your discharge teaching should include the patient's family or other caregivers to make sure the patient receives proper home care.

Special considerations

● Whenever possible, involve the patient's family in discharge planning *so they can better understand and perform patient care procedures.*
● Before the patient is discharged, perform a physical assessment. If you detect abnormal signs or if the patient develops new symptoms, notify the practitioner and delay discharge until he has seen the patient.

Nursing diagnoses

● Anxiety
● Deficient knowledge (related to discharge instructions)

Expected outcomes

The patient will:
● discuss activities that tend to decrease anxiety
● identify situations that produce anxiety
● demonstrate the desire to learn
● demonstrate an understanding of discharge instructions.

Documentation

Many health care facilities combine discharge summaries and patient instructions into one form. This form contains sections for recording patient assessment, patient education, detailed special instructions, and the circumstances of discharge. When documenting discharge instructions, be sure to include:
● date and time of discharge
● family members or caregivers present for teaching
● details of instructions given to the patient, including medications, activity, and diet as well as written instructions given to the patient
● treatments, such as dressing changes or the use of medical equipment
● signs and symptoms to report to the practitioner
● patient, family, or caregiver understanding of instructions or ability to give a return demonstration of procedures
● whether the patient or caregiver requires further instruction
● practitioner's name and telephone number
● date, time, and location of follow-up appointments.

Supportive references

Joint Commission on Accreditation of Healthcare Organizations. "Standards, Rationales, Elements of Performance Scoring," PC 15(10):202, 2005.

Naylor, M.D., et al. "Comprehensive Discharge Planning and Home Follow-up of Hospitalized Elders: A Randomized Clinical Trial," *JAMA* 281(7):613-20, February 1999. **EB1**

Naylor, M.D. "A Decade of Transitional Care Research with Vulnerable Elders," *Journal of Cardiovascular Nursing* 14(3):1-14, 88-89, April 2000.

Shaw, M.C. "Discharge Planning and Home Follow Up by Advanced Practice Nurses Reduced Hospital Readmissions of Elderly Patients," *Evidence Based Nursing* 2:125, October 1999. **EB2**

Fall prevention and management

Falls are a major cause of injury and death among elderly people. In fact, the older the person is, the more likely he'll die as a result of a fall or its complications. In people age 75 or older, falls account for three times as many accidental deaths as motor vehicle accidents.

Factors that contribute to falls include lengthy convalescent periods in elderly patients, higher risks of incomplete recovery, and increasing physical disability. After it's impaired, equilibrium takes longer to restore in elderly people than in younger adults. Naturally, loss of balance increases the risk of falling. Besides causing physical harm, injuries from falls can trigger psychological problems, leading to losses in self-confidence and hastening dependency and a move to a long-term care facility or nursing home.

Falls may be caused by environmental factors, such as poor lighting, slippery throw rugs, or highly waxed floors. However, they also may result from physiologic factors, such as temporary muscle paralysis, vertigo, orthostatic hypotension, central nervous system lesions, dementia, failing eyesight, or decreased strength or coordination.

In a hospital or other health care facility, an accidental fall can change a short stay for a minor problem into a prolonged stay for serious, possibly life-threatening problems. The risk of falling is highest during the first week of a hospital or nursing home

Determining a patient's risk for falling

The Morse Fall Scale is one method of rapidly assessing a patient's likelihood of falling. It's widely used in hospital and long-term care inpatient settings.

To use the scale, score each item and total the number of points. A score between 0 and 24 indicates no risk, 25 to 50 indicates low risk, and a score greater than 50 indicates a high risk for falling.

Item		Scale	Scoring
History of falling; immediate or within 3 months	No Yes	0 25	0
Secondary diagnosis	No Yes	0 15	0
Ambulatory aid ● Bed rest/nurse assist ● Crutches/cane/walker ● Furniture		0 15 30	15
I.V./Heparin lock	No Yes	0 20	20
Gait/Transferring ● Normal/bedrest/immobile ● Weak ● Impaired		0 10 20	20
Mental status ● Oriented to own ability ● Forgets limitations		0 15	0
TOTAL			55

Adapted with permission from Morse, J.M. *Preventing Patient Falls.* Thousand Oaks, Calif.: Sage Pubs, 1997.

stay, commonly occurring during transfers such as to and from a bed to a chair. The adage "an ounce of prevention is worth a pound of cure" is worth remembering when working with elderly patients. (See *Determining a patient's risk for falling.*)

Recommendations from the Centers for Disease Control and Prevention for preventing falls in elderly patients include:
● physical conditioning, rehabilitation, or physical therapy that includes exercise to improve endurance and strength
● environmental assessments and modifications to improve mobility such as installing handrails in hallways, raised toilet seats, and grab bars in showers
● review of prescribed medications to assess potential risks and benefits
● technological devices, such as alarm systems, that are activated when patients get out of bed. **CDC**

Nursing interventions to reduce falls should follow the clinical practice guidelines endorsed by the American Geriatrics Society, British Geriatrics Society, and

Clinical practice guideline: Preventing falls

The following guideline was developed by a panel of health care professionals to help you assess the risk of falls in elderly patients.

Assessment
As part of routine care for older persons, ask patients (or caregivers) about falls in the past year.

For the patient who reports a single fall:
- have the patient stand up from a chair without using his arms, walk several paces, turn, return to the chair, and sit down
- if the patient has no difficulty, he needs no further assessment.

For the patient who reports more than one fall or has an abnormal gait or balance, perform a fall evaluation, including:
- a history of fall circumstances, medical problems, and mobility
- a medication review and modification, as needed, especially when the patient is taking more than four drugs
- examination of vision, gait, balance, lower extremity function, neurologic function, cerebellar function, and cardiovascular status
- a home environmental assessment.

Recommended interventions
For patients living in their own homes:
- gait training and advice on assistive devices
- medication review and modification, as needed
- exercise programs with balance training
- treatment of postural hypotension
- correction of environmental hazards
- treatment of cardiovascular disorders and arrhythmias.

For patients in long-term care or assisted-living settings:
- staff education programs
- gait training and advice on assistive devices
- medication review and modification, as needed.

For patients in acute hospital settings, evidence is insufficient to recommend interventions.

Adapted from American Geriatrics Society, British Geriatrics Society, and American Academy of Orthopaedic Surgeons Panel on Falls Prevention. "Guideline for the Prevention of Falls in Older Persons," *Journal of the American Geriatrics Society* 49(5):664-72, May 2001, with permission of the publisher.

the American Academy of Orthopaedic Surgeons. (See *Clinical practice guideline: Preventing falls.*)

Equipment
Stethoscope • sphygmomanometer • analgesics • cold and warm compresses • pillows • blankets • emergency resuscitation equipment (crash cart), if needed • electrocardiograph (ECG) monitor, if needed

Preparation of equipment
If you're helping a patient who has fallen, send an assistant to collect the assessment or resuscitation equipment you need.

Implementation
- Whether your care plan focuses on preventing a fall or managing one in an elderly patient, you'll need to proceed with patience and caution.

Preventing falls
- Assess the patient's risk of falling on admission and regularly thereafter using a standardized assessment tool. (See *Reducing the risk of falls.*) Note any changes in his condition — such as decreased mental status — that increase his risk of falling. If you decide that he's at risk, take steps to reduce the danger. **EB1**
- Orient the patient to the room and nursing unit. Show him how to use the call button and assess his ability to use it. Place the call button within reach. **EB1**

● Correct potential dangers in the patient's room. Provide adequate nighttime lighting.
● Place the patient's personal belongings and aids (purse, wallet, books, tissues, urinal, commode, or cane or walker) within easy reach.
● Instruct the patient to rise slowly from a supine position *to avoid possible dizziness and loss of balance.* **EB1**
● Lower the bed to its lowest position *so the patient can easily reach the floor when he gets out of bed. This also reduces the distance to the floor in case he falls.* Place the bed against the wall, if possible. Lock the bed's wheels. If side rails are raised, observe the patient frequently.
● Advise the patient to wear nonskid footwear.
● Respond promptly to the patient's call light *to help limit the number of times he gets out of bed without help.* **EB2**
● Check the patient at least every 2 hours. Check a high-risk patient every 15 to 30 minutes.
● Alert other caregivers to the patient's risk of falling and to the interventions you've implemented.
● Frequently assess high-risk patients, such as those with urgency and those who are receiving laxatives or diuretics, and assist them with toileting on a regular schedule.
● Encourage the patient to perform active range-of-motion (ROM) exercises *to improve flexibility and coordination.*
● Educate the patient and his family about mobility limitations and fall reduction measures.

Managing falls

If you're with the patient as he falls:
● Try to break his fall with your body.
● As you gently guide him to the floor, support his body — especially his head and trunk. If possible, help him to a supine position.
● While guiding the patient, concentrate on maintaining your own body alignment to keep the center of gravity within your support base. Spread your feet to widen your support base. Remember, *the wider the base, the better your balance will be.* Bend your knees — not your back — *to support the patient and to avoid injuring yourself.* **Science**
● Remain calm and stay with the patient *to prevent further injury.*

CONTROVERSIAL ISSUE

Reducing the risk of falls

Although falls in elderly people increase morbidity, mortality, and health care costs and reduce functional level, the best approaches to reduce the risk of falls remain controversial. What's more, preventive interventions that reduce the risk of falls in one elderly population may not be effective in another. For example, research indicates that individualized exercise programs in elderly people over age 80 and in elderly people with mild deficits in strength, balance, and range of motion reduce the risk of falls but not in the general elderly population. T'ai chi, however, which provides balance training, is effective in reducing falls in the general elderly population. **EB3**

Researchers have also found that interventions, such as assistive devices and the use of behavioral and educational programs, reduce the risk of falls when implemented as part of a multifactorial program but not when used as single interventions.

Many nurses continue to use side rails to maintain safety while a patient is in bed. However, research indicates that side rails don't prevent injuries from falling out of bed nor do they prevent patients from getting out of bed on their own. In fact, the use of side rails has been shown to increase the risk of injury when patients attempt to climb out of bed without assistance. Deaths due to entrapment by side rails have been reported. Other physical consequences of the use of side rails include incontinence, bruises, skin tears, lacerations, increased dependence, and limited visual field. **EB4 EB5**

● Ask another nurse to collect any equipment you may need, such as a stethoscope, a sphygmomanometer and, if necessary, an ECG monitor.
● Assess the patient's airway, breathing, and circulation *to make sure the fall wasn't caused by respiratory or cardiac arrest.* If you don't detect respirations or a pulse, call for help and begin emergency resuscitation measures. Also note the patient's level of consciousness (LOC) **Science** and assess pupil size, equality, and reaction to light.

Medications associated with falls

This chart highlights some classes of drugs that are commonly prescribed for older patients and the possible adverse effects of each that may increase a patient's risk of falling.

Drug class	Adverse effects
Antidiabetic agents	• Acute hypoglycemia
Antihypertensives	• Hypotension
Antihistamines and benzodiazepines	• Orthostatic hypotension • Muscle rigidity • Sedation
Antipsychotics	• Excessive sedation • Confusion • Paradoxical agitation • Loss of balance
Diuretics	• Hypovolemia • Orthostatic hypotension • Electrolyte imbalance • Urinary incontinence
Hypnotics	• Excessive sedation • Ataxia • Poor balance • Confusion • Paradoxical agitation
Opioids	• Hypotension • Sedation • Motor incoordination • Agitation
Tricyclic antidepressants	• Orthostatic hypotension

• *To determine the extent of injuries,* look for lacerations, abrasions, and obvious deformities. Note any deviations from the patient's baseline condition. Notify the practitioner.

If you weren't present during the fall:
• Ask the patient or a witness what happened. Ask if the patient experienced pain or a change in his LOC.
• Don't move the patient until you evaluate his status fully. Provide reassurance as needed, and observe for such signs and symptoms as confusion, tremor, weakness, pain, and dizziness. **Science**
• Assess the patient's limb strength and motion. Don't perform ROM exercises if you suspect a fracture or if the patient complains of odd sensations or limited movement. If you suspect a disorder, don't move the patient until a practitioner examines him. **Science** Spinal cord injuries from patient falls are rare, *but if injury has occurred, movement may cause irreversible spinal damage.*
• If you suspect a spinal cord injury, however, don't place a pillow under his head.

If you don't detect problems:
• Return the patient to his bed with the help of another staff member. Never try to lift a patient alone *because you may injure yourself or the patient.*
• Take steps to control bleeding (if indicated) and to obtain an X-ray if you suspect a fracture. Provide first aid for minor injuries as needed. Then monitor the patient's status for the next 24 hours.
• Even if the patient shows no signs of distress or has sustained only minor injuries, monitor his vital signs every 15 minutes for 1 hour, every 30 minutes for 1 hour, and then every hour for 2 hours or until his condition stabilizes. Notify the practitioner if you note a change from the baseline.
• Perform necessary measures to relieve the patient's pain and discomfort. Give analgesics as ordered. Apply cold compresses for the first 24 hours and warm compresses thereafter, as ordered. **Science**
• Reassess the patient's environment and his risk of falling. Talk to him about the fall. Discuss why it occurred and how he thinks it could have been prevented. Review the events that preceded the fall. Did the patient change position abruptly? Does he wear corrective lenses, and was he wearing them when he fell? Had he been drinking alcohol? Review medications that may have contributed to the fall, such as tranquilizers and opioids. (See *Medications associated with falls.*) In addition, assess gait disturbances or the improper use of canes, crutches, or a walker. **EB1**
• Notify the patient's family if the patient has an appointed caregiver. Follow confidentiality guidelines. **JCAHO** **HIPAA**

Special considerations

• After a fall, review the patient's medical history *to determine whether he's at risk for other complications.*

For example, if he hit his head, check his history to see whether he takes anticoagulants. If he does, he's at greater risk for intracranial bleeding, and you'll need to monitor him accordingly. **JCAHO**

● Develop an individualized fall prevention program with multiple interventions.

● Consider beginning a fall prevention program in your facility if you don't already have one.

● Devise an alternative to restraints for a high-risk patient; for example, a pressure-pad alarm. The pressure sensor pad lies under the bed linens, and the reduced pressure that results as the patient gets out of bed triggers an alarm at the nurses' station. One such system, consisting of a lightweight plastic sensor sheet and a control unit, adapts to a bed and chair, and setting it up according to the manufacturer's directions prevents false alarms. **MFR** An alternative alarm device can be worn by the patient just above the knee. The alarm sounds when the patient moves his leg to a vertical position. Research is still needed to evaluate the effectiveness of alarms in reducing falls. **JCAHO**

● To promote patient safety, consider drawing a red arrow next to the patient's room number on the call-light console and making a red dot on the AT RISK card on the patient's door. Also add an appropriate notation to the Kardex and chart.

● Provide emotional support, whether you're managing a fall or preventing one. Let the elderly patient know that you recognize his limitations and acknowledge his fears. Point out measures that you'll take to provide a safe environment.

● Teach the patient how to fall safely. Show him how to protect his hands and face. If he uses a walker or a wheelchair, demonstrate how to cope with and recover from a fall. Instruct him to survey the room for a low, sturdy, supportive piece of furniture such as a coffee table. Then review the proper procedure for lifting himself off the floor and either standing up with the walker or getting into the wheelchair.

● Regularly attend continuing education programs on fall assessment and prevention.

TEACHING *Before discharge, teach the patient and his family how to prevent accidental falls at home by correcting common household hazards. Encourage them to take steps to ensure the patient's safety. (See Promoting safety in the home.)*

Promoting safety in the home

Before your patient leaves the health care facility, review these tips with him and his family.

● Secure all carpets and floor coverings around the edges, and tack down worn spots. Never use lightweight, loose mats or rugs on bare floors.

● Make sure that potential hazards, such as stairs, are well-lighted. White paint on either side of a staircase and on the edges of steps can enhance visibility.

● Install strong banisters along all indoor and outdoor steps.

● Use a bedside lamp or low-wattage night-light in the bedroom to avoid the patient's having to grope around in the dark when getting out of bed.

● Fit secure handrails in convenient places in the shower, bathtub, and toilet. Use nonskid mats inside and alongside the tub or shower.

● Minimize clutter. Store children's toys, especially those on wheels, when not in use.

● Walk carefully if a pet, such as a dog or a cat, is present.

● Secure wires from electrical appliances to walls or moldings.

● Store frequently used clothing and other items in places where they can be reached without standing on a stool or chair.

● Reduce the risk of accidental slips and falls by selecting well-fitting shoes with nonskid soles, avoiding wearing long robes, and wearing eyeglasses, if needed.

● Sit on the edge of a bed or chair for a few minutes before rising.

● Use a walking stick or cane, if necessary.

As needed, refer the patient to the home care coordinator so that nursing services can continue after discharge and during convalescence.

Nursing diagnoses
● Deficient knowledge (related to safety issues)
● Risk for injury

Expected outcomes
The patient will:
● identify and apply safety measures to prevent falls
● remain free from injury

- identify risk factors for injury.

Documentation

After a fall, complete an incident report in case the patient takes legal action. Don't file the incident report in the medical record; it isn't legally part of the patient's record. Instead, forward it to the designated person in the facility's administration. The incident report alerts the facility's insurance carrier about the possibility of a liability claim and the need for further investigation.

The report should note where and when the fall occurred, who found the patient, how he was found, and in what position. Include the events preceding the fall, the names of witnesses, the patient's reaction to the fall, and a detailed description of his condition, based on assessment findings. Note interventions taken and the names of staff members who helped care for him after the fall. Record the practitioner's name and the date and time that he was notified. Include a copy of the practitioner's report. Note whether the patient was sent for diagnostic tests or transferred to another unit.

Include all of this information in the patient's record. Also, note the patient's vital signs. If you're monitoring the patient for a severe complication, record this as well. Record the details of the fall objectively. Avoid offering opinions, assumptions, or blame. Don't include in the medical record the fact that an incident report was filed.

Supportive references

A Guide to Bed Safety: Bed Rails in Hospitals, Nursing Homes and Home Health Care: The Facts. U.S. Food and Drug Administration, March 25, 2005. *www.fda.gov/cdrh/beds/.* **EB4**

American Geriatrics Society, British Geriatrics Society, and American Academy of Orthopaedic Surgeons Panel on Falls Prevention. "Guideline for the Prevention of Falls in Older Persons," *Journal of the American Geriatrics Society* 49(5):664-72, May 2001. **EB1**

"Charting Tips: Documenting a Patient's Fall Risk," *Nursing2000* 30(11):14, November 2000.

Feder, G., et al. "Guidelines for the Prevention of Falls in People Over 65. The Guidelines Development Group," *British Medical Journal* 321(7267):1007-11, October 2000. **EB3**

Gillespie, L.D., et al. "Interventions for Preventing Falls in Elderly People," *Cochrane Database of Systematic Reviews* 3:CD000340, 2001.

Joanna Briggs Institute for Evidence Based Nursing and Midwifery. "Best Practice: Falls in the Hospital," 2(2), 1998. *www.joannabriggs.edu.au/bpmenu.html.*

Joint Commission on Accreditation of Healthcare Organizations. "National Patient Safety Goals," 2005. *www.jcaho.org.*

Kimbell, S. "Before the Fall: Keeping Your Patient on His Feet," *Nursing2001* 31(8):44-45, August 2001. **EB2**

Rogers, P.D., and Bocchino, N.L. "Restraint-Free Care: Is it Possible?" *AJN* 99(10):26-33, October 1999.

Talerico, K.A., and Capezuti, E. "Myths and Facts about Siderails," *AJN* 101(7):43-48, July 2001. **EB5**

Fecal occult blood test

Fecal occult blood tests are valuable for determining the presence of occult blood (hidden GI bleeding) and for distinguishing true melena from melena-like stools. Certain medications, such as iron supplements and bismuth compounds, can darken stools so that they resemble melena.

Two common occult blood screening tests are Hematest (an orthotolidine reagent tablet) and the Hemoccult slide (filter paper impregnated with guaiac). Both tests use a chemical reagent that produces a blue reaction in the presence of the enzyme peroxidase in the hemoglobin molecule in a fecal smear if occult blood loss exceeds 5 ml in 24 hours.

Certain foods, medications, and vitamin C can produce inaccurate test results. False-positive results can occur if the patient has recently ingested red meat, poultry, fish, certain types of raw vegetables and fruits (for example, radishes, turnips, and melons), horseradish, or certain medications that irritate the gastric mucosa and cause bleeding (such as aspirin, nonsteroidal anti-inflammatory drugs, steroids, iron preparations, and anticoagulants). False-negative results can occur if the patient has taken more than 250 mg per day of vitamin C total from all sources up to 3 days before the test — even if bleeding is present.

If the patient performs the test at home, the nurse should advise the patient to:
- avoid the restricted foods and medications to get an accurate result

- avoid performing the test during the menstrual cycle and for at least 3 days thereafter
- empty the bladder before the test to avoid contaminating the specimen.

Occult blood tests are particularly important for early detection of colorectal cancer because 80% of patients with this disorder test positive. However, a single positive test result doesn't necessarily confirm GI bleeding or indicate colorectal cancer. To confirm a positive result, the test must be repeated at least three times while the patient follows a meatless, high-residue diet. To ensure accuracy, two specimens should be taken from different areas of the stool.

Findings of occult blood are more conclusive for GI bleeding when the entire specimen is found to contain blood. Even then, a confirmed positive test doesn't necessarily indicate colorectal cancer. It does indicate the need for further diagnostic studies; GI bleeding can result from many causes other than cancer, such as ulcers and diverticula. These tests are easily performed on collected specimens or smears from digital rectal examination. (See *Guidelines for colorectal cancer screening*.)

Equipment

Test kit • glass or porcelain plate • tongue blade or other wooden applicator • gloves

Implementation

- Confirm the patient's identity using two patient identifiers according to facility policy. **JCAHO**
- Put on gloves and collect a stool specimen.
- Review the manufacturer's directions for use. **MFR**

Hematest reagent tablet test

- Use a wooden applicator to smear a bit of the stool specimen on the filter paper supplied with the test kit. Or, after performing a digital rectal examination, wipe the finger you used for examination on a square of the filter paper.
- Place the filter paper with the stool smear on a glass plate.
- Remove a reagent tablet from the bottle, and immediately replace the cap tightly. Then place the tablet in the center of the stool smear on the filter paper.
- Add one drop of water to the tablet, and allow it to soak in for 5 to 10 seconds. Add a second drop, letting it run from the tablet onto the specimen and fil-

CONTROVERSIAL ISSUE

Guidelines for colorectal cancer screening **ACS**

To help detect colorectal cancer early, the American Cancer Society (ACS) recommends one of five screening options beginning at age 50: yearly fecal occult blood test (FOBT), flexible sigmoidoscopy every 5 years, combination of yearly FOBT and flexible sigmoidoscopy every 5 years, double contrast barium enema every 5 years, or colonoscopy every 5 years. The ACS prefers the combined FOBT and flexible sigmoidoscopy option.

Screening would begin earlier for people with colorectal risk factors, such as a family history of colorectal cancer or polyps or a personal history of adenomatous polyps or chronic inflammatory bowel disease. Furthermore, a positive FOBT should be followed up with colonoscopy. The ACS is adamant that there's no reason to repeat the FOBT after a positive finding.

The National Cancer Institute recommends guaiac-based fecal occult blood testing annually or biennially in people ages 50 to 80. When occult bleeding is identified, a colonoscopy is recommended. **EB1**

A study found that even the combined yearly FOBT and flexible sigmoidoscopy every 5 years missed nearly one-fourth of all patients with advanced colorectal cancer. Colonoscopy detects these cancers; however, the test is invasive and expensive, and many practitioners consider it to be more complicated than necessary.

ter paper. If necessary, tap the plate gently to dislodge any water from the top of the tablet.
- After 2 minutes, the filter paper will turn blue if the test is positive. Don't read the color that appears on the tablet itself or develops on the filter paper after the 2-minute period.
- Note the results, and discard the filter paper.
- Remove and discard your gloves, and wash your hands thoroughly.

Home test for fecal occult blood MFR

Most fecal occult blood tests require the patient to collect a specimen of his stool and smear some of it on a slide. In contrast, some new tests don't require the patient to handle stool, making the procedure safer and simpler. One example is a test called ColoCARE.

If the patient will perform the ColoCARE test at home, tell him to avoid red meat and vitamin C supplements for 2 days before the test. He should check with his practitioner about discontinuing medications before the test. Some drugs that may interfere with test results include aspirin, indomethacin, corticosteroids, phenylbutazone, reserpine, dietary supplements, anticancer drugs, and anticoagulants.

Tell the patient to flush the toilet twice just before performing the test to remove toilet-cleaning chemicals from the tank. Tell him to defecate into the toilet but not throw toilet paper into the bowl. Within 5 minutes, he should remove the test pad from its pouch and float it printed side up on the surface of the water. Tell him to watch the pad for 15 to 30 seconds for any evidence of blue or green color changes, and have him record the result on the reply card.

Emphasize that he should perform this test with three consecutive bowel movements and then send the completed card to his physician. However, he should call his practitioner immediately if he notes a positive color change in the first test.

Hemoccult slide test

● Open the flap on the slide packet, and use a wooden applicator to apply a thin smear of the stool specimen to the guaiac-impregnated filter paper exposed in box A. Or, after performing a digital rectal examination, wipe the finger you used for the examination on a square of the filter paper.
● Apply a second smear from another part of the specimen to the filter paper exposed in box B *because some parts of the specimen may not contain blood.*
● Allow the specimen to dry for 3 to 5 minutes.
● Open the flap on the reverse side of the slide package, and place 2 drops of Hemoccult developing solution on the paper over each smear. A blue reaction will appear in 30 to 60 seconds if the test is positive.
● Record the results and discard the slide package.

● Remove and discard your gloves, and wash your hands thoroughly.

Special considerations

● Make sure that stool specimens aren't contaminated with urine, soap solution, or toilet tissue, and test them as soon as possible after collection.
● Test samples from several different portions of the same specimen *because occult blood from the upper GI tract isn't always evenly dispersed throughout the formed stool; also, blood from colorectal bleeding may occur mostly on the outer stool surface.* **EB2**
● Check the condition of the reagent tablets and note their expiration date. Use only fresh tablets and discard outdated ones. Protect Hematest tablets from moisture, heat, and light.
● If repeated testing is necessary after a positive screening test, explain the test to the patient. Instruct him to maintain a high-fiber diet and to refrain from eating red meat, poultry, fish, turnips, and horseradish for 48 to 72 hours before the test as well as throughout the collection period *because these substances may alter test results.*
● As ordered, have the patient discontinue the use of iron preparations, bromides, iodides, rauwolfia derivatives, indomethacin, colchicine, salicylates, potassium, phenylbutazone, oxyphenbutazone, bismuth compounds, steroids, and ascorbic acid for 48 to 72 hours before the test and during it *to ensure accurate test results and to avoid possible bleeding, which some of these compounds may cause.*

TEACHING *If the patient will be using the Hemoccult slide packet at home, advise him to complete the label on the slide packet before collecting the specimen. If he'll be using a ColoCARE test packet, inform him that this test is a preliminary screen for occult blood in his stool. Tell him he won't have to obtain a stool specimen to perform the test but that he should follow your instructions carefully. (See* Home test for fecal occult blood.*)*

Nursing diagnoses

● Deficient knowledge (test procedure or outcome)
● Fear

Expected outcomes

The patient will:
● communicate the need to know information

- demonstrate an understanding of the information taught
- identify the source of his fear
- use available support systems to assist in coping with his fear.

Documentation

Record the time and date of the test, the result, and any unusual characteristics of the stool tested. Report positive results to the practitioner.

Supportive references

American College of Physicians. "Clinical Guideline: Parts I and II. Suggested Technique for Fecal Occult Blood Testing and Interpretation in Colorectal Cancer Screening," *Annals of Internal Medicine* 126(10):808-10, May 1997. **EB2**

Gates, T. "Cancer Screening in Perspective," *American Family Physician* 63(6):1039-40, 1042, March 2001.

Geddie, P., et al. "Colorectal Cancer: How Nurses Can Help Patients Reduce their Risk and Detect the Disease at its Earliest Stages," *Advance for Nurses* 3(13):21-22, July 2001.

Lieberman, D.A., and Weiss, D.G. "One-Time Screening for Colorectal Cancer with Combined Fecal Occult Blood Testing and Examination of the Distal Colon," *New England Journal of Medicine* 345(8):555-60, August 2001.

National Cancer Institute. "Screening for Colorectal Cancer." *http://cis.nci.nih.gov/fact/5_31.htm.* **EB1**

Ransohoff, D.F., and Lang, C.A. "Screening for Colorectal Cancer with the Fecal Occult Blood Test: A Background Paper," *Annals of Internal Medicine* 126(10):811-22, May 1997.

Passive range-of-motion exercises

Passive range-of-motion (PROM) exercises improve or maintain joint mobility and help prevent contractures. Performed by a nurse, physical therapist, or caregiver, these exercises are indicated for the patient with temporary or permanent loss of mobility, sensation, or consciousness. To ensure the best outcome for the patient, PROM exercises require recognition of the patient's limits of motion and support of all joints during movement.

Whether the cause of immobility is permanent or temporary, the patient must receive some type of exercise to prevent muscle atrophy and joint contractures. The total amount of activity required to prevent disuse syndrome (bone demineralization and muscle atrophy) is 2 hours for every 24-hour period; but this activity must be scheduled throughout the day to avoid long periods of inactivity. **Science**

Because joint contractures can begin shortly after the onset of immobility, PROM exercises should be started as soon as possible. Contracted or immobile joints make nursing care difficult and make protective positioning of a patient impossible. Relieving pressure over bony prominences to reduce the patient's risk of developing pressure ulcers is difficult. Hygiene becomes difficult because the skin folds are hard to separate. Contractures can affect other body systems. For example, a contracture that keeps the patient in the fetal position restricts chest expansion, increasing the risk of respiratory disorders, and changes abdominal pressure, making elimination difficult.

Exercises performed in the bed help with joint mobility, strength, and endurance, and they prepare the patient for ambulating. During PROM exercises, another person moves the patient's extremities so that the joints move through a complete range of movement, maximally stretching all muscle groups within each plane over each joint.

PROM exercises are contraindicated in patients with septic joints, acute thrombophlebitis, severe arthritic joint inflammation, or recent trauma with possible hidden fractures or internal injuries.

Implementation

- Determine the joints that need PROM exercises, and consult the practitioner or physical therapist about limitations or precautions for specific exercises. The exercises described here treat all joints, but they don't have to be performed in the order given or all at once. You can schedule them over the course of a day, whenever the patient is in the most convenient position. Remember to perform all exercises slowly, gently, and fully (to the end of the normal ROM, when you meet resistance to further motion). Hold this position for 1 to 2 seconds, then slowly release. **Science** (See *Glossary of joint movements,* page 50.)
- Before you begin, raise the bed to a comfortable working height. **Science**

Glossary of joint movements

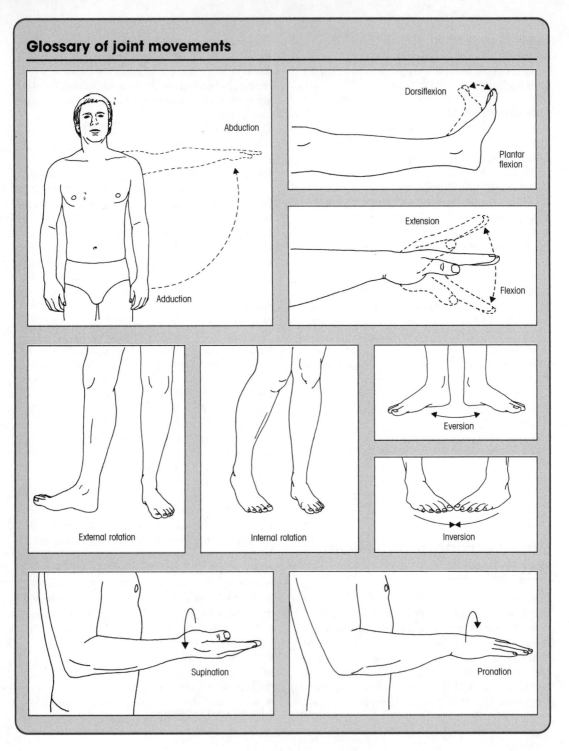

Abduction

Adduction

Dorsiflexion

Plantar flexion

Extension

Flexion

External rotation

Internal rotation

Eversion

Inversion

Supination

Pronation

● Confirm the patient's identity using two patient identifiers according to facility policy. **JCAHO**

Exercising the neck
● Support the patient's head with your hands and extend the neck, flex the chin to the chest, and tilt the head laterally toward each shoulder.
● Rotate the head from right to left.

Exercising the shoulders
● Support the patient's arm in an extended, neutral position; then extend the forearm and flex it back.
● Abduct the arm outward from the side of the body, and adduct it back to the side.
● Rotate the shoulder so that the arm crosses the midline, and bend the elbow so that the hand touches the opposite shoulder and then touches the mattress of the bed for complete internal rotation.
● Return the shoulder to a neutral position with the elbow bent, and push the arm backward so that the back of the hand touches the mattress for complete external rotation.

Exercising the elbow
● Place the patient's arm at his side with his palm facing up.
● Flex and extend the arm at the elbow.

Exercising the forearm
● Stabilize the patient's elbow, and then twist the hand to bring the palm up (supination).
● Twist it back again to bring the palm down (pronation).

Exercising the wrist
● Stabilize the forearm and flex and extend the wrist. Then rock the hand sideways for lateral flexion, and rotate the hand in a circular motion.

Exercising the fingers and thumb
● Extend the patient's fingers, and then flex the hand into a fist; repeat extension and flexion of each joint of each finger and thumb separately.
● Spread two adjoining fingers apart (abduction), and then bring them together (adduction).
● Oppose each fingertip to the thumb, and rotate the thumb and each finger in a circle.

Exercising the hip and knee
● Fully extend the patient's leg, and then bend the hip and knee toward the chest, attempting full joint flexion.
● Next, move the straight leg sideways, out and away from the other leg (abduction), and then back, over, and across it (adduction).
● Rotate the straight leg internally toward the midline and then externally away from the midline.

Exercising the ankle
● Bend the patient's foot so that the toes push upward (dorsiflexion), and then bend the foot so that the toes push downward (plantar flexion).
● Rotate the ankle in a circular motion.
● Invert the ankle so that the sole faces the midline, then evert the ankle so that the sole faces away from the midline.

Exercising the toes
● Flex the patient's toes toward the sole, then extend them back toward the top of the foot.
● Two by two, spread adjoining toes apart (abduction), and bring them together (adduction).

Special considerations
● Because joints begin to stiffen within 24 hours of disuse, start PROM exercises as soon as possible, and perform them at least once per shift, particularly while bathing or turning the patient. Use proper body mechanics, and repeat each exercise at least three times.
● Patients who experience prolonged bed rest or limited activity without profound weakness can also be taught to perform ROM exercises on their own (called active ROM), or they may benefit from isometric exercises. (See *Teaching isometric exercises,* pages 52 and 53.)
● If the disabled patient requires long-term rehabilitation after discharge, consult with a physical therapist and teach a family member or caregiver to perform PROM exercises.

Nursing diagnoses
● Activity intolerance
● Impaired physical mobility

Expected outcomes
The patient will:

Teaching isometric exercises

The patient can strengthen and increase muscle tone by contracting muscles against resistance (from other muscles or from a stationary object, such as a bed or a wall) without joint movement. These exercises require only a comfortable position — standing, sitting, or lying down — and proper body alignment. For each exercise, instruct the patient to hold each contraction for 2 to 5 seconds and to repeat it three to four times daily, below peak contraction level for the first week and at peak level thereafter.

Neck rotators

The patient places the heel of his hand above one ear. Then he pushes his head toward the hand as forcefully as possible, without moving the head, neck, or hand. He repeats the exercise on the other side.

Neck flexors

The patient places both palms on his forehead. Without moving his neck, he pushes the head forward while resisting with the palms.

Neck extensors

The patient clasps his fingers behind his head, then pushes the head back against the clasped hands without moving his neck.

Shoulder elevators

Holding the right arm straight down at the side, the patient grasps his right wrist with his left hand. He then tries to shrug his right shoulder, but prevents it from moving by holding the arm in place. He repeats this exercise, alternating arms.

Shoulder, chest, and scapular musculature

The patient places his right fist in his left palm and raises both arms to shoulder height. He pushes the fist into the palm as forcefully as possible without moving either arm. Then with his arms in the same position, he clasps the fingers and tries to pull the hands apart. He repeats the pattern, beginning with the left fist in the right palm.

Elbow flexors and extensors

With his right elbow bent 90 degrees and his right palm facing upward, the patient places his left fist against his right palm. He tries to bend the right elbow farther while resisting with the left fist. He repeats the pattern, bending the left elbow.

Abdomen

The patient assumes a sitting position and bends slightly forward, with his hands in front of the middle of his thighs. He tries to bend forward farther, resisting by pressing his palms against his thighs. Alternatively, in the supine position, he clasps his hands behind his head. Then he raises his shoulders about 1" (2.5 cm), holding this position for a few seconds.

- regain and maintain muscle mass and strength
- perform isometric exercises
- display increased mobility
- attain the highest degree of mobility within the confines of his disease.

Documentation

Record the joints exercised, the presence of edema or pressure areas, pain resulting from the exercises, limitation of ROM, and the patient's tolerance of the exercises.

Supportive references

Dawe, D., and Curran-Smith, J. "Going Through the Motions," *Canadian Nurse* 90(1):31-33, January 1994.

Koch, S., et al. "Effect of Passive Range of Motion on Intracranial Pressure in Neurosurgical Patients," *Journal of Critical Care* 11(4):176-79, December 1996.

"Performing Passive Range-of-Motion Exercises," *Nursing2006* 36(3):50-51, March 2006.

Verderber, A., et al. "The Effect of Nursing Interventions on Transcutaneous Oxygen and Carbon Dioxide Tensions," *Western Journal of Nursing Research* 17(1):76-90, February 1995.

Back extensors

In a sitting position, the patient bends forward and places his hands under his buttocks. He tries to stand up, resisting with both hands.

Hip abductors

While standing, the patient squeezes his inner thighs together as tightly as possible. Placing a pillow between the knees supplies resistance and increases the effectiveness of this exercise.

Hip extensors

The patient squeezes his buttocks together as tightly as possible.

Knee extensors

The patient straightens his knee fully. Then he vigorously tightens the muscle above the knee so that it moves the kneecap upward. He repeats this exercise, alternating legs.

Ankle flexors and extensors

The patient pulls his toes upward, holding briefly. Then he pushes them down as far as possible, again holding briefly.

Postmortem care

Postmortem care usually begins after a physician certifies the patient's death. After the patient dies, care includes preparing him for family viewing, arranging transportation to the morgue or funeral home, and determining the disposition of his belongings.

Nurses should check for the presence of family, identify the next of kin, and determine if the family has been informed of the patient's death. Postmortem care entails supporting the patient's family and friends. The nurse should observe the family's response, realize that there's no "right" way to grieve, and decide whether the family needs time alone with the patient or would feel more comfortable with a staff member in the room. Respect of ethnic and cultural differences toward death aids in the grieving process. Discussing and inquiring about cultural or spiritual practices in regard to preparation of the body helps increase the family's sense of control.

If the patient died under mysterious or violent circumstances, it's important for the nurse to explain that an autopsy must be performed. If it has already been done, she should prepare the family for the appearance of the body before viewing.

Families that wish to be involved in postmortem care should be encouraged to participate. *Allowing the family to assist can facilitate the grieving process and acknowledgment of death.*

Equipment

Gauze or soft string ties • gloves • chin straps • ABD pads • cotton balls • plastic shroud or body wrap • three identification tags • adhesive bandages to cover wounds or punctures • plastic bag for patient's belongings • water-filled basin • soap • towels • washcloths • morgue stretcher • protective equipment

A commercial morgue pack usually contains gauze or string ties, chin straps, a shroud, and identification tags.

Implementation

● Document auxiliary equipment, such as a mechanical ventilator, still present. Put on gloves.
● Put on protective equipment according to standard precautions. **JCAHO**
● Place the body in the supine position, arms at sides and head on a pillow. Then elevate the head of the bed slightly *to prevent discoloration caused by blood settling in the face.* **Science**
● If the patient wore dentures and your facility's policy permits, gently insert them; then close the mouth. Close the eyes by gently pressing on the lids with your fingertips. If they don't stay closed, place moist cotton balls on the eyelids for a few minutes, and then try again to close them. Place a folded towel under the chin to keep the jaw closed.
● Remove all indwelling urinary catheters, tubes, and tape, and apply adhesive bandages to puncture sites. Replace soiled dressings.
● Collect all the patient's valuables *to prevent loss.* If you can't remove a ring, cover it with gauze, tape it

in place, and tie the gauze to the wrist *to prevent slip-page and subsequent loss.*

● Clean the body thoroughly, using soap, a basin, and washcloths. Place one or more ABD pads between the buttocks *to absorb rectal discharge or drainage.*

● Cover the body up to the chin with a clean sheet.

● Offer comfort and emotional support to the family and intimate friends. Ask if they wish to see the body. If they do, allow them to do so in privacy. Ask if they would prefer to leave the patient's jewelry on the body. **PCP**

● After the family leaves, remove the towel under the chin, pad the chin, wrap straps under it, and tie the straps loosely on top of the head. Then pad the wrists and ankles *to prevent bruises,* and tie them together with gauze or soft string ties. **Science**

● Fill out the three identification tags. Each tag should include the deceased patient's name, room and bed numbers, date and time of death, and physician's name. Tie one tag to the deceased patient's hand or foot, but don't remove his identification bracelet *to ensure correct identification.*

● Place the shroud or body wrap on the morgue stretcher and, with assistance, transfer the body to the stretcher. Wrap the body, and tie the shroud or wrap with the string provided. Then attach another identification tag, and cover the shroud or wrap with a clean sheet. If a shroud or wrap isn't available, dress the deceased patient in a clean gown and cover the body with a sheet.

● Place the deceased patient's personal belongings, including valuables, in a bag and attach the third identification tag to it.

● If the patient died of an infectious disease, label the body according to facility policy. **JCAHO**

● Close the doors of adjoining rooms if possible. Then take the body to the morgue. Use corridors that aren't crowded and, if possible, use a service elevator.

Special considerations

● Give the deceased patient's personal belongings to his family or take them to the morgue. If you give the family jewelry or money, make sure that a coworker is present as a witness. Obtain the signature of an adult family member *to verify receipt of valuables or to state their preference that jewelry remain on the patient.*

● Offer emotional support to the deceased patient's family and friends and to the patient's roommate, if appropriate.

Documentation

Although the extent of documentation varies among facilities, always record the disposition of the patient's possessions, especially jewelry and money. Also note the date and time the deceased patient was transported to the morgue.

Supportive references

Harvey, J. "Debunking Myths about Postmortem Care," *Nursing2001* 31(7):44-45, July 2001.

Jenkins, C., and Bruera, E. "Assessment and Management of Medically Ill Patients Who Refuse Life-Prolonging Treatment: Two Case Reports and Proposed Guidelines," *Journal of Palliative Care* 14(1):18-24, Spring 1998.

Quill, T., and Byock, I. "Responding to Intractable Terminal Suffering: The Role of Terminal Sedation and Voluntary Refusal of Food and Fluids. ACP-ASIM End-of-Life Care Consensus Panel," *Annals of Internal Medicine* 132(5):408-14, March 2000.

Postoperative care

Postoperative care begins when the patient arrives in the postanesthesia care unit (PACU) and continues as he moves on to the short procedure unit, medical-surgical unit, or critical care area. Postoperative care aims to minimize complications by early detection and prompt treatment of the condition, such as postoperative pain, inadequate oxygenation, or other adverse physiologic effects.

Recovery from general anesthesia takes longer than induction because the anesthetic is retained in fat and muscle. Fat has a meager blood supply; thus, it releases the anesthetic slowly, providing enough anesthesia to maintain adequate blood and brain levels during surgery. The patient's recovery time varies with his amount of body fat, his overall condition, his premedication regimen, and the type, dosage, and duration of anesthesia. The effects of anesthesia and surgery can place the patient at risk for various physiologic disorders.

During the postoperative phase, the nurse is initially responsible for assessing the patient's physical status and monitoring changes that occur during the recovery process. When the patient's condition stabilizes, nursing care focuses on returning the patient to a functional level of wellness as soon as possible within the limitations created by surgery. The speed of a patient's recovery depends on how effectively the nurse can anticipate potential complications, begin the necessary preventive and supportive measures, and involve the patient's family in the recovery process. Facilitating communication among the patient, family, and members of the health care team is also the nurse's responsibility.

If the patient is discharged home after surgery, it's the nurse's responsibility to help the patient and his family translate instructions on the discharge sheet into useful ways to deal with practical matters at home. Areas to be discussed include food, bowel movements, resumption of sexual activity, wound care, driving, return to work, and medications. Each patient's care plan should be individualized to improve wellness and to maximize independence.

Equipment

Thermometer • watch with second hand • stethoscope • sphygmomanometer • postoperative flowchart or other documentation tool

Preparation of equipment

Assemble the necessary equipment needed at the patient's bedside.

Implementation

● Obtain the patient's record from the PACU nurse. **JCAHO** This should include a summary of operative procedures and pertinent findings, type of anesthesia, vital signs (preoperative, intraoperative, and postoperative), medical history, medication history (including preoperative, intraoperative, and postoperative medications), fluid therapy (including estimated blood loss, type and number of drains, catheters, and characteristics of drainage), and notes on the condition of the surgical wound. *If the patient had vascular surgery, for example, knowing the location and duration of blood vessel clamping can prevent postoperative complications.*

● Confirm the patient's identity using two patient identifiers according to facility policy. **JCAHO**

● Transfer the patient from the PACU stretcher to the bed and position him properly. Get coworkers to help. Never try to move a patient alone; it's best to have 3 or 4 people assisting, with one supporting the patient's head. If the patient has had orthopedic surgery, one person should move only the affected extremity. If the patient is in skeletal traction, you may receive special orders for moving him. If this occurs, have one coworker move the weights as you and another coworker move the patient. **Science**

● When moving the patient, keep transfer movements smooth *to minimize pain and postoperative complications and avoid back strain among team members.* **Science**

● Make the patient comfortable and raise the bed's side rails *to ensure his safety.*

● Assess the patient's level of consciousness, skin color, and mucous membranes.

● Monitor the patient's respiratory status by assessing his airway. Note breathing rate and depth, and auscultate for breath sounds. Administer oxygen, and initiate oximetry *to monitor oxygen saturation,* if ordered.

● Monitor the patient's pulse rate. It should be strong and easily palpable. The heart rate should be within 20% of the preoperative rate.

● Compare postoperative blood pressure to preoperative blood pressure. It should be within 20% of the preoperative level unless the patient suffered a hypotensive episode during surgery.

● Assess the patient's temperature *because anesthesia lowers body temperature.* Body temperature should be at least 95° F (35° C). If it's lower, apply blankets *to warm the patient.* **Science**

● Assess the patient's infusion sites for redness, pain, swelling, or drainage.

● Assess surgical wound dressings; they should be clean and dry. If they're soiled, assess the characteristics of the drainage and outline the soiled area. Note the date and time of assessment on the dressing. Assess the soiled area frequently; if it enlarges, reinforce the dressing and alert the physician.

● Note the presence and condition of any drains and tubes. Note the color, type, odor, and amount of drainage. Make sure that all drains are properly connected and free from kinks and obstructions.

● If the patient has had vascular or orthopedic surgery, assess the appropriate extremity or all extremities, depending on the surgical procedure. Assess color, temperature, sensation, movement, and presence and quality of pulses, and notify the practitioner of any abnormalities.

● As the patient recovers from anesthesia, monitor his respiratory and cardiovascular status closely. Stay alert for signs of airway obstruction and hypoventilation caused by laryngospasm or for sedation, which can lead to hypoxemia. Cardiovascular complications — such as arrhythmias or hypotension — may result from the anesthetic agent or the operative procedure.

● Encourage coughing and deep-breathing exercises. However, don't encourage them if the patient has just had nasal, ophthalmic, or neurologic surgery *to avoid increasing intracranial pressure.* **Science**

● Administer postoperative medications, such as antibiotics, analgesics, antiemetics, or reversal agents, as ordered and as appropriate.

● Remove all fluids from the patient's bedside until he's alert enough to eat and drink. Before giving him liquids, assess his gag reflex *to prevent aspiration.* To do this, lightly touch the back of his throat with a cotton swab — the patient will gag if the reflex has returned. Do this test quickly *to prevent a vagal reaction.* **Science**

Special considerations

● Fear, pain, anxiety, hypothermia, confusion, and immobility can upset the patient and jeopardize his safety and postoperative status. Offer emotional support to the patient and his family. Keep in mind that the patient who has lost a body part or who has been diagnosed with an incurable disease will need ongoing emotional support. Refer him and his family for counseling as needed.

● As the patient recovers from general anesthesia, reflexes appear in reverse order to that in which they disappeared. Hearing recovers first, so avoid holding inappropriate conversations. **Science**

● The patient under general anesthesia can't protect his own airway because the muscles are relaxed. As he recovers, cough and gag reflexes return. If he can lift his head without assistance, he's usually able to breathe on his own.

● If the patient received spinal anesthesia, he'll need to remain in a supine position with the bed adjusted to between 0 and 20 degrees for at least 6 hours *to reduce the risk of headache from leakage of cerebrospinal fluid.* The patient won't be able to move his legs, so be sure to reassure him that sensation and mobility will return.

● If the patient has had epidural anesthesia for postoperative pain control, monitor his respiratory status closely. *Respiratory arrest may result from paralysis of the diaphragm by the anesthetic.* He may also suffer nausea, vomiting, or itching.

● If the patient will be using a patient-controlled analgesia (PCA) unit, make sure he understands how to use it. Caution him to activate it only when he has pain, not when he feels sleepy or is pain-free. Review your facility's criteria for PCA use.

Nursing diagnoses

● Acute pain
● Hypothermia

Expected outcomes

The patient will:
● express feelings of comfort and relief from pain
● maintain body temperature within the normal range
● maintain heart rate and blood pressure within the normal range.

Complications

Possible postoperative complications include arrhythmias, hypotension, hypovolemia, septicemia, septic shock, atelectasis, pneumonia, thrombophlebitis, pulmonary embolism, urine retention, wound infection, wound dehiscence, evisceration, abdominal distention, paralytic ileus, constipation, altered body image, or postoperative psychosis.

Documentation

Document the patient's vital signs on the appropriate flowchart. Record the condition of dressings, drains, and characteristics of drainage. Document all interventions taken to alleviate pain and anxiety and the patient's responses to them. Document complications and interventions taken.

Supportive references

American Association for Respiratory Care. "Clinical Practice Guideline: Directed Cough," *Respiratory Care* 38(5):495-99, May 1993 [reviewed 2000].

Fox, V. "Postoperative Education that Works," *AORN Journal* 67(5):1010, 1012-17, May 1998.

Leinonen, T., and Leino-Kilpi, H. "Research in Perioperative Nursing Care," *Journal of Clinical Nursing* 8(2):123-38, March 1999.

Preoperative care

Preoperative care begins when surgery is planned and ends with the administration of anesthesia. This phase of care includes a preoperative interview and assessment to collect baseline subjective and objective data from the patient and his family; diagnostic tests, such as urinalysis, electrocardiogram, and chest radiography; preoperative teaching; securing informed consent from the patient; and physical preparation.

During the preoperative phase, the nurse performs a thorough assessment of the patient's emotional and physical status, to determine teaching needs and to identify patients at risk for surgery, and documents baseline data for future comparisons. The nursing goals in preparing the patient for surgery are reducing his anxiety, ensuring his safety, and identifying and decreasing the potential risks of complications of surgery.

Anxiety can interfere with the effectiveness of anesthesia and the patient's ability to actively participate in his care. Providing information about what will occur during surgery and sensations the patient can expect to feel helps to decrease anxiety. Demonstrating a caring attitude toward the patient and his family increases trust, reduces fear, and establishes a therapeutic relationship.

Many interventions and activities contribute to patient safety. According to the Patient Care Partnership, patients have the right to be informed by physicians and other direct caregivers of relevant, current, and understandable information concerning diagnosis, treatment, and progress. **PCP**

Informed consent is required by law to help protect the patient's rights, autonomy, and privacy. Failure to obtain informed consent can result in assault and battery or negligence charges against the health care providers. The surgeon should provide the patient with information regarding the extent and type of surgery, alternative therapies, and usual risks and benefits. A consent form that includes all of this information must be signed by the patient and a witness, verifying that the patient has received the required information.

The nurse is usually responsible for making sure the consent form is signed. The nurse also promotes patient safety by restricting activity after administration of sedatives and by completing a preoperative

checklist to make sure that all procedures are carried out.

Equipment

Thermometer • sphygmomanometer • stethoscope • watch with second hand • weight scale • tape measure

Preparation of equipment

Assemble all equipment needed at the patient's bedside or in the admission area.

Implementation

● Confirm the patient's identity using two patient identifiers according to facility policy. **JCAHO**
● If the patient is having same-day surgery, make sure that he knows ahead of time not to eat or drink anything before surgery. Follow your facility's policy for the time frame that the patient may not eat or drink before the procedure, which can range from 4 to 8 hours. Confirm with him what time he's scheduled to arrive at the health care facility, and tell him to leave all jewelry and valuables at home. Also make sure that the patient has arranged for someone to accompany him home after surgery.
● Obtain a health history and assess the patient's knowledge, perceptions, and expectations about the surgery. Ask about previous medical and surgical interventions. Also determine the patient's psychosocial needs; ask about occupational well-being, financial matters, support systems, mental status, and cultural beliefs. Use your facility's preoperative surgical assessment database, if available, to gather this information. Obtain a drug history. Ask about current prescription and over-the-counter medications and about known allergies to foods, drugs, and latex.
● Obtain the patient's height, weight, and vital signs.
● Identify risk factors that may interfere with a positive expected outcome. Be sure to consider age, general health, medications, mobility, nutritional status, fluid and electrolyte disturbances, and lifestyle. Also consider the primary disorder's duration, location, and nature and the extent of the surgical procedure.
● Explain preoperative procedures to the patient. Include typical events that he can expect and the sensations he can expect to experience. Discuss equipment that may be used postoperatively, such as nasogastric tubes and I.V. equipment. Explain the typical incision, dressings, and staples or sutures that will be used. *Preoperative teaching can help reduce postopera-*

tive anxiety and pain, increase patient compliance, hasten recovery, and decrease length of stay. **EB**

● Talk the patient through the sequence of events from operating room to recovery room (postanesthesia care unit [PACU]) and back to the patient's room. He may be transferred from the PACU to an intensive care unit or surgical care unit. The patient may also benefit from a tour of the areas he'll see during the perioperative events. **PCP**

● Tell the patient that when he goes to the operating room, he may have to wait a short time in the holding area. Explain that the surgeons and nurses will wear surgical dress, and even though they'll be observing him closely, they won't talk to him very much. Explain that minimal conversation will help the preoperative medication take effect.

● When discussing transfer procedures and techniques, describe sensations the patient will experience. Tell him that he'll be taken to the operating room on a stretcher and transferred from the stretcher to the operating room table. *For his own safety,* he'll be held securely to the table with soft restraints. The operating room nurses will check his vital signs frequently.

● Warn the patient that the operating room may feel cool. Electrodes may be put on his chest to monitor his heart rate during surgery. Describe the drowsy floating sensation he'll feel as the anesthetic takes effect. Tell him it's important that he relax at this time. **EB**

● Tell the patient about exercises that he may be expected to perform after surgery, such as deep breathing, coughing (while splinting the incision if necessary), limb exercises, and movement and ambulation *to minimize respiratory and circulatory complications.* If the patient will undergo ophthalmic or neurologic surgery, he won't be asked to cough *because coughing increases intracranial pressure.* **Science**

● On the day of surgery, important interventions include giving morning care, verifying that the patient has signed an informed consent form, administering ordered preoperative medications, completing the preoperative checklist and chart, and providing support to the patient and his family.

● Make sure that the surgical site has been verified by the surgeon and witnessed by the patient. The surgeon should identify the site by placing his initials with a permanent marker on the appropriate site with the assistance of the patient. **JCAHO**

● Other immediate preoperative interventions may include preparing the GI tract (restricting food and fluids before surgery) *to reduce vomiting and the risk of aspiration,* cleaning the lower GI tract of fecal material by enemas before abdominal or GI surgery, or giving antibiotics for 2 or 3 days preoperatively *to prevent contamination of the peritoneal cavity by GI bacteria.* **Science**

● Just before the patient is moved to the surgical area, make sure he's wearing a hospital gown, his identification band is in place, and his vital signs have been recorded. Check to see that hairpins, nail polish, and jewelry have been removed. Note whether dentures, contact lenses, or prosthetic devices have been removed or left in place.

Special considerations

● Preoperative medications must be given on time *to enhance the effect of ordered anesthesia.* The patient should take nothing by mouth preoperatively. Don't give oral medications unless ordered. Be sure to raise the bed's side rails immediately after giving preoperative medications.

● If family or others are present, direct them to the appropriate waiting area and offer support as needed.

Nursing diagnoses

● Anxiety
● Deficient knowledge (disease process and surgical outcome)

Expected outcomes

The patient will:
● cope with his present medical situation without demonstrating signs of anxiety
● demonstrate or verbalize an understanding of what has been taught
● communicate the need to know about the surgical outcome or disease process and prognosis.

Documentation

Complete the preoperative checklist used by your facility. Record all nursing care measures and preoperative medications, results of diagnostic tests, and the time the patient is transferred to the surgical area. The chart and the surgical checklist must accompany the patient to surgery.

Supportive references

Centers for Disease Control and Prevention Hospital Infection Control Practices Advisory Committee. "Guideline for Prevention of Surgical Site Infection, 1999," *Infection Control and Hospital Epidemiology* 20(4):250-78, April 1999. *www.cdc.gov/ncidod/hip/ SSI/SSI_guideline.htm.*

Chapman, A. "Current Theory and Practice: A Study of Pre-operative Fasting," *Nursing Standard* 10(18):33-36, January 1996.

Joint Commission on Accreditation of Healthcare Organizations. "Patient Safety Goals 2006." *www.jcaho.org.*

Matiti, M., and Sharman, J. "Dignity: A Study of Pre-operative Patients," *Nursing Standard* 14(13-15):32-35, December 1999-January 2000.

Shuldham, C. "Pre-operative Education: A Review of the Research Design," *International Journal of Nursing Studies* 36(2):179-87, April 1999.

Shuldham, C. "A Review of the Impact of Pre-operative Education on Recovery from Surgery," *International Journal of Nursing Studies* 36(2):171-77, April 1999. **EB**

Smith, J., and Rudd, C. "Streamlining Pre-operative Assessment in Orthopaedics," *Nursing Standard* 13(1):45-47, September 1998.

Pulse assessment

The pulse is a recurring wave of blood created by contraction of the left ventricle. It can be palpated where an artery crosses over bone on firm tissue. In a healthy person, pulse reflects the heartbeat, meaning that the pulse rate and the rate of ventricular contractions are the same.

In adults and children older than age 3, the radial artery in the wrist is the most common palpation site. A pulse is normally palpated by applying moderate pressure with the three middle fingers of the hand. Using the thumb is contraindicated because the thumb has its own pulse that might be mistaken for the patient's pressure. Gentle pressure should be applied to the wrist when taking the pulse. **EB1** Excessive pressure may obliterate the pulse; inadequate pressure may not detect it. In infants and children younger than age 3, the best practice is to listen to the heart itself rather than palpate a pulse. Because auscultation is done at the heart's apex, this is called the apical pulse. **Science**

An apical-radial pulse is taken by simultaneously counting apical and radial beats by auscultation at the apex of the heart and palpation at the radial artery. Some heartbeats detected at the apex can't be detected at peripheral sites. The apical pulse rate is higher than the radial, and the difference is the *pulse deficit.* An apical pulse should be taken if the patient's peripheral pulse is irregular or if he has known cardiovascular, pulmonary, or renal disease.

Assessment of the pulse should include the rate (number of beats per minute), rhythm (pattern or regularity of the beats), and volume (amount of blood pumped with each beat). If the pulse is faint or weak, use a Doppler ultrasound blood flow detector, if available. (See *Using a Doppler device,* page 60.) If the pulse is regular, count the rate for 30 seconds and multiply by two; however, if the pulse is irregular, the best practice is to count the rate for a full minute. (See *Accuracy of pulse count method,* page 61.)

Equipment

Watch with second hand • stethoscope (for auscultating apical pulse) • Doppler ultrasound blood flow detector, if necessary • alcohol pad

Preparation of equipment

If you aren't using your own stethoscope, disinfect the earpieces with an alcohol pad before and after use *to prevent cross-contamination.*

Implementation

● Wash your hands, and tell the patient you intend to take his pulse. **CDC**

● Make sure that the patient is comfortable and relaxed *because an awkward, uncomfortable position may affect the heart rate.* **Science**

Taking a radial pulse

● Place the patient in a sitting or supine position, with his arm at his side or across his chest.

● Gently press your index, middle, and ring fingers on the radial artery, inside the patient's wrist. You should feel a pulse with only moderate pressure; *excessive pressure may obstruct blood flow distal to the pulse site.* Don't use your thumb to take the patient's pulse *because you may mistake your thumb's own strong pulse for the patient's pulse.* **Science**

● After locating the pulse, count the beats for 60 seconds, or count for 30 seconds and multiply by 2.

Using a Doppler device EB2

More sensitive than palpation for determining pulse rate, the Doppler ultrasound blood flow detector is especially useful when a pulse is faint or weak. Unlike palpation, which detects arterial wall expansion and retraction, this instrument detects the motion of red blood cells (RBCs).

● Apply a small amount of coupling gel or transmission gel (not water-soluble lubricant) to the ultrasound probe.
● Position the probe on the skin directly over the selected artery. In the illustration below left, the probe is over the posterior tibial artery.
● When using a Doppler model like the one shown below left, turn the instrument on and, moving counterclockwise, set the volume control to the lowest setting. If your model doesn't have a speaker, plug in the earphones and slowly raise the volume. The Doppler ultrasound stethoscope shown below right, is basically a stethoscope fitted with an audio unit, volume control, and transducer, which amplifies the movement of RBCs.

● To obtain the best signals with either device, tilt the probe 45 degrees from the artery, making sure that there's gel between the skin and the probe. Slowly move the probe in a circular motion to locate the center of the artery and the Doppler signal — hissing noise at the heartbeat. Avoid moving the probe rapidly because this distorts the signal.
● Count the signals for 60 seconds to determine the pulse rate.
● After you've measured the pulse rate, clean the probe with a soft cloth soaked in antiseptic solution or soapy water. Don't immerse the probe or bump it against a hard surface. Wipe the gel off the patient's skin.

Doppler ultrasound blood flow detector

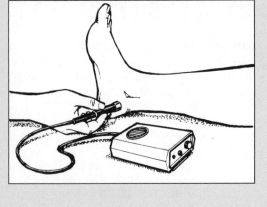

Doppler ultrasound stethoscope

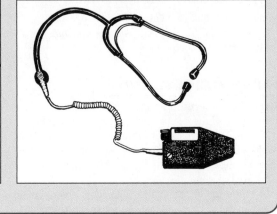

Counting for a full minute provides a more accurate picture of irregularities.
● While counting the rate, assess pulse rhythm and volume by noting the pattern and strength of the beats. If you detect an irregularity, repeat the count, and note whether it occurs in a pattern or randomly. If you're still in doubt, take an apical pulse. (See *Identifying pulse patterns.*)

Taking an apical pulse
● Help the patient to a supine position and drape him if necessary.
● Warm the diaphragm or bell of the stethoscope in your hand. *Placing a cold stethoscope against the skin may startle the patient and momentarily increase his heart rate.* Keep in mind that the bell transmits low-pitched sounds more effectively than the diaphragm.
● Place the diaphragm or bell of the stethoscope over the apex of the heart (normally located at the fifth intercostal space left of the midclavicular line). Count

CONTROVERSIAL ISSUE

Accuracy of pulse count method EB1

When a patient has atrial fibrillation, nurses have traditionally counted the apical rate for 60 seconds, using a stethoscope. However, research on the most accurate count period is contradictory. For example, three different studies produced the following three different conclusions:

- A 60-second count provides the most accurate pulse rate. (The researchers also found that many nurses underestimate the apical rate and that the margin of error increased as the apical rate increased.)

- A 30-second count is the best way to evaluate pulse rate, and the 15-second count is least accurate.
- Using a 15- or 30-second count is just as effective as using a 60-second count.

Identifying pulse patterns

Type	Rate	Rhythm (per 3 seconds)	Causes and incidence
Normal	60 to 80 beats/ minute; in neonates, 120 to 140 beats/ minute	• • • •	• Varies with such factors as age, physical activity, and gender (men usually have lower pulse rates than women)
Tachycardia	More than 100 beats/ minute	• • • • • • •	• Accompanies stimulation of the sympathetic nervous system by emotional stress (such as anger, fear, or anxiety) or the use of certain drugs such as caffeine • May result from exercise and from certain health conditions, such as heart failure, anemia, and fever (which increases oxygen requirements and therefore the pulse rate)
Bradycardia	Less than 60 beats/ minute	• • •	• Accompanies stimulation of the parasympathetic nervous system by use of certain drugs, especially digoxin, and such conditions as cerebral hemorrhage and heart block • May also be present in fit athletes
Irregular	Uneven time intervals between beats (for example, periods of regular rhythm interrupted by pauses or premature beats)	• • • • • • •	• May indicate cardiac irritability, hypoxia, digoxin toxicity, potassium imbalance, or sometimes more serious arrhythmias if premature beats occur frequently • Occasionally premature beats occurring, which are normal

the beats for 60 seconds, and note their rhythm, volume, and intensity (loudness). **Science**

● Remove the stethoscope and make the patient comfortable.

Taking an apical-radial pulse

● Two nurses work together to obtain the apical-radial pulse; one palpates the radial pulse while the other nurse auscultates the apical pulse with a stethoscope. Both must use the same watch when counting beats.

● Help the patient to a supine position and drape him if necessary.

● Locate the apical and radial pulses.

● Determine a time to begin counting. Then each nurse counts beats for 60 seconds.

Special considerations

● When the peripheral pulse is irregular, take an apical pulse to measure the heartbeat more directly. If the pulse is faint or weak, use a Doppler ultrasound blood flow detector if available.

● If another nurse isn't available for an apical-radial pulse assessment, hold the stethoscope in place with the hand that holds the watch while palpating the radial pulse with the other hand. You can then feel any discrepancies between the apical and radial pulses.

Nursing diagnoses

● Decreased cardiac output

Expected outcomes

The patient will:

● maintain a pulse rate that doesn't exceed or go below normal limits.

Documentation

Record the site, pulse rate, rhythm, and volume as well as the time of measurement. "Full" or "bounding" describes a pulse of increased volume; "weak" or "thready," decreased volume. When recording the apical pulse, include intensity of heart sounds. When recording the apical-radial pulse, chart the rate according to the pulse site—for example, apical-radial pulse of 80/76.

Supportive references

Craven, R.F., and Hirnle, C.J. *Fundamentals of Nursing Human Health and Function,* 5th ed. Philadelphia: Lippincott Williams & Wilkins, 2006. **EB1**

Thomas, J., and Feliciano, C. "Measuring BP with a Doppler Device," *Nursing2003* 33(7):52-53, July 2003. **EB2**

Respiration assessment

Respiration is the interchange of gases between an organism and the medium in which it lives. External respiration, or breathing, is the exchange of oxygen and carbon dioxide between the atmosphere and the body. Internal respiration takes place throughout the body at the cellular level.

Four measures of respiration — rate, rhythm, depth, and sound—reflect the body's metabolic state, diaphragm and chest-muscle condition, and airway patency. Respiratory rate is recorded as the number of cycles (one inspiration and one expiration) per minute; rhythm, as the regularity of these cycles; depth, as the volume of air inhaled and exhaled with each respiration; and sound, as the audible digression from normal, effortless breathing. Breathing that's normal in rate and depth is called *eupnea;* abnormally slow respiration, bradypnea, and abnormally fast respiration, tachypnea. Apnea is the absence of respiration.

Equipment

Watch with a second hand

Implementation

● The best time to assess your patient's respirations is immediately after taking the pulse rate. Keep your fingertips over the radial artery, and don't tell the patient you're counting respirations. *If you tell him, he'll become conscious of his respirations and the rate may change.* **EB**

● Count respirations by observing the rise and fall of the patient's chest as he breathes. Alternatively, position the patient's opposite arm across his chest and count respirations by feeling its rise and fall. Consider one rise and one fall as one respiration.

● Count respirations for 30 seconds and multiply by 2 or count for 60 seconds if respirations are irregular

Monitoring respiratory rate ⓔⒷ

Although nurses routinely monitor respiratory rate, little research exists on the best way to count respirations or the clinical significance of abnormal respiratory rates. One study of children under age 5 found that counting respirations for a full minute resulted in less variability than a 30-second count. Although 60 seconds appears to be a more accurate measure of respiratory rate, nurses rarely count respiration for a full minute. Moreover, researchers studying the measurement of respiratory rates in infants found that rates obtained listening to the chest with a stethoscope were 20% to 50% higher than rates obtained by visual inspection of the chest.

Nurses routinely obtain respiratory rates with vital signs to detect lung disorders. However, in several studies, researchers have found that respiratory rate didn't correlate with respiratory impairment. In one study set in an emergency room, only one-third of people with an oxygen saturation of less than 90% presented with an increased respiratory rate. Another study showed respiratory rate to be a poor indicator of serious respiratory illness in infants under age 6 months.

to account for variations in respiratory rate and pattern. (See *Monitoring respiratory rate*.) Science

● As you count respirations, stay alert for and record such breath sounds as stertor, stridor, wheezing, or an expiratory grunt. *Stertor* is a snoring sound resulting from secretions in the trachea and large bronchi; listen for it in patients who are comatose or have a neurologic disorder. *Stridor* is an inspiratory crowing sound associated with upper airway obstruction in laryngitis, croup, or the presence of a foreign body.

ALERT *When listening for stridor in infants and children with croup, also observe for sternal, substernal, or intercostal retractions.*

● *Wheezing* is caused by partial obstruction in the smaller bronchi and bronchioles. This high-pitched, musical sound is common in patients with emphysema or asthma.

ALERT *In infants, an expiratory grunt indicates imminent respiratory distress. In older patients, an expiratory grunt may result from partial airway obstruction or neuromuscular reflex.*

● Watch the patient's chest movements and listen to breathing *to determine the rhythm and sound of respirations.* (See *Identifying respiratory patterns*, page 64.)

● Use a stethoscope to detect other breath sounds — such as crackles or rhonchi — or the lack of sound in the lungs.

● Observe chest movements for depth of respirations. If the patient inhales a small volume of air, record this as shallow; if he inhales a large volume, record this as deep.

● Observe the patient for accessory muscle use, such as the scalene, sternocleidomastoid, trapezius, and latissimus dorsi. Using these muscles reflects a weakness of the diaphragm and the external intercostal muscles — the major muscles of respiration.

Special considerations

● Respiratory rates of less than 8 or more than 40 breaths/minute are usually considered abnormal; report the sudden onset of such rates promptly. Observe the patient for signs of dyspnea, such as an anxious facial expression, flaring nostrils, a heaving chest wall, or cyanosis. To detect cyanosis, look for characteristic bluish discoloration in the nail beds or the lips, under the tongue, in the buccal mucosa, or in the conjunctiva.

● In assessing the patient's respiratory status, consider his personal and family history. Ask if he smokes and, if so, for how many years and how many packs per day.

ALERT *A child's respiratory rate may double in response to exercise, illness, or emotion. Normally, the rate for neonates is 30 to 80 breaths/ minute; for toddlers, 20 to 40; and for children of school age and older, 15 to 25. Children usually reach the adult rate (12 to 20) at about age 15.*

Nursing diagnoses

● Deficient knowledge (procedure)
● Ineffective breathing pattern

Identifying respiratory patterns

Type	Characteristics	Pattern	Possible causes
Apnea	Periodic absence of breathing		• Mechanical airway obstruction • Conditions affecting the brain's respiratory center in the lateral medulla oblongata
Apneustic respirations	Prolonged, gasping inspiration followed by extremely short, inefficient expiration		• Lesions of the respiratory center
Bradypnea	Slow, regular respirations of equal depth		• Conditions affecting the respiratory center: tumors, metabolic disorders, respiratory decompensation; use of opiates and alcohol
Cheyne-Stokes respirations	Fast, deep respirations punctuated by periods of apnea lasting 20 to 60 seconds		• Increased intracranial pressure, severe heart failure, renal failure, meningitis, drug overdose, cerebral anoxia
Eupnea	Normal rate and rhythm		• Normal respiration
Kussmaul's respirations	Fast (over 20 breaths/ minute), deep (resembling sighs), labored respirations without pause		• Renal failure or metabolic acidosis, particularly diabetic ketoacidosis
Tachypnea	Rapid respirations (Rate rises with body temperature: about 4 breaths/minute for every degree Fahrenheit above normal.)		• Pneumonia, compensatory respiratory alkalosis, respiratory insufficiency, lesions of the respiratory center, salicylate poisoning

Expected outcomes

The patient will:
• demonstrate or verbalize an understanding of what has been taught
• maintain a respiratory rate within 5 breaths per minute of baseline.

Documentation

Record the rate, depth, rhythm, and sound of the patient's respirations.

Supportive references

Craven, R.F., and Hirnle, C.J. *Fundamentals of Nursing Human Health and Function*, 5th ed. Philadelphia: Lippincott Williams & Wilkins, 2006.

LeGrand, T.S., et al. "Inconsistency in Identification of Breath Sounds among Physicians, Nurses, and Respiratory Therapists," *Chest* 118(4), October 2000. *www.findarticles.com/cf_0/m0984/4_118/71127541/p1.* **EB**

Restraint application

Restraint is a method of physically restricting a person's freedom of movement, physical activity, or normal access to his body. This includes not only traditional restraints, such as limb or vest restraints, but also tightly tucked sheets or the use of side rails to prevent a patient from getting out of bed.

The Joint Commission on Accreditation of Healthcare Organizations (JCAHO) has issued standards regarding the use of restraints. According to these standards, restraints are to be limited to emergencies in which the patient is at risk for harming himself or others and when other less restrictive measures have proved ineffective. One purpose of the revisions is to reduce the use of restraints. (See *Alternatives to restraints*.) Restraints can cause numerous problems, including limited mobility, skin breakdown, impaired circulation, incontinence, psychological distress, and strangulation. (See *Patient injuries with restraints*, page 66.)

Equipment
Soft restraints
Restraint (vest, limb, mitt, belt, or body, as needed) • padding, if needed • restraint flow sheet

Leather restraints
Two wrist and two ankle leather restraints • four straps • key • large gauze pads to cushion each extremity • restraint flow sheet

Preparation of equipment
● Before entering the patient's room, make sure that the restraints are the correct size for the patient's build and weight.
● If you use leather restraints, make sure that the straps are unlocked and that the key fits the locks.

Implementation
● Follow JCAHO and Centers for Medicare & Medicaid Services (CMS) standards for applying restraints. Make sure that less restrictive measures have been tried before applying restraints.
● When all other methods have failed to keep the patient from harming himself or others, apply restraints only as a last resort and for as short a time as possible. Choose a restraint that's the least restrictive to the patient.
● Explain the need for restraints to the patient, and inform him of the conditions necessary for his release from restraints. Assure him that they're being used to

Alternatives to restraints JCAHO

Restraints must be used only as a last resort after all other measures have failed to keep the patient from harming himself or others. They should be applied in the least restrictive manner and for as short a time as possible.

To reduce the need for restraints, take an individualized approach that seeks to prevent behavior problems. Look for an underlying problem that may be causing your patient's behavior — such as adverse drug effects, infection, electrolyte imbalance, or hypoxia — and take measures to correct the problem.

Look for "agenda behaviors" in which the patient's behavior may be an attempt to correct a problem, such as pain, hunger, fatigue, heat, cold, or the need for toileting.

Create an environment that's free from restraints and encourages patient mobility. This requires a unit and facility commitment because policy changes and even structural changes may be required.

If the problem behavior continues after you've identified and corrected conditions that may be the cause, consider alternatives to restraints, such as:
● reorienting the patient as needed
● providing explanations for procedures
● keeping the patient warm, dry, and comfortable
● establishing eye contact and talking to the patient
● listening and validating the patient's concerns
● determining the patient's routines and habits and trying to adhere to them
● wrapping elastic compression bandages around I.V. sites, other tubing, or dressings
● switching to a capped I.V. line, if possible
● determining whether equipment or treatment is really necessary
● moving tubing or equipment out of the patient's sight
● using an abdominal binder to cover abdominal drains, tubes, and dressings and urinary catheters.

protect him from injury rather than to punish him. **PCP**
● If necessary, obtain adequate assistance to manually restrain the patient before entering his room to apply restraints. Enlist the aid of several coworkers and

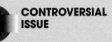

CONTROVERSIAL ISSUE

Patient injuries with restraints

Despite research showing the dangers of the use of restraints, many health care workers believe that restraints prevent falls and other injuries. However, studies show that patients who are restrained have a longer hospital stay and an increased mortality. Moreover, patients who are restrained for long periods are at risk for nosocomial infection, pressure ulcers, functional decline, depression, and incontinence.

Studies also show that restraints aren't effective in preventing the adverse events they're used to deter. In fact, restraints are more likely to be the *cause* of injury. Most patients who pull out their endotracheal tubes do so while wearing wrist restraints. Moreover, as many as 47% of patients who fall are restrained at the time of the fall.

As a result of the growing knowledge that restraints increase the risk of patient injury and death and that assessment and alternative strategies reduce the need for restraints, agencies such as the Joint Commission on Accreditation of Healthcare Organizations and the Centers for Medicare & Medicaid Services, formerly the Health Care Financing Administration, have set strict standards for the use of restraints. Many health care facilities are also developing and implementing restraint reduction programs. **CMS** **JCAHO**

organize their effort, giving each person a specific task — for example, one person explains the procedure to the patient and applies the restraints while the others immobilize the patient's arms and legs.
- Within 1 hour of placing a patient in restraints, the patient should be evaluated by a licensed independent practitioner and an order written for restraints. If restraints are still necessary, obtain an order to renew restraints every 4 hours. If a patient requires the use of restraints for at least two separate episodes in a 24-hour period, JCAHO requires that the chief medical officer or chief executive officer be notified.
- *To ensure safety*, assess the patient every 15 minutes.

- If the patient consented to have his family informed of his care, notify them of the use of restraints.

Applying a vest restraint
- Assist the patient to a sitting position if his condition permits. Then slip the vest over his gown. Crisscross the cloth flaps at the front, placing the V-shaped opening at the patient's throat. Never crisscross the flaps in the back *because this may cause the patient to choke if he tries to squirm out of the vest.*
- Pass the tab on one flap through the slot on the opposite flap. Then adjust the vest for the patient's comfort. You should be able to slip your fist between the vest and the patient. Avoid wrapping the vest too tightly *because it may restrict respiration.*
- Tie all restraints securely to the frame of the bed, chair, or wheelchair and out of the patient's reach. Use a bow or a knot that can be released quickly and easily in an emergency. (See *Knots for securing soft restraints.*) Never tie a regular knot to secure the straps. Leave 1″ to 2″ (2.5 to 5 cm) of slack in the straps *to allow room for movement.*
- After applying the vest, check the patient's respiratory rate and breath sounds regularly. Stay alert for signs of respiratory distress. Also, make sure that the vest hasn't tightened with the patient's movement. Loosen the vest frequently, if possible, *so the patient can stretch, turn, and breathe deeply.*

Applying a limb restraint
- Wrap the patient's wrist or ankle with a padded restraint.
- Pass the strap on the narrow end of the restraint through the slot in the broad end, and adjust for a snug fit, or fasten the buckle or hook-and-loop cuffs to fit the restraint. You should be able to slip one or two fingers between the restraint and the patient's skin. Avoid applying the restraint too tightly *because it may impair circulation distal to the restraint.*
- Tie the restraint as described under "Applying a vest restraint."
- After applying limb restraints, stay alert for signs of impaired circulation, movement, or sensation in the restrained extremity. If the skin appears blue or feels cold or if the patient complains of a tingling sensation or numbness, loosen the restraint. Perform range-of-motion (ROM) exercises regularly to stimulate circula-

tion and prevent contractures and resultant loss of mobility.

Applying a mitt restraint

● Roll up a washcloth or gauze pad, and place it in the patient's palm. Have him form a loose fist, if possible; then pull the mitt over it and secure the closure.

● *To restrict the patient's arm movement*, attach the strap to the mitt and tie it securely, using a bow or a knot that can be released quickly and easily in an emergency.

● When using mitts made of transparent mesh, check hand movement and skin color frequently *to assess circulation.* Remove the mitts regularly *to stimulate circulation,* and perform passive ROM exercises *to prevent contractures.*

Applying a belt restraint

● Center the flannel pad of the belt on the bed. Then wrap the short strap of the belt around the bed frame and fasten it under the bed.

● Position the patient on the pad. Then have him roll slightly to one side while you guide the long strap around his waist and through the slot in the pad.

● Wrap the long strap around the bed frame and fasten it under the bed.

● After applying the belt, slip your hand between the patient and the belt *to ensure a secure but comfortable fit. The belt is too loose if it can be raised to chest level; a belt that's too tight can cause abdominal discomfort.*

Special considerations

● Know the latest JCAHO and CMS (formerly the Health Care Financing Administration [HCFA]) standards for restraint applications. Implement alternative strategies to reduce the need for restraints. Choose the least restrictive restraint, if necessary, for your patient.

● Provide for continuous patient monitoring in which a designated person can directly observe the patient at all times.

● Assess and assist the restrained patient every 15 minutes, including injuries caused by the restraint, nutrition, hydration, circulation, ROM, vital signs, hygiene, elimination, comfort, and physical and psychosocial status. Also assess whether the patient is ready to have restraints discontinued.

Knots for securing soft restraints

When securing soft restraints, use knots that can be released quickly and easily such as those shown below. Remember, never secure restraints to the bed's side rails.

Magnus hitch

Loop

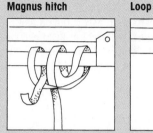

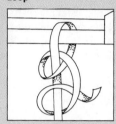

Clove hitch

Reverse clove hitch

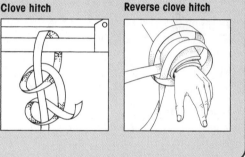

● When the patient is at risk for aspiration, restrain him on his side. Never secure all four restraints to one side of the bed *because the patient may fall out of bed.*

● When loosening restraints, have a coworker on hand to assist in manually restraining the patient if necessary.

● Don't apply a limb restraint above an I.V. site *because the constriction may occlude the infusion or cause infiltration into surrounding tissue.* **Science**

● Never secure restraints to the side rails *because someone might inadvertently lower the rail before noticing the attached restraint. This could jerk the patient's limb or body, causing him discomfort and trauma.* Never secure restraints to the fixed frame of the bed if the patient's position is to be changed.

● Don't restrain a patient in the prone position. This position limits his field of vision, intensifies feelings of helplessness and vulnerability, and impairs respiration, especially if the patient has been sedated.

● Because the restrained patient has limited mobility, his nutrition, elimination, and positioning become your responsibility. *To prevent pressure ulcers,* reposition the patient regularly, and pad bony prominences and other vulnerable areas. **Science**

● The condition of the restrained patient must be continually monitored, assessed, and evaluated. Release the restraints every hour; assess the patient's pulse and skin condition, and perform ROM exercises. A restraint flow sheet must be used with hourly notations.

Nursing diagnoses

● Risk for injury

Expected outcomes

The patient will:

● remain free from injury

● identify and acknowledge factors that increase the potential for injury

● help identify and apply safety measures to prevent injury.

Complications

● *Because excessively tight limb restraints can reduce peripheral circulation and tight vest restraints can impair respiration,* apply restraints carefully and check them according to standards.

● *To prevent skin breakdown under limb restraints,* pad the patient's wrists and ankles, loosen or remove the restraints frequently, and provide regular skin care.

● *Long periods of immobility can predispose the patient to pneumonia, urine retention, constipation, and sensory deprivation.* Reposition the patient and attend to his elimination requirements as needed.

Documentation

● Document each episode of the use of restraints, including the date and time they were initiated.

● Record the circumstances resulting in the use of restraints and nonphysical interventions used first. Describe the rationale for the specific type of restraint used.

● Chart the name of the licensed independent practitioner who ordered the restraint.

● Include the conditions or behaviors necessary for discontinuing the restraint and whether these conditions were communicated to the patient.

● Document each in-person evaluation by the licensed independent practitioner.

● Record 15-minute assessments of the patient, including signs of injury, nutrition, hydration, circulation, ROM, vital signs, hygiene, elimination, comfort, physical and psychological status, and readiness for removing restraints.

● Record your interventions to help the patient meet the conditions for removing restraints. Note that the patient was continuously monitored.

● Document any injuries or complications, the time and name of the practitioner notified of your interventions, and your actions.

Supportive references

"JCAHO and HCFA now Agree on Restraint Standards," *RN* 64(1):14, January 2001.

"JCAHO Revises Restraints Standards," *Contemporary Longterm Care* 23(8):9, August 2000.

Lusis, S. "Update on Restraint Use in Acute Care Settings," *Plastic Surgical Nursing* 20(3):145-50, Fall 2000.

McConnell, E.A. "Applying a Vest Restraint," *Nursing2000* 30(10):22, October 2000.

McConnell, E.A. "Applying a Wrist Restraint," *Nursing2000* 30(9):22, September 2000.

Spiritual care

Religious beliefs can profoundly influence a patient's recovery rate, attitude toward treatment, and overall response to hospitalization. In certain religious groups, beliefs can preclude diagnostic tests and therapeutic treatments, require dietary restrictions, and prohibit organ donation and artificial prolongation of life. (See *Beliefs and practices of selected religions.*)

Consequently, effective patient care requires identification, recognition of, and respect for the patient's religious beliefs. Data about a patient's spiritual beliefs are obtained from the patient's history, a thorough nursing history, and close attention to his nonverbal cues or to seemingly casual remarks that express his spiritual concerns. The nurse should never assume that a patient follows all the practices of his stated religion.

Beliefs and practices of selected religions

A patient's religious beliefs can affect his attitudes toward illness and traditional medicine. By trying to accommodate the patient's religious beliefs and practices in your care plan, you can increase his willingness to learn and comply with treatment regimens. Because religious beliefs may vary within particular sects, individual practices may differ from those described here.

Religion	Birth and death rituals	Dietary restrictions	Practices in health crisis
Adventist	None (baptism of adults only)	Alcohol, coffee, tea, opioids, stimulants; in many groups, meat prohibited also	Communion and baptism performed. Some members believe in divine healing, anointing with oil, and prayer. Some regard Saturday as the Sabbath.
Baptist	At birth, none (baptism of believers only); before death, counseling by clergy member and prayer	Alcohol; in some groups, coffee and tea prohibited also	Some believe in healing by laying on of hands. Resistance to medical therapy occasionally approved.
Christian Science	At birth, none; before death, counseling by a Christian Science practitioner	Alcohol, coffee, and tobacco prohibited	Many members refuse all treatment, including drugs, biopsies, physical examination, and blood transfusions and permit vaccination only when required by law. Alteration of thoughts is believed to cure illness. Hypnotism and psychotherapy are prohibited. (Christian Scientist nurses and nursing homes honor these beliefs.)
Church of Christ	None (baptism at age 8 or older)	Alcohol discouraged	Communion, anointing with oil, laying on of hands, and counseling performed by a minister.
Eastern Orthodox	At birth, baptism and confirmation; before death, last rites (For members of the Russian Orthodox Church, arms are crossed after death, fingers set in cross, and unembalmed body clothed in natural fiber.)	For members of the Russian Orthodox Church and usually the Greek Orthodox Church, no meat or dairy products on Wednesday, Friday, and during Lent	Anointing of the sick. For members of the Russian Orthodox Church, cross necklace is replaced immediately after surgery and shaving of male patients is prohibited except in preparation for surgery. For members of the Greek Orthodox Church, communion and Sacrament of Holy Unction.
Episcopal	At birth, baptism; before death, occasional last rites	For some members, abstention from meat on Friday, fasting before communion (which may be daily)	Communion, prayer, and counseling performed by a minister.
Jehovah's Witnesses	None	Abstention from foods to which blood has been added	Typically, no blood transfusions are permitted; a court order may be required for emergency transfusion.

(continued)

Beliefs and practices of selected religions *(continued)*

Religion	Birth and death rituals	Dietary restrictions	Practices in health crisis
Judaism	Ritual circumcision on eighth day after birth; burial of dead fetus; ritual washing of dead; burial (including organs and other body tissues) occurs as soon as possible; no autopsy or embalming	For Orthodox and Conservative Jews, kosher dietary laws (for example, pork and shellfish prohibited); for Reform Jews, usually no restrictions	Donation or transplantation of organs requires rabbinical consultation. For Orthodox and Conservative Jews, medical procedures may be prohibited on the Sabbath — from sundown Friday to sundown Saturday — and specific holidays.
Lutheran	Baptism usually performed 6 to 8 weeks after birth	None	Communion, prayer, and counseling performed by a minister.
Jesus Christ of Latter Day Saints (Mormon)	At birth, none (baptism at age 8 or older); before death, baptism and gospel preaching	Alcohol, tobacco, tea, and coffee prohibited; meat intake limited	Belief in divine healing through the laying on of hands; communion on Sunday; some members may refuse medical treatment. Many wear a special undergarment.
Islam	If spontaneous abortion occurs before 130 days, fetus treated as discarded tissue; after 130 days, as a human being; before death, confession of sins with family present; after death, only relatives or friends may touch the body	Pork prohibited; daylight fasting during ninth month of Islamic calendar	Faith healing for the patient's morale only; conservative members reject medical therapy.
Orthodox Presbyterian	Infant baptism; scripture reading and prayer before death	None	Communion, prayer, and counseling performed by a minister.
Pentecostal Assembly of God, Foursquare Church	None (baptism only after age of accountability)	Abstention from alcohol, tobacco, meat slaughtered by strangling, any food to which blood has been added, and sometimes pork	Divine healing through prayer, anointing with oil, and laying on of hands.
Roman Catholicism	Infant baptism, including baptism of aborted fetus without sign of clinical death (tissue necrosis); before death, anointing of the sick	Fasting or abstention from meat on Ash Wednesday and on Fridays during Lent; this practice usually waived for the hospitalized	Burial of major amputated limb (sometimes) in consecrated ground; donation or transplantation of organs allowed if the benefit to recipient outweighs the donor's potential harm. Sacrament of the Sick also performed when patients are ill, not just before death. Sometimes performed shortly after admission.
United Methodist	Baptism of children and adults	None	Communion before surgery or similar crisis; donation of body parts encouraged.

Respecting a patient's beliefs may require the nurse to set aside her own beliefs to help the patient follow his. This aids in cooperation and improved response to treatment and expected outcomes for the patient. Providing spiritual care may require contacting an appropriate member of the clergy in the facility or community, gathering equipment needed to help the pastor perform rites and administer sacraments, and preparing him for a pastoral visit.

Equipment

As appropriate: Clean towels (one or two) • teaspoon or 1-oz (30-ml) medicine cup (for baptism), if appropriate • container of water (for emergency baptism), if appropriate • other supplies specific to the patient's religious affiliation

Some health care facilities, particularly those with a religious affiliation, provide baptismal trays. The clergy member may bring holy water, holy oil, or other religious articles to minister to the patient.

Preparation of equipment

● For baptism, cover a small table with a clean towel. Fold a second towel and place it on the table, along with the teaspoon or medicine cup.
● For communion and anointing, cover the bedside stand with a clean towel.

Implementation

● Check the patient's admission record to determine his religious affiliation. Remember that some patients may claim no religious beliefs. However, even an agnostic may wish to speak with a clergy member, so watch and listen carefully for subtle expressions of this desire.
● Remember that a patient may feel acutely distressed because of his inability to participate in religious observances. Help such a patient verbalize his beliefs *to relieve stress.* Listen to him and let him express his concerns, but carefully refrain from imposing your beliefs on him *to avoid conflict and further stress.* If the patient requests, arrange a visit by an appropriate member of the clergy. Consult this clergy member if you need more information about the patient's beliefs. **EB**
● Evaluate the patient's behavior for signs of loneliness, anxiety, or fear — *emotions that may signal his need for spiritual counsel.* Commonly patients experi-

ence these feelings at night when they feel especially alone. Stay alert for comments or behaviors that indicate a need to verbalize those feelings.
● If your patient faces the possibility of abortion, amputation, transfusion, or other medical procedures with important religious implications, try to discover the spiritual attitude. Also, try to determine your patient's attitude toward the importance of laying on of hands, confession, communion, observance of holy days (such as the Sabbath), and restrictions in diet or physical appearance. *Helping the patient continue his normal religious practices during hospitalization can help reduce stress.*
● If the patient is pregnant, find out her beliefs concerning infant baptism and circumcision, and comply with them after delivery.
● If a neonate is in critical condition, call an appropriate clergy member immediately. To perform an emergency baptism, the minister or priest pours a small amount of water into a teaspoon or a medicine cup and sprinkles a few drops over the infant's head while saying, "(Name of child), I baptize you in the name of the Father, the Son, and the Holy Spirit. Amen." In an extreme emergency, you can perform a Roman Catholic baptism, using a container of available water. If you do so, be sure to notify the priest *because this sacrament must be administered only once.*
● If a Jewish woman delivers a male infant prematurely or by cesarean birth, ask her whether she plans to observe the rite of circumcision (*bris*), a significant ceremony performed on the eighth day after birth. (Because a patient who delivers a healthy, full-term baby vaginally is usually discharged quickly, this ceremony is normally performed outside the facility.) For a bris, ensure privacy and, if requested, sterilize the instruments.
● If the patient requests communion, prepare him for it before the clergy member arrives. First, place him in Fowler's or semi-Fowler's position if his condition permits. Otherwise, allow him to remain in a supine position. Tuck a clean towel under his chin and straighten the bed linens.
● If a terminally ill patient requests the Sacrament of the Sick (Last Rites) or special treatment of his body after death, call an appropriate clergy member. For the Roman Catholic patient, call a Roman Catholic priest to administer the sacrament, even if the patient

is unresponsive or comatose. To prepare the patient for this sacrament, uncover his arms and fold back the top linens to expose his feet. After the clergy member anoints the patient's forehead, eyes, nose, mouth, hands, and feet, straighten and retuck the bed linens.

Special considerations

● Handle the patient's religious articles carefully to avoid damage or loss. Become familiar with religious resources in your facility. Some facilities employ one or more clergy members who counsel patients and staff and link patients to other pastoral resources.
● If the patient tries to convert you to his personal beliefs, tell him that you respect his beliefs but are content with your own. Similarly, avoid attempts to convert the patient to your personal beliefs.

Nursing diagnoses

● Risk for impaired religiosity

Expected outcomes

The patient will:
● discuss his beliefs about religious practices
● express feelings about his usual and current religious beliefs.

Documentation

Complete a baptismal form and attach it to the patient's record; send a copy of the form to the appropriate clergy member. Record the rites of circumcision and last rites in your notes. Also record last rites in red on the Kardex so it won't be repeated unnecessarily.

Supportive references

Govier, I. "Spiritual Care in Nursing: A Systematic Approach," *Nursing Standard* 14(17):32-36, January 2000. **EB**
Page, M. "How Well Do We Care for People's Spiritual Needs?" *The Australian and New Zealand Journal of Mental Health Nursing,* 11(10):18-19, November 2005.

Surgical site verification

Wrong site surgery is a general term referring to a surgical procedure performed on the wrong body part or side of the body, or even on the wrong patient. This error may occur in the operating room or in other settings, such as in ambulatory care or interventional radiology.

Several factors that may contribute to an increased risk of wrong site surgery include inadequate patient assessment, inadequate medical review, inaccurate communication among health care team members, multiple surgeons involved in the procedure, failure to include the patient in the site verification process, and relying solely on the practitioner for surgical site verification.

Because serious consequences can result from wrong site surgery, the nurse must confirm that the correct site has been verified before surgery begins.

Equipment

Surgical consent form ● medical record ● procedure schedule ● hypoallergenic, non-latex permanent marker

Implementation

● Confirm the patient's identity using two patient identifiers according to facility policy. **JCAHO**
● Before the surgical procedure, check the patient's chart for documentation and compare the information using the medical history and physical examination form, nursing assessment, preprocedure verification checklist, signed surgical consent form with exact procedure site verified, surgical procedure scheduled, and the patient's verbal communication of the correct site.
● After verbally confirming the site with the patient, the surgeon performing the procedure or another member of the surgical team who's fully informed about the patient and the intended procedure marks the site with a permanent marker. The mark needs to be placed so that it's visible after the patient has been prepped and draped. **JCAHO**
● Make sure that the surgical team (surgeon, operating room or procedure staff, and anesthesia personnel) identifies the patient and verifies the correct procedure and correct site before beginning the surgery.

Special considerations

● If the patient's condition prevents him from verifying the correct site, the surgeon will identify and mark the site using the medical history and physical examination forms, signed surgical consent form, preprocedure verification checklist, surgical procedure scheduled, X-rays, and other diagnostic imaging studies.

Nursing diagnoses

● Risk for injury

Expected outcomes

The patient will:
● remain free from injury
● verify that the correct surgical site was identified.

Documentation

Complete the preprocedure verification checklist used by your facility, record that the correct site was verified, and note that the patient, a family member, or the surgeon has marked the site with a permanent marker.

Supportive references

Canale, S. "Wrong-Site Surgery: A Preventable Complication," *Clinical Orthopaedics & Related Research* (433):26-29, April 2005.

Joint Commission on Accreditation of Healthcare Organizations. "National Patient Safety Goals," 2005. *www.jcaho.org.*

Wimbush, S., et al. "National Audit of 'Wrong-Site' Neurosurgery," *Journal of Neurosurgical Anesthesiology* 17(3):160-61, July 2005.

Temperature assessment

Body temperature represents the balance between heat produced by metabolism, muscular activity, and other factors and heat lost through the skin, lungs, and body wastes. A stable temperature pattern promotes proper function of cells, tissues, and organs; a change in this pattern usually signals the onset of illness. Research supports observations that rectal temperature is the most accurate, followed by oral temperature, and then axillary temperature.

Temperature can be measured with an electronic digital or infrared thermometer. Oral temperature in adults normally ranges from 97° to 99.5° F (36.1° to 37.5° C); rectal temperature is usually 1° F higher; axillary temperature reads 1° to 2° F lower; and tympanic temperature reads 0.5° to 1° F higher.

ALERT *Use caution with rectal thermometers in an infant and a young child to help pre-*

vent injury. Don't leave the patient alone until the thermometer has been removed.

Temperature normally fluctuates with rest and activity. Lowest readings typically occur between 4 and 5 a.m.; the highest readings, between 4 and 8 p.m. Other factors that influence temperature include gender, age, emotional conditions, and environment. Women normally have higher temperatures than men, especially during ovulation. Normal temperature is highest in neonates and lowest in elderly persons. Heightened emotions raise temperature; depressed emotions lower it. A hot external environment can raise temperature; a cold environment can lower it. **Science**

Equipment

Electronic digital or infrared thermometer or tympanic thermometer ● water-soluble lubricant or petroleum jelly (for rectal temperature) ● gloves (for rectal temperature) ● facial tissue ● disposable thermometer sheath or probe cover ● alcohol pad

Preparation of equipment

● If you use an electronic digital or infrared thermometer, make sure that it has been recharged.

Implementation

● Confirm the patient's identity using two patient identifiers according to facility policy. **JCAHO**
● Explain the procedure to the patient, and wash your hands. If the patient has had hot or cold liquids, chewed gum, or smoked, wait 15 minutes before taking an oral temperature. **PCP** **Science**
● To use a disposable sheath or probe cover, disinfect the thermometer with an alcohol pad. Insert it into the disposable sheath opening, and then twist to tear the seal at the dotted line. Pull it apart.

Using an electronic digital thermometer

● Insert the probe into a disposable probe cover. If taking a rectal temperature, lubricate the probe cover to reduce friction and ease insertion. Leave the probe in place until the maximum temperature appears on the digital display. (See *Taking an accurate temperature,* page 74.)

CLINICAL IMPACT

Taking an accurate temperature

To take a temperature accurately with an electronic thermometer, first verify that the thermometer is set in the correct mode. In the normal mode, the thermometer will predict the temperature based on the rate of temperature change; when set in the monitor mode, the thermometer obtains an actual temperature.

Also check that the correct probe is being used at the correct site. For example, using an oral probe to obtain a rectal temperature can cause an inaccurate result.

When using a tympanic thermometer, know whether it's set to convert the temperature to rectal, oral, or core temperature. An elevated temperature in the rectal mode may be normal but be considered a fever if obtained in the oral mode. Always check the manufacturer's recommendations before using the equipment. **MFR**

Using a tympanic thermometer

● Make sure that the lens under the probe is clean and shiny. Attach a disposable probe cover.
● Examine the patient's ears. They should be free from cerumen *to obtain an accurate reading.*
● Stabilize the patient's head, and then gently pull the ear straight back (for children up to age 1) or up and back (for children age 1 and older to adult) *to straighten the external auditory canal. This technique ensures that the probe tip is directed at the tympanic membrane.* **Science**
● Insert the thermometer until the ear canal is sealed. The thermometer should be inserted toward the tympanic membrane in the same way that an otoscope is inserted. Then press the activation button and hold it for 1 second. The temperature will appear on the display.

ALERT *For infants younger than age 3 months, take three temperature readings and use the highest reading.*

Taking an oral temperature

● Position the tip of the thermometer under the patient's tongue, as far back as possible on either side of the frenulum linguae. *Placing the tip in this area promotes contact with superficial blood vessels and contributes to an accurate reading.*
● Instruct the patient to close his lips but to avoid biting down with his teeth. *Biting can break the thermometer, cutting the mouth or lips or causing ingestion of broken glass or mercury.*
● Leave an electronic thermometer in place until the maximum temperature is displayed.
● For an electronic thermometer, note the temperature, and then remove and discard the probe cover.

Taking a rectal temperature

● Position the patient on his side with his top leg flexed, and drape him to provide privacy. Then fold back the bed linens to expose the anus.
● Squeeze lubricant onto a facial tissue *to prevent contamination of the lubricant supply.* Put on gloves.
● Lubricate about ½″ (1.3 cm) of the thermometer tip for an infant, 1″ (2.5 cm) for a child, and 1½″ (3.8 cm) for an adult. **EB** *Lubrication reduces friction and thus eases insertion.* This step may be unnecessary when using disposable rectal sheaths *because they're prelubricated.*
● Lift the patient's upper buttock, and insert the thermometer about ½″ for an infant or 1½″ for an adult. Gently direct the thermometer along the rectal wall toward the umbilicus. *This will avoid perforating the anus or rectum or breaking the thermometer. It also will help ensure an accurate reading because the thermometer will register hemorrhoidal artery temperature instead of fecal temperature.*
● Hold the electronic thermometer until the maximum temperature is displayed. *Holding the thermometer prevents damage to rectal tissues caused by displacement or loss of the thermometer into the rectum.*
● Carefully remove the thermometer, wiping it as necessary. Then wipe the patient's anal area to remove lubricant or stool. Remove and dispose of the rectal sheath. Remove and discard your gloves. Wash your hands.

Taking an axillary temperature

● Position the patient with the axilla exposed.

- Gently pat the axilla dry with a facial tissue *because moisture conducts heat.* Avoid harsh rubbing, *which generates heat.*
- Ask the patient to reach across his chest and grasp his opposite shoulder, lifting his elbow.
- Position the thermometer in the center of the axilla, with the tip pointing toward the patient's head.
- Tell him to keep grasping his shoulder and to lower his elbow and hold it against his chest. *This promotes skin contact with the thermometer.*
- Remove an electronic thermometer when it displays the maximum temperature. Axillary temperature takes longer to register than oral or rectal temperature *because the thermometer isn't enclosed in a body cavity.*
- Grasp the end of the thermometer and remove it from the axilla.

Special considerations

- Oral measurement is contraindicated in patients who are unconscious, disoriented, or seizure-prone; in young children and infants; and in patients who must breathe through their mouths. Rectal measurement is contraindicated in patients with diarrhea, recent rectal or prostate surgery or injury *because it may injure inflamed tissue,* or recent myocardial infarction *because anal manipulation may stimulate the vagus nerve, causing bradycardia or another rhythm disturbance.*
- Use the same thermometer for repeated temperature taking to avoid spurious variations caused by equipment differences.
- Don't avoid taking an oral temperature when the patient is receiving nasal oxygen because oxygen administration raises oral temperature by only about 0.3° F (0.2° C).

Nursing diagnoses

- Ineffective thermoregulation

Expected outcomes

The patient will:
- maintain body temperature at normothermic levels
- have warm, dry skin
- maintain heart rate and blood pressure within normal limits.

Documentation

Record the time, route, and temperature on the patient's chart.

Supportive references

Craig, J.V., et al. "Temperature Measured at the Axilla Compared with Rectum in Children and Young People: A Systematic Review," *British Medical Journal* 320:1174-178, April 2000.

Craven, R.F., and Hirnle, C.J. *Fundamentals of Nursing Human Health and Function,* 5th ed. Philadelphia: Lippincott Williams & Wilkins, 2006. **EB**

Greenes, D.S., and Fleisher, G.R. "Accuracy of a Noninvasive Temporal Artery Thermometer for Use in Infants," *Archives of Pediatrics and Adolescent Medicine* 155(3):376-81, March 2001.

Lanham, D.M., et al. "Accuracy of Tympanic Temperature Readings in Children under 6 Years of Age," *Pediatric Nursing* 25(1):39-42, January 1999.

Pidwell, W.B., et al. "Accuracy of the Temporal Artery Thermometer," *Annals of Emergency Medicine* 36(4):S5, October 2000.

Transfer from bed to stretcher

Transfer from bed to stretcher, one of the most common transfers, can require the help of one or more coworkers, depending on the patient's size and condition and the primary nurse's physical abilities. Techniques for achieving this transfer include the straight lift, carry lift, lift sheet, and sliding board. The nurse should always remember to maintain good body mechanics — a wide base of support and bent knees — when transferring a patient, to reduce the risk of injury to the patient and herself. To reduce the risk of injury to the patient during transfer, the nurse should make sure that the patient maintains proper body alignment — back straight, head in neutral position, and extremities in a functional position. **Science**

In the straight (or patient-assisted) lift — used to move a child, a very light patient, or a patient who can assist transfer — the transfer team members place their hands and arms under the patient's buttocks and, if necessary, his shoulders. Other patients may require a four-person straight lift, detailed below. In the carry lift, team members roll the patient onto their upper arms and hold him against their chests. In the lift sheet transfer, they place a sheet under the patient and lift or slide him onto the stretcher. In the sliding-board transfer, two team members slide him onto the stretcher.

Equipment
Stretcher • sliding board or lift sheet, if necessary

Preparation of equipment
Adjust the bed to the same height as the stretcher.

Implementation
● Tell the patient that you're going to move him from the bed to the stretcher, and place him in the supine position.
● Ask team members to remove watches and rings *to avoid scratching the patient during transfer.*

Four-person straight lift
● Place the stretcher parallel to the bed, and lock the wheels of both *to ensure the patient's safety.*
● Stand at the center of the stretcher, and have another team member stand at the patient's head. The two other team members should stand next to the bed, on the other side — one at the center and the other at the patient's feet.
● Slide your arms, palms up, beneath the patient, while the other team members do the same. In this position, you and the team member directly opposite support the patient's buttocks and hips; the team member at the head of the bed supports the patient's head and shoulders; the one at the foot supports the patient's legs and feet.
● On a count of three, the team members lift the patient several inches, move him onto the stretcher, and slide their arms out from under him. Keep movements smooth *to minimize patient discomfort and avoid muscle strain by team members.*

Four-person carry lift
● Place the stretcher perpendicular to the bed, with the head of the stretcher at the foot of the bed. Lock the bed and stretcher wheels *to ensure the patient's safety.*
● Raise the bed to a comfortable working height.
● Line up all four team members on the same side of the bed as the stretcher, with the tallest member at the patient's head and the shortest at his feet. The

member at the patient's head is the leader of the team and gives the lift signals.
● Tell the team members to flex their knees and slide their hands, palms up, under the patient until he rests securely on their upper arms. Make sure that the patient is adequately supported at the head and shoulders, buttocks and hips, and legs and feet. **EB**
● On a count of three, the team members straighten their knees and roll the patient onto his side, against their chests. *This positioning reduces strain on the lifters and allows them to hold the patient for several minutes, if necessary.* **EB**
● Together, the team members step back, with the member supporting the feet moving the farthest. The team members move forward to the stretcher's edge and, on a count of three, lower the patient onto the stretcher by bending at the knees and sliding their arms out from under the patient.

Four-person lift sheet transfer
● Position the bed, stretcher, and team members for the straight lift. Then instruct the team to hold the edges of the sheet under the patient, grasping them close to the patient *to obtain a firm grip, provide stability, and spare the patient undue feelings of instability.*
● On a count of three, the team members lift or slide the patient onto the stretcher in a smooth, continuous motion *to avoid muscle strain and minimize patient discomfort.* **Science**

Sliding-board transfer
● Place the stretcher parallel to the bed, and lock the wheels of both *to ensure the patient's safety.*
● Stand next to the bed, and instruct a coworker to stand next to the stretcher.
● Reach over the patient and pull the far side of the bedsheet toward you to turn the patient slightly on his side. Your coworker then places the sliding board beneath the patient, making sure the board bridges the gap between the stretcher and the bed.
● Ease the patient onto the sliding board and release the sheet. Your coworker then grasps the near side of the sheet at the patient's hips and shoulders and pulls him onto the stretcher in a smooth, continuous motion. She then reaches over the patient, grasps the far side of the sheet, and logrolls him toward her.

● Remove the sliding board as your coworker returns the patient to the supine position.

After all transfers
● Position the patient comfortably on the stretcher, apply safety straps, and raise and secure the side rails.

Special considerations
● When transferring a helpless or markedly obese patient from the bed to a stretcher, begin by lifting and moving him, in increments, to the edge of the bed. Then rest for a few seconds, repositioning the patient if necessary, and lift him onto the stretcher. If the patient can bear weight on his arms or legs, two or three coworkers can perform this transfer: One can support the buttocks and guide the patient, another can stabilize the stretcher by leaning over it and guiding the patient into position, and a third can transfer any attached equipment. If a team member isn't available to guide equipment, move I.V. lines and other tubing first *to make sure that they're out of the way and not in danger of pulling loose,* or disconnect tubes if possible. If the patient is light, three coworkers can perform the carry lift; however, no matter how many team members are present, someone must stabilize the patient's head if he can't support it himself, has cervical instability or injury, or has undergone surgery.
● Depending on the patient's size and condition, a lift sheet transfer can require 2 to 7 people.

Nursing diagnoses
● Risk for injury

Expected outcomes
The patient (and family members) will:
● remain free from injury
● develop strategies to prevent injury
● identify and apply safety measures to prevent injury.

Documentation
Record the time and, if necessary, the type of transfer in your notes. Complete other required forms.

Supportive references
Collins, J., and Owen, B. "NIOSH Research Initiatives to Prevent Back Injuries to Nursing Assistants, Aides and Orderlies in Nursing Homes," *American Journal of Industrialized Medicine* 29(4):421-24, April 1996.

Owen, B. "Preventing Injuries Using an Ergonomic Approach," *AORN Journal* 72(6):1031-36, December 2000.

Owen, B., et al. "What Are We Teaching about Lifting and Transferring Patients?" *Research in Nursing and Health* 22(1):3-13, February 1999. **EB**

Owen, B., and Fragala, G. "Reducing Perceived Physical Stress While Transferring Patients," *AAOHN Journal* 47(7):316-23, July 1999.

Transfer from bed to wheelchair

For the patient with diminished or absent lower-body sensation or one-sided weakness, immobility, or injury, transfer from the bed to a wheelchair may require partial support to full assistance — initially by at least two health care team members. Subsequent transfer of the patient with generalized weakness may be performed by one nurse. After transfer, proper positioning and body alignment helps prevent excessive pressure on bony prominences, which predisposes the patient to skin breakdown.

Equipment
Wheelchair with locks (or sturdy chair) ● pajama bottoms (or robe) ● shoes or slippers with nonslip soles ● watch with a second hand ● stethoscope ● sphygmomanometer ● optional: transfer board if appropriate (see *Teaching use of a transfer board,* page 78)

Implementation
● Explain the procedure to the patient and demonstrate his role. **PCP**
● Place the wheelchair parallel to the bed, facing the foot of the bed, and lock its wheels. Make sure that the bed wheels are also locked. Raise the footrests *to avoid interfering with the transfer.*
● Check pulse rate and blood pressure with the patient supine *to obtain a baseline.* Then help him put on the pajama bottoms and slippers or shoes with nonslip soles *to prevent falls.* **Science**

Teaching use of a transfer board

For the patient who can't stand, a transfer board allows safe transfer from his bed to a wheelchair. To perform this transfer, take the following steps.

- First, explain and demonstrate the procedure. Eventually, the patient may become proficient enough to transfer himself independently or with some supervision.
- Help the patient put on pajama bottoms or a robe and shoes or slippers.
- Place the wheelchair angled slightly and facing the foot of the bed. Lock the wheels, and remove the armrest closest to the patient. Make sure that the bed is flat, and adjust its height so that it's level with the wheelchair seat.
- Assist the patient to a sitting position on the edge of the bed, with his feet resting on the floor. Make sure that the front edge of the wheelchair seat is aligned with the back of the patient's knees, as shown below left. *Although it's important that the patient have an even surface on which to transfer, he may find it easier to transfer to a slightly lower surface.*
- Ask the patient to lean away from the wheelchair while you slide one end of the transfer board under him.

- Now place the other end of the transfer board on the wheelchair seat, and help the patient return to the upright position.
- Stand in front of the patient *to prevent him from sliding forward.* Tell him to push down with both arms, lifting the buttocks up and onto the transfer board. The patient then repeats this maneuver, edging along the board, until he's seated in the wheelchair. If the patient can't use his arms to assist with the transfer, stand in front of him, put your arms around him, and — if he's able — have him put his arms around you. Gradually slide him across the board until he's safely in the chair, as shown below right.
- When the patient is in the wheelchair, fasten a seat belt, if necessary, *to prevent falls.*
- Then remove the transfer board, replace the wheelchair armrest, and reposition the patient in the wheelchair.

Positioning the transfer board

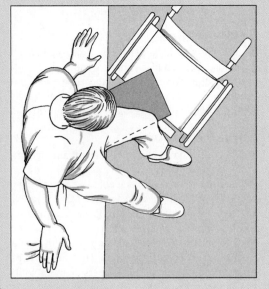

Assisting the patient

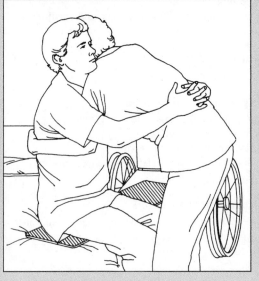

- Raise the head of the bed and allow the patient to rest briefly *to adjust to posture changes.* Then bring him to the dangling position. Recheck his pulse rate and blood pressure if you suspect cardiovascular instability. Don't proceed until the patient's pulse rate and blood pressure are stabilized *to prevent falls.* `Science`

- Tell the patient to move toward the edge of the bed and, if possible, to place his feet flat on the floor. Stand in front of the patient, blocking his toes with your feet and his knees with yours *to prevent his knees from buckling.*

- Flex your knees slightly, place your arms around the patient's back above the waist but below the level of the axilla, and tell him to place his hands on the edge of the bed. Avoid bending at your waist *to prevent back strain.* `Science`

- Ask the patient to push himself off the bed and to support as much of his own weight as possible. At the same time, straighten your knees and hips, raising the patient as you straighten your body.

- Supporting the patient as needed, pivot toward the wheelchair, keeping your knees next to his. Tell the patient to grasp the farthest armrest of the wheelchair with his closest hand.

- Help the patient lower himself into the wheelchair by flexing your hips and knees, but not your back. Instruct him to reach back and grasp the other wheelchair armrest as he sits *to avoid abrupt contact with the seat.* Fasten the seat belt *to prevent falls* and, if necessary, check his pulse rate and blood pressure *to assess cardiovascular stability.* If the pulse rate is 20 beats or more above baseline, stay with the patient and monitor him closely until it returns to normal *because he's experiencing orthostatic hypotension.*

- If the patient can't position himself correctly, help him move his buttocks against the back of the chair *so that the ischial tuberosities, not the sacrum, provide the base of support.*

- Place the patient's feet flat on the footrests, pointed straight ahead. Then position the knees and hips with the correct amount of flexion and in appropriate alignment. If appropriate, use elevating leg rests to flex the patient's hips at more than 90 degrees; *this position relieves pressure on the popliteal space and places more weight on the ischial tuberosities.*

- Position the patient's arms on the wheelchair's armrests with shoulders abducted, elbows slightly flexed, forearms pronated, and wrists and hands in the neutral position. If necessary, support or elevate the patient's hands and forearms with a pillow *to prevent dependent edema.*

Special considerations

- If the patient starts to fall during transfer, ease him to the closest surface — bed, floor, or chair. Never stretch to finish the transfer. *Doing so can cause loss of balance, falls, muscle strain, and other injuries to you and to the patient.*

- If the patient has one-sided weakness, follow the preceding steps, but place the wheelchair on the patient's unaffected side. Instruct the patient to pivot and bear as much weight as possible on the unaffected side. Support the affected side *because the patient will tend to lean to this side.* Use pillows to support the hemiplegic patient's affected side *to prevent slumping in the wheelchair.*

Nursing diagnoses

- Risk for injury

Expected outcomes

The patient (and family members) will:
- remain free from injury
- develop strategies to prevent injury
- identify and apply safety measures to prevent injury.

Documentation

Record the time of transfer and the extent of assistance in your notes, and note how the patient tolerated the activity.

Supportive references

Owen, B. "Preventing Injuries Using an Ergonomic Approach," *AORN Journal* 72(6):1031-36, December 2000.

Owen, B., et al. "What Are We Teaching about Lifting and Transferring Patients?" *Research in Nursing and Health* 22(1):3-13, February 1999.

Owen, B., and Fragala, G. "Reducing Perceived Physical Stress While Transferring Patients," *AAOHN Journal* 47(7):316-23, July 1999.

Using a hydraulic lift

After placing the patient in a supine position in the center of the sling, position the hydraulic lift above him, as shown here. Then attach the chains to the hooks on the sling.

Turn the lift handle clockwise to raise the patient to the sitting position. If he's positioned properly, continue to raise him until he's suspended just above the bed.

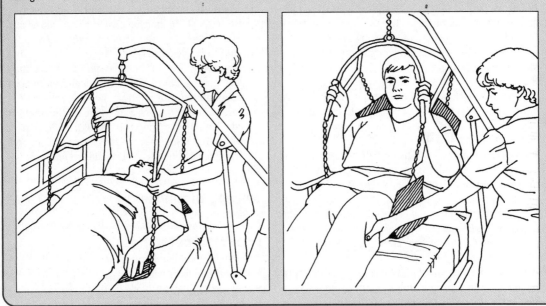

Transfer with a hydraulic lift

Using a hydraulic lift to raise the immobile patient from the supine to the sitting position permits a safe, comfortable transfer between the bed and a chair. It's indicated for the obese or immobile patient for whom manual transfer poses the potential for nurse or patient injury. Although one person can operate most hydraulic lift models, it's better to have two staff members present during transfer to stabilize and support the patient. To reduce the risk of harm to a patient, it's important to maintain the patient's body alignment during transfer. (See *Using a hydraulic lift*.)

Equipment

Hydraulic lift, with sling, chains or straps, and hooks
• chair or wheelchair

Preparation of equipment

● Because hydraulic lift models may vary in weight capacity, check the manufacturer's specifications before attempting patient transfer. **MFR**
● Make sure that the bed and wheelchair wheels are locked before beginning the transfer.

Implementation

● Explain the procedure to the patient, and reassure him that the hydraulic lift can safely support his weight and won't tip over. **PCP**
● Ensure the patient's privacy. If the patient has an I.V. line or urinary drainage bag, move it first. Arrange tubing securely *to prevent dangling during transfer*. If the tubing of the urinary drainage bag isn't long enough to permit the transfer, clamp the tubing and drainage bag and place it on the patient's abdomen during transfer. After the transfer, replace the drainage bag in a dependent position and unclamp the tubing. **PCP** **Science**

After positioning the patient above the wheelchair, turn the lift handle counterclockwise to lower him onto the seat. When the chains become slack, stop turning and unhook the sling from the lift.

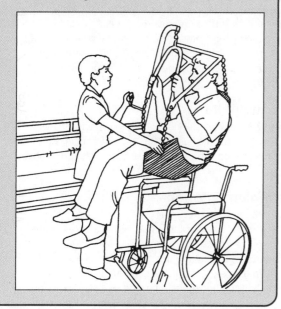

● Make sure that the side rail opposite you is raised and secure. Then roll the patient toward you, onto his side, and raise the side rail. Walk to the opposite side of the bed and lower the side rail.
● Place the sling under the patient's buttocks with its lower edge below the greater trochanter. Then fanfold the far side of the sling against the back and buttocks.
● Roll the patient toward you onto the sling, and raise the side rail. Then lower the opposite side rail.
● Slide your hands under the patient and pull the sling from beneath him, smoothing out all wrinkles. Then roll the patient onto his back and center him on the sling.
● Place the appropriate chair next to the head of the bed, facing the foot.
● Lower the side rail next to the chair, and raise the bed only until the base of the lift can extend under the bed. *To avoid alarming and endangering the patient,* don't raise the bed completely.

● Set the lift's adjustable base to its widest position *to ensure optimal stability.* Then move the lift so that its arm lies perpendicular to the bed, directly over the patient.
● Connect one end of the chains (or straps) to the side arms on the lift; connect the other, hooked end to the sling. Face the hooks away from the patient *to prevent them from slipping and to avoid the risk of their pointed edges injuring the patient.* The patient may place his arms inside or outside the chains (or straps) or he may grasp them when the slack is gone *to avoid injury.*
● Tighten the turnscrew on the lift. Then depending on the type of lift you're using, pump the handle or turn it clockwise until the patient has assumed a sitting position and his buttocks clear the bed surface by 1″ or 2″ (2.5 or 5 cm). Momentarily suspend the patient above the bed *until he feels secure in the lift and sees that it can bear his weight.*
● Steady the patient as you move the lift or, preferably, have another coworker guide the patient's body while you move the lift. Depending on the type of lift you're using, the arm should now rest in front or to one side of the chair.
● Release the turnscrew. Then depress the handle or turn it counterclockwise *to lower the patient into the chair.* While lowering the patient, push gently on his knees *to maintain the correct sitting posture.* After lowering the patient into the chair, fasten the seat belt *to ensure his safety.*
● Remove the hooks or straps from the sling, but leave the sling in place under the patient so you'll be able to transfer him back to the bed from the chair. Then move the lift away from the patient.
● To return the patient to bed, reverse the procedure.

Special considerations
● If the patient has an altered center of gravity (caused by a halo vest or a lower-extremity cast, for example), obtain help from a coworker before transferring him with a hydraulic lift.
● If the patient will require the use of a hydraulic lift for transfers after discharge, teach his family how to use this device correctly and allow them to practice with supervision.

Nursing diagnoses
● Risk for injury

Expected outcomes

The patient (and family members) will:
● remain free from injury
● recognize and apply measures to ensure their safety.

Documentation

Record the time of transfer in your notes, and note how the patient tolerated the activity.

Supportive references

Collins, J., and Owen, B. "NIOSH Research Initiatives to Prevent Back Injuries to Nursing Assistants, Aides and Orderlies in Nursing Homes," *American Journal of Industrial Medicine* 29(4):421-24, April 1996.

Owen, B. "Preventing Injuries Using an Ergonomic Approach," *AORN Journal* 72(6):1031-36, December 2000.

Owen, B., et al. "What Are We Teaching about Lifting and Transferring Patients?" *Research in Nursing and Health* 22(1):3-13, February 1999.

Owen, B., and Fragala, G. "Reducing Perceived Physical Stress While Transferring Patients," *AAOHN Journal* 47(7):316-23, July 1999.

Transfer to other health care facilities

Patients may be transferred to receive different forms of therapy, to receive continuity of care, or to receive or continue care elsewhere when financial resources prohibit remaining in the current health care facility. Patient transfer — either within the health care facility or to another — requires thorough preparation and careful documentation.

Preparation includes an explanation of the transfer to the patient and his family, discussion of the patient's condition and care plan with the staff at the receiving unit or facility, and arrangements for transportation if necessary. Nursing preparation should include assessing the patient's physical condition to determine if he's stable for transfer and to consult on the appropriate vehicle for transportation. Transfers are sometimes planned quickly. To protect the patient's rights, the nurse should determine his level of understanding of the reason for transfer and feelings about the change in care setting. The nurse should

also assess whether the patient's family has been informed about the transfer; their support aids in the patient's emotional and psychological adjustment to the transfer. **PCP**

Documentation of the patient's condition before and during transfer and adequate communication between nursing staffs ensure continuity of nursing care and provide legal protection for the transferring facility and its staff. To protect the patient's right to privacy, the nurse should confirm that the patient or family member has signed a release form because information in the patient record is confidential and its use requires a signed release.

Equipment

Admission inventory of patient's belongings ● patient's chart, medication record, and nursing Kardex ● medications ● bag or suitcase ● wheelchair or stretcher, as necessary ● transfer order form

Implementation

● Obtain a transfer order.
● Explain the transfer to the patient and his family. (See *Reducing anxiety about transfers.*) If the patient's condition precludes patient teaching, be sure to explain the reason for transfer to family members, especially if the transfer is the result of a serious change in the patient's condition. **EB1** Assess his physical condition *to determine the means of transfer,* such as a wheelchair or stretcher.
● Using the admissions inventory of belongings as a checklist, collect the patient's property. Be sure to check the entire room, including the closet, bedside stand, overbed table, and bathroom. If the patient is being transferred to another facility, don't forget valuables or personal medications that have been stored.
● Gather the patient's medications from the cart and the refrigerator. If the patient is being transferred to another unit, send the medications to the receiving unit; if he's being transferred to another health care facility, return them to the pharmacy.
● Notify the business office and other appropriate departments of the patient's transfer.
● Have a staff person notify the dietary department, pharmacy, and the facility's telephone operator about the transfer (if the transfer is within the facility).
● Report to the nurses on the receiving unit about the patient's condition and drug regimen and review

the patient's nursing care plan with them *to ensure continuity of care.*

Transfer within the health care facility

● If the patient is being transferred from or to an intensive care unit, your facility may require new care orders from the patient's physician. If so, review the new orders with the nursing staff at the receiving unit.

● Send the patient's chart, laboratory request forms Kardex, special equipment, and other required materials to the receiving unit.

● Use a wheelchair to transport the ambulatory patient to the newly assigned room unless it's on the same unit as his present one, in which case he may be allowed to walk. Use a stretcher to transport the bedridden patient.

● Introduce the patient to the nursing staff at the receiving unit. Then take the patient to his room and, depending on his condition, place him in the bed or seat him in a chair. Introduce him to his new roommate, if appropriate, and tell him about any unfamiliar equipment such as the call bell.

Transfer to an extended-care facility

● Make sure that the patient's physician has written the transfer order on his chart and has completed the special transfer form. This form should include the patient's diagnosis, care summary, drug regimen, and special care instructions, such as diet and physical therapy.

● Complete the nursing summary, including the patient's assessment, progress, required nursing treatments, and special needs, *to ensure continuity of care.*
JCAHO

● Keep one copy of the transfer order form and the nursing summary with the patient's chart, and forward the other copies to the receiving facility. However, don't send the patient's medications, Kardex, or chart.

Transfer to an acute-care facility

● Make sure that the physician has written the transfer order on the patient's chart and has completed the transfer form as previously described. Then complete the nursing summary.

● Depending on the physician's instructions, send one copy of the transfer form and the nursing sum-

---

Reducing anxiety about transfers **EB2**

Several studies have documented the stresses experienced by parents of children hospitalized in a pediatric intensive care unit (PICU). However, there's a lack of research on the anxiety experienced by parents when their child is transferred from the PICU to a general unit. In one study, researchers investigated whether better parent preparation would help reduce anxiety about their child's transfer. They found parents who received a transfer preparation letter, a verbal explanation of the procedure and positive aspects of the transfer, and a chance to ask questions had lower anxiety levels than parents who received a standard transfer protocol without being prepared in advance.

---

mary and photocopies of the pertinent excerpts from the patient's chart — such as laboratory test and X-ray results, patient history and physical progress notes, and vital signs records — to the receiving facility with the patient. Or, following your facility's policy, substitute a written summary of the patient's condition and facility history for the excerpts from the patient's chart. Make sure that this information is complete.
JCAHO

Special considerations

● If the patient requires an ambulance to take him to another health care facility, arrange transportation with the social services department. Make sure that the necessary equipment is assembled to provide care during transport.

● Be especially careful that all documentation is complete when the patient is being transferred to another health care facility. *A communications breakdown can hurt the patient's chances for recovery.*

● If the patient is being transferred to a different health care facility, make sure that none of the following patient care measures have been omitted: suctioning of airway, administering prescribed medications, changing soiled dressing, bathing an incontinent patient, and emptying drainage collection devices.

Nursing diagnoses
- Anxiety
- Fear

Expected outcomes
The patient will:
- cope with the current medical situation and the need for transfer
- state an understanding of the need for transfer.

Documentation
Record the reason for the transfer, time and date of transfer, the patient's condition before and during transfer (if the nurse accompanies the patient), the name of the receiving unit or health care facility, and the means of transportation. Include equipment accompanying the patient, such as I.V. lines and pumps, surgical drains, and oxygen therapy. Note the name and title of the person to whom you gave report; also include the names of staff or family members accompanying the patient.

Supportive references
Bouve, L.R., et al. "Preparing Patients for their Child's Transfer from the PICU to the Pediatric Floor," *Applied Nursing Research* 12(3):114-20, August 1999. **EB2**

Miles, M.S. "Parents who Received Transfer Preparation had Lower Anxiety about their Children's Transfer from the Pediatric Intensive Care Unit to a General Patient Ward," *Evidence-Based Nursing* 3:17, January 2000. **EB1**

Urine collection

A random urine specimen, usually collected as part of the physical examination or at various times during hospitalization, permits laboratory screening for urinary and systemic disorders as well as for drug use. A clean-catch midstream specimen is replacing random collection because it provides a virtually uncontaminated specimen without the need for catheterization.

When the patient can void voluntarily, a midstream specimen is commonly collected for culture and sensitivity testing. To protect the patient's rights, the nurse should assess the patient's level of understanding for the purpose of the test and the method of collection. This allows for clarification of any misunderstanding and promotes patient cooperation. Reference to the medical record for indications of infection will explain the purpose of the specimen procedure to the patient. **PCP**

Research has shown that the best time to perform urine collection is in the morning because the bacterial count is highest after overnight incubation in the bladder. Forced fluids or random specimens can dilute the specimens and may reduce colony counts, making the test results inaccurate.

Specimens should always be covered and refrigerated. Covering the specimen prevents carbon dioxide from diffusing into the air, which could result in the urine becoming alkaline and fostering bacterial growth. If a sample isn't refrigerated for over 2 hours, it should be discarded. If the patient is menstruating, the nurse should make a note of this on the laboratory request form. **Science**

An indwelling catheter specimen — obtained either by clamping the drainage tube and emptying the accumulated urine into a container or by aspirating a specimen with a syringe — requires sterile collection technique to prevent catheter contamination and urinary tract infection. This method is contraindicated after genitourinary surgery.

Equipment
Random specimen
Bedpan or urinal with cover, if necessary • gloves • graduated container • specimen container with lid • label • laboratory request form

Clean-catch midstream specimen
Soap and water • gloves • graduated container • three sterile 2″ × 2″ gauze pads • povidone-iodine solution • sterile specimen container with lid • label • bedpan or urinal, if necessary • laboratory request form (Commercial clean-catch kits containing antiseptic towelettes, sterile specimen container with lid and label, and instructions for use in several languages are widely used.)

Indwelling catheter specimen
Gloves • alcohol pad • 10-ml syringe • 21G or 22G 1½″ needle • tube clamp • sterile specimen container with lid • label • laboratory request form

Implementation
- Confirm the patient's identity using two patient identifiers according to facility policy. **JCAHO**

● Tell the patient that you need a urine specimen for laboratory analysis. Explain the procedure to him and his family, if necessary, *to promote cooperation and prevent accidental disposal of specimens.*

Collecting a random specimen

● Provide privacy. Instruct the patient on bed rest to void into a clean bedpan or urinal, or ask the ambulatory patient to void into either one in the bathroom.
● Put on gloves. **CDC**
● Pour at least 120 ml of urine into the specimen container, and cap the container securely. If the patient's urine output must be measured and recorded, pour the remaining urine into the graduated container. Otherwise, discard the remaining urine. If you inadvertently spill urine on the outside of the container, clean and dry it *to prevent cross-contamination.*
● After you label the sample container with the patient's name and room number and the date and time of collection, attach the request form and send it to the laboratory immediately. *Delayed transport of the specimen may alter test results.*
● Clean the graduated container and urinal or bedpan, and return them to their proper storage. Discard disposable items. **CDC**
● Wash your hands thoroughly *to prevent cross-contamination.* Offer the patient a washcloth and soap and water to wash his hands. **CDC**

Collecting a clean-catch midstream specimen

● *Because the goal is a virtually uncontaminated specimen,* explain the procedure to the patient carefully. Provide illustrations *to emphasize the correct collection technique,* if possible.
● Tell the male patient to remove all clothing from the waist down and to stand in front of the toilet as for urination; tell the female patient to sit far back on the toilet seat and spread her legs. Then have the patient clean the periurethral area (tip of the penis or labial folds, vulva, and urethral meatus) with soap and water and then wipe the area three times, each time with a fresh 2″ × 2″ gauze pad soaked in povidone-iodine solution, or with the wipes provided in a commercial kit. For the uncircumcised male patient, emphasize the need to retract his foreskin *to effectively clean the meatus* and to keep it retracted during voiding.

● Instruct the female patient to separate her labial folds with her thumb and forefinger. Tell her to wipe down one side with the first pad and discard it, to wipe the other side with the second pad and discard it and, finally, to wipe down the center over the urinary meatus with the third pad and discard it. Stress the importance of cleaning from front to back *to avoid contaminating the genital area with fecal matter.* **Science** Tell her to straddle the bedpan or toilet *to allow labial spreading.* She should continue to keep her labia separated while voiding.
● Instruct the patient to begin voiding into the bedpan, urinal, or toilet. Then without stopping the urine stream, the patient should move the collection container into the stream, collecting about 30 to 50 ml at the midstream portion of the voiding. He can then finish voiding into the bedpan, urinal, or toilet.
● Put on gloves before discarding the first and last portions of the voiding, and measure the remaining urine in a graduated container for intake and output records, if necessary. Be sure to include the amount in the specimen container when recording the total amount voided.
● Take the sterile container from the patient, and cap it securely. Avoid touching the inside of the container or the lid. If the outside of the container is soiled, clean it and wipe it dry. Remove gloves and discard them properly.
● Wash your hands thoroughly. Tell the patient to wash his hands also. **CDC**
● Label the container with the patient's name and room number, name of test, type of specimen, collection time, and suspected diagnosis, if known. If a urine culture has been ordered, note current antibiotic therapy on the laboratory request form. Send the container to the laboratory immediately, or place it on ice *to prevent specimen deterioration and altered test results.*

Collecting an indwelling catheter specimen

● About 30 minutes before collecting the specimen, clamp the drainage tube *to allow urine to accumulate.*
● Put on gloves. If the drainage tube has a built-in sampling port, wipe the port with an alcohol pad. Uncap the needle on the syringe, and insert the needle into the sampling port at a 90-degree angle to the tubing. Aspirate the specimen into the syringe. (See *Aspirating a urine specimen,* page 86.)

Aspirating a urine specimen [EB]

If the patient has an indwelling urinary catheter in place, clamp the tube distal to the aspiration port for about 30 minutes. Wipe the port with an alcohol pad, and insert a needle and a 20- or 30-ml syringe into the port perpendicular to the tube. Aspirate the required amount of urine, and expel it into the specimen container. Remove the clamp on the drainage tube.

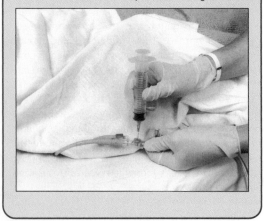

● If the drainage tube doesn't have a sampling port and the catheter is made of rubber, obtain the specimen from the catheter. *Other types of catheters will leak after you withdraw the needle.* To withdraw the specimen from a rubber catheter, wipe it with an alcohol pad just above where it connects to the drainage tube. Insert the needle into the rubber catheter at a 45-degree angle and withdraw the specimen. Never insert the needle into the shaft of the catheter *because this may puncture the lumen leading to the catheter balloon.* [EB]
● Transfer the specimen to a sterile container, label it, and send it to the laboratory immediately or place it on ice. If a urine culture is to be performed, be sure to list current antibiotic therapy on the laboratory request form.
● If the catheter isn't made of rubber or has no sampling port, wipe the area where the catheter joins the drainage tube with an alcohol pad. Disconnect the catheter, and allow urine to drain into the sterile specimen container. Avoid touching the inside of the sterile container with the catheter, and don't touch anything with the catheter drainage tube *to avoid*

contamination. When you have collected the specimen, wipe both connection sites with an alcohol pad and join them. Cap the specimen container, label it, and send it to the laboratory immediately or place it on ice.

⚠ **ALERT** *Make sure that you unclamp the drainage tube after collecting the specimen to prevent urine backflow, which may cause bladder distention and infection.*

📋 **TEACHING** *Instruct the patient to collect the specimen in a clean container with a tight-fitting lid and to keep it on ice or in the refrigerator (separating it from food items) for up to 24 hours.*

Nursing diagnoses
● Risk for infection

Expected outcomes
The patient will:
● remain free from pathogens in his urine culture
● have urine that remains clear, yellow, odorless, and free from sediment.

Documentation
Record the times of specimen collection and transport to the laboratory. Specify the test as well as the appearance, odor, color, and any unusual characteristics of the specimen. If necessary, record the urine volume on the intake and output record.

Supportive references
Craven, R.F., and Hirnle, C.J. *Fundamentals of Nursing Human Health and Function,* 5th ed. Philadelphia: Lippincott Williams & Wilkins, 2006. [EB]
Roberts, K. "The AAP Practice Parameter on Urinary Tract Infections in Febrile Infants and Young Children," *American Family Physician* 62(8):1815-22, October 2000.
*Smith-Temple, J., and Johnson, J. *Nurses' Guide to Clinical Procedures,* 4th ed. Philadelphia: Lippincott Williams & Wilkins, 2002.

Venipuncture

Venipuncture is the primary method for acquiring blood samples for laboratory testing and involves inserting a hollow-bore needle into the lumen of a large vein to obtain a sample.

Typically, venipuncture is performed at the antecubital fossa. If necessary, however, it can be performed on a vein in the wrist, the dorsum of the hand or foot, or another accessible location. Although laboratory personnel usually perform this procedure in the hospital setting, nurses commonly perform it.

Before attempting venipuncture, the nurse should inform the patient of the need for venipuncture and its possible risks and assess the patient's understanding of the procedure. This will reduce the patient's anxiety and promote cooperation during venipuncture.

Every upper-extremity venipuncture carries the risk of inadvertently puncturing or nicking a nerve. To avoid this complication, the Infusion Nurses Society recommends limiting the number of attempts of venipuncture on a patient. After two unsuccessful tries, the nurse should either ask another colleague to try or consult the I.V. team, nurse-anesthetist, or anesthesiologist.

For most adults, the hand is the common site for I.V. access. Using the patient's hand — preferably the nondominant one — leaves more proximal sites available for subsequent venipunctures. The nurse should avoid using the hands with elderly patients, who have lost subcutaneous tissue surrounding the veins; they're at increased risk for hematoma.

The nurse should also determine if special conditions exist before venipuncture. It's important that the patient be assessed for possible risks of venipuncture, such as anticoagulant therapy, low platelet count, bleeding disorders, and other abnormalities that increase the risk of bleeding and hematoma formation.

When selecting a catheter, the nurse should consider the patient's condition and the type of solution to be infused over the next 48 to 72 hours. Using the smallest-gauge catheter in the largest vein possible diminishes chemical and mechanical irritation to the vein wall. **INS**

Equipment

Tourniquet • gloves • syringe or evacuated tubes and needle holder • alcohol or chlorhexidine pads **CDC** • 20G or 21G needle for the forearm or 25G needle for the wrist, hand, and ankle and for children • color-coded collection tubes containing appropriate additives • labels • laboratory request form • 2″ × 2″ gauze pads • adhesive bandage

Preparation of equipment

● If you're using evacuated tubes, open the needle packet, attach the needle to its holder, and select the appropriate tubes.
● If you're using a syringe, attach the appropriate needle to it. Be sure to choose a syringe large enough to hold all the blood required for the test.
● Label all collection tubes clearly with the patient's name and room number, the practitioner's name, and the date and time of collection.

Implementation

● Wash your hands thoroughly and put on gloves. **CDC**
● Confirm the patient's identity using two patient identifiers according to facility policy. **JCAHO**
● Tell the patient that you're about to take a blood sample, and explain the procedure *to ease his anxiety and ensure his cooperation.* Ask him if he has ever felt faint, sweaty, or nauseated when having blood drawn. If the patient is a child, try using distraction with a toy or game to reduce anxiety. **PCP**
● If the patient is on bed rest, ask him to lie supine, with his head slightly elevated and his arms at his sides. Ask the ambulatory patient to sit in a chair and support his arm securely on an armrest or table.
● Assess the patient's veins *to determine the best puncture site.* (See *Common venipuncture sites,* page 88.)
● Observe the patient's skin for the vein's blue color, or palpate the vein for a firm rebound sensation.
● Tie a tourniquet 2″ (5 cm) proximal to the area chosen. *By impeding venous return to the heart while still allowing arterial flow, a tourniquet produces venous dilation.* If arterial perfusion remains adequate, you'll be able to feel the radial pulse. (If the tourniquet fails to dilate the vein, have the patient open and close his fist repeatedly. Then ask him to close his fist as you insert the needle and to open it again when the needle is in place.)
● Clean the venipuncture site with an alcohol or chlorhexidine pad. **CDC** Wipe in a circular motion, spiraling outward from the site *to avoid introducing potentially infectious skin flora into the vessel during the procedure.* If you use alcohol, apply it with fric-

Common venipuncture sites

These illustrations show the anatomic locations of veins commonly used for venipuncture. The most commonly used sites are on the forearm, followed by those on the hand.

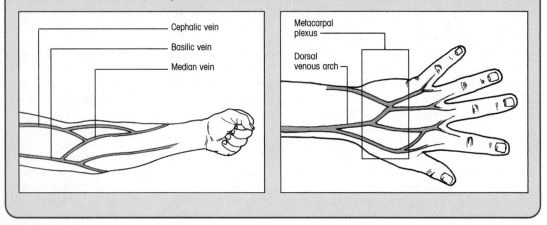

Cephalic vein
Basilic vein
Median vein

Metacarpal plexus
Dorsal venous arch

tion for 30 seconds, or until the final pad comes away clean. Allow the skin to dry before performing venipuncture. **Science**

● Immobilize the vein by pressing just below the venipuncture site with your thumb and drawing the skin taut.

● Position the needle holder or syringe with the needle bevel up and the shaft parallel to the path of the vein and at a 30-degree angle to the arm. Insert the needle into the vein. If you're using a syringe, venous blood will appear in the hub; withdraw the blood slowly, pulling the plunger of the syringe gently *to create steady suction* until you obtain the required sample. *Pulling the plunger too forcibly may collapse the vein.* If you're using a needle holder and an evacuated tube, grasp the holder securely to stabilize it in the vein, and push down on the collection tube until the needle punctures the rubber stopper. Blood will flow into the tube automatically. **INS**

● Remove the tourniquet as soon as blood flows adequately *to prevent stasis and hemoconcentration, which can impair test results.* If the flow is sluggish, leave the tourniquet in place longer, but always remove it before withdrawing the needle. **INS**

● Continue to fill the required tubes, removing one and inserting another. Gently rotate each tube as you remove it *to help mix the additive with the sample.*

● After you've drawn the sample, place a gauze pad over the puncture site, and slowly and gently remove the needle from the vein. When using an evacuated tube, remove it from the needle holder *to release the vacuum* before withdrawing the needle from the vein.

● Apply gentle pressure to the puncture site for 2 or 3 minutes or until bleeding stops. *This prevents extravasation into the surrounding tissue, which can cause a hematoma.* **INS**

● After bleeding stops, apply an adhesive bandage.

● If you've used a syringe, transfer the sample to a collection tube. Detach the needle from the syringe, open the collection tube, and gently empty the sample into the tube, being careful to avoid foaming, *which can cause hemolysis.*

● Finally, check the venipuncture site *to see if a hematoma has developed.* If it has, apply pressure to the site.

● Discard syringes, needles, and used gloves in the appropriate containers. **CDC**

Special considerations

● Never draw a venous sample from an arm or leg that's already being used for I.V. therapy or blood administration *because this may affect test results; I.V. fluids may dilute blood.*

● Don't collect a venous sample from an infection site *because this may introduce pathogens into the vascular system.* Similarly, avoid drawing blood from edematous areas or sites of previous hematoma or vascular injury *because the vessel wall may be damaged* . **INS**

● Don't use an arm on the side of a mastectomy *because reduced lymphatic drainage increases the risk of infection at the site.* **INS**

● Never use an arm with an arteriovenous fistula *because of the increased risk of clotting and bleeding.* **INS**

● If the patient has large, distended, highly visible veins, perform venipuncture without a tourniquet *to minimize the risk of hematoma formation.* If the patient has a clotting disorder or is receiving anticoagulant therapy, maintain firm pressure on the venipuncture site for at least 5 minutes after withdrawing the needle *to prevent hematoma formation.*

● Avoid using veins in the patient's legs for venipuncture, if possible, *because this increases the risk of thrombophlebitis.*

● If a large-bore catheter is necessary, consider using a topical or subcutaneous anesthetic agent *to reduce pain.*

Nursing diagnoses
● Risk for infection
● Risk for injury

Expected outcomes
The patient will:
● have no signs and symptoms of infection at the venipuncture site
● remain free from injury.

Complications
● A hematoma at the needle insertion site is the most common complication of venipuncture.
● Infection may result from poor technique.

Documentation
Record the date, time, and site of venipuncture; name of the test; the time the sample was sent to the laboratory; the amount of blood collected; the patient's temperature; and any adverse reactions to the procedure.

Supportive references

Carlson, K., et al. "Using Distraction to Reduce Reported Pain, Fear and Behavioral Distress in Children and Adolescents: A Multisite Study," *Journal of the Society of Pediatric Nurses* 5(2):75-85, April-June 2000.

Centers for Disease Control and Prevention. Hospital Infection Control Practices Advisory Committee. *Guideline for Prevention of Intravascular Device-Related Infections.* 1996; last reviewed May 2001. *www.cdc.gov/ncidod/hip/IV/IV.htm.*

"Infusion Nursing Standards of Practice," *Journal of Intravenous Nursing* 29(1S), January-February 2006.

Millam, D.A., and Hadaway, L.C. "On the Road to Successful I.V. Starts," *Nursing2000* 30(4):34-48, April 2000.

Patterson, P., et al. "Comparison of 4 Analgesic Agents for Venipuncture," *AANA Journal* 68(1)43-51, February 2000.

Infection control

The task of preventing and controlling infectious disease became far easier in the 19th century, when Louis Pasteur and other microbiologists discovered the link between bacteria and infection. Yet, health care-associated infections (HAIs) continue to cast a shadow over patients in health care facilities.

Approximately 2 million HAIs occur annually in the United States. Their substantial morbidity and mortality cause about 80,000 patient deaths per year, raise health care costs by about $4.5 billion, and significantly prolong hospital stays. **CDC** For example, hospitalization for a urinary tract infection secondary to an HAI has been estimated to be about 1 to 4 days; for surgical site infections, 7 to 8½ days; and for bloodstream infection, 7 to 21 days.

Studies have shown that strict adherence to infection control principles, practices, and guidelines can prevent one-third of HAIs. **EB** However, patients whose immune systems are compromised or suppressed might succumb to an HAI despite precautions.

In this chapter, you'll find recommendations of best practice techniques and precautions for maintaining the highest quality infection control. Many of these recommendations are evidence-based **EB**. Others come from the American Hospital Association **AHospA** and its Patient Care Partnership **PCP**, the Centers for Disease Control and Prevention **CDC** and its Advisory Committee on Immunization Practices **ACIP**, the Occupational Safety and Health Administration **OSHA**, and the Association for Professionals in Infection Control and Epidemiology **APIC**. Others are from specific manufacturers' recommendations for the use of their products. **MFR**

The goal of infection control is to prevent the transmission of disease among patients, health care workers, and visitors to the health care facility. Although many factors contribute to the development of HAIs,

strict adherence to your facility's infection control policies and the practices outlined in this chapter can significantly reduce the rate of HAIs and help provide the best outcome for your patients.

Causes and incidence

Health care-associated infections (HAIs) are infections that patients acquire during the course of receiving treatment for other conditions. Health care workers can also get HAIs while performing their duties within the health care setting. HAIs result from aerobic or anaerobic bacteria, viruses, parasites, or fungi. (See *Infectious diseases possibly acquired in health care facilities*.) They occur most commonly in the urinary and lower respiratory tracts, bloodstream, and surgical sites. Urinary tract infections most commonly result from catheter insertion, urogenital surgery, or instrumentation. Respiratory tract infections usually result from aspiration of oropharyngeal secretions, inhalation of airborne pathogens from other patients or caregivers, contaminated ventilation equipment, or lung seeding from blood-borne pathogens. Surgical site infection may result from contamination during surgery, preexisting medical conditions, skin damage during preoperative preparation (such as shaving), or impaired blood supply.

The risk of HAIs increases with the patient's age, underlying medical condition, length of hospitalization, and use of invasive devices.

Evolution of infection control

Infection control practices have evolved continuously since JCAHO and the American Hospital Association issued a statement in 1958 advising that every accred-

Infectious diseases possibly acquired in health care facilities

The Division of Healthcare Quality Promotion, a division of the Centers for Disease Control and Prevention, has identified these diseases that may be acquired by patients or health care professionals in health care facilities:

- Bloodborne pathogens
- *Clostridium difficile*
- *C. sordellii*
- Creutzfeldt-Jakob disease
- Ebola (viral hemorrhagic fever)
- GI infections
- Hepatitis A
- Hepatitis B
- Hepatitis C
- Human immunodeficiency virus/acquired immunodeficiency syndrome
- Influenza

- Methicillin-resistant *Staphylococcus aureus*
- Norovirus
- Parvovirus
- Poliovirus
- Pneumonia
- Rubella
- Severe acute respiratory syndrome
- *Streptococcus pneumoniae* (drug resistant)
- Tuberculosis
- Vancomycin intermediate *S. aureus*
- Vancomycin-resistant enterococci
- Varicella (chickenpox)

Infection control timeline

This time line describes when infection control practices were implemented in hospitals and provides a brief description of various isolation categories.

- 1958: The Joint Commission on the Accreditation of Healthcare Organizations recommends that all accredited hospitals must have an infection control committee and implement a formal infection control program.
- 1970: The Centers for Disease Control and Prevention (CDC) publishes *Isolation Techniques for Use in Hospitals.*
- 1975: CDC releases an update to its 1970 isolation techniques publication.

- 1980: CDC releases its *Guidelines for Prevention and Control of Nosocomial Infections.* This guideline outlines ways to prevent or control hospital-borne pathogens.
- 1983: CDC releases an update to its 1975 isolation techniques publication.
- 1985: CDC publishes *Universal Precautions.*
- 1987: CDC establishes its recommendations for body substance isolation.
- 1996: CDC institutes *Standard Precautions* and further updates the isolation precautions.

ited health care facility must have an infection control committee and a monitoring system as part of a formal infection control program. **AHospA** **OSHA**

Twelve years later, in 1970, the Centers for Disease Control and Prevention (CDC) published a guide to isolation techniques in hospitals; the guide was updated in 1975, 1983, and again in 1996. In 1980, the CDC released *Guidelines for the Prevention and Control of Nosocomial Infections.* The guidelines had two purposes: to disseminate advice on prevention or

control of specific nosocomial infection problems and to cover the questions most frequently asked of the CDC's Division of Healthcare Quality Promotion staff. (See *Infection control timeline.*)

An atmosphere of concern regarding the transmission of human immunodeficiency virus brought about the expansion of isolation guidelines to include protective measures, such as wearing gloves, masks, gowns, and goggles to guard against exposure to blood and body fluids. The expanded guidelines, re-

Indications for airborne precautions

Airborne precautions are designed to reduce the risk of airborne transmission of the following infectious agents.

Disease	Precautionary period
Chickenpox (varicella)	Until lesions are crusted and no new lesions appear
Herpes zoster (disseminated)	Duration of illness
Herpes zoster (localized in an immunocompromised patient)	Duration of illness
Measles (rubeola)	Duration of illness
Severe acute respiratory syndrome	Duration of illness; gown, gloves, and eye goggles must be worn
Tuberculosis (TB) — pulmonary or laryngeal, confirmed or suspected	Depends on clinical response; patient must be on effective therapy, be improving clinically (decreased cough and fever and improved findings on chest radiograph), and have three consecutive negative sputum smears collected on different days, or TB must be ruled out

leased in 1985, were called universal precautions. Body substance isolation guidelines, concerning the handling and disposal of potentially infectious body substances, were introduced in 1987.

In 1996, the CDC instituted standard precautions, which combined major features of blood and body fluid precautions with practices regarding body substance isolation. Standard precautions recommend that health care workers wear appropriate protective clothing or use appropriate protective equipment when the duty being performed requires or may involve contact with any body substance, mucous membrane, or broken skin. The CDC also added three other categories called transmission-based precautions — airborne precautions, droplet precautions, and contact precautions.

Supportive references

Centers for Disease Control and Prevention. *Isolation Techniques for Use in Hospitals,* 2nd ed. Washington, D.C.: U.S. Department of Health and Human Services, 1975. HHS publication no. (CDC) 76-8314.

Garner, J.S. "Hospital Infection Control Practices Advisory Committee Guideline for Isolation Precautions in Hospitals," *Infection Control and Hospital Epidemiology* 17:53-80, January 1996. *www.cdc.gov/ncidod/hip/isolat/isopart2.htm.* **EB**

Joint Commission on Accreditation of Healthcare Organizations. *Comprehensive Accreditation Manual for Hospitals.* Oakbrook Terrace, Ill.: JCAHO, 2005. *www.jcaho.gov.*

Airborne precautions
CDC **EB1**

Airborne precautions, used in addition to standard precautions, prevent the spread of infectious diseases transmitted by droplet nuclei 5 µm or smaller that are breathed, sneezed, or coughed into the environment. (See *Indications for airborne precautions.*) Diseases in this category include the former categories of acid-fast bacillus isolation and respiratory isolation.

To effectively guard against the spread of infection from an airborne transmitted infection, an isolation patient requires a monitored negative-pressure room with the door kept closed *to maintain the proper air pressure balance* in the isolation room, the anteroom, and the adjoining hallway or corridor. The air should undergo 12 air exchanges per hour for new construction and 6 air exchanges per hour for construction before 2001. **EB2** It should be appropriately discharged directly to the outside of the building or filtered through high-efficiency particulate air (HEPA) filtration before it's circulated to other areas of the health care facility. If for some reason a private room isn't available, patients infected with the same disease can share a room, but consultation with infection control professionals is advised before patient placement.

All persons who enter the room must wear respiratory protection. In 1993, the Centers for Disease Control and Prevention (CDC) published tuberculosis guidelines recommending the use of a disposable respirator, such as an N95 respirator or HEPA respirator; a reusable respirator, such as a HEPA respirator; or a powered air-purifying respirator (PAPR) that provides protection against microorganisms transmitted by airborne droplet nuclei. Regardless of the type of respirator used, the health care worker must make sure that the respirator properly fits her face, covering the mouth and nose, each time she wears it. Fit testing of all respirators ensures proper fit. **OSHA** If the patient must leave the room for an essential procedure, he should wear a surgical mask to cover his nose and mouth while out of the room, and personnel in the area where the patient is going should be notified and instructed to take airborne precautions.

Equipment

Respirators (either disposable N95 or HEPA respirators or reusable HEPA respirators or PAPRs) • surgical masks • isolation door card • other personal protective equipment as needed for standard precautions

Gather additional supplies needed for routine patient care, such as a thermometer, stethoscope, and blood pressure cuff.

Preparation of equipment

Keep airborne precaution supplies outside the patient's room in a cart or anteroom.

Implementation

● Situate the patient in a negative-pressure room with the door closed. If possible, the room should have an anteroom, and it should be possible to monitor the negative pressure. If necessary, two patients with the same infection may share a room. Explain isolation precautions to the patient and his family.
● Keep the patient's door (and the anteroom door) closed at all times *to maintain the negative pressure*

Checking the respirator seal

Before using a respirator, always check the respirator seal. To do this, place your hands over the respirator and exhale. If you feel air leaking around your nose, adjust the nosepiece. If air leaks at the respirator's edges, adjust the straps along the side of your head. Recheck respirator fit after this adjustment.

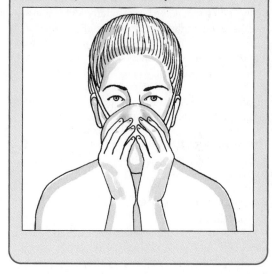

---

and contain the airborne pathogens. Put an airborne precautions sign on the door *to notify anyone entering the room.*
● Put your respirator on according to the manufacturer's directions. **MFR** Adjust the straps for a firm but comfortable fit. Check the fit. (See *Checking the respirator seal.*)
● Instruct the patient to cover his nose and mouth with a facial tissue while coughing or sneezing.
● Tape an impervious bag to the patient's bedside *so the patient can dispose of facial tissues correctly.*
● Make sure that visitors wear respiratory protection while in the patient's room.
● Limit the patient's movement from the room. If he must leave the room for essential procedures, make sure he wears a surgical mask over his nose and mouth. Notify the receiving department or area of the patient's isolation precautions *so that the precautions will be maintained and the patient can be returned to his room promptly.*

● All negative-pressure rooms require constant monitoring usually via electronic devices. **CDC** When the monitor's alarm sounds, it indicates a problem with negative pressure. **MFR**

Special considerations

● Before leaving the room, remove gloves (if worn), and wash your hands. Remove your respirator outside the patient's room after closing the door.
● Depending on the type of respirator and recommendations from the manufacturer, follow your facility's policy and either discard your respirator or store it until the next use. If your respirator is to be stored until the next use, store it in a dry, well-ventilated place (not a plastic bag) *to prevent microbial growth.* Nondisposable respirators must be cleaned according to the manufacturer's recommendations. **MFR**

Nursing diagnoses

● Risk for injury
● Risk for loneliness

Expected outcomes

The patient will:
● help identify and apply safety measures to prevent injury
● develop strategies to maintain safety
● identify feelings of loneliness
● identify ways to socialize within the confines of isolation.

Documentation

Record the need for airborne precautions on the nursing care plan and as otherwise indicated by your facility. Document initiation and maintenance of the precautions, the patient's tolerance of the procedure, and any patient or family teaching. Also document the date airborne precautions were discontinued.

Supportive references

Garner, J.S. "Hospital Infection Control Practices Advisory Committee Guideline for Isolation Precautions in Hospitals," *Infection Control and Hospital Epidemiology* 17(1):53-80, January 1996. *www.cdc.gov/ncidod/hip/isolat/isopart2.htm.* **EB1**
"Guidelines for Environmental Infection Control in Health Care Facilities," *MMWR Morbidity and Mortality Weekly Report* 52(RR-10):1-42, June 2003. **EB2**

Contact precautions **CDC**

Contact precautions prevent the spread of infectious diseases transmitted by direct or indirect contact with the patient (skin-to-skin), patient-care items (bedpans, urinals), or indirect contact with surfaces in the patient's room that are contaminated with the infectious microorganism. (See *Indications for contact precautions.*)

The Centers for Disease Control and Prevention (CDC) recommends that contact precautions apply to patients who are known or suspected to be infected or colonized (presence of microorganism without obvious clinical signs and symptoms of infection) with epidemiologically important organisms that can be transmitted by direct or indirect contact. Effective contact precautions require a private room. If no private room is available, two patients infected with the same (but no other) microorganism can share a room.

CDC guidelines advise considering the epidemiology of the microorganism and the patient population and consulting infection control professionals before patient placement.

Anyone having contact with the patient, the patient's support equipment, or items soiled with the patient's bodily fluids should wear clean, nonsterile gowns and gloves. Gloves should be changed after contact with infective material that may contain high concentrations of the microorganism, such as fecal material or wound drainage. A gown and gloves should be removed before leaving the patient's room. Thorough hand washing with an antimicrobial agent or waterless antiseptic agent and proper handling and disposal of contaminated items are also essential in maintaining contact precautions.

Patient transport should be limited to essential purposes only. If the patient is transported, make sure that precautions are maintained *to decrease the risk of transmission to other patients and contamination of environmental surfaces.*

When possible, medical and noncritical patient-care equipment (I.V. pumps, monitors) should be used for only one patient. If sharing equipment is unavoidable, then items must be properly cleaned or disinfected before use with another patient.

Indications for contact precautions

Contact precautions are designed to reduce the risk of transmitting infectious agents, by direct or indirect contact, such as the ones listed here.

Disease	Precautionary period
Acute viral (acute hemorrhagic) conjunctivitis	Duration of illness
Clostridium difficile enteric infection	Duration of illness
Diphtheria (cutaneous)	Duration of illness
Enteroviral infection, in diapered or incontinent patient	Duration of illness
Escherichia coli disease, in diapered or incontinent patient	Duration of illness
Hepatitis A, in diapered or incontinent patient	Duration of illness
Herpes simplex virus infection (neonatal or mucocutaneous)	Duration of illness
Impetigo	Until 24 hours after initiation of effective therapy
Infection or colonization with multidrug-resistant bacteria	Until off antibiotics and culture is negative
Major abscesses, cellulitis, or decubiti	Until 24 hours after initiation of effective therapy
Parainfluenza virus infection, in diapered or incontinent patient	Duration of illness
Pediculosis (lice)	Until 24 hours after initiation of effective therapy
Respiratory syncytial virus infection, in infants and young children	Duration of illness
Rotavirus infection, in diapered or incontinent patient	Duration of illness
Rubella, congenital syndrome	Precautions during any admission until infant is age 1, unless nasopharyngeal and urine cultures negative for virus after age 3 months
Scabies	Until 24 hours after initiation of effective therapy
Shigellosis, in diapered or incontinent patient	Duration of illness
Smallpox	Duration of Illness; requires airborne and contact precautions
Staphylococcal furunculosis in infants and young children	Duration of illness
Viral hemorrhagic infections (Ebola, Lassa, Marburg)	Duration of illness
Zoster (chickenpox, disseminated zoster, or localized zoster in immunodeficient patient)	Until all lesions are crusted; requires airborne precautions

Equipment

Gloves • gowns or aprons • masks, if necessary • isolation door card • plastic bags

Gather additional supplies, such as a thermometer, stethoscope, and blood pressure cuff.

Preparation of equipment

Keep contact precaution supplies outside the patient's room in a cart or anteroom.

Implementation CDC

● Situate the patient in a single room with private toilet facilities and an anteroom, if possible. If necessary, two patients with the same (but no other) infection may share a room. Explain isolation procedures to the patient and his family.
● Instruct visitors to wear gloves and a gown while visiting the patient and to wash their hands after removing the gown and gloves.
● Place a contact precautions card on the door *to notify anyone entering the room.*
● Wash your hands before entering and after leaving the patient's room and after removing gloves.
● Place laboratory specimens in impervious, labeled containers, and send them to the laboratory at once. Attach requisition slips to the outside of the container.
● Place items that have come in contact with the patient in a single impervious bag, and arrange for disposal or disinfection and sterilization. OSHA
● Limit the patient's movement from the room. If the patient must be moved, cover draining wounds with clean dressings. Notify the receiving department or area of the patient's isolation precautions *so that the precautions will be maintained and the patient can be returned to the room promptly.*

Special considerations

● Clean and disinfect equipment between uses by different patients.
● Try to dedicate certain reusable equipment (thermometer, stethoscope, blood pressure cuff) for the patient in contact precautions *to reduce the risk of transmitting infection to other patients.*
● Remember to change gloves during patient care as indicated by the procedure or task. Wash your hands after removing gloves and before putting on new gloves.

Nursing diagnoses

● Social isolation

Expected outcomes

The patient will:
● express feelings of isolation
● interact with his family members and friends
● interact with caregivers.

Documentation

Record the need for contact precautions on the nursing care plan and as otherwise indicated by your facility. Document initiation and maintenance of the precautions, the patient's tolerance of the procedure, and patient or family teaching. Also document the date contact precautions were discontinued.

Supportive references

Garner, J.S. "Hospital Infection Control Practices Advisory Committee Guidelines for Isolation Precautions in Hospitals," *Infection Control and Hospital Epidemiology* 17(1):53-80, January 1996. *www.cdc.gov/ncidod/hip/isolat/isopart2.htm.*

Droplet precautions CDC

Droplet precautions prevent the transmission and spread of infectious diseases caused by large-particle droplets (larger than 5 mm in size) from the infected patient to the susceptible host. Infection occurs when droplets come in contact with the mucous membranes of a host. (See *Indications for droplet precautions.*)

The Centers for Disease Control and Prevention (CDC) guidelines state that droplet transmission is theoretically a form of contact transmission. This type of transmission is very distinct from indirect or direct transmission and can occur during talking, coughing, or sneezing and during the performance of certain procedures, such as suctioning and bronchoscopy. Because the droplets of moisture are heavy and don't remain suspended in the air, special air handling and ventilation aren't required to prevent transmission or infection.

Effective droplet precautions require a private room (the door may remain open). If a private room isn't available, the CDC and the Occupational Safety and Health Administration guidelines state that the pa-

Indications for droplet precautions

Droplet precautions are designed to reduce the risk of droplet transmission of the following diseases. Also listed are the precautionary periods for each disease.

Disease	Precautionary period
Adenovirus infection in infants and young children	Duration of illness
Diphtheria (pharyngeal)	Until off antibiotics and two cultures taken at least 24 hours apart are negative
Influenza	Duration of illness
Invasive *Haemophilus influenzae* type b disease, including meningitis, pneumonia, and sepsis	Until 24 hours after initiation of effective therapy
Invasive *Neisseria meningitidis* disease, including meningitis, pneumonia, epiglottiditis, and sepsis	Until 24 hours after initiation of effective therapy
Mumps	For 9 days after onset of swelling
Mycoplasma pneumoniae infection	Duration of illness
Parvovirus B19	Maintain precautions for duration of hospitalization when chronic disease occurs in an immunodeficient patient (For patients with transient aplastic crisis or red cell crisis, maintain precautions for 7 days.)
Pertussis	Until 5 days after initiation of effective therapy
Pneumonic plague	Until 72 hours after initiation of effective therapy
Rubella (German measles)	Until 7 days after onset of rash
Streptococcal pharyngitis, pneumonia, or scarlet fever in infants and young children	Until 24 hours after initiation of effective therapy

tient may be placed in a room with another patient who has the same active (but no other) infection. All persons — including visitors — who may be in close contact with the patient should maintain a distance of at least 3′ (1 m) from the patient and should wear a surgical mask covering the nose and mouth. **OSHA**

During handling of infants and young children who require droplet precautions, gloves and a gown should be worn *to prevent soiling clothing from nasal and oral secretions*.

Equipment

Masks • gowns, if necessary • gloves • plastic bags • droplet precautions door card

Gather additional supplies needed for routine patient care, such as a thermometer, stethoscope, and blood pressure cuff.

Preparation of equipment

Keep droplet precaution supplies outside the patient's room in a cart or anteroom.

Implementation

- Situate the patient in a single room with private toilet facilities and an anteroom, if possible. If necessary, two patients with the same infection (but no other infections) may share a room. Explain isolation procedures to the patient and his family. **PCP**
- Make sure that visitors wear masks (and, if necessary, gowns and gloves) within 3′ (1 m) of the patient.
- Put a droplet precautions sign on the door *to notify anyone entering the room.*
- Wash your hands before entering and after leaving the room and during patient care, as indicated.
- Pick up your mask by the top strings, adjust it around your nose and mouth, and tie the strings for a comfortable fit. If the mask has a flexible metal nose strip, adjust it to fit firmly but comfortably.
- Instruct the patient to cover his nose and mouth with a facial tissue while coughing or sneezing.
- Tape a plastic bag to the patient's bedside *so the patient can dispose of facial tissues correctly.*
- Limit the patient's movement from the room. If he must leave the room for essential procedures, make sure that he wears a surgical mask over his nose and mouth. Notify the receiving department or area of the patient's isolation precautions *so that the precautions will be maintained and the patient can be returned to the room promptly.*
- Some health care facilities have added contact precautions to droplet precautions because the patient's environment is contaminated.

Special considerations

- Before removing your mask, remove your gloves (if worn), and wash your hands.
- Untie the strings and dispose of the mask, handling it by the strings only.

Nursing diagnoses

- Social isolation

Expected outcomes

The patient will:
- express feelings of isolation
- interact with his family members and friends
- interact with caregivers.

Documentation

Record the need for droplet precautions on the nursing care plan and as otherwise indicated by your facility. Document initiation and maintenance of the precautions, the patient's tolerance of the procedure, and patient or family teaching. Also document the date droplet precautions were discontinued.

Supportive references

Garner, J.S. "Hospital Infection Control Practices Advisory Committee Guidelines for Isolation Precautions in Hospitals," *Infection Control and Hospital Epidemiology* 17(1):53-80, January 1996. *www.cdc.gov/ncidod/hip/isolat/isopart2.htm.*

Hughes, J.M. "Guideline for Handwashing and Hospital Environmental Control, 1985," *MMWR Morbidity and Mortality Weekly Report* 37(24), June 1988. *www.cdc.gov/ncidod/hip/guide/handwash.htm.*

Hand hygiene

The success of infection control in the United States has been due in a large part to recognizing the individual as a primary source of health care-associated infections (HAIs). *The hands are the conduits for almost every transfer of potential pathogens* from one patient to another, from a contaminated object to the patient, or from a staff member to the patient. Each year approximately 2 million patients in U.S. hospitals develop HAIs and roughly 80,000 die as a result. *Hand hygiene is the single most important effective measure for preventing infection,* yet it's commonly neglected. A study discovered that one way to increase compliance of hand hygiene in hospitals is to equip hospital units with dispensers filled with a rinse-free, alcohol-based gel. **EB1**

To protect patients from HAIs, hand hygiene must be performed routinely and thoroughly.

The Centers for Disease Control and Prevention guidelines define hand hygiene as handwashing, antiseptic handwashing, antiseptic hand rub, or surgical hand antisepsis. Plain soap, detergents, or antimicrobial-containing products may be used to wash the hands. Hand hygiene can be broken down into two processes. *Mechanical removal of microorganisms* occurs when the hands are washed with plain soap or detergent; in this process, microorganisms are removed from the hands, which are then rinsed. *Chemical removal of microorganisms* occurs when the hands are washed with an antimicrobial agent; this process kills or inhibits the growth of microorgan-

isms. The decision as to when hand hygiene should occur depends on four factors:
- intensity of contact with patients or fomites
- degree of contamination that's likely to occur with contact
- susceptibility of patients to infection
- procedure to be performed. **CDC**

Washing hands thoroughly and promptly between patients is the best way to reduce the risk of contamination and an important part of maintaining any type of isolation precautions. *Artificial nails may serve as a reservoir for microorganisms;* therefore, they shouldn't be worn in health care facilities. **EB2** Naturally long nails may also harbor more microorganisms; keep nails trimmed short, no more than ¼″ beyond the edge of the finger. It's also important to keep hands soft and use lotion between washings *because microorganisms are more difficult to remove from rough or chapped hands.*

Equipment

Handwashing: Antibacterial or antimicrobial soap or detergent • warm running water • paper towels • optional: antiseptic cleaning agent, fingernail brush, disposable sponge brush or plastic cuticle stick
Hand-sanitizing: Alcohol-based hand rub

Implementation
Handwashing
- Remove rings as your facility policy dictates *because they harbor dirt and skin microorganisms.* Remove your watch or wear it well above the wrist.
- Wet your hands and wrists with warm water and apply soap from a dispenser. Don't use bar soap *because it allows cross-contamination.* Hold your hands below elbow level *to prevent water from running up your arms and back down, thus contaminating clean areas.* (See *Proper hand hygiene technique.*)
- Work up a generous lather by rubbing your hands together vigorously for about 10 seconds. *Soap and warm water reduce surface tension and this, aided by friction, loosens surface microorganisms, which wash away in the lather.* **EB1**
- Pay special attention to the area under the fingernails and around the cuticles and to the thumbs, knuckles, and sides of the fingers and hands *because microorganisms thrive in these protected or overlooked areas.* If you don't remove your wedding band, move it up and down your finger to clean beneath it.

Proper hand hygiene technique

To minimize the spread of infection, follow these basic hand hygiene instructions. With your hands angled downward under the faucet, adjust the water temperature until it's comfortably warm.

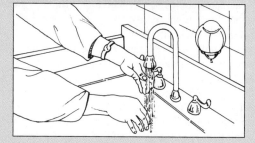

Work up a generous lather by scrubbing vigorously for 10 seconds. Be sure to clean beneath your fingernails, around your knuckles, and along the sides of your fingers and hands.

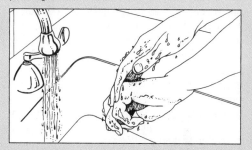

Rinse your hands completely *to wash away suds and microorganisms.* Pat dry with a paper towel. *To prevent recontaminating your hands on the faucet handles,* cover each one with a dry paper towel before turning off the water.

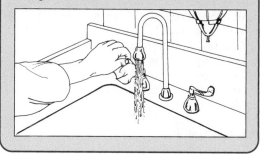

- Avoid splashing water on yourself or the floor *because microorganisms spread more easily on wet surfaces and because slippery floors are dangerous.* Avoid touching the sink or faucets *because they're considered contaminated.*
- Rinse hands and wrists well *because running water flushes suds, soil, and microorganisms away.*
- Pat hands and wrists dry with a paper towel. Avoid rubbing, *which can cause abrasion and chapping.*
- If the sink isn't equipped with knee or foot controls, turn off the faucets by gripping them with a dry paper towel *to avoid recontaminating your hands.*

Hand sanitizing
- Apply a small amount of the alcohol-based hand rub to all surfaces of the hands.
- Rub hands together until all of the product has dried (usually 30 seconds).

Special considerations
- Wash your forearms as well as your hands before participating in a sterile procedure, or whenever your hands are grossly contaminated. Clean under the fingernails as well and in and around the cuticles with a fingernail brush, disposable sponge brush, or plastic cuticle stick. Use these softer implements *because brushes, metal files, or other hard objects may injure your skin and, if reused, may be a source of contamination.*
- Follow your facility's policy concerning when to wash with soap and when to use an antiseptic cleaning agent. Typically, you'll wash with soap before coming on duty, before and after direct or indirect patient contact, before preparing or serving food, before preparing or administering medications, before and after performing any bodily functions (such as blowing your nose or using the bathroom), after direct or indirect contact with a patient's excretions, secretions, or blood, and after completing your shift.
- Use an antiseptic cleaning agent before performing invasive procedures, wound care, and dressing changes, and after contamination. Antiseptics are also recommended for hand hygiene in isolation rooms, neonate nurseries, and before caring for a highly susceptible patient.
- If your hands aren't visibly soiled, an alcohol-based hand rub is preferred for routine decontamina-

tion. Always wash your hands after removing gloves. **CDC**
- If you're providing care in the patient's home, bring your own supply of soap and disposable paper towels. If there's no running water, use an alcohol-based hand sanitizer.
- Don't use an alcohol-based hand sanitizer if you contact items contaminated with Clostridium difficile or Bacillus anthracis (Anthrax). These organisms can form spores and alcohol won't kill them. Wash your hands with soap and water or antiseptic soap and water if either of these organisms is known or suspected to be present.

Nursing diagnoses
- Risk for infection

Expected outcomes
The patient will:
- remain free from infection
- maintain temperature within normal range
- maintain a white blood cell count and differential within normal range.

Complications
- Frequent hand hygiene strips the skin of natural oils, causing dryness, cracking, and irritation. However, these effects are probably more common after repeated use of antiseptic cleaning agents, especially in someone with sensitive skin. *To help minimize irritation,* rinse your hands thoroughly, making sure that they're free from residue.

Supportive references
Earl, M.L., et al. "Improved Rates of Compliance with Hand Antisepsis Guidelines: A Three-Phase Observational Study," *AJN* 101(3):26-33, March 2001. **EB1**

Garner, J.S. "Hospital Infection Control Practices Advisory Committee Guidelines for Isolation Precautions in Hospitals," *Infection Control and Hospital Epidemiology* 17(1):53-80, January 1996. *www.cdc.gov/ncidod/hip/isolat/isopart2.htm.*

"Guidelines for Hand Hygiene in Health-Care Settings," *MMWR Morbidity and Mortality Weekly Report* 51(RR-16):1-144, October 2002. **EB2**

Pittet, D. "Infection Control and Quality Health Care in the New Millenium," *American Journal of Infection Control* 33(5):258-67, June 2005.

Childhood immunization schedule ACIP

This chart shows the immunization schedule that the Centers for Disease Control and Prevention's Advisory Committee on Immunization Practices recommends for children.

Vaccine	Schedule
Diphtheria/tetanus/acellular pertussis (DtaP)	Should be given at ages 2, 4, 6, and 15 to 18 months, and then at ages 4 to 6; child should receive a tetanus booster shot every 10 years
Hepatitis B virus (HBV)	At birth only if mother is hepatitis B surface antigen-negative
Haemophilus influenzae type B (Hib)	Should be given at ages 2, 4, 6, and 12 to 15 months
Inactivated polio vaccine (IPV)	Should be given at ages 2, 4, and 6 to 18 months, and then at ages 4 to 6
Measles/mumps/rubella (MMR)	Should receive two vaccinations, the first at age 2 months to 18 months and the second at ages 4 to 6
Varicella (chickenpox)	One vaccination at 12 to 18 months
Pneumococcal conjugate vaccine	Should be given at ages 2, 4, 6, and 12 to 15 months; consult physician if child is older than age 23 months

Adapted from recommendations of the Advisory Committee on Immunization Practices, Centers for Disease Control and Prevention.

"Public Health Focus: Surveillance, Prevention, and Control of Nosocomial Infections," *MMWR Morbidity and Mortality Weekly Report* 41(42):783-87, October 1992.

Immunization guidelines

Vaccines have reduced, and in some cases eliminated, numerous diseases that once injured or killed many infants, children, and adults. Although the United States has a low incidence of vaccine-preventable childhood diseases, not all such diseases have disappeared. That's why it's especially important that children, especially infants and young children, receive recommended immunizations on time. (See *Childhood immunization schedule*. Also see *Adolescent immunization schedule*, page 102.)

Although immunization is common in the pediatric setting, it's unusual in the treatment of adults, despite the fact that morbidity and mortality from vaccine-preventable disease occur largely in adults.

Many factors have influenced the use of vaccines among adults, such as a lack of knowledge about safe vaccines, unsubstantiated concerns about adverse reactions, and missed opportunities by health care workers to vaccinate adults during hospital or office visits.

The National Coalition for Adult Immunization was formed in 1988 to improve immunization practices for adult patients. The coalition consists of professional, private, public, and volunteer organizations with the common goal of improving vaccine use among adults by educating health care providers and patients. *To further reduce the unnecessary occurrence of vaccine-preventable diseases,* the Advisory Committee on Immunization Practices (ACIP) recommends that health care providers for adults provide vaccinations as a routine part of their practice. (See *Adult immunization schedule,* page 103, and *Recommended vaccines for adults,* page 104.)

Adolescent immunization schedule ACIP

This chart shows the immunization schedule that the Centers for Disease Control and Prevention's Advisory Committee on Immunization Practices recommends for adolescents ages 11 to 18.

Immunization	Indications	Timing
Hepatitis A	Adolescents who are at increased risk for hepatitis A infection or its complications	Two doses: 6 to 18 months apart
Hepatitis B virus (HBV)	Adolescents not vaccinated previously for HBV	Three doses: second dose 1 to 2 months after first dose; third dose 4 months after first dose
Influenza (flu)	Adolescents who are at risk for complications caused by influenza or who have contact with persons at increased risk for these complications	Annually (September to December); now available in intranasal form
Measles-mumps-rubella (MMR)	Adolescents not vaccinated previously with two doses of MMR vaccine at age 12 months or older	One dose*
Meningococcal	Some academic universities require as part of admission process, especially those who live in dormitories	One dose
Pneumococcal	Adolescents who are at increased risk for pneumococcal disease or its complications	One dose (may repeat dose 5 years later for those at highest risk)
Tetanus-diphtheria (Td)	Adolescents not vaccinated within previous 5 years	A booster dose, and then one dose every 10 years through age 50, and as needed
Varicella (chickenpox)	Adolescents not vaccinated previously and who have no reliable history of chickenpox	Ages 11 to 12 receive one dose; age 13 and older receive 2 doses: second dose 1 month after first dose+

*Shouldn't be given to pregnant adolescents or those considering pregnancy within 3 months of vaccination.
+ Shouldn't be given to pregnant adolescents or those considering pregnancy within 1 month of vaccination.
Excluding typhoid, never restart a series.
Ensure at least 1 month between doses, excluding typhoid. Early dosing is more significant (if dose is given within 1 month, it may not boost immunity and so may need repeating). Extra doses aren't contraindicated.
All vaccines can be given simultaneously but not in the same syringe.
If the patient is on pulse steroids, wait 1 month to immunize (inhaled and topical steroids have no impact). For long-term steroid use, consult with a pediatric infectious disease specialist.
DtaP-Hib (TriHIBit) vaccine only used as a fourth dose in United States because of possibly lower immunity conferred.

Adapted from recommendations of the Advisory Committee on Immunization Practices, Centers for Disease Control and Prevention.

Adults ages 18 to 24 ACIP

A complete series of diphtheria and tetanus vaccinations is recommended for anyone who didn't receive these immunizations in infancy or childhood. In young adults, a primary series consists of three doses of preparations containing diphtheria and tetanus toxoids. The first two doses should be given at least 4 weeks apart and the third dose 6 to 12 months after the second dose. After the series is completed, a booster dose should be given every 10 years. If the person's history is unknown or he's uncertain about having received diphtheria and tetanus toxoids, he

Adult immunization schedule ACIP

This chart shows the immunizations that the Centers for Disease Control and Prevention's Advisory Committee on Immunization Practices recommends for individuals over age 18.

Vaccine	Timing and considerations
Hepatitis A for those at risk	Two doses: 6 to 12 months apart for long-term protection, first dose 4 weeks before departure to endemic countries
Hepatitis B virus (HBV) if never had initial series	Three doses: second dose at least 1 month after first dose; third dose 5 months after first dose
Influenza (flu)	Annually before flu season (September to December), especially for those age 65 or older, those with medical problems (heart or lung disease, diabetes, chronic conditions), and those who work or live with hish-risk individuals; now available in intranasal form
Measles-mumps-rubella (MMR)	Two doses: 1 month apart if born after 1957 or if immunity can't be proved* Ages 50 to 65 = 1 dose
Pneumococcal	One dose at age 65; also recommended for persons with chronic disease, kidney disorders, and sickle cell anemia; booster dose recommended 6 years after first dose
Tetanus-diphtheria (Td) if never had initial series	Three doses: second dose after 1 month, third dose 6 to 12 months after second; booster needed every 10 years
Varicella (chickenpox)	Two doses for every patient who hasn't had chickenpox; second dose 1 month after first dose**

*Shouldn't be given to pregnant patients or those considering pregnancy within 3 months of vaccination.
**Shouldn't be given to pregnant patients or those considering pregnancy within 1 month of vaccination.
All vaccines can be given simultaneously but not in the same syringe or site.
If patient is on pulse steroids, wait 1 month to immunize (inhaled or long-term steroids have no impact). For long-term steroid use, consult an infectious disease specialist.

Adapted from recommendations of the Advisory Committee on Immunization Practices, Centers for Disease Control and Prevention.

should be considered unvaccinated and receive a full three-dose primary series.

Most young adults should be immune to measles, mumps, and rubella. However, as a result of the 1989 outbreak of measles in schools and colleges, recommendations were made to implement a routine two-dose schedule for the measles-mumps-rubella (MMR) vaccine. The first dose usually occurs in early childhood and the second before entry into middle or junior high school.

Young adults who are attending college or newly employed in an environment with a high risk of measles, mumps, or rubella transmission (a hospital or day care center, for example) should present documentation that they received two doses of live MMR or evidence of immunity, such as physician-diagnosed measles or laboratory evidence of immunity. If the person was vaccinated with killed-measles-virus vaccine (available in the United States from 1963 until 1967) or with a measles vaccine of unknown type, he should receive two doses of live-measles-virus vaccine at least 1 month apart.

Adults ages 25 to 64

Adults ages 25 to 64 should have completed a primary series of diphtheria and tetanus and should receive a booster dose every 10 years. If needed, a primary series should be given.

Recommended vaccines for adults ACIP

This chart shows the immunization schedule that the Centers for Disease Control and Prevention's Advisory Committee on Immunization Practices recommends for the various adult age-groups.

Age-group (years)	Tetanus-diphtheria	Measles	Mumps	Rubella	Influenza	Pneumococcal polysaccharide
18 to 24	Yes	Yes	Yes	Yes	Not necessary	Not necessary
25 to 64	Yes	Yes	Yes	Yes	Not necessary	Not necessary
≥ 65	Yes	Yes	Yes	Yes	Yes	Yes

Adapted from recommendations of the Advisory Committee on Immunization Practices, Centers for Disease Control and Prevention.

A serologic study of hospital workers indicated that 10% of persons born before 1957 weren't immune to measles. **EB** The study also found that 97 of the 341 health care workers who had measles between 1985 through 1990 were born before 1957. A person born in 1957 or later, who has no contraindications, should receive one dose of measles vaccine unless he has documented evidence of MMR vaccination, measles infection, or laboratory evidence of immunity.

Unless proof of vaccination with rubella vaccine or laboratory evidence is available, rubella vaccine is recommended for adults, especially women of child-bearing age. The vaccine of choice is MMR if recipients are likely to be susceptible to more than one of the three diseases.

Adults age 65 and older ACIP

Older adults should receive an influenza vaccine annually, in addition to a single dose of the pneumococcal polysaccharide vaccine. According to the ACIP, revaccination is suggested 6 years after the first dose for those at highest risk for fatal pneumococcal disease (such as asplenic patients), or a rapid decline in antibody levels (such as patients who have had a transplant or patients with chronic renal failure).

Special occupations

Persons in specific occupations with an increased risk of exposure to certain vaccine-preventable diseases need specific vaccines in addition to those recommended for their age-group. Health and public safety

workers are particularly at risk for exposure to, and possible transmission of, vaccine-preventable diseases because of their contact with patients or infectious materials from patients.

Because of the increased risk of exposure to hepatitis B, all health care workers should receive the hepatitis B virus (HBV) vaccine. Serologic evidence of HBV infection is present in approximately 15% to 30% of health care personnel with frequent exposure to blood; the incidence in the public is 5%. The HBV vaccine provides protection against HBV for 7 years or more after vaccination; booster doses aren't needed during this interval. **CDC**

An influenza vaccine is recommended yearly for physicians, nurses, and other personnel in hospitals and chronic-care and outpatient-care settings who have contact with high-risk patients in all age-groups. **ACIP**

Pregnancy

The ACIP recommends that any vaccine given during pregnancy should be delayed, when possible, until the second or third trimester. Pregnant women not previously vaccinated against tetanus and diphtheria should receive two doses of the vaccine. Those who received one or two doses of tetanus-diphtheria toxoid should complete their primary series during pregnancy. Pregnant women who have completed a primary series 10 years or more previously should receive a booster dose. *Because of a theoretical risk to the developing fetus,* pregnant women or those likely to become pregnant within 3 months shouldn't be given live virus vaccines.

The ACIP strongly recommends that an MMR and varicella vaccine be administered in the postpartum period to women not known to be immune, preferably before discharge from the hospital.

Nursing diagnoses
● Health-seeking behaviors (immunization)

Expected outcomes
The patient will:
● adhere to recommended immunization schedules
● state an understanding of the need to seek immunization.

Supportive references
"Immunization of Adolescents: Recommendations of the Advisory Committee on Immunization Practices, the American Academy of Pediatrics, the American Academy of Family Physicians, and the American Medical Association," *MMWR Morbidity and Mortality Weekly Report* 45(RR-13):1-16, November 1996.

"Immunization of Healthcare Workers: Recommendations of the Advisory Committee on Immunization Practices and the Hospital Infection Control Practices Advisory Committee (HICPAC)," *MMWR Morbidity and Mortality Weekly Report* 46(RR-18):1-42, December 1997.

Nurse Practitioner's Clinical Companion. Springhouse, Pa.: Springhouse Corp., 2000.

"Recommended Adult Immunization Schedule," *MMWR Morbidity and Mortality Weekly Report* 54:(40), October 2005. **EB**

Standard precautions

Standard precautions were developed by the Centers for Disease Control and Prevention (CDC) to provide the broadest possible protection against the transmission of infection. The CDC recommends that health care workers handle blood, body fluids (including secretions, excretions, and drainage), tissues, and contact with mucous membranes and broken skin as if they contain infectious agents, regardless of the patient's diagnosis.

Standard precautions encompass much of the isolation precautions previously recommended by the CDC for patients with known or suspected bloodborne pathogens as well as the precautions previously known as body substance isolation. These precautions are to be used in conjunction with the airborne, contact, and droplet precautions that will be discussed in greater detail below. (See "Airborne precautions," page 92; "Contact precautions," page 94; and "Droplet precautions," page 96.)

Standard precautions include wearing gloves for known or anticipated contact with blood, body fluids, tissue, mucous membrane, and nonintact skin. (See *Choosing the right glove,* page 106.) If the task or procedure being performed may result in splashing or splattering of blood or body fluids to the face, a mask and goggles or face shield should be worn. If the task or procedure being performed may result in splashing or splattering of blood or body fluids to the body, a fluid-resistant gown or apron should be worn. Additional protective clothing, such as shoe covers, may be appropriate to protect the caregiver's feet in situations that may expose him to large amounts of blood or body fluids (or both) such as care of a trauma patient in the operating room or emergency department. **CDC**

Equipment
Gloves ● masks ● goggles, glasses, or face shields ● gowns or aprons ● resuscitation bag ● bags for specimens ● Environmental Protection Agency (EPA)-registered tuberculocidal disinfectant or diluted bleach solution (diluted between 1:10 and 1:100, mixed fresh daily), or both, or EPA-registered disinfectant labeled effective against hepatitis B virus (HBV) and human immunodeficiency virus (HIV)

Implementation **CDC**
● Wash your hands immediately if they become contaminated with blood or body fluids, excretions, secretions, or drainage; wash your hands before and after patient care and after removing gloves. *Hand hygiene removes microorganisms from your skin.*
● Wear gloves if you will or could come in contact with blood, specimens, tissue, body fluids, secretions or excretions, mucous membranes, broken skin, or contaminated surfaces or objects.
● Change your gloves and wash your hands between patient contacts *to avoid cross-contamination*.
● Wear a fluid-resistant gown, a mask, goggles and, if necessary, a face shield (*for added protection*) during procedures, such as surgery, endoscopic procedures, dialysis, assisting with intubation or manipula-

Choosing the right glove

Health care workers may develop allergic reactions as a result of their exposure to latex gloves and other products containing natural rubber latex. Patients may also have latex sensitivity. (See "Latex allergy protocol," page 314.) Take the following steps to protect yourself and your patient from allergic reactions to natural rubber latex.

● Use nonlatex (for example, vinyl or synthetic) gloves for activities that aren't likely to involve contact with infectious materials (such as food preparation and routine cleaning).

● Use appropriate barrier protection when handling infectious materials. If you choose latex gloves, use powder-free gloves with reduced protein content.

● After wearing and removing gloves, wash your hands with soap and dry them thoroughly.

● When wearing latex gloves, don't use oil-based hand creams or lotions (which can cause gloves to deteriorate) unless they've been shown to maintain glove-barrier protection.

● Refer to the material safety data sheet for the appropriate glove to wear when handling chemicals. **OSHA**

● Learn procedures for preventing latex allergy, and learn how to recognize symptoms of latex allergy, such as skin rashes, hives, flushing, itching, asthma, shock, and nasal, eye, or sinus symptoms.

● If you have (or suspect you have) a latex sensitivity, use nonlatex gloves, avoid contact with latex gloves and other latex-containing products, and consult a physician experienced in treating latex allergy.

For latex allergy

If you have a latex allergy, consider these precautions:

● Avoid contact with latex gloves and other products containing latex.

● Avoid areas where you might inhale the powder from latex gloves worn by other workers.

● Tell your employers and your health care providers (physicians, nurses, dentists, and others).

● Wear a medical identification bracelet.

● Follow your physician's instructions for dealing with allergic reactions to latex.

tion of arterial lines, or other procedure with the potential for splashing or splattering body fluids.

● Handle used needles and other sharp instruments carefully. Don't bend, break, reinsert them into their original sheaths, remove needles from syringes, or unnecessarily handle them. Discard them intact immediately after use into a puncture-resistant disposal box. Use tools to pick up broken glass or other sharp objects. *These measures reduce the risk of accidental injury or infection.* **OSHA**

● Immediately notify your employer's health care provider of needle-stick or other sharp-object injuries, mucosal splashes, or contamination of open wounds or nonintact skin with blood or body fluids *to allow investigation of the incident and appropriate care and documentation.* **OSHA**

● Properly label specimens collected from patients and place them in plastic bags at the collection site. Attach requisition slips to the outside of the bags.

● Place items — such as nondisposable utensils or instruments — that have come in direct contact with the patient's secretions, excretions, blood, drainage, or body fluids in a single impervious bag or container before removal from the room. Place linens and trash in single bags of sufficient thickness to contain the contents. **OSHA**

● While wearing the appropriate personal protective equipment (PPE), promptly clean blood and body-fluid spills with detergent and water followed by an EPA-registered tuberculocidal disinfectant or diluted bleach solution (diluted between 1:10 and 1:100, mixed daily), or both, or an EPA-registered disinfectant labeled effective against HBV and HIV *provided that the surface hasn't been contaminated with agent — or volumes of or concentrations of — agents for which higher-level disinfection is recommended.*

● Disposable food trays and dishes aren't necessary.

● If you have an exudative lesion, avoid direct patient contact until the condition has resolved and you've been cleared by your employer's health care provider.

● If you have dermatitis or other conditions resulting in broken skin on your hands, avoid situations where you may have contact with blood and body fluids (even though gloves could be worn) until the condition has resolved and you've been cleared by your employer's health care provider.

Special considerations
● Standard precautions, such as hand hygiene and appropriate use of PPE, should be routine infection-control practices.
● Keep mouthpieces, resuscitation bags, and other ventilation devices nearby *to minimize the need for emergency mouth-to-mouth resuscitation, thus reducing the risk of exposure to body fluids.*

▲ **ALERT** *Because you may not always know what organisms may be present in every clinical situation, you must use standard precautions for every contact with blood, body fluids, secretions, excretions, drainage, mucous membranes, and nonintact skin. Use your judgment in individual cases about whether to implement additional isolation precautions, such as airborne, droplet, or contact precautions, or a combination of precautions. What's more, if your work requires you to be exposed to blood, you should receive the HBV vaccine series.* **CDC**

Nursing diagnoses
● Risk for infection
● Risk for injury

Expected outcomes
The patient will:
● have no pathogens appear in cultures
● have a white blood cell count and differential within normal limits
● remain free from signs and symptoms of infection
● identify factors that increase the risk of injury
● identify and apply safety measures to prevent injury.

Complications
Failure to follow standard precautions may lead to exposure to blood-borne diseases or other infections and to the complications they may cause.

Documentation
Record special needs for isolation precautions on the nursing care plan and as otherwise indicated by your facility.

Supportive references
Garner, J.S. "Hospital Infection Control Practices Advisory Committee Guidelines for Isolation Precautions in Hospitals," *Infection Control and Hospital Epidemiology* 17(1):53-80, January 1996. *www.cdc.gov/ncidod/hip/isolat/isopart2.htm.*

Perry, J. "The Bloodborne Pathogen Standards, 2001: What's Changed?" *Nursing Management* 32(6 Pt 1): 25-26, June 2001.

Rebmann, T. "Management of Patients Infected with Airborne-spread Diseases: An Algorithrm for Infection Control Professionals," *American Journal of Infection Control* 33(10):571-79, December 2005.

4

Intravascular therapy

More than 80% of patients require some form of I.V. therapy. Although nurses may not be required to insert all types of I.V. lines, they're responsible for maintaining the lines and preventing complications throughout the patient's therapy. Nurses also assist in minor surgical procedures, such as the insertion of central venous and arterial lines.

This chapter explains the types, administration, methods, and primary indications for I.V. therapy. You'll review how to prepare I.V. therapy: how to insert, maintain, and remove specific lines and devices, how to control infection and maintain I.V. flow rates, and how to monitor the patient's response to therapy. After reading this chapter, you'll also know what various organizations recommend as best practices for I.V. therapy. Some of those practices rely on basic principles of science **Science** or are evidence-based **EB**, representing research data. Many are endorsed by professional groups, such as the Infusion Nurses Society **INS**, the Oncology Nurses Society **ONS**, the American Society for Parenteral and Enteral Nutrition **ASPEN**, and the Institute of Medicine **IOM**. Practices relating to medication risks stem from the Institute for Safe Medication Practices **ISMP** and the American Association of Blood Banks **AABB**. Other practices derive from such organizations as the AABB, the American Heart Association **AHA**, the American Hospital Association and its Patient Care Partnership **PCP**, the Joint Commission on Accreditation of Healthcare Organizations **JCAHO**, the National Institutes of Health **NIH**, and the Centers for Disease Control and Prevention **CDC**. Still others are mandated by JCAHO, the Occupational Safety and Health Administration **OSHA**, and from specific manufacturers' **MFR** recommendations for the use of their products.

I.V. delivery methods

The factors involved in choosing a specific type of I.V. therapy include the therapy's purpose and duration, the condition of the patient's veins, and his diagnosis, age, and health history. Peripheral I.V. therapy, for example, typically involves intermittent or short-term administration of solutions given through the hands, arms, legs, or feet. In central venous (CV) therapy, a method used for patients requiring a large volume of fluid, hypertonic solution, caustic drug, or high-calorie parenteral nutrition solution, administration occurs through a central vein, such as the subclavian vein or the internal or external jugular veins. Implanted vascular access devices provide a variation on CV infusion. The infused solution enters the vein through a surgically implanted device, usually in the subcutaneous pocket. This method is used for patients requiring I.V. therapy for 6 months or longer. Midline and peripherally inserted catheters are used in home care and in health care facilities.

Uses of I.V. therapy

The most common uses for I.V. therapy are maintaining and restoring fluid and electrolyte balance, administering drugs, transfusing blood, and providing nutrition.

The I.V. route allows for rapid, effective drug administration. Commonly infused drugs include antibiotics, thrombolytics, antineoplastic drugs, cardiovascular drugs, anticonvulsants, and patient-controlled analgesics. Drugs can be given over time or can be infused rapidly (I.V. push). Blood transfusion is used to maintain adequate blood volume, increase the blood's oxygen-carrying capacity, and maintain homeostasis. In caring for patients receiving blood transfusions, your responsibilities include administering blood and blood components and monitoring patients receiving therapy.

Parenteral nutrition is the administration of nutrients by I.V. route. Low-concentration parenteral nutrition solutions are given through a peripheral vein, while highly concentrated ones are given via a central vein. If you're caring for a patient receiving parenteral nutrition, you'll need to monitor his response to the therapy as well as his fluid and electrolyte balance, glucose tolerance, and acid, mineral, and vitamin levels. You'll also need to detect and prevent complications from the therapy.

Patient teaching

Many patients are apprehensive about I.V. therapy. *To reduce a patient's anxiety,* it's important that you provide information *to allay his fears and clarify misconceptions* he may have about the therapy. If possible, show the patient the equipment and explain how it will be used during therapy. You can also use pamphlets and videotapes if available.

Always allow the patient to express his fears and concerns and reassure him by answering his questions fully. Also, involve his family members or caregivers *to provide more reassurance to the patient.*

Home I.V. therapy

Home I.V. therapy benefits the patient *by making him feel more comfortable and allowing him to perform many of his normal activities.* The lower cost of home I.V. therapy, in addition to benefiting the patient, *helps to keep costs down for health care facilities.*

Home care patients may receive fluids or such medications as antibiotics, antifungals, chemotherapeutic agents, insulin, and analgesics. In some situations, blood products may also be given at home after the initial therapy.

Candidates for home I.V. therapy should be selected carefully. These patients and families must be willing and able to administer therapy safely, learn potential complications and interventions, understand the basics of asepsis, and obtain the necessary supplies.

Teaching the patient about home I.V. therapy requires you to demonstrate the procedures and answer questions. Have the patient or family members give return demonstrations whenever possible. It's important to include family members or caregivers during the teaching process. Teaching should begin in the health care facility and be completed before the patient is discharged.

Blood transfusion

Whole blood transfusion replenishes the volume and the oxygen-carrying capacity of the circulatory system by increasing the mass of circulating red cells. Transfusion of packed red blood cells (RBCs), from which 80% of the plasma has been removed, restores only the oxygen-carrying capacity. After plasma is removed, the resulting component has a hematocrit of 65% to 80% and a usual volume of 250 to 300 ml.

Each unit of whole blood or RBCs contains enough hemoglobin to raise the hemoglobin concentration in an average-sized adult 1 g/dl. Both types of transfusion treat decreased hemoglobin level and hematocrit. Whole blood is usually used only when decreased levels result from hemorrhage; packed RBCs are used when such depressed levels accompany normal blood volume to avoid possible fluid and circulatory overload. (See *Transfusing blood and selected components,* pages 110 to 112.) Whole blood and packed RBCs contain cellular debris, requiring in-line filtration during administration.

Before starting the transfusion, positive patient identification, the therapy's appropriateness, blood compatibility, physician's order, and signed consent form should be verified by the nurse. **AABB** **INS** In addition to confirming patient identity with the appropriate blood or blood component identification numbers, the patient's identity must also also be verified using two patient identifiers, aside from the patient's room number, according to your facility's policy. **JCAHO**

✓ **CLINICAL IMPACT** *To prevent errors and a potentially fatal reaction, two nurses should identify the patient and blood products before administering a transfusion.* **JCAHO** *If the patient is a Jehovah's Witness, a transfusion requires special written permission.*

Blood and blood components should be filtered and transfused through an appropriate blood administration set. Straight-line and Y-type blood administration sets are commonly used. Although filters come in mesh and microaggregate types, the latter type is preferred, especially when transfusing multiple units of blood. Highly effective leukocyte removal filters are available for use when transfusing blood and packed RBCs. *The use of these filters can postpone sensitization to transfusion therapy.* **AABB** **INS**

(Text continues on page 112.)

Transfusing blood and selected components

Blood component	Indications	Compatibility	Nursing considerations
Whole blood Complete (pure) blood	• To restore blood volume lost from hemorrhaging, trauma, or burns • Exchange transfusion in sickle cell disease	• ABO identical: Group A receives A; group B receives B; group AB receives AB; group O receives O • Rh type must match	• Remember that whole blood is seldom administered. • Use blood administration tubing to infuse within 4 hours. • Closely monitor patient volume status for volume overload. • Warm blood if giving a large quantity. • Use only with normal saline solution.
Packed red blood cells (RBCs) Same RBC mass as whole blood but with 80% of the plasma removed	• To restore or maintain oxygen-carrying capacity • To correct anemia and surgical blood loss • To increase RBC mass • Red cell exchange	• Group A receives A or O • Group B receives B or O • Group AB receives AB, A, B, or O • Group O receives O • Rh type must match	• Use blood administration tubing to infuse over more than 4 hours. • Use only with normal saline solution. • Avoid administering packed RBCs for anemic conditions correctable by nutritional or drug therapy.
Leukocyte-poor RBCs Same as packed RBCs with about 70% of the leukocytes removed	• Same as packed RBCs • To prevent febrile reactions from leukocyte antibodies • To treat immunocompromised patients • To restore RBCs to patients who have had two or more nonhemolytic febrile reactions	• Same as packed RBCs • Rh type must match	• Use blood administration tubing. • May require a 40-micron filter suitable for hard-spun, leukocyte-poor RBCs. • Other considerations are same as those for packed RBCs. • Cells expire 24 hours after washing.

Transfusing blood and selected components *(continued)*

Blood component	Indications	Compatibility	Nursing considerations
White blood cells (leukocytes) Whole blood with all the RBCs and about 80% of the plasma removed	• To treat sepsis that's unresponsive to antibiotics (especially if patient has positive blood cultures or a persistent fever exceeding 101° F [38.3° C]) and life-threatening granulocytopenia (granulocyte count less than 500/μl)	• Same as packed RBCs • Compatibility with human leukocyte antigen (HLA) preferable but not necessary unless patient is sensitized to HLA from previous transfusions • Rh type must match	• Use a blood administration set. Give 1 unit daily for 4 to 6 days or until infection resolves. • As prescribed, premedicate with antihistamines, acetaminophen (Tylenol), or steroids. • If fever occurs, administer an antipyretic, don't discontinue transfusion; instead, reduce flow rate, as ordered, *for patient comfort.* • Because reactions are common, administer slowly over 2 to 4 hours. Check patient's vital signs and assess him every 15 minutes throughout transfusion. • Give transfusion with antibiotics *to treat infection.*
Platelets Platelet sediment from RBCs or plasma platelets	• To treat bleeding caused by decreased circulating platelets or functionally abnormal platelets • To improve platelet count preoperatively in a patient whose count is 50,000/μl or less	• ABO compatibility identical; Rh-negative recipients should receive Rh-negative platelets	• Use a blood filter or leukocyte-reduction filter. • As prescribed, premedicate with antipyretics and antihistamines if patient's history includes a platelet transfusion reaction or to reduce chills, fever, and allergic reactions. • Use single doner platelets if patient has a need for repeated transfusions. • Platelets aren't used to treat autoimmune thrombocytopenia or thrombocytopenic purpura unless patient has a life-threatening hemorrhage.
Fresh frozen plasma (FFP) Uncoagulated plasma separated from RBCs and rich in coagulation factors V, VIII, and IX	• To treat postoperative hemorrhage • To correct an undetermined coagulation factor deficiency • To replace a specific factor when that factor isn't available • Warfarin reversal	• ABO compatibility required • Rh match not required	• Use a blood administration set and administer infusion rapidly. • Keep in mind that large-volume transfusions of FFP may require correction for hypocalcemia because citric acid in FFP binds calcium. • Must be infused within 24 hours of being thawed.

(continued)

Transfusing blood and selected components *(continued)*

Blood component	Indications	Compatibility	Nursing considerations
Albumin 5% (buffered saline); albumin 25% (salt-poor)			
A small plasma protein prepared by fractionating pooled plasma	• To replace volume lost because of shock from burns, trauma, surgery, or infections • To treat hypoproteinemia (with or without edema)	• Not required	• Use administration set supplied by manufacturer and set rate based on patient's condition and response. • Keep in mind that albumin is contraindicated in severe anemia. • Administer cautiously in cardiac and pulmonary disease *because heart failure may result from circulatory overload.*
Factor VIII concentrate (antihemophilic factor)			
Cold insoluble portion of plasma recovered from FFP	• To treat a patient with hemophilia A • To treat a patient with von Willebrand's disease	• ABO compatibility not required	• Administer by I.V. injection using a filter needle, or use administration set supplied by manufacturer.
Cryoprecipitate			
• Insoluble plasma portion of FFP containing fibrinogen, factor VIIIc, factor VIIvWF, factor XIII and fibronectin	• To treat factor VIII deficiency and fibrinogen disorders • To treat significant factor XIII deficiency	• ABO compatibility required • Rh match not required	• Administer with a blood administration set. • Add normal saline solution to each bag of cryoprecipitate, as necessary, *to facilitate infusion.* • Keep in mind that cryoprecipitate must be administered within 6 hours of thawing. • Before administration, check laboratory studies to confirm a deficiency of one of specific clotting factors present in cryoprecipitate. • Be aware that patients with hemophilia A or von Willebrand's disease should only be treated with cryoprecipitate when appropriate factor VIII concentrates aren't available.

Administer packed RBCs with a Y-type set. Using a straight-line set forces you to piggyback the tubing so you can stop the transfusion if necessary but still keep the vein open. *Piggybacking increases the chance of harmful microorganisms entering the tubing as you're connecting the blood line to the established line.*

Single units of whole blood or blood components should be transfused within a 4-hour period. The start of the transfusion should begin within 30 minutes from the time the blood is released from the blood bank. No medications should be added to the blood other than normal saline solution. Patients should also be monitored 15 minutes after the start of therapy and at 15- to 30-minute intervals throughout the transfusion. **AABB** **INS**

Multiple-lead tubing minimizes the risk of contamination, especially when transfusing multiple units of blood (a straight-line set would require multiple piggybacking). A Y-type set gives you the option of adding normal saline solution to packed cells — decreasing their viscosity — if the patient can tolerate the added fluid volume.

CONTROVERSIAL ISSUE *Hemoglobin replacement products (or blood substitutes) may be an alternative to blood transfusions. The replacement product is derived from human RBCs. It carries the benefits of decreased viral and bacterial* *transmission, reduced risk of allergic or immune reactions, universal compatibility with all blood types, efficient oxygen delivery to vital organs and tissues, and an extended shelf life of at least 1 year (compared with 42 days for donor blood). Successful transfusions have been performed in clinical trials with cardiac bypass patients. However, these products don't provide blood cells with clotting factors or the ability to fight infection.* **AABB**

Equipment

Blood recipient set (170- to 260-micron filter and tubing with drip chamber for blood, or combined set) • I.V. pole • gloves • gown • face shield • multiple-lead tubing • whole blood or packed RBCs • 250 ml of normal saline solution • venipuncture equipment, if necessary (should include 20G or larger catheter) • optional: ice bag, warm compresses

Preparation of equipment

● Avoid obtaining either whole blood or packed RBCs until you're ready to begin the transfusion.
● Prepare the equipment when you're ready to start the infusion.

Implementation

● Confirm the patient's identity using two patient identifiers according to facility policy. **JCAHO**
● Explain the procedure to the patient. Explain possible signs and symptoms of a transfusion reaction (chills, rash, fever, flank or back pain, dizziness, or blood in urine) and to report these possible signs and symptoms to the nurse. **NIH** Make sure that he has signed an informed consent form before transfusion therapy is initiated. **AABB** **INS** **PCP**
● Record the patient's baseline vital signs.
● Obtain whole blood or packed RBCs from the blood bank within 30 minutes of the transfusion start time. Check the expiration date on the blood bag, and observe for abnormal color, RBC clumping, gas bubbles, and extraneous material. Return outdated or abnormal blood to the blood bank. **AABB** **INS**
● Compare the patient's confirmed identity with that on the blood bag label. Check the blood bag identification number, ABO blood group, and Rh compatibility. Also, compare the patient's blood bank identification number, if present, with the number on the blood bag. Identification of blood and blood products

is performed at the patient's bedside by two licensed professionals, according to your facility's policy.
● Put on gloves, a gown, and a face shield. **CDC** **OSHA**
● Using a blood administration set, close all the clamps on the set. Then insert the spike of the line you're using for the normal saline solution into the bag of saline solution. Next, open the port on the blood bag, and insert the spike of the line you're using to administer the blood or cellular component into the port. Hang the bag of normal saline solution and blood or cellular component on the I.V. pole, open the clamp on the line of saline solution, and squeeze the drip chamber until it's half full. Then remove the adapter cover at the tip of the blood administration set, open the main flow clamp, and prime the tubing with saline solution. **AABB** **CDC** **INS** **OSHA**
● If you're administering packed RBCs with a blood administration set, you can add normal saline solution to the bag *to dilute the cells* by closing the clamp between the patient and the drip chamber and opening the clamp from the blood. Then lower the blood bag below the saline container and let 30 to 50 ml of normal saline solution flow into the packed cells. Finally, close the clamp to the blood bag, rehang the bag, rotate it gently *to mix the cells and normal saline solution,* and close the clamp to the saline container.
● If the patient doesn't have an I.V. line in place, perform a venipuncture, using a 20G or larger-diameter catheter. Avoid using an existing line if the needle or catheter lumen is smaller than 20G. Central venous access devices may also be used for transfusion therapy. **AABB** **INS**
● If you're administering whole blood, gently invert the bag several times *to mix the cells.*
● Attach the prepared blood administration set to the venipuncture device, and flush it with normal saline solution. Then close the clamp to the saline solution, and open the clamp between the blood bag and the patient. Adjust the flow rate to no greater than 5 ml/minute for the first 15 minutes of the transfusion *to observe for a possible transfusion reaction.* **Science**
● Remain with the patient and watch for signs of a transfusion reaction. If such signs develop, record his vital signs and stop the transfusion. Infuse saline solution at a moderately slow infusion rate, and notify the physician at once. If no signs of a reaction appear

within 15 minutes, you'll need to adjust the flow clamp to the ordered infusion rate. The rate of infusion should be as rapid as the patient's circulatory system can tolerate. **AABB** **INS**

● It's undesirable for RBC preparations to remain at room temperature for more than 4 hours. If the infusion rate must be so slow that the entire unit can't be infused within 4 hours, it may be appropriate to divide the unit and keep one portion refrigerated until it can be safely administered. **AABB** **INS**

● After completing the transfusion, you'll need to put on gloves and remove and discard the used infusion equipment. Then remember to reconnect the original I.V. fluid, if necessary, or discontinue the I.V. infusion. **CDC** **OSHA**

● Return the empty blood bag to the blood bank, if facility policy dictates, and discard the tubing and filter. **CDC**

● Record the patient's vital signs.

Special considerations

● Although some microaggregate filters can be used for up to 10 units of blood, always replace the filter and tubing if more than 1 hour elapses between transfusions. When administering multiple units of blood under pressure, use a blood warmer *to avoid hypothermia.* Blood components may be warmed to no more than 107.6° F (42° C).

● For rapid blood replacement, you may need to use a pressure bag. Be aware that excessive pressure may develop, leading to broken blood vessels and extravasation, with hematoma and hemolysis of the infusing RBCs.

● If the transfusion stops, take the following steps as needed:
– Check that the I.V. container is at least 3′ (1 m) above the insertion device.
– Make sure that the flow clamp is open and that the blood completely covers the filter. If it doesn't, squeeze the drip chamber until it does.
– Gently rock the bag back and forth, agitating blood cells that may have settled.
– Untape the dressing over the I.V. site to check needle placement. Reposition the needle if necessary.
– Flush the line with saline solution and restart the transfusion. Using a Y-type set, close the flow clamp to the patient and lower the blood bag. Next, open the saline clamp and allow some saline solution to

flow into the blood bag. Rehang the blood bag, open the flow clamp to the patient, and reset the flow rate.
– If a hematoma develops at the I.V. site, immediately stop the infusion. Remove the I.V. cannula. Notify the physician and expect to place ice on the site intermittently for 8 hours; then apply warm compresses. Follow your facility's policy.
– If the blood bag empties before the next one arrives, administer normal saline solution slowly. If you're using a Y-type set, close the blood-line clamp, open the saline clamp, and let the saline run slowly until the new blood arrives. Decrease the flow rate or clamp the line before attaching the new unit of blood.

Nursing diagnoses

● Impaired gas exchange
● Risk for injury

Expected outcomes

The patient will:
● have his hemoglobin level and hematocrit return to normal
● have no signs of active bleeding
● show no signs and symptoms of a transfusion reaction
● identify possible complications and notify the nurse if they occur.

Complications

● Despite improvements in crossmatching precautions, transfusion reactions can still occur. Unlike a transfusion reaction, an infectious disease transmitted during a transfusion may go undetected until days, weeks, or even months later, when it produces signs and symptoms. Measures to prevent disease transmission include laboratory testing of blood products and careful screening of potential donors, neither of which is guaranteed.

● Hepatitis C accounts for most posttransfusion hepatitis cases. The tests that detect hepatitis B and C can produce false-negative results and may allow some hepatitis cases to go undetected.

● When testing for antibodies to human immunodeficiency virus (HIV), keep in mind that antibodies don't appear until 6 to 12 weeks after exposure. The estimated risk of acquiring HIV from blood products varies from 1 in 40,000 to 1 in 153,000.

● Many blood banks screen blood for cytomegalovirus (CMV). Blood with CMV is especially dangerous for an immunosuppressed, seronegative patient. Blood banks also test blood for syphilis, but refrigerating blood virtually eliminates the risk of transfusion-related syphilis.

● Circulatory overload and hemolytic, allergic, febrile, and pyogenic reactions can result from any transfusion. Coagulation disturbances, citrate intoxication, hyperkalemia, acid-base imbalance, loss of 2,3-diphosphoglycerate, ammonia intoxication, and hypothermia can result from massive transfusion.

Documentation

Record the date and time of the transfusion, the type and amount of transfusion product, the patient's vital signs, your check of all identification data, and the patient's response. Document any transfusion reaction and treatment. (See *Documenting blood transfusions*.)

Supportive references

American Association of Blood Banks. *Technical Manual*, 13th ed. Vengelen-Tyler, V., ed. Bethesda, Md.: AABB, 1999.

Joint Commission on Accreditation of Healthcare Organizations. *Comprehensive Accreditation Manual for Home Care*. Oakbrook Terrace, Ill.: JCAHO, 2005. *www.jcaho.gov.*

Joint Commission on Accreditation of Healthcare Organizations. *Comprehensive Accreditation Manual for Hospitals*. Oakbrook Terrace, Ill.: JCAHO, 2005.

"Standard 32. Filters. Infusion Nursing Standards of Practice," *Journal of Infusion Nursing* 29(1S):S33-34, January-February 2006.

"Standard 34. Blood and Fluid Warmers. Infusion Nursing Standards of Practice," *Journal of Infusion Nursing* 29(1S):S35, January-February 2006.

"Standard 48. Administration Set Change. Infusion Nursing Standards of Practice," *Journal of Infusion Nursing* 29(1S):S48-50, January-February 2006.

"Standard 70. Transfusion Therapy. Infusion Nursing Standards of Practice," *Journal of Infusion Nursing* 29(1S):S76-77, January-February 2006.

Weinstein, S.M. *Plumer's Principles and Practice of Intravenous Therapy*, 7th ed. Philadelphia: Lippincott Williams & Wilkins, 2001.

Documenting blood transfusions AABB INS

Whether you administer blood or blood components, you must use proper identification and crossmatching procedures.

After matching the patient's name, medical record number, blood group (or type) and Rh factor (the patient's and the donor's), the cross match data, and the blood bank identification number with the label on the blood bag, you'll need to clearly record that you did so. The blood or blood component must be identified and documented properly by two health care professionals as well.

On the transfusion record, document:
● date and time the transfusion was started and completed
● name of the health care professional who verified the information
● catheter type and gauge
● total amount of the transfusion
● patient's vital signs before and after the transfusion
● any infusion device used
● flow rate and if blood warming unit was used.

If the patient receives his own blood, document in the intake and output records:
● amount of autologous blood retrieved
● amount of autologous blood infused
● laboratory data during and after the autotransfusion
● patient's pretransfusion and posttransfusion vital signs.

Pay particular attention to:
● patient's coagulation profile
● hemoglobin level, hematocrit, and arterial blood gas and calcium levels.

Central venous catheters

A central venous (CV) catheter is a sterile catheter that's inserted through a large vein, such as the subclavian vein (or, less commonly, the internal jugular vein), and terminates in the superior vena cava. CV catheters allow long-term administration in situations requiring safe, repeated access to the venous system for administration of drugs, fluids and nutrition, and blood products. (See *Central venous catheter pathways*, page 116.)

Central venous catheter pathways

The illustrations below show several common pathways for central venous (CV) catheter insertion. Typically, a CV catheter is inserted in the subclavian vein or internal jugular vein. The catheter usually terminates in the superior vena cava. The CV catheter is tunneled when long-term placement is required.

Insertion: Subclavian vein
Termination: Superior vena cava

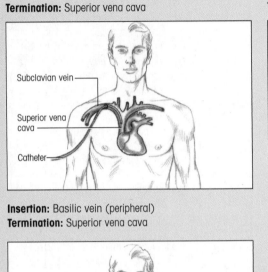

Insertion: Internal jugular vein
Termination: Superior vena cava

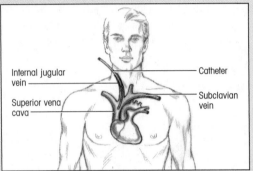

Insertion: Basilic vein (peripheral)
Termination: Superior vena cava

Insertion: Through a subcutaneous tunnel to the subclavian vein (Dacron cuff helps hold catheter in place)
Termination: Superior vena cava

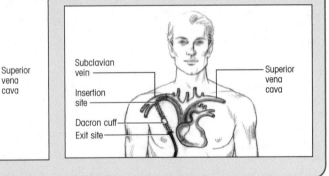

Other benefits of CV therapy include ease in monitoring CV pressure, drawing blood samples, administering large fluid volumes and irritating substances (such as total parenteral nutrition), and providing long-term venous access. Because multiple blood samples can be drawn through it without repeated venipuncture, the use of a CV catheter *decreases the patient's anxiety and preserves or restores peripheral veins.*

CV therapy increases the risk of complications, such as pneumothorax, sepsis, thrombus formation, and vessel and adjacent organ perforation (all life-threatening conditions). Also, the CV catheter may decrease patient mobility, is difficult to insert, and costs more than a peripheral I.V. catheter.

✔ **CLINICAL IMPACT** *In 2002, the Centers for Disease Control and Prevention revealed evidence-based guidelines to prevent I.V. catheter-related infections. Based on these guidelines, prevention begins before the catheter is inserted and proper education of caregivers is essential.* **EB1**

According to the Infusion Nurses Society (INS), site selection for a CV catheter should be considered a medical act. A catheter should be chosen with the minimum number of lumens needed for patient care. **EB2** There also seems to be a lower incidence of infection when the subclavian route is chosen over the internal jugular or femoral sites. **EB3** The femoral vein should be used with caution, with the distal tip terminating in the inferior vena cava. Nursing assessment should include the patient's condition, infusion history, and duration and type of therapy. **INS**

The type of catheter (tunneled, implanted, or percutaneously inserted) to be used is determined by the patient's condition, length of therapy, and type of medication to be infused. INS standards also recommend that a single lumen catheter be used unless additional therapies are required. An X-ray should be taken before initiation of therapy *to confirm proper catheter placement* and intermittently *to verify that the catheter tip is in the superior vena cava.* **INS**

A sterile dressing, either gauze or transparent semipermeable membrane should be applied and maintained on the CV catheter. Topical antibiotic ointment or cream isn't recommended for use on the insertion site due to the potential of promoting a fungal infection or antimicrobial resistance. **CDC** The edges of the gauze dressing should be covered with an occlusive material and should routinely be changed every 48 hours and immediately if the integrity of the dressing is compromised. The optimal interval for changing transparent semipermeable dressings depends on the dressing material's age and the patient's condition. Gauze used in conjunction with a transparent membrane should be changed every 48 hours. **INS** Good hand hygiene and aseptic technique during insertion and care decreases the risk of catheter-related infection. **CDC**

ALERT *If a catheter-related infection is suspected, the catheter should be cultured. If a complication is suspected, the catheter should be removed immediately. A physician or nurse usually performs CV catheter removal, either at the end of therapy or at the onset of complications. Caution should be used in the removal of a CV catheter, including precautions to prevent air embolism. Pressure should be applied to the site until bleeding stops, antiseptic ointment should be applied, and the site covered with a sterile occlusive dressing.*

Equipment

Inserting a CV catheter

Shave preparation kit, if necessary • sterile gloves and gowns • blanket • linen-saver pad • sterile towel • sterile drape • masks • 2% chlorhexidine swabs **CDC** **INS** • normal saline solution • 3-ml syringe with 25G 1″ needle • 1% or 2% injectable lidocaine • dextrose 5% in water (D_5W) • syringes for blood sample collection • suture material • two 14G or 16G CV catheters • I.V. solution with administration set prepared for use • infusion pump or controller, as needed • sterile 4″ × 4″ gauze pads • 1″ adhesive tape • sterile scissors • heparin or normal saline flushes, as needed • sterile marker • sterile labels • optional: transparent semipermeable dressing

Flushing a catheter

Normal saline solution or heparin flush solution • 2% chlorhexidine **ASPEN** **CDC** **INS**

Changing an injection cap

Alcohol pad • injection cap • padded clamp

Removing a CV catheter

Clean gloves and sterile gloves • sterile suture removal set • 2% chlorhexidine **ASPEN** **CDC** **INS** • alcohol pads • sterile 4″ × 4″ gauze pads • forceps • tape • sterile, plastic adhesive-backed dressing or transparent semipermeable dressing • agar plate or culture tube, if necessary for culture

Some facilities have prepared trays containing most of the equipment for catheter insertion. The type of catheter selected depends on the type of therapy to be used. (See *Guide to central venous catheters,* pages 118 to 120.)

CONTROVERSIAL ISSUE *The decision to use heparin lock flush solution depends on the facility's protocol, the manufacturer's recommendations, and the patient's situation. The literature contains articles supporting and discouraging its use. Heparin may not be necessary if flushing with saline solution is performed regularly.* **MFR**

Preparation of equipment

● Before inserting a CV catheter, confirm catheter type and size with the practitioner; the most commonly used sizes are 14G and 16G.

(Text continues on page 120.)

Guide to central venous catheters

Types of central venous (CV) catheters differ in their design, composition, and indications for use. This chart outlines the advantages, disadvantages, and nursing considerations for several commonly used catheters.

Catheter description and indications	Advantages and disadvantages	Nursing considerations

Short-term, single-lumen catheter

Description
- Polyurethane or silicone rubber (Silastic)
- Approximately 8″ (20 cm) long
- Variety of lumen gauges

Indications
- Short-term CV access
- Emergency access
- Patient who requires only a single lumen

Advantages
- It can be inserted at the bedside.
- It's easily removed.
- Stiffness aids CV pressure monitoring.

Disadvantages
- Catheter has limited functions.
- Catheter should be changed every 3 to 7 days (depending on facility policy).

- Assess frequently for signs and symptoms of infection and clot formation.

Short-term, multilumen catheter

Description
- Polyurethane or silicone rubber
- Double, triple, or quadruple lumen at ¾″ (1.9-cm) intervals
- Variety of lumen gauges

Indications
- Short-term CV access
- Patient with limited insertion sites who requires multiple infusions

Advantages
- It can be inserted at the bedside.
- It's easily removed.
- Stiffness aids CV pressure monitoring.
- It allows infusion of multiple solutions through the same catheter — even for the same task (for example, incompatible solutions).

Disadvantages
- Catheter has limited functions.
- Catheter needs to be changed every 3 to 7 days.

- Know the gauge and purpose of each lumen.
- Use the same lumen for the same task (for example, to administer total parenteral nutrition (TPN) or to collect a blood sample).

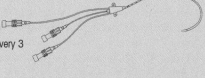

Groshong catheter

Description
- Silicone rubber
- Approximately 35″ (89 cm) long
- Closed end with pressure-sensitive three-way valve
- Dacron cuff
- Available with single or double lumen
- Tunneled

Indications
- Long-term CV access
- Patient with heparin allergy

Advantages
- It's less thrombogenic than catheters made with polyvinylchloride.
- Pressure-sensitive three-way valve eliminates heparin flushes.
- Dacron cuff anchors catheter and prevents bacterial migration.

Disadvantages
- It requires surgical insertion.
- It tears and kinks easily.
- Blunt end makes it difficult to clear substances from its tip.

- Two surgical sites require dressing after insertion.
- Handle the catheter gently.
- Check the external portion frequently for kinks or leaks. (Repair kit is available.)
- Observe frequently for kinks or tears.
- Remember to flush the lumen with enough saline solution to clear the catheter, especially after drawing or administering blood.
- Change the end caps weekly.

Guide to central venous catheters *(continued)*

Catheter description and indications	Advantages and disadvantages	Nursing considerations

Hickman catheter

Description
- Silicone rubber
- Approximately 35" (89 cm) long
- Open end with clamp
- Dacron cuff 11¾" (30 cm) from hub
- Tunneled

Indications
- Long-term CV access
- Home therapy

Advantages
- Dacron cuff prevents excess motion and organism migration.
- Clamps eliminate need for Valsalva's maneuver.

Disadvantages
- It requires surgical insertion.
- Catheter has an open end.
- It requires a physician for removal.
- It tears and kinks easily.

- Two surgical sites require dressing after insertion.
- Handle the catheter gently.
- Observe frequently for kinks or tears. (Repair kit is available.)
- Clamp the catheter whenever it becomes disconnected or open, using a clamp on the catheter.
- Flush the catheter daily when not in use with 3 to 5 ml of heparin (10 units/ml) and before and after each use using the SASH (S = saline; A = additive; S = saline; H = heparin) protocol.

Broviac catheter

Description
- Silicone rubber
- Approximately 35" long
- Open end with clamp
- Dacron cuff 11¾" from hub
- Tunneled

Indications
- Long-term CV access
- Patient with small central vessels (pediatric, elderly)

Advantages
- Small lumen ensures better comfort.

Disadvantages
- Small lumen may limit its uses.
- It has a single lumen, which limits its functions (can't infuse multiple solutions at once).
- In children, growth may cause the catheter tip to move its position outside the superior vena cava.

- Check facility policy before drawing or administering blood products.
- Flush the catheter daily when not in use with 3 to 5 ml of heparin (10 units/ml) and before and after each use using the SASH protocol.

Hickman-Broviac catheter

Description
- Hickman and Broviac catheters combined in one catheter

Indications
- Long-term CV access
- Patient who needs multiple infusions

Advantages
- Double-lumen Hickman catheter allows sampling and administration of blood.
- Broviac lumen delivers I.V. fluids, including TPN fluids.

Disadvantages
- It requires surgical insertion.
- Catheter has an open end.
- It requires a physician for removal.
- It tears and kinks easily.

- Know the purpose and function of each lumen.
- Label lumens to prevent confusion.
- Flush the catheter when not in use with 3 to 5 ml of heparin (10 units/ml), and before and after each use using the SASH protocol.

(continued)

Guide to central venous catheters *(continued)*

Catheter description and indications	Advantages and disadvantages	Nursing considerations
Long-line catheter		
Description ● Peripherally inserted central catheter ● Silicone rubber ● 20″ to 24″ (51 to 61 cm) long; available in 14G, 16G, 18G, 20G, 22G, and 24G **Indications** ● Long-term CV access ● Patient with poor central access ● Patient at high risk for complications from insertion at central access sites ● Patient who needs CV access but faces or has had head and neck surgery	**Advantages** ● It's peripherally inserted. ● It can be inserted at the bedside with minimal complications. ● It may be inserted by a trained, skilled, competent registered nurse in most states. ● Single or double lumen is available. **Disadvantages** ● Catheter may occlude smaller peripheral vessels. ● It may be difficult to keep immobile.	● Check frequently for signs of phlebitis and thrombus formation. ● Insert the catheter above the antecubital fossa. ● Use an arm board if necessary. ● The catheter may alter CV pressure measurements.

● Set up the I.V. solution and prime the administration set using strict sterile technique.

● Attach the line to the infusion pump or controller, if ordered.

● Recheck all connections *to make sure that they're tight.*

● Label all medications, medication containers, and other solutions on and off the sterile field. **JCAHO**

● As ordered, notify the radiology department that a chest X-ray machine will be needed.

Implementation
Inserting a CV catheter

● Confirm the patient's identity using two patient identifiers according to facility policy. **JCAHO**

● Wash your hands thoroughly *to prevent the spread of microorganisms.* **CDC**

● Reinforce the practitioner's explanation of the procedure, and answer the patient's questions. Make sure that the patient has signed a consent form, if necessary, and check his history for hypersensitivity to iodine, latex, or the local anesthetic. **PCP**

● Place the patient in Trendelenburg's position *to dilate the veins and reduce the risk of air embolism.*

● For subclavian vein insertion, place a rolled blanket lengthwise between the shoulders *to increase venous distention.* For jugular insertion, place a rolled blanket under the opposite shoulder *to extend the neck, making anatomic landmarks more visible.* Place a linen-saver pad under the patient *to prevent soiling the bed.* **INS**

● Turn the patient's head away from the site *to prevent possible contamination from airborne pathogens and to make the site more accessible.* Place a mask on the patient if required by your facility's policy, unless doing so increases his anxiety or is contraindicated due to his respiratory status.

● Prepare the insertion site. You may need to wash the skin with soap and water first. Make sure that the skin is free from hair *because hair can harbor microorganisms.* Infection-control practitioners recommend clipping the hair close to the skin rather than shaving, *which may cause skin irritation and create multiple small open wounds, increasing the risk of infection.* (If the physician orders that the area be shaved, try shaving it the evening before catheter insertion *to allow partial healing of minor skin irritations.*) **AABB** **INS**

● Establish a sterile field on a table, using a sterile towel or the wrapping from the instrument tray.

● Put on a mask and sterile gloves and gown, and clean the area around the insertion site with a clorhexidine swab using a vigorous back-and-forth motion. If the patient is sensitive to chlorhexidine, use an alcohol applicator. **CDC** **INS**

● After the physician puts on a sterile mask, a gown, and gloves and drapes the area to create a sterile field, open the packaging of the 3-ml syringe and 25G needle and hand it to him, using sterile technique. **CDC**

CLINICAL IMPACT *Studies show that infections and sepsis present a major problem in CV catheter usage. Complications of infection may be minimized through the use of maximum sterile barriers (while inserting CV catheters) and highly permeable transparent dressings. In addition, the use of real-time ultrasound guidance during CV catheter insertion may help prevent complications of misplaced lines.*

● Wipe the top of the lidocaine vial with an alcohol pad and invert it. The physician will then fill the 3-ml syringe and inject the anesthetic into the site.
● Open the catheter package and give the catheter to the physician, using sterile technique. The physician should inspect the catheter for leaks before inserting the catheter.
● Prepare the I.V. administration set for immediate attachment to the catheter hub. Ask the patient to perform Valsalva's maneuver while the physician attaches the I.V. line to the catheter hub. *Valsalva's maneuver increases intrathoracic pressure, reducing the possibility of an air embolus.* (See *Teaching Valsalva's maneuver.*) **Science**
● After the physician attaches the I.V. line to the catheter hub, set the flow rate at a keep-vein-open rate *to maintain venous access.* (Alternatively, the catheter may be capped and flushed with heparin.) The physician then sutures the catheter in place.
● After an X-ray confirms correct catheter placement in the midsuperior vena cava, set the flow rate as ordered.
● Use normal saline solution *to remove dried blood that could harbor microorganisms.* Secure the catheter with adhesive tape, and apply a sterile 4″ × 4″ gauze pad. You may also use a transparent semipermeable dressing, either alone or placed over the gauze pad. Expect some serosanguineous drainage during the first 24 hours.
● Place the patient in a comfortable position and reassess his status. Label the dressing with the time and date of catheter insertion and catheter length and gauge (if not imprinted on the catheter). **INS**

Teaching Valsalva's maneuver

Increased intrathoracic pressure reduces the risk of air embolus during insertion and removal of a central venous catheter. A simple way to achieve this is to ask the patient to perform Valsalva's maneuver: forced exhalation against a closed airway. Instruct the patient to take a deep breath and hold it, and then bear down for 10 seconds. Then tell the patient to exhale and breathe quietly.

Valsalva's maneuver raises intrathoracic pressure from its normal level of 3 to 4 mm Hg to levels of 60 mm Hg or higher. It also slows the pulse rate, decreases the return of blood to the heart, and increases venous pressure.

This maneuver is contraindicated in patients with increased intracranial pressure. It shouldn't be taught to patients who aren't alert or cooperative.

Flushing the catheter

● *To maintain patency,* flush the catheter routinely according to your facility's policy. If the system is being maintained as a heparin lock and the infusions are intermittent, the flushing procedure will vary according to your facility's policy, the medication administration schedule, and the type of catheter used.
● All lumens of a multilumen catheter must be flushed regularly. Most facilities use a heparin flush solution available in premixed 10-ml multidose vials. Recommended concentrations vary from 10 to 100 units of heparin per milliliter. Use normal saline solution instead of heparin to maintain patency in two-way valved devices, such as the Groshong type, *because research suggests that heparin isn't always needed to keep the line open.* **INS**
● The recommended frequency for flushing CV catheters varies from once every 8 hours to once weekly.
● The recommended amount of flushing solution also varies. Some facilities recommend using twice the volume of the cannula and the add-on devices if this volume is known. If the volume is unknown, most facilities recommend 3 to 5 ml of solution to flush the catheter, although some call for as much as 10 ml of solution. Different catheters require different amounts of solution.

- To perform the flushing procedure, start by cleaning the cap with an alcohol pad. Allow the cap to dry. If using the needleless system, follow the manufacturer's guidelines. **MFR**
- Access the cap and aspirate until blood appears *to confirm the CV catheter patency.* **INS**
- Inject the recommended type and amount of flush solution.
- After flushing the catheter, maintain positive pressure by keeping your thumb on the plunger of the syringe while withdrawing the needle. *This prevents blood backflow and clotting in the line.* If flushing a valved catheter, close the clamp just before the last of the flush solution leaves the syringe. **INS**

Changing the injection cap

- CV catheters used for intermittent infusions have needle-free injection caps (short luer-lock devices similar to the heparin lock adapters used for peripheral I.V. infusion therapy). These caps must be luer-lock types *to prevent inadvertent disconnection and air embolism.* Unlike heparin lock adapters, however, these caps contain a minimal amount of empty space, so you don't have to preflush the cap before connecting it.
- The frequency of cap changes varies according to your facility's policy and how often the cap is used; however, if the integrity of the product is compromised, it should be changed immediately. Use strict sterile technique when changing the cap. **INS**
- Clean the connection site with an alcohol pad or clorhexidine.
- Instruct the patient to perform Valsalva's maneuver while you quickly disconnect the old cap and connect the new cap using sterile technique. If he can't perform this maneuver, use a padded clamp *to prevent air from entering the catheter.*

Removing a CV catheter

- If you're removing the CV catheter, first check the patient's record for the most recent placement (confirmed by an X-ray) *to trace the catheter's path as it exits the body.* Make sure that assistance is available if a complication, such as uncontrolled bleeding, occurs during catheter removal. (Some vessels, such as the subclavian vein, can be difficult to compress.) Confirm the patient's identity using two patient identifiers according to facility policy. **JCAHO** Before you

remove the catheter, explain the procedure to the patient. **INS**
- Place the patient in a supine position *to prevent emboli.*
- Wash your hands, and put on clean gloves and a mask. **CDC**
- Turn off all infusions and prepare a sterile field, using a sterile drape.
- Remove and discard the old dressing, and change to sterile gloves.
- Clean the site with an alcohol pad or a gauze pad soaked in clorhexidine. Inspect the site for signs of drainage or inflammation.
- Clip the sutures and, using forceps, remove the catheter in a slow, even motion. Have the patient perform Valsalva's maneuver as the catheter is withdrawn *to prevent an air embolism.* **INS** **Science**
- Apply pressure with a sterile gauze pad immediately after removing the catheter.
- Apply clorhexidine to the insertion site *to seal it.* Cover the site with a gauze pad, and place a transparent semipermeable dressing over the gauze. Label the dressing with the date and time of the removal and your initials. The site should be assessed every 24 hours until epithetization occurs. **INS**
- Inspect the catheter tip and measure the length of the catheter *to ensure that the catheter has been completely removed.* If you suspect that the catheter hasn't been completely removed, notify the practitioner immediately and monitor the patient closely for signs of distress. If you suspect an infection, swab the catheter on a fresh agar plate, or clip the tip of the catheter, place it in a sterile container, and send it to the laboratory for culture. **INS**
- Dispose of the I.V. tubing and equipment properly. **CDC** **OSHA**

Special considerations

- While you're awaiting chest X-ray confirmation of proper catheter placement, infuse an I.V. solution, such as D_5W or normal saline solution, at a keep-vein-open rate until correct placement is assured. Or use heparin to flush the line. *Infusing an isotonic solution avoids the risk of vessel wall thrombosis.*

 ALERT *Stay alert for such signs of air embolism as sudden onset of pallor, cyanosis, dyspnea, coughing, and tachycardia, progressing to syncope and shock. If any of these signs occur,* *place the patient on his left side in Trendelenburg's position and notify the physician.*

● After insertion, watch for signs and symptoms of pneumothorax, such as shortness of breath, uneven chest movement, tachycardia, and chest pain. Notify the physician immediately if such signs and symptoms appear.

● Change the dressing every 48 hours if a gauze dressing is used or every 7 days if a transparent semipermeable dressing is used, according to your facility's policy, or whenever it becomes moist or soiled. While the CV catheter is in place, change the tubing every 72 hours and the solution every 24 hours **CDC** or according to your facility's policy. Dressing, tubing, and solution changes for a CV catheter should be performed using sterile technique. (See *Changing a central venous catheter dressing.*) Assess the site for signs and symptoms of infection, such as discharge, inflammation, and tenderness. **INS**

● *To prevent an air embolism*, close the catheter clamp or have the patient perform Valsalva's maneuver each time the catheter hub is open to air. (A Groshong catheter doesn't require clamping because it has an internal valve.)

TEACHING *Long-term use of a CV catheter allows patients to receive caustic fluids and blood infusions at home. These catheters have a much longer life because they're less thrombogenic and less likely to cause infection than short-term devices.*

A candidate for home therapy must have a family member or friend who can safely and competently administer I.V. fluids, a backup helper, a suitable home environment, a telephone, transportation, adequate reading skills, and the ability to prepare, handle, store, and dispose of the equipment. The care procedures used in the home are the same as those used in the facility, except that the home therapy patient uses clean instead of sterile technique.

The overall goal of home therapy is patient safety, so your patient teaching must begin well before discharge. After discharge, a home therapy coordinator will provide follow-up care until the patient or someone close to him can independently provide catheter care and infusion therapy. Many home therapy patients learn to care for the catheter themselves and infuse their own medications and solution.

Changing a central venous catheter dressing

Expect to change your patient's central venous catheter dressing every 7 days. Many health care facilities specify dressing changes whenever the dressing becomes soiled, moist, or loose. The following illustrations show the key steps you'll perform.

First, use proper hand hygiene with water and antiseptic soap or a waterless alcohol-based gel or foam. **CDC** Put on clean gloves, and remove the old dressing by pulling it toward the exit site of a long-term catheter or toward the insertion site of a short-term catheter. *This technique helps you avoid pulling out the line.* Remove and discard your gloves.

Next, put on sterile gloves, and clean the skin around the site three times, using a new alcohol pad each time. Start at the center and move outward. Allow the skin to dry and clean the site with chlorhexidine swabs using a vigorous back-and-forth motion (as shown).

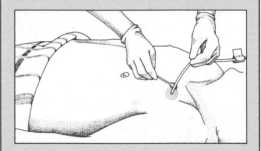

After the solution has dried, cover the site with a dressing, such as a gauze dressing or the transparent semipermeable dressing shown here. Topical antibiotic ointments or creams aren't recommended for use on insertion sites because of the risk of fungal infections or antimicrobial resistance. **CDC** Write the time and date on the dressing.

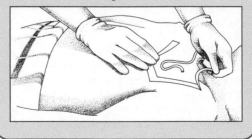

Nursing diagnoses

- Risk for imbalanced fluid volume
- Risk for infection

Expected outcomes

The patient will:
- maintain fluid intake and output at appropriate levels
- maintain urine specific gravity of 1.005 to 1.015
- have mucous membranes that appear pink and moist
- maintain vital signs and laboratory values within normal limits
- maintain temperature within normal limits
- maintain white blood cell and differential counts within normal range
- have culture results that show no evidence of pathogens.

Complications

- Complications can occur at any time during infusion therapy. Traumatic complications, such as pneumothorax, typically occur on catheter insertion but may not be noticed until after the procedure is completed.
- Systemic complications, such as sepsis, typically occur later during infusion therapy.
- Other complications include phlebitis (especially in peripheral CV therapy), thrombus formation, and air embolism.

Documentation

Record the time and date of insertion, length and location of the catheter, solution infused, practitioner's name, and patient's response to the procedure. Document the time of the X-ray, its results, and your notification of the physician.

Record the time and date of removal and the type of antimicrobial ointment and dressing applied. Note the condition of the catheter insertion site and collection of a culture specimen.

Supportive references

Andris, D.A., and Krzywda, E.A. "Central Venous Access: Clinical Practice Issues," *Nursing Clinics of North America* 32(4):719-40, December 1997.

Centers for Disease Control and Prevention. "Guidelines for Prevention of Intravascular Catheter-Related Infections," *Morbidity and Mortality Monthly Report* 51(RR-10):1-29, August 2002. **EB1**

Ely, E.W., et al. "Venous Air Embolism from Central Venous Catheterization: A Need for Increased Physician Awareness," *Critical Care Medicine* 27(10):2113-17, October 1999.

Kim, D.K., et al. "The CVC Removal Distress Syndrome: An Unappreciated Complication of Central Venous Catheter Removal," *American Journal of Surgery* 64(4):344-47, April 1998.

Merrer, J., et al. "Complications of Femoral and Subclavian Venous Catheterization in Critically Ill Patients: A Randomized Controlled Trial," *JAMA* 286(6):700-707, 2001. **EB3**

Pearson, M.L. "Guideline for Prevention of Intravascular Device-Related Infections. Part I. Intravascular Device-Related Infections: An Overview. The Hospital Infection Control Practices Advisory Committee. *American Journal of Infection Control* 24(4):262-77, August 1996.

Pearson, M.L. "Guideline for Prevention of Intravascular Device-Related Infection. Part II. Recommendations for Prevention of Nosocomial Intravascular Device-Related Infections. Hospital Infection Control Practices Advisory Committee. *American Journal of Infection Control* 24(4):277-93, August 1996.

"Standard 29. Add-on Devices and Junction Securement. Infusion Nursing Standards of Practice," *Journal of Infusion Nursing* 29(1S):S32, January-February 2006.

"Standard 37. Site Selection. Infusion Nursing Standards of Practice," *Journal of Infusion Nursing* 29(1S): S37-39, January-February 2006.

"Standard 38. Catheter Selection. Infusion Nursing Standards of Practice," *Journal of Infusion Nursing* 29(1S):S39-40, January-February 2006.

"Standard 39. Hair Removal. Infusion Nursing Standards of Practice," *Journal of Infusion Nursing* 29(1S):S40-41, January-February 2006.

"Standard 40. Local Anesthesia. Infusion Nursing Standards of Practice," *Journal of Infusion Nursing* 29(1S):S41, January-February 2006.

"Standard 41. Access Site Preparation. Infusion Nursing Standards of Practice," *Journal of Infusion Nursing* S29(1S):S41-42, January-February 2006.

"Standard 42. Catheter Placement. Infusion Nursing Standards of Practice," *Journal of Infusion Nursing* 29(1S):S42-44, January-February 2006.

"Standard 49. Catheter Removal. Infusion Nursing Standards of Practice," *Journal of Infusion Nursing* 29(1S):S51-55, January-February 2006.

Treston-Aurand, J., et al. "Impact of Dressing Materials on Central Venous Catheter Infection Rates," *Journal of Intravenous Nursing* 20(4):201-206, July-August 1997.

U.S. Department of Health and Human Services. "Public Health Service. Centers for Disease Control and Prevention. Guidelines for Prevention of Intravascular Device-Related Infections," *American Journal of Infection Control* 24(4):262-77, August 1996.

Weinstein, S.M. *Plumer's Principles and Practice of Intravenous Therapy*, 7th ed. Philadelphia: Lippincott Williams & Wilkins, 2001.

Wojcik, J. "Central Venous Catheters," *Advance for Nurses* 7(23):25-28, October 2005. **EB2**

Chemotherapeutic drug administration

Administration of chemotherapeutic drugs requires specific skills in addition to those used when giving other drugs.

Only specially trained nurses and physicians should give chemotherapeutic drugs. The Infusion Nurses Society recommends that the nurse administering antineoplastic agents have knowledge of:

- disease processes
- drug classifications
- pharmacologic indications
- actions and adverse effects
- adverse reactions
- method of administration
- rate of delivery
- treatment goals
- drug properties
- dosage calculations related to height, weight, and body surface area. **INS**

Chemotherapeutic drugs may be administered through various routes. Although the I.V. route (using peripheral or central veins) is used most commonly, these drugs may also be given orally, subcutaneously, I.M., intra-arterially, into a body cavity, through a central venous (CV) catheter, through an Ommaya reservoir into the spinal canal, or through a device implanted in a vein or subcutaneously such as through a patient-controlled analgesia device. (See *Understanding patient-controlled analgesia,* page 126.) They may also be administered into an artery, the peritoneal cavity, or the pleural space. (See *Intraperitoneal chemotherapy: An alternative approach,* page 127.)

Before administering chemotherapy, laboratory data (electrolyte levels and white blood cell count) should be reviewed, the patient should be assessed for the appropriateness of the prescribed therapy, and the drug order should be validated by two clinicians with special attention to medication concentration and the infusion rate. **INS**

The administration route depends on the drug's pharmacodynamics and the tumor's characteristics. For example, if a malignant tumor is confined to one area, the drug may be administered through a localized, or regional, method. Regional administration allows delivery of a high drug dose directly to the tumor. This is particularly advantageous because many solid tumors don't respond to drug levels that are safe for systemic administration.

If the drug to be administered is a vesicant, the nurse should remember two key factors: a low-pressure infusion device should be the instrument of choice, and a new access site should be initiated before vesicant administration. **INS**

Chemotherapy may be administered to a patient whose cancer is believed to have been eradicated through surgery or radiation therapy. This treatment, called adjuvant chemotherapy, helps *to ensure that no undetectable metastasis exists*. A patient may also receive chemotherapy, or neoadjuvant or synchronous chemotherapy, before surgery or radiation therapy. Induction chemotherapy helps improve survival rates *by shrinking a tumor* before surgical excision or radiation therapy.

In general, chemotherapeutic drugs prove more effective when given in higher doses, although their adverse effects commonly limit the dosage. An exception to this rule is methotrexate, which is particularly effective against rapidly growing tumors but toxic to normal tissues that grow and divide rapidly. *Folinic acid halts the effects of methotrexate;* therefore, it's administered after the methotrexate has destroyed the cancer cells but before it damages vital organs. **EB**

Equipment

Prescribed drug • aluminum foil or a brown paper bag (if the drug is photosensitive) • normal saline solution • syringes and needleless adapters • infusion pump or controller • gloves • impervious containers labeled CAUTION: BIOHAZARD

Understanding patient-controlled analgesia

In patient-controlled analgesia (PCA), the patient controls I.V. delivery of an analgesic (usually morphine) by pressing the button on a delivery device. In this way, he receives analgesia at the level he needs and at the time he needs it. The PCA device prevents the patient from accidentally overdosing by imposing a lockout time between doses — usually 6 to 10 minutes. During this interval, the patient won't receive any analgesic, even if he pushes the button.

The device shown below is a reusable, battery-operated peristaltic action pump that delivers a drug dose when the patient presses a call button at the end of a cord.

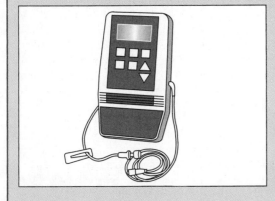

Indications and advantages

Indicated for patients who need parenteral analgesia, PCA therapy is typically given to trauma patients postoperatively and to terminal cancer patients and others with chronic diseases. To receive PCA therapy, patients must be mentally alert and able to understand and comply with instructions and procedures and have no history of allergy to the analgesic. Patients ineligible for therapy include those with limited respiratory reserve, a history of drug abuse or chronic sedative or tranquilizer use, or a psychiatric disorder. PCA therapy's advantages include:
- no need for I.M. analgesics

- pain relief tailored to each patient's size and pain tolerance
- a sense of control over pain
- ability to sleep at night with minimal daytime drowsiness
- lower opioid use compared with patients not on PCA
- improved postoperative deep breathing, coughing, and ambulation.

PCA setup

To set up a PCA system, the practitioner's order should include:
- medication to be dosed
- the appropriate lockout interval
- the amount the patient will receive when he activates the device
- the maximum amount the patient can receive within a specified time (if an adjustable device is used).

Occasionally the practitioner may order a loading dose and sometimes a base rate will be prescribed.

Nursing considerations

Because the primary adverse effect of analgesics is respiratory depression, monitor the patient's respiratory rate routinely. Also, check for infiltration into the subcutaneous tissues and for catheter occlusion, which may cause the drug to back up in the primary I.V. tubing. If the analgesic nauseates the patient, you may need to administer an antiemetic.

Before the patient starts using the PCA device, teach him how it works. Then have the patient practice with a sample device. Explain that he should take enough analgesic to relieve acute pain but not enough to induce drowsiness.

During therapy, monitor and record the amount of analgesic infused, the patient's respiratory rate, and the patient's assessment of pain relief. If the patient reports insufficient pain relief, notify the physician.

Preparation of equipment
- Verify the drug, dosage, and administration route by checking the medication record against the practitioner's order.
- Make sure that you know the immediate and delayed adverse effects of the ordered drug.

- Follow administration guidelines for appropriate procedures.

Implementation
- Confirm the patient's identity using two patient identifiers according to facility policy. **JCAHO**

• Assess the patient's physical condition and review his medical history.

• Make sure that you understand what needs to be given and by what route, and provide the necessary teaching and support to the patient and his family.

• Determine the best site to administer the drug. When selecting the site, consider drug compatibilities, frequency of administration, and the vesicant potential of the drug. (See *Risks of tissue damage*, page 128.) For example, if the physician has ordered the intermittent administration of a vesicant drug, you can give it by either instilling the drug into the side port of an infusing I.V. line or by direct I.V. push. If the vesicant drug is to be infused continuously, you should administer it only through a CV line or vascular access device. On the other hand, nonvesicant agents (including irritants) may be given by direct I.V. push, through the side port of an infusing I.V. line, or as a continuous infusion. **INS**

• Check your facility's policy before administering a vesicant. *Because vein integrity decreases with time,* some facilities require that vesicants be administered *before* other drugs. Conversely, *because vesicants increase vein fragility,* other facilities require that vesicants be given after other drugs.

• Evaluate your patient's condition, paying particular attention to the results of recent laboratory studies, specifically the complete blood count, blood urea nitrogen level, platelet count, urine creatinine level, and liver function studies. **INS** **ONS**

• Determine whether the patient has received chemotherapy before, and note the severity of any adverse effects.

• Check his drug history for medications that might interact with chemotherapy. As a rule, you shouldn't mix chemotherapeutic drugs with other medications. If you have questions or concerns about giving the chemotherapeutic drug, talk with the practitioner or pharmacist before you give it. **ONS**

• Next, double-check the patient's chart for the complete chemotherapy protocol order, including the patient's name, drug's name and dosage, and the route, rate, and frequency of administration. See if the drug's dosage depends on certain laboratory values. Be aware that some facilities require two nurses to read the dosage order and to check the drug and the amount being administered. **ONS** **INS**

• Check to see whether the physician has ordered an antiemetic, fluids, a diuretic, or electrolyte supple-

Intraperitoneal chemotherapy: An alternative approach

Administering chemotherapeutic drugs into the peritoneal cavity has several benefits for patients with malignant ascites or ovarian cancer that has spread to the peritoneum. This technique passes drugs directly to the tumor area in the peritoneal cavity, exposing malignant cells to high concentrations of chemotherapy — up to 1,000 times the amount that could be safely given systemically. Furthermore, the semipermeable peritoneal membrane permits prolonged exposure of malignant cells to the drug.

Typically, intraperitoneal chemotherapy is performed using a peritoneal dialysis kit, but drugs can also be administered directly to the peritoneal cavity by way of a Tenckhoff catheter (as shown in the illustration below). This method can be performed on an outpatient basis, if necessary, and uses equipment that's readily available on most units with oncology patients.

In this technique, the chemotherapy bag is connected directly to the Tenckhoff catheter with a length of I.V. tubing, the solution is infused, and the catheter and I.V. tubing are clamped. Then the patient is asked to change positions every 10 to 15 minutes for 1 hour *to move the solution around in the peritoneal cavity.* After the prescribed dwell time, the chemotherapeutic drugs are drained into an I.V. bag. The patient is encouraged to change positions *to facilitate drainage.* Then the I.V. tubing and catheter are clamped, the I.V. tubing is removed, and a new intermittent infusion cap is fitted to the catheter. Finally, the catheter is flushed with a syringe of heparin flush solution.

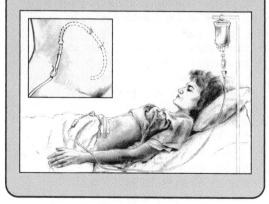

Risks of tissue damage

To administer chemotherapy safely, you need to know each drug's potential for damaging tissue. In this regard, chemotherapeutic drugs are classified as vesicants, nonvesicants, or irritants.

Vesicants

Vesicants cause a reaction so severe that blisters form and tissue is damaged or destroyed. Chemotherapeutic vesicants include:
- dactinomycin (Cosmegen)
- daunorubicin (Cerubidine)
- doxorubicin (Adriamycin)
- idarubicin (Indamycin)
- mechlorethamine (Mustargen)
- mitomycin (Mutamycin)
- mitoxantrone (Novantrone)
- vinblastine (Velban)
- vincristine (Oncovin)
- vinorelbine (Navelbine).

Nonvesicants

Nonvesicants don't cause irritation or damage. Chemotherapeutic nonvesicants include:
- asparaginase (Elspar)
- bleomycin (Blenoxane)
- cyclophosphamide (Cytoxan)
- cytarabine (Cytosar-u)
- floxuridine (FUDR)
- fluorouracil (Efudex).

Irritants

Irritants can cause a local venous response, with or without a skin reaction. Chemotherapeutic irritants include:
- carboplatin (Paraplatin)
- carmustine (BiCNU)
- dacarbazine (DTIC-Dome)
- etoposide (VePesid)
- ifosfamide (Ifex)
- irinotecan (Camptosar)
- streptozocin (Zanosar)
- topotecan (Hycamtin).

ments to be given before, during, or after chemotherapy administration.
- Evaluate the patient's and his family's understanding of chemotherapy, and make sure that the patient or a responsible family member has signed the consent form. **PCP**
- Next, put on gloves. Keep them on through all stages of handling the drug, including preparation, priming the I.V. tubing, and administration. **CDC** **ONS** **OSHA**
- Before administering the drug, perform a new venipuncture proximal to the old site. Avoid giving chemotherapeutic drugs through an existing I.V. line. To identify an administration site, examine the patient's veins, starting with his hand and proceeding to his forearm. **INS**
- After an appropriate line is in place, infuse 10 to 20 ml of normal saline solution to test vein patency. *Never test vein patency with a chemotherapeutic drug.* Next, administer the drug as appropriate: nonvesicants by I.V. push or admixed in a bag of I.V. fluid; vesicants by I.V. push through a piggyback set connected to a rapidly infusing I.V. line.
- During I.V. administration, closely monitor the patient for signs of a hypersensitivity reaction or extravasation. Check for adequate blood return after

5 ml of the drug has been infused or according to your facility's guidelines. **ONS**
- After infusion of the medication, infuse 20 ml of normal saline solution. Do this between administrations of different chemotherapeutic drugs and before discontinuing the I.V. line. **INS**
- Dispose of used needles and syringes carefully. *To prevent aerosol dispersion of chemotherapeutic drugs,* don't clip needles. Place them intact in an impervious container for incineration. Dispose of I.V. bags, bottles, gloves, and tubing in a properly labeled and covered trash container. **OSHA**
- Wash your hands thoroughly with soap and warm water after giving a chemotherapeutic drug, even though you've worn gloves. **OSHA**

Special considerations

- Observe the I.V. site frequently for signs of extravasation and allergic reaction (swelling, redness, urticaria). If you suspect extravasation, *stop the infusion immediately.* Leave the I.V. catheter in place and notify the physician. A conservative method for treating extravasation involves aspirating any residual drug from the tubing and I.V. catheter, instilling an I.V. antidote, and then removing the I.V. catheter. Afterward, you may apply heat or cold to the site and elevate the affected limb.

ALERT *Extravasation — the infiltration of a vesicant drug into the surrounding tissue — is a rare occurrence resulting from a punctured vein or leakage around a venipuncture site. Vesicant extravasation can result in significant pain, prolonged healing, infection, cosmetic disfigurement, and loss of function and may necessitate multiple debridements and, possibly, amputation. Extravasation of vesicant drugs requires emergency treatment. Follow your facility's protocol. Essential steps may include the following:*

Stop the I.V. flow, aspirate the remaining drug in the catheter, and remove the I.V. line, unless you need the needle to infiltrate the antidote. Estimate the amount of extravasated solution and notify the practitioner.

Instill the appropriate antidote according to your facility's protocol then elevate the extremity.

Record the extravasation site, the patient's symptoms, estimated amount of infiltrated solution, and treatment. Include the time you notified the physician and the physician's name. Continue documenting the appearance of the site and associated symptoms.

Ice is typically applied to all extravasated areas, with the exception of etoposide and vinca alkaloids, for 15 to 20 minutes every 4 to 6 hours for about 3 days. For etoposide (Toposar) and vinca alkaloids, heat is applied.

If skin breakdown occurs, apply dressings as ordered. If severe tissue damage occurs, plastic surgery and physical therapy may be needed.

● During infusion, some drugs need protection from direct sunlight *to avoid possible drug breakdown.* If this is the case, cover the vial with a brown paper bag or aluminum foil.

● When giving vesicants, avoid sites where damage to underlying tendons or nerves may occur (for example, veins in the antecubital fossa, near the wrist, or in the dorsal surface of the hand).

● If you can't stay with the patient during the entire infusion, use an infusion pump or controller *to ensure drug delivery within the prescribed time and rate.*

● Observe the patient at regular intervals and after treatment for adverse reactions. Monitor his vital signs throughout the infusion *to assess any changes during chemotherapy administration.*

● Maintain a list of the types and amounts of drugs the patient has received. This is especially important if he has received drugs that have a cumulative effect and that can be toxic to such organs as the heart or kidneys.

Nursing diagnoses
● Deficient fluid volume
● Nausea

Expected outcomes
The patient will:
● maintain electrolyte levels within normal limits
● maintain adequate fluid volume
● produce an adequate urine volume
● ingest sufficient nutrients to maintain health
● take steps to manage episodes of nausea and vomiting.

Complications
● Common adverse effects of chemotherapy are nausea and vomiting, ranging from mild to debilitating.
● Another major complication is bone marrow suppression, leading to neutropenia and thrombocytopenia.
● Other adverse effects include intestinal irritation, stomatitis, pulmonary fibrosis, cardiotoxicity, nephrotoxicity, neurotoxicity, hearing loss, anemia, alopecia, urticaria, radiation recall (if drugs are given with, or soon after, radiation therapy), anorexia, esophagitis, diarrhea, and constipation. I.V. administration of chemotherapeutic drugs may also lead to extravasation, causing inflammation, ulceration, necrosis, and loss of vein patency.

CONTROVERSIAL ISSUE *Neutropenia can vary in occurrence and depends on the agents used, dose given, and frequency of administration. Prevention methods, which are controversial and not well documented, include avoiding people recently vaccinated with live organisms or viruses (such as polio), avoiding pet excreta (including cleaning fish tanks), and avoiding exposure to fresh fruits, vegetables, flowers, and live plants.*

Documentation
Record the location and description of the I.V. site before treatment, or the presence of blood return during bolus administration. Also record the drugs and dosages administered, sequence of drug administration, needle type and size used, amount and type of

flushing solution, and the site's condition after treatment. Document adverse reactions, the patient's tolerance of the treatment, and the topics discussed with the patient and his family.

Supportive references

Baker, E.S., and Connor, T.H. "Monitoring Occupational Exposure to Cancer Chemotherapy Drugs," *American Journal of Health System Pharmacists* 53(22):2713-23, November 1996.

Brown, K., et al., eds. *Chemotherapy and Biotherapy Guidelines and Recommendations for Practice.* Pittsburgh, Pa.: Oncology Nursing Society, 2001. **EB**

Camp-Sorrel, D. "Developing Extravasation Protocols and Monitoring Outcomes," *Journal of Infusion Nursing* 21(4):232-39, July-August 1998.

Connor, T.H. "Permeability of Nitrile Rubber, Latex, Polyurethane Neoprene Gloves to 18 Antineoplastic Drugs," *American Journal of Health System Pharmacists* 56:2450-53, 1999.

Fischer, D.S., et al. *The Cancer Chemotherapy Book,* 5th ed. St. Louis: Mosby–Year Book, Inc., 1997.

Infusion Nurses Society. "Position Paper: The Administration of Neoplastic Agents," *Journal of Intravenous Nursing* 19:72-73, 1996.

"Standard 37. Site Selection. Infusion Nursing Standards of Practice," *Journal of Infusion Nursing* 29(1S):S37-39, January-February 2006.

"Standard 54. Infiltration. Infusion Nursing Standards of Practice," *Journal of Infusion Nursing* 29(1S):S59-60, January-February 2006.

"Standard 55. Extravasation. Infusion Nursing Standards of Practice," *Journal of Infusion Nursing* 29(1S):S61-62, January-February 2006.

"Standard 69. Antineoplastic and Biologic Therapy. Infusion Nursing Standards of Practice," *Journal of Infusion Nursing* 29(1S):S69-71, January-February 2006.

Weinstein, S.M. *Plumer's Principles and Practice of Intravenous Therapy,* 7th ed. Philadelphia: Lippincott Williams & Wilkins, 2001.

Chemotherapeutic drug preparation

Preparation of chemotherapeutic drugs requires extra care for the safety of the patient and the health care provider. The patient receiving chemotherapy and the people who prepare and handle the drugs are at risk for teratogenic, mutagenic, and carcinogenic effects of the drugs. (See *Chemotherapy effects on reproduction.*)

CLINICAL IMPACT *Although little research has been done on the long-term risks at the levels of exposure encountered by unprotected health care workers, these drugs have been associated with human cancers at high (therapeutic) levels of exposure and are carcinogens and teratogens in many animal species. As a result of the research, most health care facilities developed policies, procedures, and such protocols as protective clothing, spill kits, and isolation precautions to reduce health care workers' exposure to these drugs.*

The nurse handling and mixing antineoplastic agents should strictly adhere to protective protocols, such as mixing drugs under vertical laminar flow hoods or biological safety cabinets, and wearing protective clothing. Pregnant nurses (actual or suspected) should be advised of the potential risks associated with handling chemotherapy drugs and should be given the option not to prepare or administer such products. **ONS INS**

Occupational Safety and Health Administration (OSHA) guidelines for handling chemotherapeutic drugs have two basic requirements; first, all health care workers who handle chemotherapeutic drugs must be educated and trained. A key element of such training involves learning how to reduce your exposure when handling the drugs. The second requirement states that the drugs should be prepared in a class II biological safety cabinet. If a biological safety cabinet isn't available, OSHA recommends that a respirator be worn while mixing the drugs. **OSHA**

OSHA guidelines recommend that chemotherapeutic drugs be mixed in a properly enclosed and ventilated work area and that respiratory and skin protection be worn. Smoking, drinking, applying cosmetics, and eating where these drugs are prepared, stored, or used should be strictly prohibited, and sterile technique should be used while mixing the drugs. **OSHA**

Gloves, gowns, syringes or vials, and other materials that have been used in chemotherapy preparation and administration present a possible source of exposure or injury to the facility's staff, patients, and visitors. Therefore, use of properly labeled, sealed, and covered containers, handled only by trained and protected personnel, should be routine practice. Spills also represent a hazard, and all employees should be familiar with appropriate spill procedures for their own protection. **OSHA**

Equipment

Prescribed drug or drugs • patient's medication record and chart • long-sleeved gown • latex surgical gloves • face shield or goggles • eyewash • plastic absorbent pad • alcohol pads • sterile gauze pads • shoe covers • impervious container with the label CAUTION: BIO-HAZARD for the disposal of unused drugs or equipment • I.V. solution • diluent (if necessary) • compatibility reference source • medication labels • class II biological safety cabinet • disposable towel • hydrophobic filter or dispensing pin • 18G needle • syringes and needles of various sizes • I.V. tubing with luer-lock fittings • I.V. controller pump (if available)

Have a chemotherapeutic spill kit available that includes: water-resistant, nonpermeable, long-sleeved gown with cuffs and back closure • shoe covers • two pairs of gloves (for double gloving) • goggles • mask • disposable dustpan • plastic scraper (for collecting broken glass) • plastic-backed or absorbent towels • container of desiccant powder or granules (to absorb wet contents) • two disposable sponges • puncture-proof, leakproof container labeled BIOHAZARD WASTE • container of 70% alcohol for cleaning the spill area

Implementation

● Remember to wash your hands before and after drug preparation and administration. **CDC**

● Prepare the drugs in a class II biological safety cabinet. **OSHA**

● Wear protective garments (such as a long-sleeved gown, gloves, a face shield or goggles, and shoe covers), as indicated by your facility's policy. Don't wear the garments outside the preparation area. **OSHA**

● Don't eat, drink, smoke, or apply cosmetics in the drug preparation area.

● Before you prepare the drug (and after you finish), clean the internal surfaces of the cabinet with 70% alcohol and a disposable towel. Discard the towel in a leakproof chemical waste container. **OSHA**

● Cover the work surface with a clean plastic absorbent pad *to minimize contamination by droplets or spills*. Change the pad at the end of the shift or whenever a spill occurs.

Chemotherapy effects on reproduction

Recently, studies have been conducted on the effect chemotherapy drugs have during pregnancy and the outcomes on the fetus. According to the *Journal of the National Cancer Institute*, chemotherapy and radiotherapy increase the genetic defects in germ cells, but this increase depends on the agent used and the state of the fetal development. The potential teratogenic effects of the cancer treatment also depends on the developmental stage of the fetus at the time of exposure and on what chemotherapeutic drug was used.

It was found that during the first trimester, malformation and abortion rates increased. During the second and third trimesters, chemotherapy may increase the risk of fetal growth retardation, stillbirth occurrence, and premature birth. Maternal myelosuppression was also increased, which can be detrimental to the fetus because it increases maternal bleeding and infection. Research about the effects of chemotherapy on reproductive outcomes continues.

Adapted with permission from Meiron, A., and Schiff, E. "Appraisal of Chemotherapy Effects on Reproductive Outcome According to Animal Studies and Clinical Date," *Journal of the National Cancer Institute Monographs* 34:21-25, 2005.

● Consider all of the equipment used in drug preparation as well as any unused drug as hazardous waste. Dispose of them according to your facility's policy.

● Place all chemotherapeutic waste products in labeled, leakproof, sealable plastic bags or other appropriate impervious containers. **OSHA**

Special considerations

● Prepare the drugs according to current product instructions, paying attention to compatibility, stability, and reconstitution technique. Label the prepared drug with the patient's name, dosage strength, and date and time of preparation.

● Take precautions to reduce your exposure to chemotherapeutic drugs. Systemic absorption can occur through ingestion of contaminated materials, contact with the skin, or inhalation. You can inhale a drug without realizing it, such as while opening a vial, clipping a needle, expelling air from a syringe, or discarding excess drug. You can also absorb a drug from handling contaminated stools or body fluids.

● *For maximum protection,* mix all chemotherapeutic drugs in an approved class II biological safety cabinet. Also, prime all I.V. bags that contain chemotherapeutic drugs under the hood. Leave the hood blower on 24 hours per day, 7 days per week. **OSHA**

● If a hood isn't available, prepare drugs in a well-ventilated work space, away from heating or cooling vents and other personnel. Vent vials with a hydrophobic filter, or use negative-pressure techniques. Also, use a needle with a hydrophobic filter to remove the solution from a vial. To break an ampule, wrap a sterile gauze pad or alcohol pad around the neck of the ampule *to decrease the risk of contamination.* **OSHA**

● Make sure that the biological safety cabinet is examined every 6 months, or any time the cabinet is moved by a company specifically qualified to perform this work. If the cabinet passes certification, the certifying company will affix a sticker to the cabinet attesting to its approval. **OSHA**

● Use only syringes and I.V. sets that have luer-lock fittings. Label all chemotherapeutic drugs with a chemotherapy hazard label.

● Don't clip needles, break syringes, or remove the needles from the syringes. Use a gauze pad when removing chemotherapy syringes and needles from I.V. bags of chemotherapeutic drugs. **OSHA**

● Place used syringes or needles in a puncture-proof container, along with other sharp or breakable items.

● When mixing chemotherapeutic drugs, wear latex surgical gloves and a gown of low-permeability fabric with a closed front and cuffed long sleeves. When working steadily with chemotherapeutic drugs, change gloves every 30 minutes. If you spill a drug solution or puncture or tear a glove, remove your gloves immediately. Wash your hands before putting on new gloves and any time you remove your gloves. **OSHA**

● If some of the drug comes in contact with your skin, wash the involved area thoroughly with soap (not a germicidal agent) and water. If eye contact occurs, flood the eye with water or an isotonic eyewash for at least 5 minutes while holding the eyelid open. Obtain a medical evaluation as soon as possible after accidental exposure. **OSHA**

● If a major spill occurs, use a chemotherapeutic spill kit to clean the area.

● Discard disposable gowns and gloves in an appropriately marked, waterproof receptacle when contaminated or when you leave the work area.

● Don't place food or drinks in the same refrigerator as chemotherapeutic drugs.

● Become familiar with drug excretion patterns, and take appropriate precautions when handling a chemotherapy patient's body fluids.

● Provide male patients with a urinal with a tight-fitting lid. Wear disposable latex surgical gloves when handling body fluids. Before flushing the toilet, place a waterproof pad over the toilet bowl *to avoid splashing.* Wear gloves and a gown when handling linens soiled with body fluids. Place soiled linens in isolation linen bags designated for separate laundering. **INS** **OSHA**

● Women who are pregnant, trying to conceive, or breast-feeding should exercise caution when handling chemotherapeutic drugs.

TEACHING *When teaching your patient about handling chemotherapeutic drugs, discuss appropriate safety measures. If the patient will be receiving chemotherapy at home, teach him how to dispose of contaminated equipment. Tell the patient and his family to wear gloves whenever handling chemotherapy equipment or contaminated linens or gowns and pajamas. Instruct them to place soiled linens in a separate washable pillowcase and to launder the pillowcase twice, with the soiled linens inside, separately from other linens.*

When providing home care, empty waste products into the toilet close to the water to minimize splashing. *Close the lid and flush three times.*

All materials used for the treatment should be placed in a leakproof container and taken to a designated disposal area. The patient or his family should make arrangements with either a hospital or a private company for pickup and proper disposal of contaminated waste.

Nursing diagnoses
● Deficient knowledge (procedure)
● Risk for injury

Expected outcomes
The patient will:

- state an understanding of the procedure
- demonstrate proper procedure for handling chemotherapeutic drugs
- remain free from injury and complications.

Complications

- Chemotherapeutic drugs may be mutagenic. Chronic exposure to chemotherapeutic drugs may damage the liver or chromosomes.
- Direct exposure to these drugs may burn and damage the skin.

Documentation

Document each incident of exposure according to your facility's policy.

Supportive references

Brown, K., et al., eds. *Chemotherapy and Biotherapy Guidelines and Recommendations for Practice.* Pittsburgh, Pa.: Oncology Nursing Society, 2001.

"Standard 25. Disposal of Sharps, Hazardous Materials, and Hazardous Waste. Infusion Nursing Standards of Practice," *Journal of Infusion Nursing* 29(1S):S30, January-February 2006.

"Standard 26. Laminar Flow Hood. Infusion Nursing Standards of Practice," *Journal of Intravenous Nursing* 23(6S):S28, November-December 2000.

"Standard 54. Infiltration. Infusion Nursing Standards of Practice," *Journal of Infusion Nursing* 29(1S):S59-60, January-February 2006.

"Standard 55. Extravasation. Infusion Nursing Standards of Practice," *Journal of Infusion Nursing* 29(1S):S61-62, January-February 2006.

"Standard 65. Antineoplastic and Biologic Therapy. Infusion Nursing Standards of Practice," *Journal of Infusion Nursing* 29(1S):S69-71, January-February 2006.

U.S. Department of Labor. Occupational Safety & Health Administration. "Controlling Occupational Exposure to Harmful Drugs." In: TED 1-0.15A, Section VI, chapter 2. OSHA Technical Manual. Washington, D.C.: OSHA, January 1999. *www.osha.gov/dts/osta_vi/otm_vi_2.htm.*

Valanis, B.G., et al. "Occupational Exposure to Antineoplastic Agents and Self-Reported Infertility among Nurses and Pharmacists," *Journal of Occupational and Environmental Medicine* 39(6):574-80, June 1997.

Endotracheal drug administration

When an I.V. line isn't readily available, drugs can be administered into the respiratory system through an endotracheal (ET) tube. This route *allows uninterrupted resuscitation efforts and can save precious moments in an emergency* while waiting for venous access. This route also *avoids complications from direct cardiac administration of drugs, such as cardiac tamponade, pneumothorax, and coronary artery laceration.*

Drugs given endotracheally usually have a longer duration of action than when given I.V. because they're absorbed in the alveoli. For this reason, repeat doses and continuous infusions must be adjusted to prevent adverse effects.

Epinephrine, lidocaine, atropine, naloxone (Narcan), and vasopressin (Pitressin) can be absorbed via the trachea, the I.V. route, or the intraosseous route, which is preferred. The American Heart Association (AHA) recommends administering all ET medication at 2 to $2\frac{1}{2}$ times the recommended I.V. dose. **AHA**

In an emergency, a physician, a critical care nurse, or an emergency medical technician usually administers these drugs. Although guidelines may vary, depending on state, county, or city regulations, the basic administration method is the same. (See *Administering endotracheal drugs,* page 134.)

ET drugs may be given using the syringe method or adapter method. Usually used for bronchoscopy suctioning, the swivel adapter can be placed on the end of the ET tube and, while ventilation continues through a bag-valve device, the drug can be delivered with a needle through the closed stopcock.

Equipment

ET tube or swivel adapter • gloves • CO_2 detector or an esophageal detector device • handheld resuscitation bag • prescribed drug • syringe or adapter • sterile water or normal saline solution

Preparation of equipment

- Verify the order on the patient's medication record by checking it against the physician's order. Wash your hands. **CDC** Check ET tube placement by using an exhaled CO_2 detector or an esophageal detector device. **AHA**

Administering endotracheal drugs

In an emergency, some drugs may be given through an endotracheal (ET) tube if I.V. access isn't available. The syringe method or the adapter method may be used.

Before injecting any drug, use your stethoscope to check for proper placement of the ET tube. Make sure that the patient is supine and that her head is level with or slightly higher than her trunk.

Syringe method
Remove the needle before injecting medication into the ET tube. Insert the tip of the syringe into the ET tube, and inject the drug deep into the tube (as shown below).

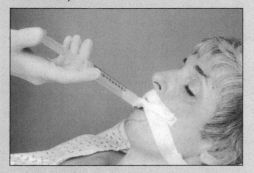

Adapter method
A device developed for ET drug administration provides a more closed system of drug delivery than the syringe method. A special adapter placed on the end of the ET tube (as shown below) allows needle insertion and drug delivery through the closed stopcock.

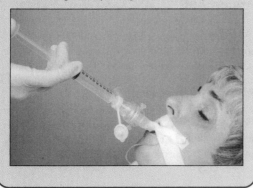

- Calculate the drug dose. Adult advanced cardiac life support guidelines recommend that the drugs be administered at 2 to 2½ times the recommended I.V. dose. Next, draw the drug up into a syringe. Dilute the dose in 5 to 10 ml of distilled water or normal saline solution. *Dilution increases drug volume and contact with the lung.* **AHA**

CONTROVERSIAL ISSUE *AHA 2005 guidelines recommend distilled water instead of normal saline solution because it allows greater tracheal absorption. However, there's insufficient evidence to recommend water dilution over normal saline solution.*

Implementation
- Put on gloves. **CDC**
- Move the patient into the supine position, and make sure that his head is level with or slightly higher than his trunk.
- Ventilate the patient three to five times with the resuscitation bag, and then remove the bag. **AHA**
- Remove the needle from the syringe and insert the tip of the syringe into the ET tube or swivel adapter. Inject the drug deep into the tube.
- After injecting the drug, reattach the resuscitation bag and ventilate the patient briskly *to propel the drug into the lungs, oxygenate the patient, and clear the tube.* **AHA**
- Discard the syringe in the sharps container. **OSHA**
- Remove and discard your gloves. **CDC**

Special considerations
Be aware that the drug's onset of action may be quicker than it would be by I.V. administration. If the patient doesn't respond quickly, the physician may order a repeat dose.

Nursing diagnoses
- Impaired gas exchange
- Ineffective tissue perfusion: Cardiopulmonary

Expected outcomes
The patient will:
- maintain respiratory rate within 5 breaths per minute of baseline
- have normal breath sounds
- maintain a heart rate within the prescribed limits
- maintain adequate cardiac output.

Complications

Potential complications of ET drug administration result from the prescribed drug, not the administration route.

Documentation

Record the date and time of the drug administered and the patient's response.

Supportive references

"2005 International Consensus on Cardiopulmonary Resuscitation and Emergency Cardiovascular Care," Part 2: Ethical Issues. *Circulation* 112(suppl IV):IV-6-IV-11, 2005.

Katz, S.H., and Falk, J.L. "Misplaced Endotracheal Tubes by Paramedics in an Urban Emergency Medical Services System," *Annals of Emergency Medicine* 37(1):32-37, January 2001.

Plaisance, P., et al. "Inspiratory Impedance during Active Compression-Decompression Cardiopulmonary Resuscitation: A Randomized Evaluation of Inpatients in Cardiac Arrest," *Circulation* 101(9):989-94, March 2000.

Intermittent infusion devices

Also called a *saline lock,* an intermittent infusion device consists of a cannula with an attached injection cap. Filled with saline solution *to prevent blood clot formation,* the device maintains venous access in patients who are receiving I.V. medication regularly or intermittently but who don't require continuous infusion.

A saline lock should be inserted using sterile technique and maintaining standard precautions. If contamination occurs or is suspected, or the integrity of the product is compromised, it should be removed immediately. **INS**

Considerations when choosing the size of an I.V. catheter include size and condition of the vein, the viscosity of the fluid to be infused, the patient's age, and the type and duration of I.V. therapy. (See *Choosing the right I.V. size.*)

An intermittent infusion device is superior to an I.V. line that's maintained at a moderately slow infusion rate because it *minimizes the risk of fluid overload and electrolyte imbalance.* It also *cuts costs, reduces the risk of contamination* by eliminating I.V. solution

---

Choosing the right I.V. size

Catheters come in various sizes (gauges). Choose the shortest catheter with the largest gauge appropriate for the type and duration of the infusion. The larger the gauge number, the smaller the catheter's bore.

- 24G — used mostly in neonates, pediatric patients, and elderly patients
- 22G — used especially in children and elderly patients
- 18G — best used for blood, blood products, and viscous medications
- 16G — (largest catheter) used in major surgeries, obstetric emergencies, and traumas

---

containers and administration sets, *increases patient comfort and mobility, reduces patient anxiety and, if inserted in a large vein, allows collection of multiple blood samples without repeated venipuncture.*

Equipment

Intermittent infusion device • needleless system device • normal saline solution • tourniquet • alcohol pad or other approved antimicrobial solution, such as 2% chlorhexidine swabs • venipuncture equipment • transparent semipermeable dressing • tape

Prefilled saline cartridges are available for use in a syringe cartridge holder.

Implementation

- Confirm the patient's identity using two patient identifiers according to facility policy. **JCAHO**
- Wash your hands thoroughly *to prevent contamination of the venipuncture site.* **CDC**
- Explain the procedure to the patient, and describe the purpose of the intermittent infusion device.
- Remove the set from its packaging, wipe the port with an alcohol pad, and inject normal saline solution to fill the tubing and needleless system. *This removes air from the system, preventing formation of an air embolus.* **INS**
- Select a venipuncture site. Put on gloves. Apply a tourniquet 2″ (5.1 cm) proximal to the chosen area. **INS**
- Clean the venipuncture site with alcohol or other approved antimicrobial solution according to your facility's policy and manufacturer's directions. **MFR**

Converting an I.V. line to an intermittent infusion device

The male adapter plug shown below allows you to convert an existing I.V. line into an intermittent infusion device. To make the conversion, follow these steps:
- Prime the male adapter plug with normal saline solution.
- Clamp the I.V. tubing, and remove the administration set from the cannula or needle hub.
- Insert the male adapter plug.
- Flush the access with the remaining solution *to prevent occlusion.*

Short male adapter
The male luer-lock adapter plug twists into place.

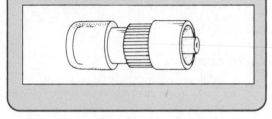

- Perform the venipuncture and ensure correct needle placement in the vein. Then release the tourniquet.
- Tape the set in place. Loop the tubing, if applicable, *so the injection port is free and easily accessible.*
- Flush the catheter with saline solution.

✔ **CLINICAL IMPACT** *The volume of flush solution should be equal to or twice that of the capacity of the catheter and add-on device. If the site is used intermittently, it will need to be flushed with normal saline solution (injectable) at established intervals to maintain patency. Flushing will also need to be performed before and after administration of incompatible medications or solutions.*

- Apply a transparent semipermeable dressing. On the dressing label, write the time, date, and your initials, and place the label on the dressing.
- Remove and discard gloves. **CDC**
- Inject normal saline solution every 8 to 24 hours or according to your facility's policy *to maintain the patency of the intermittent infusion device.* Inject the saline slowly *to prevent stinging.* **INS**

Special considerations

- When accessing an intermittent infusion device, be sure to stabilize the device *to prevent dislodging it from the vein.*
- If the patient feels a burning sensation during the injection of saline, stop the injection and check the cannula placement. If the cannula is in the vein, inject the saline at a slower rate *to minimize irritation.* If the needle isn't in the vein, remove and discard it. Then select a new venipuncture site and, using fresh equipment, restart the procedure. **INS**
- Change the intermittent infusion device every 48 to 72 hours, according to your facility's policy, using a new venipuncture site. Some facilities use a transparent semipermeable dressing. *This allows more patient freedom and better observation of the injection site.* **INS**
- If the physician orders an I.V. infusion discontinued and an intermittent infusion device inserted in its place, convert the existing line by disconnecting the I.V. tubing and inserting a male adapter plug into the device. (See *Converting an I.V. line to an intermittent infusion device.*)
- Most health care facilities require the use of luer-lock systems on all infusion cannulas and lines.

📋 **TEACHING** *If you're caring for a patient who'll be going home with a peripheral line, teach him how to care for the I.V. site and how to identify complications. If he must observe movement restrictions, make sure that he understands which movements to avoid.*

Because the patient may have special drug delivery equipment that differs from the type used in the facility, be sure to demonstrate the equipment and have the patient give a return demonstration.

Teach the patient to examine the site and to notify the nurse if the dressing becomes moist, if blood appears in the tubing, or if redness, swelling, or discomfort develops.

Also tell the patient to report problems with the I.V. line — for instance, if the solution stops infusing or if an alarm goes off on the infusion pump controller. Explain that the I.V. site will be changed at established intervals by a home care nurse.

Teach the patient or caregiver how and when to flush the device. Finally, teach the patient to document daily whether the I.V. site is free from pain, swelling, and redness.

Nursing diagnoses
- Risk for infection
- Risk for injury

Expected outcomes
The patient will:
- maintain vital signs and laboratory values with normal limits
- maintain white blood cell and differential counts within normal range
- remain free from complications or injury.

Complications
Use of an intermittent infusion device has the same potential complications as the use of a peripheral I.V. line. (See "Peripheral I.V. lines," page 152.)

Documentation
Record the date and time of insertion; type, brand, and gauge of the needle and length of the cannula; anatomic location of the insertion site; the patient's tolerance of the procedure; and the date and time of each saline flush.

Supportive references

Arduino, M.S., et al. "Microbiological Evaluation of Needleless and Needle-Access Devices," *American Journal of Infection Control* 25(5):377-80, October 1997.

Metheny, N.M. *Fluid and Electrolyte Balance: Nursing Considerations,* 4th ed. Philadelphia: Lippincott Williams & Wilkins, 2000.

"Standard 13. Keep Vein Open. Infusion Nursing Standards of Practice," *Journal of Intravenous Nursing* 23(6S):S19, November-December 2000.

"Standard 29. Add-on Devices and Junction Securement. Infusion Nursing Standards of Practice," *Journal of Infusion Nursing* 29(1S):S32, January-February 2006.

"Standard 45. Implanted Ports and Pumps. Infusion Nursing Standards of Practice," *Journal of Infusion Nursing* 29(1S):S45-46, January-February 2006.

"Standard 50. Flushing. Infusion Nursing Standards of Practice," *Journal of Infusion Nursing* 29(1S):S552, January-February 2006.

Weinstein, S.M. *Plumer's Principles and Practice of Intravenous Therapy,* 7th ed. Philadelphia: Lippincott Williams & Wilkins, 2001.

Using I.V. clamps

With a roller clamp or screw clamp, you can increase or decrease the flow through the I.V. line by turning a wheel or screw.

Roller clamp   **Screw clamp**

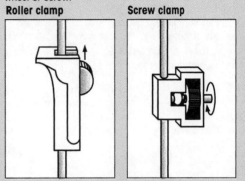

With a slide clamp, you can open or close the line by moving the clamp horizontally. However, you can't make fine adjustments to the flow rate.

Slide clamp

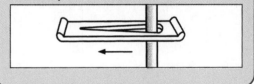

I.V. infusion rates and manual control

Infusion rates are vital to the safe administration of I.V. fluids and medications. Information necessary to calculate infusion rates includes:
- volume of fluid to be infused
- total infusion time
- calibration of the administration set—number of drops per milliliter (found on I.V. tubing package).

Many devices can regulate the infusion of I.V. solution, including clamps, controllers, the flow regulator (or rate minder), and the volumetric pump. (See *Using I.V. clamps.*)

When regulated by a clamp or controller, the infusion rate is usually measured in drops per minute; by a volumetric pump, in milliliters per hour. The infusion regulator can be set to deliver the desired amount of solution, also in milliliters per hour. Less

Calculating infusion rates

When calculating the infusion rate of I.V. solutions, remember that the number of drops required to deliver 1 ml varies with the type and manufacturer of the administration set used. The illustration on the left shows a standard (macrodrip) set, which delivers from 10 to 20 drops/ml. The illustration in the center shows a pediatric (microdrip) set, which delivers about 60 drops/ml. The illustration on the right shows a blood transfusion set, which delivers about 10 drops/ml.

To calculate the infusion rate, you must know the calibration of the drip rate for each manufacturer's product. Use this formula to calculate specific drip rates:

$$\frac{\text{volume of infusion (in ml)}}{\text{time of infusion (in minutes)}} \times \text{drip factor (in drops/ml)} = \text{drops/minute}$$

Macrodrip set   **Microdrip set**   **Blood transfusion set**

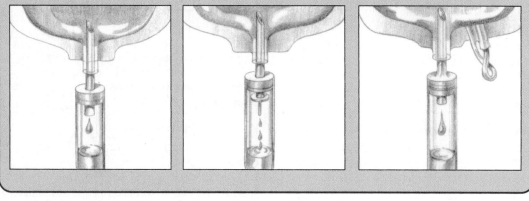

accurate than infusion pumps or controllers, infusion regulators are most reliable when used with inactive adult patients. With any device, the infusion rate can be easily monitored by using a time tape, which indicates the prescribed solution level at hourly intervals.

Equipment

I.V. administration set with clamp • 1″ paper or adhesive tape (or premarked time tape) • infusion pump and controller (if infusing medication) • watch with second hand • drip rate chart, as necessary • pen

Standard macrodrip sets deliver from 10 to 20 drops/ml, depending on the manufacturer; microdrip sets, 60 drops/ml; and blood transfusion sets, 10 drops/ml. A commercially available adapter can convert a macrodrip set to a microdrip system. **MFR**

Implementation

● The infusion rate requires close monitoring and correction *because such factors as venous spasm, ve-*
nous pressure changes, patient movement or manipulation of the clamp, and bent or kinked tubing can cause the infusion rate to vary markedly.

Calculating and setting the drip rate

● Follow the steps in *Calculating infusion rates,* to determine the proper drip rate, or use your unit's drip rate chart.
● After calculating the desired drip rate, remove your watch and hold it next to the drip chamber of the I.V. administration set *to allow simultaneous observation of the watch and the drops.* **INS**
● Release the clamp to the approximate drip rate. Then count drops for 1 minute *to account for flow irregularities.*
● Adjust the clamp, as necessary, and count drops for 1 minute. Continue to adjust the clamp and count drops until the correct rate is achieved.

Managing I.V. infusion-rate deviations

Problem	Cause	Intervention
Too fast	• Patient or visitor manipulates the clamp	• Instruct patient not to touch clamp, and place tape over it. Restrain patient or administer I.V. solution with an infusion pump or a controller, if necessary.
	• Tubing disconnected from the catheter	• Wipe distal end of tubing with alcohol, reinsert it firmly into catheter hub, and tape at connection site. Consider using tubing with luer-lock connections.
	• Change in patient position	• Administer I.V. solution with an infusion pump or a controller *to ensure correct flow rate.*
	• Bevel against vein wall (positional cannulation)	• Manipulate cannula, and place a 2″ x 2″ gauze pad over or under catheter hub to change angle. Reset flow clamp at desired rate. If necessary, remove cannula and reinsert.
	• Flow clamp drifting as a result of patient movement	• Place tape below clamp.
Too slow	• Venous spasm after insertion	• Apply warm soaks over site.
	• Venous obstruction from bending arm	• Secure with an arm board, if necessary.
	• Pressure change (decreasing fluid in bottle causes solution to run slower due to decreasing pressure)	• Readjust flow rate.
	• Elevated blood pressure	• Readjust flow rate. Use an infusion pump or a controller *to ensure correct flow rate.*
	• Cold solution	• Allow solution to warm to room temperature before hanging.
	• Change in solution viscosity from medication added	• Readjust flow rate.
	• I.V. container too low or patient's arm or leg too high	• Hang container higher or remind patient to keep his arm below heart level.
	• Bevel against vein wall (positional cannulation)	• Withdraw needle slightly, or place a folded 2″ × 2″ gauze pad over or under catheter hub to change angle.
	• Excess tubing dangling below insertion site	• Replace tubing with a shorter piece, or tape excess tubing to I.V. pole, below flow clamp (make sure tubing isn't kinked).
	• Cannula too small	• Remove cannula in use and insert a larger-bore cannula, or use an infusion pump.
	• Infiltration or clotted cannula	• Remove cannula in use and insert a new cannula.
	• Kinked tubing	• Check tubing over its entire length and unkink it.
	• Clogged filter	• Remove filter and replace it with a new one.
	• Tubing memory (tubing compressed at area clamped)	• Massage or milk tubing by pinching and wrapping it around a pencil four or five times. Quickly pull pencil out of coiled tubing.

Making a time tape

● Calculate the number of milliliters to be infused per hour. Place a piece of tape vertically on the container alongside the volume-increment markers.
● Starting at the current solution level, move down the number of milliliters to be infused in 1 hour, and mark the appropriate time and a horizontal line on the tape at this level. Then continue to mark 1-hour intervals until you reach the bottom of the container.
● Check the infusion rate every 15 minutes until stable. Then recheck it every hour or according to your facility's policy and adjust as necessary.
● With each check, inspect the I.V. site for complications, and assess the patient's response to therapy.

Special considerations

● If the infusion rate slows significantly, a slight rate increase may be necessary.
● If the rate must be increased by more than 30%, consult the physician.
● When infusing drugs, use an I.V. pump or controller, if possible, *to avoid infusion rate inaccuracies.*
● Always use a pump or controller when infusing solutions by way of a central line.
● Large-volume solution containers have about 10% more fluid than the amount indicated on the bag *to allow for tubing purges.* Thus, a 1,000-ml bag or bottle contains an additional 100 ml; similarly, a 500-ml container holds an extra 50 ml; and a 250-ml container, 25 ml.

Nursing diagnoses

● Risk for imbalanced fluid volume

Expected outcomes

The patient will:
● maintain fluid intake and output at appropriate levels
● maintain vital signs within normal range.

Complications

An excessively slow infusion rate may cause insufficient intake of fluids, drugs, and nutrients; an excessively rapid rate of fluid or drug infusion may cause circulatory overload — possibly leading to heart failure and pulmonary edema as well as adverse effects. (See *Managing I.V. infusion-rate deviations,* page 139.)

Documentation

Record the original flow rate when setting up a peripheral line. If you adjust the rate, record the change, the date and time, and your initials.

Supportive references

Joint Commission on Accreditation of Healthcare Organizations. *Comprehensive Accreditation Manual for Hospitals.* Oakbrook Terrace, Ill.: JCAHO, 2002. *www.jcaho.gov.*

Otto, S.E. *Mosby's Pocket Guide to Intravenous Therapy,* 4th ed. St. Louis: Mosby–Year Book, Inc., 2001.

"Standard 33. Flow-Control Devices. Infusion Standards of Practice," *Journal of Infusion Nursing* 29(1S):S34-35, January-February 2006.

I.V. pumps

Various types of I.V. pumps electronically regulate the flow of I.V. solutions or drugs with great accuracy.

Volumetric pumps, used for high-pressure infusion of drugs or for the accurate delivery of fluids or drugs, have mechanisms to propel the solution at the desired rate under pressure. The peristaltic pump applies pressure to the I.V. tubing to force the solution through it. (Not all peristaltic pumps are volumetric; some count drops.) These pumps are also indicated for use with arterial lines. Most volumetric pumps operate at high pressures (up to 45 psi), delivering from 1 to 999 ml/hour with about 98% accuracy. **INS**

For the administration of vesicants, a low-pressure pump — one that operates at 10 to 25 psi — is the instrument of choice. The portable syringe pump, another type of volumetric pump, delivers small amounts of fluid over a long period. It's used for administering fluids to infants and for delivering intra-arterial drugs. Other specialized devices include the controlled-release infusion system, secondary syringe converter, and patient-controlled analgesia (PCA) device. **INS**

CLINICAL IMPACT *Pumps and tubing shouldn't allow for the free flow of I.V. solution for general use and for PCA I.V. infusion pumps used in the health care facility.* **JCAHO**

Pumps have various detectors and alarms that automatically signal or respond to the completion of an infusion, air in the line, low battery power, and occlusion or inability to deliver at the set rate. Depending

Infusion pumps

Infusion pumps electronically regulate the flow of I.V. solutions and drugs. You'll use them when a precise flow rate is required—for instance, when administering total parenteral nutrition solutions and chemotherapeutic or cardiovascular agents.

Infusion pump

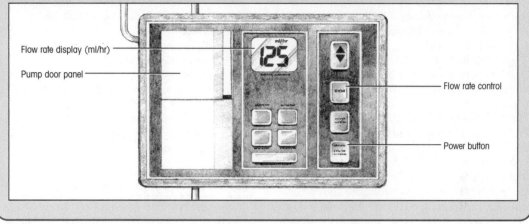

Flow rate display (ml/hr)

Pump door panel

Flow rate control

Power button

on the problem, these devices may sound or flash an alarm, shut off, or switch to a keep-vein-open rate.

Equipment

Peristaltic pump • I.V. pole • I.V. solution • sterile administration set • sterile peristaltic tubing or cassette, if needed • alcohol pads • adhesive tape

Tubing and cassettes vary with each manufacturer. (See *Infusion pumps*.)

Preparation of equipment
To set up a volumetric pump
● Attach the pump to the I.V. pole.
● Swab the port on the I.V. container with alcohol, insert the administration set spike, and fill the drip chamber *to prevent air bubbles from entering the tubing*.
● Prime the tubing and close the clamp. Follow the manufacturer's instructions for tubing placement. **MFR**

Implementation
● Position the pump on the same side of the bed as the I.V. or anticipated venipuncture site *to avoid crossing I.V. lines over the patient*. If necessary, perform the venipuncture. **INS**
● Plug in the machine and attach its tubing to the needle or catheter hub.
● Depending on the machine, turn it on and press the START button. Set the appropriate dials on the front panel to the desired infusion rate and volume. Always set the volume dial at 50 ml less than the prescribed volume or 50 ml less than the volume in the container *so that you can hang a new container before the old one empties*. **INS**
● Check the patency of the I.V. line and watch for infiltration.
● Tape all connections
● Turn on the alarm switches. Then explain the alarm system to the patient *to prevent anxiety when a change in the infusion activates the alarm*.

Special considerations
● Monitor the pump and the patient frequently *to ensure the device's correct operation and flow rate and to detect infiltration and such complications as infection and air embolism*.

● If electrical power fails, the pump will automatically switch to battery power.

● Check the manufacturer's recommendations before administering opaque fluids, such as blood, *because some pumps fail to detect opaque fluids and others may cause hemolysis of infused blood.* **MFR**

● Remove I.V. solutions from the refrigerator 1 hour before infusing them to help release small gas bubbles from the solutions. *Small bubbles in the solution can join to form larger bubbles, which can activate the pump's air-in-line alarm.*

TEACHING *Make sure that the patient and his family understand the purpose of using the pump. If necessary, demonstrate how it works. Also demonstrate how to maintain the system (tubing, solution, and site assessment and care) until you're confident that the patient and family can proceed safely. As time permits, have the patient repeat the demonstration. Discuss what complications to watch for, such as infiltration, and review the measures to take if complications occur. Schedule a teaching session with the patient or his family so you can answer questions they may have about the procedure before the patient's discharge.*

Nursing diagnoses
● Risk for infection
● Risk for injury

Expected outcomes
The patient will:
● maintain white blood cell and differential counts within normal limits
● have culture results that show no evidence of pathogens
● remain free from complications
● not develop signs and symptoms of extravasation.

Complications
● Complications associated with I.V. pumps are the same as those associated with peripheral lines. (See "Peripheral I.V. lines," page 152.)
● Keep in mind that infiltration can develop rapidly with infusion by a volumetric pump because the increased subcutaneous pressure won't slow the infusion rate until significant edema occurs.

Documentation
In addition to routine documentation of the I.V. infusion, record the use of a pump on the I.V. record and in your notes.

Supportive references
Joint Commission on Accreditation of Healthcare Organizations. *Comprehensive Accreditation Manual for Hospitals.* Oakbrook Terrace, Ill.: JCAHO, 2002. *www.jcaho.gov.*

Phillips, L.D. *Manual of I.V. Therapeutics,* 3rd ed. Philadelphia: F.A. Davis Co., 2001.

"Standard 33. Flow-Control Devices. Infusion Standards of Practice," *Journal of Infusion Nursing* 29(1S):S34-35, January-February 2006.

Weinstein, S.M. *Plumer's Principles and Practices of Intravenous Therapy,* 7th ed. Philadelphia: Lippincott Williams & Wilkins, 2001.

I.V. therapy preparation

Selection and preparation of equipment are essential for accurate delivery of an I.V. solution. Selection of an I.V. administration set depends on the rate and type of infusion and the type of I.V. solution container. There are two types of drip sets available, the macrodrip and the microdrip. The macrodrip set can deliver a solution in large quantities and at rapid rates because it delivers a larger amount of solution with each drop than the microdrip set. The microdrip set, used for pediatric patients and certain adult patients requiring small or closely regulated amounts of I.V. solution, delivers a smaller quantity of solution with each drop.

Administration tubing with a secondary injection port permits separate or simultaneous infusion of two solutions; tubing with a piggyback port and a back-check valve permits intermittent infusion of a secondary solution and, on its completion, a return to infusion of the primary solution. Vented I.V. tubing is selected for solutions in nonvented bottles; nonvented tubing is selected for solutions in bags or vented bottles. Assembly of I.V. equipment requires sterile technique *to prevent contamination, which can cause local or systemic infection.*

According to Infusion Nurses Society standards, primary and secondary sets should be changed every 72 hours, using sterile technique and immediately upon suspected contamination or when the integrity of the system has been compromised. **INS**

If a health care facility fails to maintain an ongoing phlebitis rate of 5% or less with the practice of 72-hour administration set changes, the sets should be changed every 48 hours. The same applies if there's an increased rate of catheter-related blood-stream infections. **INS**

✓ **CLINICAL IMPACT** *Patient allergies influence the selection and preparation of equipment for I.V. therapy. If the patient is allergic to latex, a life-threatening reaction may occur if you use latex-based products. It's recommended that the health care facility keep a latex-free cart to be used for a patient identified with true latex allergies to avoid hypersensitivity reactions.*

Equipment

I.V. solution • 2% chlorhexidine swabs • I.V. administration set • in-line (0.2 micron containing a membrane that's bacterial/particulate-retentive and also air-eliminating) filter, if needed • I.V. pole • medication and label, if necessary

Preparation of equipment

● Verify the type, volume, and expiration date of the I.V. solution. Discard outdated solution.
● If the solution is contained in a glass bottle, inspect the bottle for chips and cracks; if it's in a plastic bag, squeeze the bag *to detect leaks.*
● Examine the I.V. solution for particles, abnormal discoloration, and cloudiness. If present, discard the solution and notify the pharmacy or dispensing department.
● If ordered, add medication to the solution, and place a completed medication-added label on the container.
● Remove the administration set from its box, and check for cracks, holes, and missing clamps.

Implementation

● Wash your hands thoroughly *to prevent introducing contaminants during preparation.* **CDC**
● Slide the flow clamp of the administration set tubing down to the drip chamber or injection port, and close the clamp.

Setting up a bag

● Place the bag on a flat, stable surface or hang it on an I.V. pole.
● Remove the protective cap or tear the tab from the tubing insertion port.
● Remove the protective cap from the administration set spike.
● Holding the port firmly with one hand, insert the spike with your other hand.
● Hang the bag on the I.V. pole, if you haven't already, and squeeze the drip chamber until it's half full.

Setting up a nonvented bottle

● Remove the bottle's metal cap and inner disk, if present.
● Place the bottle on a stable surface and wipe the rubber stopper with an alcohol pad.
● Remove the protective cap from the administration set spike, and push the spike through the center of the bottle's rubber stopper. Avoid twisting or angling the spike *to prevent pieces of the stopper from breaking off and falling into the solution.*
● Invert the bottle. If its vacuum is intact, you'll hear a hissing sound and see air bubbles rise (this may not occur if you've already added medication). If the vacuum isn't intact, discard the bottle and begin again. **INS**
● Hang the bottle on the I.V. pole, and squeeze the drip chamber until it's half full.

Setting up a vented bottle

● Remove the bottle's metal cap and latex diaphragm *to release the vacuum.* If the vacuum isn't intact (except after medication has been added), discard the bottle and begin again.
● Place the bottle on a stable surface and wipe the rubber stopper with an alcohol pad.
● Remove the protective cap from the administration set spike, and push the spike through the insertion port next to the air vent tube opening.
● Hang the bottle on the I.V. pole, and squeeze the drip chamber until it's half full.

Priming the I.V. tubing

● If necessary, attach a filter to the opposite end of the I.V. tubing, and follow the manufacturer's instructions for filling and priming it. Purge the tubing be-

Indications for in-line filters

An in-line filter removes pathogens and particles from I.V. solutions, helping *to reduce the risk of infusion phlebitis.* Because an in-line filter is expensive and its installation is awkward and time-consuming, these filters aren't used routinely. Many health care facilities require that a filter be used only when administering an admixture. If you're unsure of whether to use a filter, check your facility's policy or follow this list of do's and don'ts.

Do's

Use an in-line filter:
- when administering solutions to an immunodeficient patient
- when administering total parenteral nutrition
- when using additives comprising many separate particles, such as antibiotics requiring reconstitution, or when administering several additives
- when using rubber injection ports or plastic diaphragms repeatedly
- when phlebitis is likely to occur.

Change the in-line filter according to the manufacturer's recommendations (and with administration set change). **MFR** *If you don't, bacteria trapped in the filter releases endotoxin, a pyrogen small enough to pass through the filter into the bloodstream.*

Use an add-on filter of larger pore size (1.2 microns) when infusing lipid emulsions or total nutrient admixtures that require filtration.

If a positive-pressure electronic infusion device is used, consider the pound per square inch (psi) rating of the filter. If the psi from the infusion device exceeds that of the filter, the filter will crack or break under the pressure.

Don'ts

Don't use an in-line filter:
- when administering solutions with large particles *that will clog a filter and stop I.V. flow,* such as blood and its components, suspensions, lipid emulsions, and high-molecular-volume plasma expanders
- when administering a drug dose of 5 mg or less *(because the filter may absorb it).*

fore attaching the filter *to avoid forcing air into the filter and, possibly, clogging some filter channels.* Most filters are positioned with the distal end of the tubing facing upward *so that the solution will completely wet the filter membrane and all air bubbles will be eliminated from the line.* (See *Indications for in-line filters.*) **MFR**
- If you aren't using a filter, aim the distal end of the tubing over a wastebasket or sink and slowly open the flow clamp. (Most distal tube coverings allow the solution to flow without having to remove the protective cover.)
- Leave the clamp open until the I.V. solution flows through the entire length of tubing *to release trapped air bubbles and force out all the air.*
- Invert all Y-ports and backcheck valves and tap them, if necessary, *to fill them with solution.*
- After priming the tubing, close the clamp. Then loop the tubing over the I.V. pole.
- Label the container with the patient's name and room number, date and time, the container number, ordered rate and duration of infusion, and your initials.

Special considerations

- Before initiation of I.V. therapy, the patient should be told what to expect. (See *Teaching about I.V. therapy.*)
- Always use sterile technique when preparing I.V. solutions. If you contaminate the administration set or container, replace it with a new one *to prevent introducing contaminants into the system.* **INS**
- If necessary, you can use vented tubing with a vented bottle. To do this, don't remove the latex diaphragm. Instead, insert the spike into the larger indentation in the diaphragm.
- Change I.V. tubing every 48 or 72 hours according to your facility's policy or more frequently if you suspect contamination. Change the filter according to the manufacturer's recommendations or sooner if it becomes clogged. **INS** **MFR**

CONTROVERSIAL ISSUE *Controversy exists regarding the reuse of single-use equipment for I.V. therapy. Regulatory, ethical, financial, and liability risks exist and must be considered when reusing equipment. If your facility allocates reuse of single-item equipment, check the policy regarding this, and consult expert resources to help determine if this use is indeed valid to practice.*

TEACHING

Teaching about I.V. therapy

Many patients are apprehensive about peripheral I.V. therapy, so before you begin to administer such therapy, tell your patient what to expect before, during, and after the procedure. Thorough patient teaching *can reduce anxiety, making therapy easier. Follow these guidelines.*

Before insertion
● Describe the procedure. Tell the patient that "intravenous" means inside the vein and that a plastic catheter or needle will be placed in his vein. Explain that fluids containing certain nutrients or medications will flow from a bag or bottle through a length of tubing and then through the plastic catheter or needle into his vein.
● Tell the patient about how long the catheter or needle will stay in place. Explain that the physician will decide how much and what type of fluid the patient needs.
● If the patient will receive a local anesthetic at the insertion site, ask him if he's allergic to lidocaine. If in doubt, use another anesthetic. Tell him that this injection will numb the site to reduce the pain of I.V. device insertion.
● If no anesthetic will be used, tell the patient that he may feel transient pain at the insertion site but that the discomfort will stop after the catheter or needle is in place.
● Tell the patient that I.V. fluid may feel cold at first but that this sensation should last only a few minutes.

During therapy
● Instruct the patient to report any discomfort after the catheter or needle has been inserted and the fluid has begun to flow.
● Explain any restrictions as ordered. As appropriate, tell the patient that he may be able to walk and, depending on the insertion site and the device, to shower or take a tub bath during therapy.
● Teach the patient how to care for the I.V. line. Tell him not to pull at the insertion site or tubing, not to remove the container from the I.V. pole, and not to kink the tubing or lie on it. Instruct him to call a nurse if the flow rate suddenly slows or speeds up.

At removal
● Explain that removing a peripheral I.V. line is a simple procedure. Tell the patient that pressure will be applied to the site until the bleeding stops. Reassure him that after the device is out and the bleeding stops, he'll be able to use the affected arm or leg as before therapy.

Nursing diagnoses
● Risk for injury

Expected outcomes
The patient will:
● remain free from injury and complications.

Documentation
Document the type of solution used and any additives to the solution. (See *Documenting insertion of a venipuncture device,* page 146.)

Supportive references
Gritter, M. "Latex Allergy: Prevention is the Key," *Journal of Intravenous Nursing* 22(5):281-85, September-October 1999.

Joint Commission on Accreditation of Healthcare Organizations. *Comprehensive Accreditation Manual for Hospitals.* Oakbrook Terrace, Ill.: JCAHO, 2002. *www.jcaho.gov.*

"Standard 11. Patient Education. Infusion Nursing Standards of Practice," *Journal of Infusion Nursing* 29(1S):S19-20, January-February 2006.

"Standard 14. Documentation. Infusion Nursing Standards of Practice," *Journal of Infusion Nursing* 29(1S):S22-23, January-February 2006.

"Standard 32. Filters. Infusion Nursing Standards of Practice," *Journal of Infusion Nursing* 29(1S):S33-34, January-February 2006.

Tan, M.W. "Reuse of Single-Use Equipment: The Intravenous Nurse Specialist's Role in Institutional Policy Development," *Journal of Intravenous Nursing* 22(1):11-13, January-February 1999.

Documenting insertion of a venipuncture device

After you establish an I.V. route, remember to document the date, time, and venipuncture site together with the equipment used, such as the type and gauge of catheter or needle. Record how the patient tolerated the procedure and any patient teaching that you performed with the patient and his family, such as explaining the purpose of I.V. therapy, describing the procedure itself, and discussing possible complications.

You'll need to update your records each time you change the insertion site and change the venipuncture device or I.V. tubing. Also document reason for changing the I.V. site, such as extravasation, phlebitis, occlusion, patient removal, or routine change according to your facility's policy.

Weinstein, S.M. *Plumer's Principles and Practices of Intravenous Therapy,* 7th ed. Philadelphia: Lippincott Williams & Wilkins, 2001.

Medication error reduction

The National Coordinating Council for Medication Error Reporting and Prevention defines a medication error as "any preventable event that may cause or lead to inappropriate medication use or patient harm while the medication is in the control of the health care professional, patient, or consumer. **NCCMERP** Such events may be related to professional practice, health care products, procedures, and systems, including prescribing; order communication; product labeling, packaging, and nomenclature; compounding; dispensing; distribution; administration; education; monitoring; and use."

A 1999 report by the Institute of Medicine (IOM) found that medication errors are the most common cause of medical errors in the hospital and affect 3.7% of patients. Medical errors accounted for 44,000 to 98,000 deaths each year, with the total cost of medical errors estimated at $17 to $29 billion annually. **IOM**

To reduce medication errors, the Institute for Safe Medication Practices (ISMP) recommends that health care facilities set up a multidisciplinary team. At a minimum, the team should be comprised of front-line practitioners — physicians, pharmacists, and nurses who have intimate knowledge of the medication use processes; a strong facilitator, such as a risk management or quality improvement professional, to handle the day-to-day team issues; a representative from high-level administration for support and quick decision-making; and another physician who's willing to help promote medication safety initiatives. The team's goals should include:
- promoting a nonpunitive approach to reducing medication errors and increasing detection and reporting of medication errors
- educating practitioners about the system-based causes of errors and their prevention and exploring the cause of medication errors
- responding to potentially hazardous situations (such as medication labeling) before errors occur
- recommending and facilitating hospitalwide, system-based changes to prevent medication errors. **ISMP**

Key nursing steps in reducing errors

Taking the following steps can help reduce the risk of medication errors.

Know your patient

Studies have shown that preventable adverse drug events occur because the practitioner doesn't know enough about the patient — for example, awareness of a patient's drug allergies — before prescribing, dispensing, and administering medications. Having information about the patient helps the primary care provider determine appropriate medications, dosages, and administration routes. Information such as height, weight, allergies, medical history, and pregnancy status as well as vital signs and laboratory values are key to monitoring the effects of medications and the underlying disease process. This information should be communicated to the pharmacist so that he can properly screen all medication orders before dispensing them.

Properly identify your patient

Knowing your patient isn't enough to prevent a medication error. Each time you administer a medication, you must confirm the patient's identity using two patient identifiers, aside from the patient's room number, according to facility policy. **JCAHO**

Know the medications

Keeping abreast of new drug therapies is important. Not knowing about current therapies can be as risky as not knowing your patient. Most serious medication errors occur because the patient receives the wrong medication or the wrong dose. Errors in medication dosing usually occur due to miscommunication or miscalculation. To get up-to-date information about medications, use various sources, such as textbooks, a controlled drug formulary, drug protocols, dosing scales and order sets, medication administration records, and communication with your in-house pharmacy.

Communicate

Miscommunication is one of the major causes of medication errors. It could result from:
● absence of a standardized prescribing vocabulary. At least 1 in 10 medication errors is directly related to the use of incorrect drug names, confusing use of dosage forms, or misunderstood abbreviations. The Joint Commission for Accreditation of Healthcare Organization's National Patient Safety Goals require the use of standardized abbreviations, acronyms, and symbols. Using a standardized prescribing vocabulary eliminates the use of acronyms, "coined names," and confusing abbreviations, which aids in preventing medication errors. (See *Commonly miscommunicated abbreviations,* page 148.)
● incorrect decimal point placement. This could cause serious harm to the patient. When the dose is less than 1, a zero should always precede the decimal, and a zero should never appear after a whole number — for example, 2 mg shouldn't appear as 2.0 mg because if the decimal point is missed, the patient could receive 10 times the prescribed dose. **JCAHO**
● verbal orders. Although convenient for the prescriber, verbal orders can easily be misheard and should only be used in an emergency. The protocol for verbal orders should include safety checks, such as having another nurse on the phone when taking a verbal order by telephone, restating the patient's name, spelling out the drug name, and repeating the dosage to the prescriber. After receiving the verbal order, you should immediately write it in the patient's chart. In instances when the prescriber attempts to give a verbal order while visiting a patient, request that he write the order in the patient's chart instead. **JCAHO**
● intimidation. This can commonly hinder effective communication between health care professionals. The problem may be compounded further if the facility doesn't have a policy on how to settle disagreements about the safety of orders. It's important to speak up and get answers about any order that doesn't seem to be right.

Watch for drugs that sound alike

Confusion over drug names that sound alike is one of the most common reasons pharmacies dispense and nurses administer the wrong drug. Adding to the problem are label packaging and confusing labels. One way to reduce the risk of dispensing and administering the wrong drug is to store drugs with similar packaging separate from one another.

Improper labeling coupled with the lack of a unit-dose system also contribute to faulty drug identification. To avoid this factor, ask the pharmacist to send up prefilled, prelabeled syringes of medications, such as heparin, sodium chloride solution flushes, and opioids. In addition, use blank labels that can be easily added to the needles, even if you intend to administer the medication right away. Otherwise, prepare the patient's medication at the bedside and administer it right away.

The IOM has developed strategies to improve medication safety. Some key strategies are:
● implementing a standard process for medication doses, dose timing, and dose scales in a given patient care unit
● standardizing prescription writing and prescribing rules (for example, including the purpose of the prescribed medication)
● using pharmaceutical software
● having a central pharmacy supply dispense high-risk I.V. medications such as chemotherapeutic drugs
● limiting the type of medications stored on patient care units

Commonly miscommunicated abbreviations JCAHO

The Joint Commission on the Accreditation of Healthcare Organizations has approved the following "minimum list" of abbreviations, acronyms, and symbols that are dangerous when handwritten imprecisely. Using this list can help to protect patients from the effects of miscommunication in clinical documentation. In addition, those abbreviations, acronyms, and symbols slated for possible future inclusion are also listed.

Do not use	Potential problem	Preferred term
U (for unit)	Mistaken as zero, four, or cc	Write out "unit"
IU (for international unit)	Mistaken as IV (intravenous) or 10 (ten)	Write out "international unit"
Q.D., QD, q.d., qd (daily) Q.O.D., QOD, q.o.d., qod (every other day)	Mistaken for each other; the period after the Q can be mistaken for an "I"; the "O" also can be mistaken for an "I"	Write out "daily" or "every other day"
Trailing zero (X.0 mg) (*Note:* Prohibited only for medication-related notations), lack of leading zero (.X mg)	Decimal point is missed	Never write a zero by itself after a decimal point (X mg), and always use a zero before a decimal point (0.X mg)
MS, MSO_4, $MgSO_4$	Confused for one another; can mean morphine sulfate or magnesium sulfate	Write out "morphine sulfate" or "magnesium sulfate"

Additional abbreviations, acronyms, and symbols (for possible future inclusion)

> (greater than) < (less than)	Misinterpreted as the number "7" (seven) or the letter "L" Confused for each another	Write "greater than" Write "less than"
Abbreviations for drug names	Misinterpreted due to similar abbreviations for multiple drugs	Write drug names in full
Apothecary units	Unfamiliar to many practitioners Confused with metric units	Use metric units
@	Mistaken for the number "2" (two)	Write "at"
cc	Mistaken for U (units) when poorly written	Write "ml" or "milliliters"
µg	Mistaken for mg (milligrams) resulting in 1,000-fold overdose	Write "mcg" or "micrograms"

● including the pharmacist on patient rounds in the units. **IOM**

In general, implementing simple strategies and working with a team to improve medication prescription, administration, and dispensing of drugs helps reduce medication errors. When medication orders don't seem quite right, pharmacists, nurses, and physicians must take the extra step to verify an order before a medication is prescribed, dispensed, or administered to a patient.

Supportive references

Bond, C.A., et al. "Medication Errors in United States Hospitals," *Pharmacotherapy* 21(9):1023-36, July 2001.

"Please Don't Sleep Through This Wake-up Call," *ISMP Medication Safety Alert!* May 2, 2001. *www.ismp.org.*

"A Multidisciplinary Team is Essential to Medication Error Reduction Education," *ISMP Medication Safety Alert!* March 8, 2000. *www.ismp.org.*

JCAHO 2005 National Patient Safety Goals. Comprehensive Accreditation Manual for Hospitals: The Official Handbook, November 2005.

Smetzer, J. "Take 10 Giant Steps to Medication Safety," *Nursing2001* 31(11):49, November 2001.

Peripheral I.V. line maintenance

Routine maintenance of I.V. sites and systems includes the regular assessment and rotation of the site and periodic changes of the dressing, tubing, and solution. **INS** These measures help prevent complications, such as thrombophlebitis and infection. They should be performed according to your facility's policy. Typically, gauze I.V. dressings are changed every 48 hours or whenever the dressing becomes wet, soiled, or nonocclusive.

Transparent semipermeable dressings are changed whenever I.V. tubing is changed (every 48 to 72 hours or according to your facility's policy), and I.V. solution is changed every 24 hours or as needed. The site should be assessed every 2 hours if a transparent semipermeable dressing is used or with every dressing change otherwise and should be rotated every 48 to 72 hours. Sometimes limited venous access will prevent frequent site changes; if so, be sure to assess the site frequently. **INS**

Equipment
Dressing changes
Sterile gloves ● antiseptic solution ● adhesive bandage, sterile 2″ × 2″ gauze pad, or transparent semipermeable dressing ● 1″ adhesive tape

Solution changes
Solution container ● alcohol pad

Tubing changes
I.V. administration set ● sterile gloves ● sterile 2″ × 2″ gauze pad ● adhesive tape for labeling ● optional: hemostats

I.V. site changes
Commercial kits containing the equipment for dressing changes are available.

Preparation of equipment
● If your facility keeps I.V. equipment and dressings in a tray or cart, have it nearby, if possible, *because you may have to select a new venipuncture site, depending on the current site's condition.*
● If you're changing the solution and the tubing, attach and prime the I.V. administration set before entering the patient's room.

Implementation
● Wash your hands thoroughly *to prevent the spread of microorganisms.* Remember to wear sterile gloves when working near the venipuncture site. **CDC**
● Confirm the patient's identity using two patient identifiers according to facility policy. **JCAHO**
● Explain the procedure to the patient *to allay his fears and ensure cooperation.* **PCP**

Changing the dressing
● Remove the old dressing, open all supply packages, and put on sterile gloves.
● Hold the cannula in place with your nondominant hand *to prevent accidental movement or dislodgment, which could puncture the vein and cause infiltration.*
● Assess the venipuncture site for signs of infection (redness and pain at the puncture site), infiltration (coolness, blanching, and edema at the site), and thrombophlebitis (redness, firmness, pain along the path of the vein, and edema). If any such signs are present, cover the area with a sterile 2″ × 2″ gauze

pad and remove the catheter or needle. Apply pressure on the area until the bleeding stops, and apply an adhesive bandage. Then using fresh equipment and solution, start the I.V. line in another appropriate site, preferably on the opposite extremity. **INS**

● If the venipuncture site is intact, stabilize the cannula and carefully clean around the puncture site with the antiseptic solution. Depending on the solution selected, follow the manufacturer's directions.

● Cover the site with a transparent semipermeable dressing. *The transparent dressing allows visualization of the insertion site and maintains sterility.* It's placed over the insertion site to halfway up the hub of the cannula.

Changing the solution

● Wash your hands. **CDC**

● Inspect the new solution container for cracks, leaks, and other damage. Check the solution for discoloration, turbidity, and particulates. Note the date and time the solution was mixed and its expiration date. **INS**

● Clamp the tubing when inverting it *to prevent air from entering the tubing.* Keep the drip chamber half full. **INS**

● If you're replacing a bag, remove the seal or tab from the new bag and remove the old bag from the pole. Remove the spike, insert it into the new bag, and adjust the flow rate.

● If you're replacing a bottle, remove the cap and seal from the new bottle and wipe the rubber port with an alcohol pad. Clamp the line, remove the spike from the old bottle, and insert the spike into the new bottle. Then hang the new bottle and adjust the flow rate.

Changing the tubing

● Reduce the I.V. flow rate, remove the old spike from the container, and hang it on the I.V. pole. Place the cover of the new spike loosely over the old one.

● Keeping the old spike in an upright position above the patient's heart level, insert the new spike into the I.V. container (as shown at top of next column).

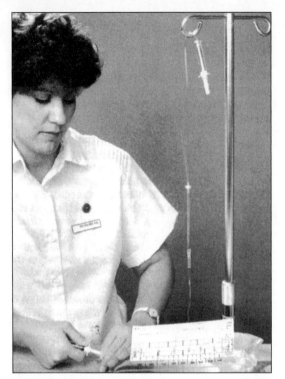

● Prime the system. Hang the new I.V. container and primed set on the pole, and grasp the new adapter in one hand. Then stop the flow rate in the old tubing.

● Put on sterile gloves. **CDC**

● Place a sterile gauze pad under the needle or cannula hub *to create a sterile field.* Press one of your fingers over the cannula *to prevent bleeding.* **INS**

● Gently disconnect the old tubing (as shown at top of next page), being careful not to dislodge or move the I.V. device. (If you have trouble disconnecting the old tubing, use a hemostat to hold the hub securely while twisting the tubing *to remove it.* Or, use one hemostat on the venipuncture device and another on the hard plastic end of the tubing. Then pull the hemostats in opposite directions. Don't clamp the hemostats shut; *this may crack the tubing adapter or the venipuncture device.*)

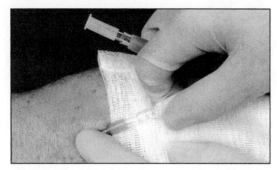

● Remove the protective cap from the new tubing, and connect the new adapter to the cannula tip. Hold the hub securely *to prevent dislodging the needle or cannula tip.*
● Observe for blood backflow into the new tubing *to verify that the needle or cannula is still in place.* (You may not be able to do this with small-gauge cannulas.)
● Adjust the clamp *to maintain the appropriate flow rate.*
● Retape the cannula hub and I.V. tubing, and recheck the I.V. flow rate *because taping may alter it.*
● Label the new tubing and container with the date and time. Label the solution container with a time strip.

Special considerations
● Check the prescribed I.V. flow rate before each solution change *to prevent errors.* If you crack the adapter or hub (or if you accidentally dislodge the cannula from the vein), remove the cannula. Apply pressure and an adhesive bandage *to stop any bleeding.* Perform a venipuncture at another site and restart the I.V.

Nursing diagnoses
● Deficient knowledge (procedure)
● Risk for injury

Expected outcomes
The patient will:
● state an understanding of the need for I.V. therapy
● remain free from injury or complications.

Documentation
Record the time, date, and rate and type of solution (and any additives) on the I.V. flowchart. Also record this information, dressing or tubing changes, and the site's appearance in your notes.

Supportive references
Calamandrei, M., et al. "Comparison of Two Application Techniques of EMLA and Pain Assessment in Pediatric Oncology Patients," *Regional Anesthesia* 21(6):557-60, November-December 1996.

Mermel, L.A. "Prevention of Intravascular Catheter-Related Infections," *Annals of Internal Medicine* 132(5):391-402, March 2000.

Metheny, N.M. *Fluid and Electrolyte Balance: Nursing Considerations,* 4th ed. Philadelphia: Lippincott Williams & Wilkins, 2000.

"Standard 36. Tourniquet. Infusion Nursing Standards of Practice," *Journal of Infusion Nursing* 29(1S):S36, January-February 2006.

"Standard 37. Site Selection. Infusion Nursing Standards of Practice," *Journal of Infusion Nursing* 29(1S):S37-39, January-February 2006.

"Standard 38. Catheter Selection. Infusion Nursing Standards of Practice," *Journal of Infusion Nursing* 29(1S):S39-40, January-February 2006.

"Standard 39. Hair Removal. Infusion Nursing Standards of Practice," *Journal of Infusion Nursing* 29(1S):S40-41, January-February 2006.

"Standard 40. Local Anesthesia. Infusion Nursing Standards of Practice," *Journal of Infusion Nursing* 29(1S):S41, January-February 2006.

"Standard 41. Access Site Preparation. Infusion Nursing Standards of Practice," *Journal of Infusion Nursing* 29(1S):S41-42, January-February 2006.

"Standard 42. Catheter Placement. Infusion Nursing Standards of Practice," *Journal of Infusion Nursing* 29(1S):S42-44, January-February 2006.

"Standard 43. Catheter Stabilization. Infusion Nursing Standards of Practice," *Journal of Infusion Nursing* 29(1S):S44, January-February 2006.

"Standard 44. Dressings. Infusion Nursing Standards of Practice," *Journal of Infusion Nursing* 29(1S):S44-45, January-February 2006.

"Standard 53. Phlebitis. Infusion Nursing Standards of Practice," *Journal of Infusion Nursing* 29(1S):S58-59, January-February 2006.

"Standard 54. Infiltration. Infusion Nursing Standards of Practice," *Journal of Infusion Nursing* 29(1S):S59-60, January-February 2006.

Weinstein, S.M. *Plumer's Principles and Practice of Intravenous Therapy,* 7th ed. Philadelphia: Lippincott Williams & Wilkins, 2001.

Welk, T. "Clinical and Ethical Considerations of Fluid and Electrolyte Management in the Terminally Ill Client," *Journal of Intravenous Nursing* 22(1):43-47, January-February 1999.

Peripheral I.V. lines

Peripheral I.V. line insertion involves the selection of a venipuncture device and an insertion site, application of a tourniquet, preparation of the site, and venipuncture. A peripheral line allows administration of fluids, medication, blood, and blood components and maintains I.V. access to the patient. If possible, choose a vein in the nondominant arm or hand.

Selection of a venipuncture device and site depends on the type of solution to be used; frequency and duration of the infusion; patency and location of accessible veins; the patient's age, size, and condition; and, when possible, the patient's preference. The same nurse should make no more than two attempts; if unsuccessful after two tries, consult the I.V. team, nurse-anesthetist, or anesthesia physician or resident. **INS**

Preferred venipuncture sites are the cephalic and basilic veins in the lower arm and the veins in the dorsum of the hand; least favorable are the leg and foot veins *because of the increased risk of thrombophlebitis and infection.* Antecubital veins can be used if no other venous access is available *to accommodate a large-bore needle* or *to administer drugs that require large-volume dilution.* **INS**

Insertion is contraindicated in a sclerotic vein, an edematous or impaired arm or hand, or a postmastectomy arm, and in patients with a mastectomy, burns, or an arteriovenous fistula. Subsequent venipunctures should be performed proximal to a previously used or injured vein. If the I.V. line has to be inserted in the mastectomy arm or one with impaired circulation, a physician should be contacted and an order written before starting therapy. **INS**

CONTROVERSIAL ISSUE *Controversy exists as to whether to provide hydration in certain* populations of patients such as the terminally ill. *Not providing hydration to patients who can no longer ingest an adequate amount of fluid may be seen as negligence in meeting a patient's basic needs and may shorten his life span. Various factors need to be considered (clinical, ethical, legal, and emotional) when you're deciding on the appropriateness or inappropriateness of using available technology to provide hydration and nutrition.*

Equipment

Antiseptic solution • gloves • tourniquet (rubber tubing or a blood pressure cuff) • I.V. access devices • I.V. solution with attached and primed administration set • I.V. pole • sharps container • sterile 2″ × 2″ gauze pads or a transparent semipermeable dressing • 1″ hypoallergenic tape • optional: arm board, roller gauze, tube gauze, warm packs, scissors

Commercial venipuncture kits come with or without an I.V. access device. (See *Comparing basic venous access devices.*) In many health care facilities, venipuncture equipment is kept on a tray or cart, allowing more choice of correct access devices and easy replacement of contaminated items.

Preparation of equipment

● Check the information on the label of the I.V. solution container, including the patient's name and room number, the type of solution, the time and date of its preparation, the preparer's name, and the ordered infusion rate.

● Compare the physician's orders with the solution label *to verify that the solution is the correct one.*

● Select the appropriate-gauge device that's best for the infusion unless subsequent therapy will require a larger one. *Smaller gauges cause less trauma to veins, allow greater blood flow around their tips, and reduce clotting risk.*

● If you're using a winged infusion set, connect the adapter to the administration set, and unclamp the line until fluid flows from the open end of the needle cover.

● Close the clamp, and place the needle on a sterile surface such as the inside of its packaging.

● If you're using a catheter device, open its package *to allow easy access.*

Comparing basic venous access devices

Use the chart below to compare the two major types of venous access devices

Over-the-needle catheter
Purpose
- Long-term therapy for the active or agitated patient

Advantages
- Inadvertent puncture of vein less likely than with a winged steel needle set
- More comfortable for the patient
- Radiopaque thread for easy location
- Syringe attached to some units that permits easy check of blood return and prevents air from entering the vessel on insertion
- Safety needles that prevent accidental needle sticks
- Activity-restricting device, such as arm board, rarely required

Disadvantages
- Difficult to insert
- Extra care required to ensure that needle and catheter are inserted into vein

Winged steel needle set
Purpose
- Short-term therapy (such as single-dose infusion) for cooperative adult patient
- Therapy of any duration for an infant or a child or for an elderly patient with fragile or sclerotic veins

Advantages
- Easiest intravascular device to insert because needle is thin-walled and extremely sharp
- Ideal for nonirritating I.V. push drugs
- Available with catheter that can be left in place like over-the-needle catheter

Disadvantage
- Infiltration easily caused if rigid needle winged infusion device is used

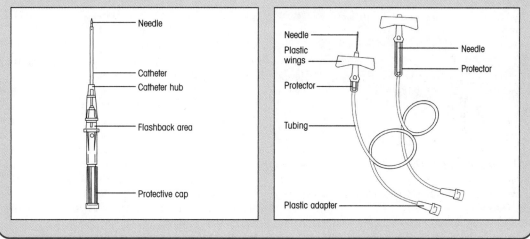

Implementation
- Place the I.V. pole in the proper slot in the patient's bed frame. If you're using a portable I.V. pole, position it close to the patient.
- Hang the I.V. solution with attached primed administration set on the I.V. pole.
- Verify the patient's identity by comparing the information on the solution container with the patient's wristband.
- Wash your hands thoroughly. **CDC**
- Explain the procedure to the patient *to ensure cooperation and reduce anxiety. Anxiety can cause a vasomotor response resulting in venous constriction.* **PCP**

Selecting the site

● Select the puncture site. If long-term therapy is anticipated, start with a vein at the most distal site *so that you can move proximally as needed for subsequent I.V. insertion sites*. To infuse an irritating medication, choose a large vein distal to a nearby joint. Make sure that the intended vein can accommodate the cannula. **INS**

● Place the patient in a comfortable, reclining position, leaving the arm in a dependent position *to increase capillary refill of the lower arms and hands*. If the patient's skin is cold, warm it by rubbing and stroking the arm, or cover the entire arm with warm packs for 5 to 10 minutes.

Applying the tourniquet

● Apply a tourniquet about 4″ to 6″ (10 to 15 cm) above the intended puncture site *to dilate the vein* (as shown below). Check for a radial pulse. If it isn't present, release the tourniquet and reapply it with less tension *to prevent arterial occlusion*. **INS**

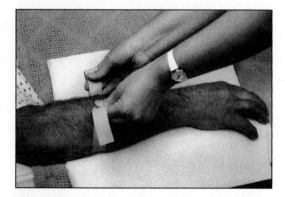

● Lightly palpate the vein with the index and middle fingers of your nondominant hand. Stretch the skin *to anchor the vein*. If the vein feels hard or ropelike, select another.

● If the vein is easily palpable but not sufficiently dilated, one or more of the following techniques may help raise the vein. Place the extremity in a dependent position for several seconds, and gently tap your finger over the vein or rub or stroke the skin upward toward the tourniquet. If you've selected a vein in the arm or hand, tell the patient to open and close his fist several times.

● Leave the tourniquet in place for no more than 3 minutes. If you can't find a suitable vein and prepare the site in that time, release the tourniquet for a few minutes. Then reapply it and continue the procedure. **INS**

Preparing the site

● Put on gloves. Clip the hair around the insertion site if needed. Clean the site with an antiseptic solution, such as 2% chlorhexidine, according to your facility's policy and manufacturer's directions.

● If ordered, administer a local anesthetic. Make sure that the patient isn't sensitive to lidocaine.

✓ CLINICAL IMPACT *Lidocaine or other injectable local anesthetics shouldn't be used routinely for insertion of a peripheral I.V. line. Other types of local anesthesia, such as iontophoresis or topical transdermal agents, may be considered and used according to your facility's policy and procedures as well as manufacturer guidelines. Topical agents (such as EMLA cream) may need to be applied up to 30 minutes before insertion of the I.V. line and may be helpful for select populations such as pediatric patients.* **MFR**

● Lightly press the vein with the thumb of your nondominant hand about 1½″ (3.8 cm) from the intended insertion site. The vein should feel round, firm, fully engorged, and resilient.

● Grasp the access cannula. If you're using a winged infusion set, hold the short edges of the wings (with the needle's bevel facing upward) between the thumb and forefinger of your dominant hand. Then squeeze the wings together. If you're using an over-the-needle cannula, grasp the plastic hub with your dominant hand, remove the cover, and examine the cannula tip. If the edge isn't smooth, discard and replace the device. If you're using a through-the-needle cannula, grasp the needle hub with one hand, and unsnap the needle cover. Then rotate the access device until the bevel faces upward.

● Using the thumb of your nondominant hand, stretch the skin taut below the puncture site *to stabilize the vein* (as shown at top of next page).

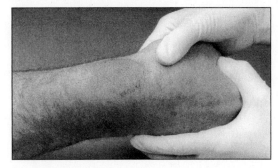

- Tell the patient that you're about to insert the device.
- Hold the needle bevel up and enter the skin directly over the vein at a 15- to 25-degree angle (as shown below).

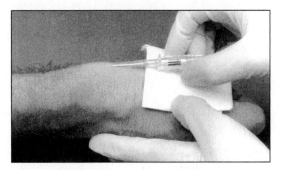

- Aggressively push the needle directly through the skin and into the vein in one motion. Check the flashback chamber behind the hub for blood return, *signifying that the vein has been properly accessed.* (You may not see a blood return in a small vein.) **INS**
- Level the insertion device slightly by lifting the tip of the device up *to prevent puncturing the back wall of the vein with the access device.*
- If you're using a winged infusion set, advance the needle fully, if possible, and hold it in place. Release the tourniquet, open the administration set clamp slightly, and check for free flow or infiltration.
- If you're using an over-the-needle cannula, advance the device 2 to 3 mm *to ensure that the cannula itself — not just the introducer needle — has entered the vein.* Then remove the tourniquet. **INS**
- Grasp the cannula hub to hold it in the vein, and withdraw the needle. As you withdraw it, press lightly on the catheter tip *to prevent bleeding* (as shown at top of next column).

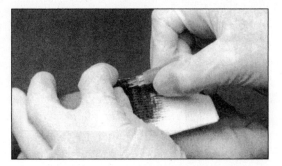

- Advance the cannula up to the hub or until you meet resistance.
- To advance the cannula while infusing I.V. solution, release the tourniquet and remove the inner needle. Using sterile technique, attach the I.V. tubing and begin the infusion. While stabilizing the vein with one hand, use the other to advance the catheter into the vein. When the catheter is advanced, decrease the I.V. flow rate. *This method reduces the risk of puncturing the vein's opposite wall because the catheter is advanced without the steel needle and because the rapid flow dilates the vein.*
- To advance the cannula before starting the infusion, first release the tourniquet. While stabilizing the vein with one hand, use the other to advance the catheter up to the hub (as shown below). Next, remove the inner needle and, using sterile technique, quickly attach the I.V. tubing. *This method typically results in less blood being spilled.*

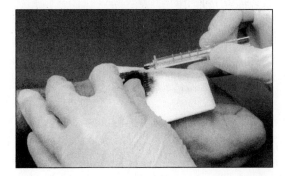

- If you're using a through-the-needle cannula, remove the tourniquet, hold the needle in place with one hand and, with your opposite hand, grasp the cannula through the protective sleeve. Then slowly thread the cannula through the needle until the hub

Applying a transparent semipermeable dressing

To secure the I.V. insertion site, you can apply a transparent semipermeable dressing as follows:

- Make sure that the insertion site is clean and dry.
- Remove the dressing from the package and, using sterile technique, remove the protective seal. Avoid touching the sterile surface.
- Place the dressing directly over the insertion site and the hub, as shown. Don't cover the tubing. Also, don't stretch the dressing; *doing so may cause itching.*

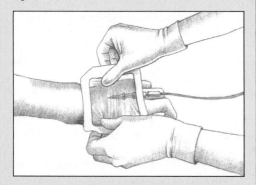

- Tuck the dressing around and under the cannula hub *to make the site impervious to microorganisms.*
- To remove the dressing, grasp one corner, and then lift and stretch it. If removal is difficult, try loosening the edges with alcohol or water.

is within the needle collar. Never pull back on the cannula without pulling back on the needle *to avoid severing and releasing the cannula into the circulation, causing an embolus.* If you feel resistance from the valve, withdraw the cannula and needle slightly and reinsert them, rotating the cannula as you pass the valve. Then withdraw the metal needle, split the needle along the perforated edge (according to the manufacturer's instructions), and carefully remove it from around the cannula. Dispose of the needle pieces appropriately. Remove the stylet and protective sleeve, and attach the administration set to the cannula hub. Open the administration set clamp slightly, and check for free flow or infiltration. **INS** **MFR**

Dressing the site

- After the venous access device has been inserted, clean the skin completely. If necessary, dispose of the stylet in a sharps container. **CDC** Then regulate the flow rate.
- You may use a transparent semipermeable dressing *to secure the device.* (See *Applying a transparent semipermeable dressing.*)
- If you don't use a transparent dressing, cover the I.V. site with a sterile gauze pad or small adhesive bandage. **INS**
- Loop the I.V. tubing on the patient's limb, and secure the tubing with tape. *The loop allows some slack to prevent dislodgment of the cannula from tension on the line.* (See *Taping a venous access site.*)
- Label the last piece of tape with the type, needle gauge, and cannula length; insertion date and time; and your initials. Adjust the flow rate as ordered.
- If the puncture site is near a movable joint, place a padded arm board under the joint and secure it with roller gauze or tape *to provide stability because excessive movement can dislodge the venous access device and increase the risk of thrombophlebitis and infection.* **INS**

Removing a peripheral I.V. line

- A peripheral I.V. line is removed on completion of therapy, for cannula site changes, and for suspected infection or infiltration; the procedure usually requires gloves, a sterile gauze pad, and an adhesive bandage. **CDC** **INS**
- To remove the I.V. line, first clamp the I.V. tubing *to stop the flow of solution.* Then gently remove the transparent dressing and all tape from the skin.
- Using sterile technique, open the gauze pad and adhesive bandage and place them within reach. Put on gloves. Hold the sterile gauze pad over the puncture site with one hand, and use your other hand to withdraw the cannula slowly and smoothly, keeping it parallel to the skin. (Inspect the cannula tip; if it isn't smooth, assess the patient immediately, and notify the physician.) **INS**
- Using the gauze pad, apply firm pressure over the puncture site for 1 to 2 minutes after removal or until bleeding has stopped. **INS**
- Clean the site and apply the adhesive bandage or, if blood oozes, apply a pressure bandage.
- If drainage appears at the puncture site, send the tip of the device and a sample of the drainage to the

Taping a venous access site

When using tape to secure the access device to the insertion site, use one of the basic methods described here. Use only sterile tape under a transparent semipermeable dressing.

Chevron method

- Cut a long strip of ½" tape and place it sticky side up under the cannula and parallel to the short strip of tape.
- Cross the ends of the tape over the cannula so that the tape sticks to the patient's skin (as shown).
- Apply a piece of 1" tape across the two wings of the chevron.
- Loop the tubing and secure it with another piece of 1" tape. After the dressing is secured, apply a label. On the label, write the date and time of insertion, type and gauge of the needle, and your initials.

U method

- Cut a 2" (5 cm) strip of ½" tape. With the sticky side up, place it under the hub of the cannula.
- Bring each side of the tape up, folding it over the wings of the cannula in a U shape (as shown). Press it down parallel to the hub.
- Now apply tape to stabilize the catheter.
- After the dressing is secured, apply a label. On the label, write the date and time of insertion, type and gauge of the needle or cannula, and your initials.

H method

- Cut three strips of 1" tape.
- Place one strip of tape over each wing, keeping the tape parallel to the cannula (as shown).
- Now place the other strip of tape perpendicular to the first two. Put it either directly on top of the wings or just below the wings, directly on top of the tubing.
- Make sure that the cannula is secure, and then apply a dressing and label. On the label, write the date and time of insertion, type and gauge of the needle or cannula, and your initials.

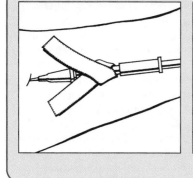
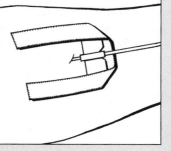
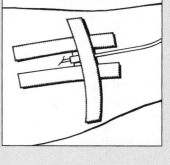

laboratory to be cultured according to your facility's policy. (A draining site may be infected.) Then clean the area, apply a sterile dressing, and notify the physician.

- Instruct the patient to restrict activity for about 10 minutes and to leave the dressing in place for at least 1 hour. If the patient feels lingering tenderness at the site, apply warm packs and notify the physician. **INS**

Special considerations

 ALERT *In the elderly patient, apply the tourniquet carefully to avoid pinching the skin. If necessary, apply it over the patient's gown. Tourniquets may not be necessary in the patient with very frail veins because the tourniquet may injure the site and result in an unsuccessful venipuncture attempt. Make sure that skin preparation materials are at room temperature to avoid vasoconstriction resulting from lower temperatures.*

- If the patient is allergic to iodine-containing compounds, clean the skin with alcohol.
- If you fail to see flashback after the needle enters the vein, pull back slightly and rotate the device. If you still fail to see flashback, remove the cannula and try again, or proceed according to facility policy.

● Change a gauze or transparent dressing whenever you change the administration set (every 48 to 72 hours or according to your facility's policy). **INS**

● Be sure to rotate the I.V. site, usually every 48 to 72 hours or according to your facility's policy. **INS**

TEACHING *The patient who receives I.V. therapy at home usually has a central venous line. But if you're caring for a patient going home with a peripheral line, you should teach him how to care for the I.V. site and identify certain complications. If the patient must observe movement restrictions, make sure that he understands them.*

Teach the patient how to examine the site, and instruct him to notify the physician or home care nurse if redness, swelling, or discomfort develops, if the dressing becomes moist, or if blood appears in the tubing.

Also tell the patient to report problems with the I.V. line — for instance, if the solution stops infusing or if an alarm goes off on an infusion pump. Explain that the I.V. site will be changed at established intervals by a home care nurse.

If the patient is using an intermittent infusion device, teach him how and when to flush it. Finally, teach the patient to document daily whether the I.V. site is free from pain, swelling, and redness.

Nursing diagnoses

● Risk for infection
● Risk for injury

Expected outcomes

The patient will:
● maintain vital signs and laboratory values within normal limits
● maintain temperature within normal limits
● remain free from injury
● not develop signs and symptoms of complications.

Complications

Peripheral line complications can result from the needle or catheter (infection, phlebitis, and embolism) or from the solution (circulatory overload, infiltration, sepsis, and allergic reaction). (See *Risks of peripheral I.V. therapy*.)

Documentation

In your notes or on the appropriate I.V. sheets, record the date and time of the venipuncture; the type, gauge, and length of the cannula or needle; the anatomic location of the insertion site; the length of the catheter; and the reason the site was changed.

Also document the number of attempts at venipuncture (if you made more than one), the type and flow rate of the I.V. solution, the name and amount of medication in the solution (if any), adverse reactions and actions taken to correct them, patient teaching and evidence of patient understanding, and your initials.

Supportive references

Mermel, L.A. "Prevention of Intravascular Catheter-Related Infections," *Annals of Internal Medicine* 132(5):391-402, March 2000.

Metheny, N.M. *Fluid and Electrolyte Balance: Nursing Considerations,* 4th ed. Philadelphia: Lippincott Williams & Wilkins, 2000.

"Standard 36. Tourniquet. Infusion Nursing Standards of Practice," *Journal of Infusion Nursing* 29(1S):S36, January-February 2006.

"Standard 37. Site Selection. Infusion Nursing Standards of Practice," *Journal of Infusion Nursing* 29(1S):S37-39, January-February 2006.

"Standard 38. Catheter Selection. Infusion Nursing Standards of Practice," *Journal of Infusion Nursing* 29(1S):S38-40, January-February 2006.

"Standard 39. Hair Removal. Infusion Nursing Standards of Practice," *Journal of Infusion Nursing* 29(1S):S40-41, January-February 2006.

"Standard 40. Local Anesthesia. Infusion Nursing Standards of Practice," *Journal of Infusion Nursing* 29(1S):S40-41, January-February 2006.

"Standard 41. Access Site Preparation. Infusion Nursing Standards of Practice," *Journal of Infusion Nursing* 29(1S):S41-42, January-February 2006.

"Standard 42. Catheter Placement. Infusion Nursing Standards of Practice," *Journal of Infusion Nursing* 29(1S):S42-44, January-February 2006.

"Standard 43. Catheter Stabilization. Infusion Nursing Standards of Practice," *Journal of Infusion Nursing* 29(1S):S44, January-February 2006.

"Standard 44. Dressings. Infusion Nursing Standards of Practice," *Journal of Infusion Nursing* 29(1S):S44-45, January-February 2006.

(Text continues on page 163.)

Risks of peripheral I.V. therapy

Complication	Signs and symptoms	Possible causes	Nursing interventions
Local complications			
Catheter dislodgment	• Catheter partly backed out of vein • Solution infiltrating	• Loosened tape, or tubing snagged in bed linens, resulting in partial retraction of catheter; pulled out by confused patient	• If no infiltration occurs, retape without pushing catheter back into vein. If pulled out, apply pressure to I.V. site with sterile dressing. *Prevention* • Tape venipuncture device securely on insertion.
Hematoma	• Tenderness at venipuncture site • Bruised area around site • Inability to advance or flush I.V. line	• Vein punctured through opposite wall at time of insertion • Leakage of blood from needle displacement	• Remove venous access device. • Apply pressure and warm soaks to affected area. • Recheck for bleeding. • Document patient's condition and your interventions. *Prevention* • Choose a vein that can accommodate size of venous access device. • Release tourniquet as soon as successful insertion achieved.
Infiltration	• Swelling at and around I.V. site (may extend along entire limb) • Discomfort, burning, or pain at site • Tight feeling at site • Decreased skin temperature around site • Blanching at site • Continuing fluid infusion even when vein is occluded (although rate may decrease) • Absent blood backflow • Slower infusion rate	• Venous access device dislodged from vein or perforated vein	• Stop infusion and remove device. • Apply warm soaks *to aid absorption*. Elevate limb. • Notify practitioner that the complication has occurred, if severe. • Check for pulse, numbness or tingling, and capillary refill periodically *to assess circulation*. • Restart infusion above infiltration site or in another limb. • Document patient's condition and your interventions. *Prevention* • Check I.V. site frequently especially when using an I.V. pump. • Don't obscure area above site with tape. • Teach patient to report discomfort pain or swelling.
Nerve, tendon, or ligament damage	• Extreme pain (similar to electrical shock when nerve is punctured) • Numbness and muscle contraction • Delayed effects, including paralysis, numbness, and deformity	• Improper venipuncture technique, resulting in injury to surrounding nerves, tendons, or ligaments • Tight taping or improper splinting with arm board	• Stop procedure and remove device. *Prevention* • Don't repeatedly penetrate tissues with venous access device. • Don't apply excessive pressure when taping; don't encircle limb with tape. • Pad arm boards and tape securing arm boards if possible.

(continued)

Risks of peripheral I.V. therapy *(continued)*

Complication	Signs and symptoms	Possible causes	Nursing interventions
Local complications (continued)			
Occlusion	• No increase in infusion rate when I.V. container is raised • Blood backflow in line • Discomfort at insertion site	• I.V. flow interrupted • Heparin lock not flushed • Blood backflow in line when patient walks • Line clamped too long • Hypercoaguable patient	• Use a low flush pressure syringe during injection. Don't force it. If resistance is met, stop immediately. If unsuccessful, remove I.V. line and insert a new one. *Prevention* • Maintain I.V. flow rate. • Flush promptly after intermittent piggyback administration. • Have patient walk with his arm bent at elbow *to reduce risk of blood backflow.*
Phlebitis	• Tenderness at tip of and proximal to venous access device • Redness at tip of cannula and along vein • Puffy area over vein • Vein hard on palpation • Elevated temperature	• Poor blood flow around venous access device • Friction from cannula movement in vein • Venous access device left in vein too long • Clotting at cannula tip (thrombophlebitis) • Drug or solution with high or low pH or high osmolarity	• Remove venous access device. • Apply warm soaks. • Notify practitioner. • Document patient's condition and your interventions. *Prevention* • Restart infusion using larger vein for irritating solution, or restart with smaller-gauge device *to ensure adequate blood flow.* • Tape device securely *to prevent movement.*
Severed catheter	• Leakage from catheter shaft	• Catheter inadvertently cut by scissors • Reinsertion of needle into catheter	• If broken part is visible, attempt to retrieve it. If unsuccessful, notify practitioner. • If portion of cannula enters bloodstream, place tourniquet above I.V. site *to prevent progression of broken part.* • Notify practitioner and radiology department. • Document patient's condition and your interventions. *Prevention* • Don't use scissors around I.V. site. • Never reinsert needle into catheter. • Remove unsuccessfully inserted catheter and needle together.
Thrombophlebitis	• Severe discomfort • Reddened, swollen, and hardened vein	• Thrombosis and inflammation	• Remove venous access device; restart infusion to opposite limb if possible. • Apply warm soaks. • Notify practitioner. • Watch for I.V. therapy-related infection. *Prevention* • Check site frequently. Remove venous access device at first sign of redness and tenderness.

Risks of peripheral I.V. therapy (continued)

Complication	Signs and symptoms	Possible causes	Nursing interventions
Local complications (continued)			
Thrombosis	• Painful, reddened, or swollen vein • Sluggish or stopped I.V. flow	• Injury to endothelial cells or vein wall allowing platelets to adhere and thrombi to form	• Remove venous access device; restart infusion to opposite limb if possible. • Apply warm soaks • Watch for I.V. therapy-related infections. *Prevention* • Use proper venipuncture technique to reduce injury to vein.
Vein irritation or pain at I.V. site	• Rapidly developing signs of phlebitis • Possible blanching if vasospasm occurs • Pain during infusion • Red skin over vein during insertion	• Solution with high or low pH or high osmolarity, such as potassium chloride, phenytoin, and some antibiotics (vancomycin [Vancocin] and nafcillin)	• Decrease infusion rate. Try using an electronic infusion device to achieve steady infusion rate. *Prevention* • Dilute solutions before administration. For example, give antibiotics in 250-ml solution rather than 100-ml solution. If drug has low pH, ask pharmacist if drug can be buffered with sodium bicarbonate. (Refer to your facility's policy.) • If long-term therapy of irritating drugs is planned, ask practitioner to use a central line.
Venous spasm	• Pain along vein • Infusion rate sluggish when clamp completely open • Blanched skin over vein	• Severe vein irritation from irritating drugs or fluids • Administration of cold fluids or blood • Very rapid infusion rate (with fluids at room temperature)	• Apply warm soaks over vein and surrounding area. • Decrease infusion rate. *Prevention* • Use a blood warmer for blood or packed red blood cells when appropriate.
Systemic complications			
Air embolism	• Respiratory distress • Unequal breath sounds • Weak pulse • Increased central venous pressure • Decreased blood pressure • Confusion, disorientation, loss of consciousness	• Solution container empty • Solution container empties, next container pushes air down the line • Tubing disconnected from venous access device or I.V. bag	• Discontinue infusion. • Place patient on his left side in Trendelenburg's position *to allow air to enter right atrium and disperse by way of pulmonary artery.* • Administer oxygen. • Notify practitioner. • Document patient's condition and your interventions. *Prevention* • Purge tubing of air completely before starting infusion. • Use air-detection device on pump or air-eliminating filter proximal to I.V. site. • Secure all connections.

(continued)

Risks of peripheral I.V. therapy *(continued)*

Complication	Signs and symptoms	Possible causes	Nursing interventions
Systemic complications (continued)			
Allergic reaction	• Itching • Watery eyes and nose • Bronchospasm • Wheezing • Urticarial rash • Edema at I.V. site • Anaphylactic reaction (flushing, chills, anxiety, agitation, generalized itching, palpitations, paresthesia, throbbing in ears, wheezing, coughing, seizures, cardiac arrest) within minutes or up to 1 hour after exposure	• Allergens such as medications	• If reaction occurs, stop infusion immediately and infuse normal saline solution. • Maintain a patent airway. • Notify practitioner. • Administer antihistaminic steroid, anti-inflammatory, and antipyretic drugs, as prescribed. • Give 0.2 to 0.5 ml of 1:1,000 aqueous epinephrine subcutaneously, as prescribed. Repeat at 3-minute intervals and as needed and prescribed. • Administer cortisone if prescribed. ***Prevention*** • Obtain patient's allergy history. Be aware of cross-allergies. • Assist with test dosing and document any new allergies. • Monitor patient carefully during first 15 minutes of administration of a new drug.
Circulatory overload	• Discomfort • Neck vein engorgement • Respiratory distress • Increased blood pressure • Crackles • Increased difference between fluid intake and output	• Roller clamp loosened to allow run-on infusion • Infusion rate too rapid • Miscalculation of fluid requirements	• Raise head of bed. • Slow infusion rate (but don't remove venous access device). • Administer oxygen as needed. • Notify practitioner. • Administer medications (probably furosemide [Lasix]) as prescribed. ***Prevention*** • Use pump, volume-control set, or rate minder for elderly or compromised patients. • Recheck calculations of fluid requirements. • Monitor infusion frequently.
Systemic infection (septicemia or bacteremia)	• Fever, chills, and malaise for no apparent reason • Contaminated I.V. site, usually with no visible signs of infection at site	• Failure to maintain sterile technique during insertion or site care • Severe phlebitis, which can set up ideal conditions for organism growth • Poor taping that permits venous access device to move, which can introduce organisms into bloodstream • Prolonged indwelling time of device • Immunocompromised patient	• Notify practitioner. • Administer medications as prescribed. • Culture site and device. • Monitor patient's vital signs. ***Prevention*** • Use scrupulous sterile technique when handling solutions and tubing, inserting venous access device, and discontinuing infusion. • Secure all connections. • Change I.V. solutions, tubing, and venous access device at recommended times. • Use I.V. filters.

"Standard 53. Phlebitis. Infusion Nursing Standards of Practice," *Journal of Infusion Nursing* 29(1S):S58-59, January-February 2006.

"Standard 54. Infiltration. Infusion Nursing Standards of Practice," *Journal of Infusion Nursing* 29(1S):S59, January-February 2006.

Weinstein, S.M. *Plumer's Principles and Practice of Intravenous Therapy,* 7th ed. Philadelphia: Lippincott Williams & Wilkins, 2001.

Welk, T. "Clinical and Ethical Considerations of Fluid and Electrolyte Management in the Terminally Ill Client," *Journal of Intravenous Nursing* 22(1):43-47, January-February 1999.

Peripherally inserted central catheters

Peripheral central venous (CV) therapy involves the insertion of a catheter into a peripheral vein instead of a central vein, but the catheter tip still lies in the CV circulation. A peripherally inserted central catheter (PICC) usually enters at the basilic vein and terminates in the subclavian vein or superior vena cava. A specially trained nurse may insert PICCs. New catheters have longer needles and smaller lumens, facilitating this procedure. For a patient who needs CV therapy for 1 to 6 months or who requires repeated venous access, a PICC may be the best option.

PICCs are commonly used in home I.V. therapy but may also be used with chest injury; chest, neck, or shoulder burns; compromised respiratory function; proximity of a surgical site to the CV line placement site; and if a physician isn't available to insert a CV line. With any of these conditions, a PICC helps avoid complications that may occur with a CV line.

Infusions commonly given by a PICC include total parenteral nutrition, chemotherapy, antibiotics, opioids, and analgesics. PICC therapy works best when introduced early in treatment; it shouldn't be considered as a last resort for patients with sclerotic or repeatedly punctured veins.

Before PICC insertion, anatomical measurements should be taken to determine the length of the catheter required *to ensure full advancement of the catheter with tip placement in the superior vena cava.* PICCs may range from 16G to 23G in diameter and from 16″ to 24″ (40.5 to 61 cm) in length. **INS**

The patient receiving PICC therapy must have a peripheral vein large enough to accept a 14G or 16G introducer needle and a 3.8G to 4.8G catheter.

Site selection should be routinely initiated in the region of the antecubital fossa; veins that should be considered for PICC insertion are the cephalic, basilic, and median cubital veins. **INS**

If your state nurse practice act permits, you may insert a PICC if you show sufficient knowledge of vascular access devices. To prove your competence in PICC insertion, it's recommended that you complete an 8-hour workshop and demonstrate three successful catheter insertions. You may have to demonstrate competence every year.

Equipment

Catheter insertion kit • antiseptic solution • 3-ml vial of heparin (100 units/ml) • injection port with short extension tubing • sterile and clean measuring tape • vial of normal saline solution • sterile gauze pads • tape • linen-saver pad • sterile drapes • tourniquet • sterile transparent semipermeable dressing • sterile marker • sterile labels • two pairs of sterile gloves • sterile gown • mask • goggles • clean gloves

Preparation of equipment

● Gather the necessary supplies.

● If you're administering PICC therapy in the patient's home, bring the equipment listed above with you.

Implementation

● Confirm the patient's identity using two patient identifiers according to facility policy. **JCAHO**

● Describe the procedure to the patient and answer her questions. **PCP**

● Wash your hands. **CDC**

● Prepare the sterile field and label all medications, medication containers, and other solutions on and off the sterile field. **JCAHO**

Inserting a PICC

● Place the tourniquet on the patient's arm, and assess the antecubital fossa. Select the insertion site.

● Remove the tourniquet.

● Determine catheter tip placement or the spot at which the catheter tip will rest after insertion.

● For placement in the superior vena cava, measure the distance from the insertion site to the shoulder and from the shoulder to the sternal notch. Then add 3″ (7.6 cm) to the measurement (as shown below). **INS**

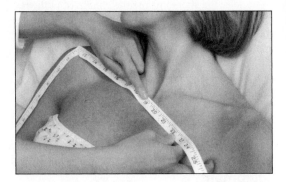

● Have the patient lie in a supine position with her arm at a 90-degree angle to her body. Place a linen-saver pad under her arm.

● Open the PICC tray and drop the rest of the sterile items onto the sterile field. Put on the sterile gown, mask, goggles, and gloves. **CDC**

● Using the sterile measuring tape, cut the distal end of the catheter according to the manufacturer's recommendations and guidelines, using the equipment provided by the manufacturer (as shown below). **MFR**

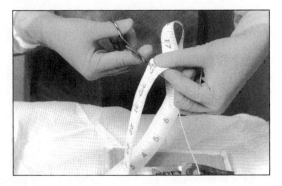

● Using sterile technique, withdraw 5 ml of the normal saline solution and flush the extension tubing and the cap (as shown at top of next column).

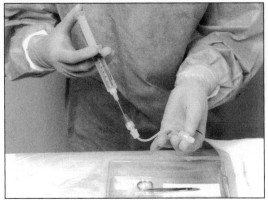

● Remove the needle from the syringe. Attach the syringe to the hub of the catheter and flush (as shown below).

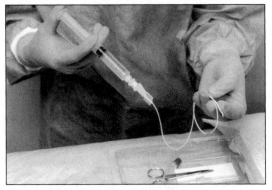

● Prepare the insertion site using an antiseptic solution. Follow manufacturer's recommendations for proper cleaning techniques depending on solution used. **MFR** Allow the area to dry. Be sure not to touch the intended insertion site. Take your gloves off. Then apply the tourniquet about 4″ (10 cm) above the antecubital fossa.

● Put on a new pair of sterile gloves. Then place a sterile drape under the patient's arm and another on top of her arm. Drop a sterile 4″× 4″ gauze pad over the tourniquet. **INS**

● Stabilize the patient's vein. Insert the catheter introducer at a 10-degree angle directly into the vein (as shown at top of next page).

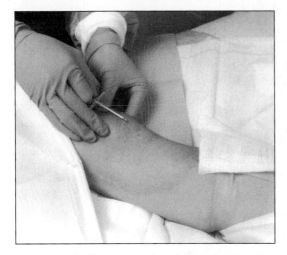

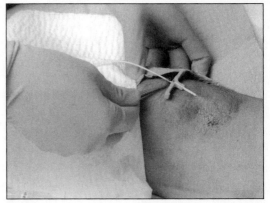

● After successful vein entry, you should see a blood return in the flashback chamber. Without changing the needle's position, gently advance the plastic introducer sheath until you're sure the tip is well within the vein. **INS**

● Carefully withdraw the needle while holding the introducer still. *To minimize blood loss,* try applying finger pressure on the vein just beyond the distal end of the introducer sheath (as shown below).

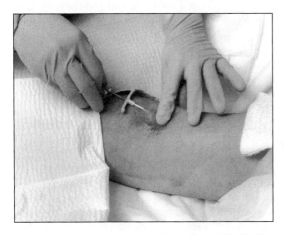

● Using sterile forceps, insert the catheter into the introducer sheath, and advance it into the vein 2″ to 4″ (5 to 10 cm) (as shown at top of next column).

● Remove the tourniquet using a sterile 4″ × 4″ gauze pad.

CONTROVERSIAL ISSUE *PICC placement may be enhanced through the use of imaging support such as ultrasonography. Studies have shown that the use of ultrasound decreases the number of needle penetrations required to successfully cannulate the vein by 42%. Risks may be minimized through ultrasound use as well, but cost-effectiveness hasn't been demonstrated.*

● When you've advanced the catheter to the shoulder, ask the patient to turn her head toward the affected arm and place her chin on her chest. *This will occlude the jugular vein and ease the catheter's advancement into the subclavian vein.*

● Advance the catheter until about 4″ remain. Then pull the introducer sheath out of the vein and away from the venipuncture site (as shown below).

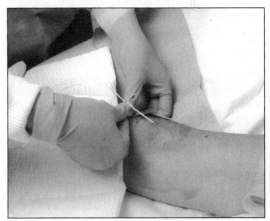

● Grasp the tabs of the introducer sheath, and flex them toward its distal end *to split the sheath.*
● Pull the tabs apart and away from the catheter until the sheath is completely split (as shown below). Discard the sheath.

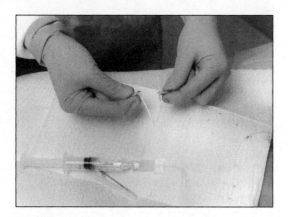

● Continue to advance the catheter until it's completely inserted. Flush with normal saline solution followed by heparin, according to facility policy.
● With the patient's arm below heart level, remove the syringe. Connect the capped extension set to the catheter hub. **Science**
● Apply a sterile 2″× 2″ gauze pad directly over the site and a sterile transparent semipermeable dressing over that. Leave this dressing in place for 24 hours. **INS**

> ✓ **CLINICAL IMPACT** *The tip of the PICC should be in the vena cava. The tip of the catheter can be determined radiologically and should be documented in the patient's medical record before starting the prescribed therapy. In addition, radiologic confirmation should be performed intermittently* because the catheter is no longer considered a central catheter if located outside the vena cava. *It will then need to be removed because the location may no longer be appropriate for the prescribed therapy.*

● After the initial 24 hours, apply a new sterile transparent semipermeable dressing. The gauze pad is no longer necessary. You can place Steri-Strips over the catheter wings. **INS**
● Flush with heparin, according to facility policy.

Administering drugs
● As with any CV line, be sure to check for blood return and flush with normal saline solution before administering a drug through a PICC line. **INS**
● Clamp the 7″ (17.8-cm) extension tubing, and connect the empty syringe to the tubing. Release the clamp and aspirate slowly *to verify blood return.* Flush with 3 ml of normal saline solution in a 10-ml syringe, then administer the drug.
● After giving the drug, flush again with 3 ml of normal saline solution in a 10-ml syringe. (Remember to flush with normal saline solution between infusions of incompatible drugs or fluids.)

Changing the dressing
● Change the dressing every 2 to 7 days and more frequently if the integrity of the dressing becomes compromised. If possible, choose a transparent semipermeable dressing, *which has a high moisture-vapor transmission rate.* Use sterile technique. **INS**
● Wash your hands and assemble the necessary supplies. Position the patient with her arm extended away from her body at a 45- to 90-degree angle so that the insertion site is below heart level *to reduce the risk of air embolism.* Put on a sterile mask. **CDC** **Science**
● Open a package of sterile gloves and use the inside of the package as a sterile field. Then open the transparent semipermeable dressing and drop it onto the field. Put on clean gloves, and remove the old dressing by holding your left thumb on the catheter and stretching the dressing parallel to the skin. Repeat the last step with your right thumb holding the catheter. Free the remaining section of the dressing from the catheter by peeling toward the insertion site from the distal end to the proximal end *to prevent catheter dislodgment.* Remove the clean gloves. **INS**
● Put on sterile gloves. Clean the area thoroughly with three alcohol swabs or other approved antimicrobial solution, starting at the insertion site and working outward from the site. Repeat the step three times with 2% chlorhexidine swabs and allow to dry. **CDC** **Science**
● Apply the dressing carefully. Secure the tubing to the edge of the dressing over the tape with ¼″ adhesive tape.

Removing a PICC

- You'll remove a PICC when therapy is complete, if the catheter becomes damaged or broken and can't be repaired or, possibly, if the line becomes occluded. Measure the catheter after you remove it *to ensure that the line has been removed intact.* **INS**
- Assemble the necessary equipment at the patient's bedside.
- Explain the procedure to the patient. Wash your hands. Place a linen-saver pad under the patient's arm. **CDC** **PCP**
- Remove the tape holding the extension tubing. Open two sterile gauze pads on a clean, flat surface. Put on clean gloves. Stabilize the catheter at the hub with one hand. Without dislodging the catheter, use your other hand to gently remove the dressing by pulling it toward the insertion site.
- Next, withdraw the catheter with smooth, gentle pressure in small increments. It should come out easily. If you feel resistance, stop. Apply slight tension to the line by taping it down. Then try to remove it again in a few minutes. If you still feel resistance, notify the physician for further instructions. **INS**
- After you successfully remove the catheter, apply manual pressure to the site with a sterile gauze pad for 1 minute.
- Measure and inspect the catheter. If a part has broken off during removal, notify the physician immediately and monitor the patient for signs of distress. **INS**
- Cover the site with antiseptic ointment, and tape a new folded gauze pad in place. Dispose of used items properly, and wash your hands. **CDC**

Special considerations

- For a patient receiving intermittent PICC therapy, flush the catheter with 6 ml of normal saline solution and 3 ml of heparin (100 units/ml) after each use. For catheters that aren't being used routinely, flushing every 12 hours with 3 ml (100 units/ml) of heparin will maintain patency.
- You can use a declotting agent to clear a clotted PICC, but make sure that you read the manufacturer's recommendations first and follow your facility's policy. **MFR**
- Remember to add an extension set to all PICCs *so you can start and stop an infusion away from the insertion site.* An extension set will also make using a PICC easier for the patient who'll be administering infusions herself.
- If a patient will be receiving blood or blood products through the PICC, use at least an 18G cannula.
- Assess the catheter insertion site through the transparent semipermeable dressing every 24 hours. Look at the catheter and cannula pathway, and check for bleeding, redness, drainage, and swelling. Ask the patient if she's having pain associated with therapy. Although oozing is common for the first 24 hours after insertion, excessive bleeding after that should be evaluated.

ALERT *If a portion of the catheter breaks during removal, immediately apply a tourniquet to the upper arm, close to the axilla,* **to prevent advancement of the catheter piece into the right atrium.** *Then check the patient's radial pulse. If you don't detect the radial pulse, the tourniquet is too tight. Keep the tourniquet in place until an X-ray can be obtained, the physician is notified, and surgical retrieval is attempted.*

Nursing diagnoses

- Risk for infection
- Risk for injury

Expected outcomes

The patient will:
- maintain vital signs and laboratory values within normal limits
- maintain temperature within normal limits
- have culture results that show no evidence of pathogens
- remain free from injury
- not develop signs and symptoms of complications.

Complications

- PICC therapy causes fewer and less severe complications than conventional CV lines. Catheter breakage on removal is probably the most common complication.
- Air embolism, always a potential risk of venipuncture, poses less danger in PICC therapy than with traditional CV lines *because the line is inserted below heart level.*
- Catheter tip migration may occur with vigorous flushing. Patients receiving chemotherapy are most vulnerable to this complication *because of frequent*

nausea and vomiting and subsequent changes in intrathoracic pressure.
● Catheter occlusion is a relatively common complication.

Documentation

Document the entire procedure, including problems with catheter placement. Also document the size, length, and type of catheter as well as the insertion location.

Supportive references

Camara, D. "Minimizing Risks Associated with Peripherally Inserted Central Catheters in the NICU," *The American Journal of Maternal/Child Nursing* 26(1):17-21, January-February 2001.

LaRue, G. "Efficacy of Ultrasonography in Peripheral Venous Cannulation," *Journal of Intravenous Nursing* 23(1):29-34, January-February 2000.

Macklin, D. "How to Manage PICCs," *AJN* 97(9):26-33, September 1997.

Sansivero, G.E. "The Microintroducer Technique for Peripherally Inserted Central Catheter Placement," *Journal of Intravenous Nursing* 23(6):345-51, November-December 2000.

"Standard 37. Site Selection. Infusion Nursing Standards of Practice," *Journal of Infusion Nursing* 29(1S):S37-39, January-February 2006.

"Standard 38. Catheter Selection. Infusion Nursing Standards of Practice," *Journal of Infusion Nursing* 29(1S):S39-40, January-February 2006.

"Standard 41. Access Site Preparation. Infusion Nursing Standards of Practice," *Journal of Infusion Nursing* 29(1S):S41-42, January-February 2006.

"Standard 42. Catheter Placement. Infusion Nursing Standards of Practice," *Journal of Infusion Nursing* 29(1S):S42-44, January-February 2006.

"Standard 43. Catheter Stabilization. Infusion Nursing Standards of Practice," *Journal of Infusion Nursing* 29(1S):S44, January-February 2006.

"Standard 44. Dressings. Infusion Nursing Standards of Practice," *Journal of Infusion Nursing* 29(1S):S44-45, January-February 2006.

"Standard 49. Catheter Removal. Infusion Nursing Standards of Practice," *Journal of Infusion Nursing* 29(1S):S51-55, January-February 2006.

"Standard 50. Flushing. Infusion Nursing Standards of Practice," *Journal of Infusion Nursing* 29(1S):S55-57, January-February 2006.

"Standard 60. Catheter Clearance. Infusion Nursing Standards of Practice," *Journal of Infusion Nursing* 29(1S):S65, January-February 2006.

Weinstein, S.M. *Plumer's Principles and Practice of Intravenous Therapy,* 7th ed. Philadelphia: Lippincott Williams & Wilkins, 2001.

Secondary I.V. lines

A secondary I.V. line is a complete I.V. set — container, tubing, and microdrip or macrodrip system — connected to the lower Y port (secondary port) of a primary line instead of to the I.V. catheter or needle. It can be used for continuous or intermittent drug infusion. When used continuously, a secondary I.V. line permits drug infusion and titration while the primary line maintains a constant total infusion rate.

When used intermittently, a secondary I.V. line is commonly called a *piggyback set.* In this case, the primary line maintains venous access between drug doses. Typically, a piggyback set includes a small I.V. container, short tubing, and a macrodrip system. This set connects to the primary line's upper Y port, also called a piggyback port. Antibiotics are most commonly administered by intermittent (piggyback) infusion. *To make this set work,* the primary I.V. container must be positioned below the piggyback container. (The manufacturer provides an extension hook for this purpose.)

To prevent needle-stick injuries the Centers for Disease Control and Prevention and the Occupational Safety and Health Administration suggest that drugs be piggybacked with a needle-free system, which consists of a blunt-tipped plastic insertion device and a rubber injection port. The port may be part of a special administration set or an adapter for existing administration sets. The rubber injection port has a preestablished slit that can open and reseal immediately. **CDC**

I.V. pumps may be used *to maintain constant infusion rates,* especially with a drug such as lidocaine. A pump allows more accurate titration of drug dosage and helps maintain venous access *because the drug is delivered under sufficient pressure to prevent clot formation in the I.V. cannula.*

Equipment

Patient's medication record and chart ● prescribed I.V. medication ● prescribed I.V. solution ● administration set with secondary injection port • needleless adapter • alcohol pads • 1″ adhesive tape • time tape • labels • infusion pump • extension hook and appropriate solution for intermittent piggyback infusion • optional: normal saline solution for infusion with incompatible solutions

For intermittent infusion, the primary line typically has a piggyback port with a backcheck valve that stops the flow from the primary line during drug infusion and returns to the primary flow after infusion. A volume-control set can also be used with an intermittent infusion line.

Preparation of equipment
● Verify the order on the patient's medication record by checking it against the physician's order.
● Wash your hands. **CDC**
● Inspect the I.V. container for cracks, leaks, and contamination, and check drug compatibility with the primary solution. Verify the expiration date. Check to see whether the primary line has a secondary injection port. If it doesn't and the medication is to be given regularly, replace the I.V. set with one that has a secondary injection port.
● If necessary, add the drug to the secondary I.V. solution. To do so, remove any seals from the secondary container and wipe the main port with an alcohol pad. Inject the prescribed medication, and gently agitate the solution *to mix the medication thoroughly.* Properly label the I.V. mixture. Insert the administration set spike and attach the needle. Open the flow clamp and prime the line. Then close the flow clamp.
● Some medications are available in vials that are suitable for hanging directly on an I.V. pole. Instead of preparing medication and injecting it into a container, you can inject diluent directly into the medication vial. Then you can spike the vial, prime the tubing, and hang the set, as directed.

Implementation
● Confirm the patient's identity using two patient identifiers according to facility policy. **JCAHO** If you're hanging an antibiotic, confirm that the patient has no history of an allergic reaction to the drug. **PCP**
● If the drug is incompatible with the primary I.V. solution, replace the primary solution with a fluid that's compatible with both solutions, such as normal saline solution, and flush the line before starting the

Assembling a piggyback set

A piggyback set is useful for intermittent drug infusion. To work properly, the secondary set's container must be positioned higher than the primary set's container.

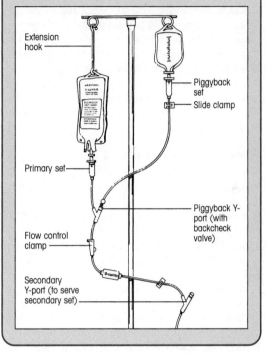

Extension hook
Piggyback set
Slide clamp
Primary set
Piggyback Y-port (with backcheck valve)
Flow control clamp
Secondary Y-port (to serve secondary set)

drug infusion. Many facility protocols require that the primary I.V. solution be removed and that a sterile I.V. plug be inserted into the container until it's ready to be rehung. *This maintains the sterility of the solution and prevents someone else from inadvertently restarting the incompatible solution before the line is flushed with normal saline solution.* **INS**
● Hang the secondary set's container and wipe the injection port of the primary line with an alcohol pad.
● Insert the needleless adapter from the secondary line into the injection port and secure it to the primary line. **CDC**
● To run the secondary set's container by itself, lower the primary set's container with an extension hook. To run both containers simultaneously, place them at the same height. (See *Assembling a piggyback set.*) **Science**

● Open the clamp and adjust the drip rate. For continuous infusion, set the secondary solution to the desired drip rate; then adjust the primary solution *to achieve the desired total infusion rate.*
● For intermittent infusion, adjust the primary drip rate, as required, on completion of the secondary solution. If the secondary solution tubing is being reused, close the clamp on the tubing and follow your facility's policy: Either remove the needleless adapter and replace it with a new one, or leave it securely taped in the injection port and label it with the time it was first used. In this case, also leave the empty container in place until you replace it with a new dose of medication at the prescribed time. If the tubing won't be reused, discard it appropriately with the I.V. container. **CDC**

Special considerations

● If your facility's policy allows, use a pump for drug infusion. Put a time tape on the secondary container *to help prevent an inaccurate administration rate.*
● When reusing secondary tubing, change it according to your facility's policy, usually every 48 to 72 hours. Similarly, inspect the injection port for leakage with each use and change it more often if needed. **INS**
● Unless you're piggybacking lipids, don't piggyback a secondary I.V. line to a total parenteral nutrition line *because of the risk of contamination.* Check your facility's policy for possible exceptions.
● After adding a medication to an administration set, the solution should be infused or discarded within a 24-hour period. **INS**

Nursing diagnoses

● Risk for infection
● Risk for injury

Expected outcomes

The patient will:
● maintain vital signs within normal limits
● have white blood cell and differential counts within normal limits
● have culture results that show no evidence of pathogens
● remain free from injury
● show no signs and symptoms of complications.

Complications

● The patient may experience an adverse reaction to the infused drug.
● Repeated punctures of the secondary injection port can damage the seal, possibly allowing leakage or contamination.

Documentation

Record the amount and type of drug and the amount of I.V. solution on the intake and output and medication records. Note the date, duration and rate of infusion, and the patient's response, when applicable.

Supportive references

Gahart, B.L., and Nazareno, A.R. *Intravenous Medication 2002s: A Handbook for Nurses and Other Allied Health Professionals*, 18th ed. St. Louis: Mosby–Year Book, Inc., 2001.
Otto, S.E. *Mosby's Pocket Guide to Intravenous Therapy*, 4th ed. St. Louis: Mosby–Year Book, Inc., 2001.
Weinstein, S.M. *Plumer's Principles and Practice of Intravenous Therapy*, 7th ed. Philadelphia: Lippincott Williams & Wilkins, 2001.

Total parenteral nutrition

When a patient can't meet his nutritional needs by oral or enteral feedings, he may require I.V. nutritional support, or parenteral nutrition. The patient's diagnosis, history, and prognosis determine the need for parenteral nutrition. Generally, this treatment is prescribed for a patient who can't absorb nutrients though the GI tract for more than 10 days. More specific indications, including those from the American Society for Parenteral and Enteral Nutrition, include:
● debilitating illness lasting longer than 2 weeks **ASPEN**
● loss of 10% or more of pre-illness weight **ASPEN**
● serum albumin level below 3.5 g/dl
● excessive nitrogen loss from wound infection, fistulas, or abscesses
● renal or hepatic failure
● a nonfunctioning GI tract for 5 to 7 days in a severely catabolic patient.

Other reasons for initiating parenteral nutrition include massive small-bowel resection, bone marrow transplantation, high-dose chemotherapy or radiation therapy, and major surgery.

Infants with congenital or acquired disorders may need parenteral nutrition *to promote growth and development.* Specific disorders that may require parenteral nutrition include tracheoesophageal fistula, gastroschisis, duodenal atresia, cystic fibrosis, meconium ileus, diaphragmatic hernia, volvulus, malrotation of the gut, and annular pancreas.

Parenteral nutrition shouldn't be given to patients with a normally functioning GI tract, and it has limited value for well-nourished patients whose GI tract will resume normal function within 10 days. It may also be inappropriate for patients with a poor prognosis or if the risks of parenteral nutrition outweigh the benefits. **ASPEN**

Parenteral nutrition may be given through a peripheral or central venous (CV) line. Depending on the solution, it may be used to boost the patient's calorie intake, to supply full calorie needs, or to surpass the patient's calorie requirements. Infusion-specific filtration and an electronic infusion device should be used to administer parenteral nutrition. **INS**

The type of parenteral solution prescribed depends on the patient's condition and metabolic needs and the administration route. The solution usually contains protein, carbohydrates, electrolytes, vitamins, and trace minerals. A lipid emulsion provides the necessary fat. (See *Types of parenteral nutrition,* pages 172 and 173.)

CLINICAL IMPACT *Total parenteral nutrition (TPN) may need to be started early in select populations. Appropriate provision of nutrition with emphasis on early enteral nutrition in critically ill and surgical patients can enhance wound healing.*

Nutritional solutions containing concentrations exceeding 10% dextrose, 5% protein, or both, such as TPN, should be given through a CV line with the distal tip in the superior vena cava or right atrium. **ASPEN** Because TPN is in a lipid emulsion, it should be filtered through a 1.2-micron filter. Peripheral parenteral nutrition (PPN) has a concentration of 10% dextrose and 5% protein or less and can be given through a peripheral line. The maximum administration period for PPN should be 7 to 10 days, unless supplemental oral or enteral feeding is also provided. **INS**

The most common delivery route for TPN is through a CV catheter into the superior vena cava. The catheter may also be placed through the infraclavicular approach or, less commonly, through the supraclavicular, internal jugular, or antecubital fossa approach.

Equipment

Bag or bottle of prescribed parenteral nutrition solution • sterile I.V. tubing with attached extension tubing • 0.22-micron filter (or 1.2-micron filter if solution contains lipids or albumin) • reflux valve • time tape • alcohol pads • electronic infusion pump • portable glucose monitor • scale • intake and output record • sterile gloves • optional: mask

Preparation of equipment

Make sure that the solution, the patient, and the equipment are ready. Remove the solution from the refrigerator at least 1 hour before use *to avoid pain, hypothermia, venous spasm, and venous constriction, which can result from delivery of a chilled solution.* Check the solution against the physician's order for the correct patient name, expiration date, and formula components. Observe the container for cracks and the solution for cloudiness, turbidity, and particles. If present, return the solution to the pharmacy. If you'll be administering a total nutrient admixture solution, look for a brown layer on the solution, which indicates that the lipid emulsion has "cracked," or separated from the solution. If you see a brown layer, return the solution to the pharmacy.

When you're ready to administer the solution, explain the procedure to the patient. Check the name on the solution container against the name on the patient's wristband. **INS** Confirm the patient's identity using two patient identifiers according to facility policy. **JCAHO** Then put on gloves and, if specified by your facility's policy, a mask. Throughout the procedure, use strict sterile technique. **CDC**

In sequence, connect the pump tubing, the micron filter with attached extension tubing (if the tubing doesn't contain an in-line filter), and the reflux valve. Insert the filter as close to the catheter site as possible. If the tubing doesn't have luer-lock connections, tape all connections *to prevent accidental separation, which could lead to air embolism, exsanguination, and sepsis.* Next, squeeze the I.V. drip chamber and, holding the drip chamber upright, insert the tubing spike into the I.V. bag or bottle. Then release the drip chamber. Squeezing the drip chamber before spiking an I.V. bottle *prevents accidental dripping of the parenteral nutrition solution.* An I.V. bag, however, shouldn't drip.

Types of parenteral nutrition

Type	Solution components/liter	Uses	Special considerations
Total parenteral nutrition (TPN) by way of central venous (CV) line	• $D_{15}W$ to $D_{25}W$ (1 L dextrose 25% = 850 nonprotein calories) • Crystalline amino acids 2.5% to 8.5% • Electrolytes, vitamins, trace elements, and insulin, as ordered • Lipid emulsion 10% to 20% (usually infused as a separate solution)	• 2 weeks or more • For patients with large calorie and nutrient needs • Provides calories, restores nitrogen balance, and replaces essential vitamins, electrolytes, minerals, and trace elements • Promotes tissue synthesis, wound healing, and normal metabolic function • Allows bowel rest and healing; reduces activity in the gallbladder, pancreas, and small intestine • Improves tolerance of surgery	*Basic solution* • Nutritionally complete • Requires minor surgical procedure for CV line insertion (can be done at bedside by physician) • Highly hypertonic solution • May cause metabolic complications (glucose intolerance, electrolyte imbalance, essential fatty acid deficiency) *I.V. lipid emulsion* • May not be used effectively in severely stressed patients (especially burn patients) • May interfere with immune mechanisms; in patients suffering respiratory compromise, reduces carbon dioxide buildup • Given by way of CV line; irritates peripheral vein in long-term use
Total nutrient admixture	• 1 day's nutrients are contained in a single, 3-L bag (also called 3:1 solution) • Combines lipid emulsion with other parenteral solution components	• 2 weeks or more • For relatively stable patients because solution components can be adjusted just once daily • For other uses, see TPN (above)	• See TPN (above) • Reduces need to handle bag, reducing risk of contamination • Decreases nursing time and reduces need for infusion sets and electronic devices, lowering facility costs, increasing patient mobility, and allowing easier adjustment to home care • Has limited use because not all types and amounts of components are compatible • Precludes use of certain infusion pumps *because they can't accurately deliver large volumes of solution;* precludes use of standard I.V. tubing filters *because a 0.22-micron filter blocks lipid and albumin molecules*

(continued)

Next, prime the tubing. Invert the filter at the distal end of the tubing, and open the roller clamp. Let the solution fill the tubing and the filter. Gently tap it *to dislodge air bubbles trapped in the Y-ports.* If indicated, attach a time tape to the parenteral nutrition container for accurate measurement of fluid intake. Record the date and time you hung the fluid, and initial the parenteral nutrition solution container. Next, attach the setup to the infusion pump, and prepare it according to the manufacturer's instructions. Remove and discard your gloves. **CDC**

With the patient in the supine position, flush the catheter with normal saline solution, according to your facility's policy. Then put on gloves, and clean the catheter injection cap with an alcohol pad.

Types of parenteral nutrition *(continued)*

Type	Solution components/liter	Uses	Special considerations
Peripheral parenteral nutrition (PPN)	• D_5W to $D_{10}W$ • Crystalline amino acids 2.5% to 5% • Electrolytes, minerals, vitamins, and trace elements, as ordered • Lipid emulsion 10% or 20% (1 L of dextrose 10% and amino acids 3.5% infused at the same time as 1 L of lipid emulsion = 1,440 nonprotein calories) • Heparin or hydrocortisone, as ordered	• 2 weeks or less • Provides up to 2,000 calories/day • Maintains adequate nutritional status in patients who can tolerate relatively high fluid volume, in those who usually resume bowel function and oral feedings after a few days, and in those who are susceptible to infections associated with the CV catheter	*Basic solution* • Nutritionally complete for short time • Can't be used in nutritionally depleted patients • Can't be used in volume-restricted patients *because PPN requires large fluid volume* • Doesn't cause weight gain • Avoids insertion and care of CV line but requires adequate venous access; site must be changed every 72 hours • Delivers less hypertonic solutions than CV line TPN • May cause phlebitis and increases risk of metabolic complications • Less chance of metabolic complications than with CV line TPN *I.V. lipid emulsion* • As effective as dextrose for calorie source • Diminishes phlebitis if infused at same time as basic nutrient solution • Irritates vein in long-term use • Reduces carbon dioxide buildup when pulmonary compromise is present

Implementation

• Confirm the patient's identity using two patient identifiers according to facility policy. **JCAHO**
• If you're attaching the container of parenteral nutrition solution to a CV line, clamp the CV line before disconnecting it *to prevent air from entering the catheter*. If a clamp isn't available, ask the patient to perform Valsalva's maneuver just as you change the tubing, if possible. Or, if the patient is being mechanically ventilated, change the I.V. tubing immediately after the machine delivers a breath at peak inspiration. *Both of these measures increase intrathoracic pressure and prevent air embolism.* **AABB** **INS** **Science**
• Using sterile technique, attach the tubing to the designated luer-lock port. After connecting the tubing, remove the clamp, if applicable.
• Set the infusion pump at the ordered flow rate, and start the infusion. Check to make sure that the catheter junction is secure.
• Tag the tubing with the date and time of change.

Starting the infusion

• *Because parenteral nutrition solution usually contains a large amount of glucose,* you may need to start the infusion slowly *to allow the patient's pancreatic beta cells time to increase their output of insulin.* Depending on the patient's tolerance, parenteral nutrition is usually initiated at a rate of 40 to 50 ml/hour and then advanced by 25 ml/hour every 6 hours (as tolerated) until the desired infusion rate is achieved. However, when the glucose concentration is low, as occurs in most PPN formulas, you can initiate the rate necessary to infuse the complete 24-hour volume and discontinue the solution without tapering. **Science**
• You may allow a parenteral nutrition solution container to hang for 24 hours.

Changing solutions

• Prepare the new solution and I.V. tubing as described earlier. Put on gloves. Remove the protective caps from the solution containers, and wipe the tops of the containers with alcohol pads.

• Turn off the infusion pump and close the flow clamps. Using strict sterile technique, remove the spike from the solution container that's hanging and insert it into the new container. **INS**

• Hang the new container and tubing alongside the old. Turn on the infusion pump, set the flow rate, and open the flow clamp completely.

• If you're attaching the solution to a peripheral line, examine the skin above the insertion site for redness and warmth and assess for pain. If you suspect phlebitis, remove the existing I.V. line and start a line in a different vein. Also insert a new line if the I.V. catheter has been in place for 72 hours or more *to reduce the risk of phlebitis and infiltration.* **INS**

• Turn off the infusion pump and close the flow clamp on the old tubing. Disconnect the tubing from the catheter hub, and connect the new tubing. Open the flow clamp on the new container to a moderately slow rate.

• Remove the old tubing from the infusion pump, and insert the new tubing according to the manufacturer's instructions. Then turn on the infusion pump, set it to the desired flow rate, and open the flow clamp completely. Remove the old equipment and dispose of it properly. **MFR**

Special considerations

• Always infuse a parenteral nutrition solution at a constant rate without interruption *to avoid blood glucose fluctuations.* If the infusion slows, consult the physician before changing the infusion rate.

• Monitor the patient's vital signs every 4 hours or more often if necessary. Watch for an increased temperature, *an early sign of catheter-related sepsis.*

• Check the patient's blood glucose every 6 hours. He may require supplementary insulin, which the pharmacist may add directly to the solution. The patient may require additional subcutaneous doses.

• *Because most patients receiving PPN are in a protein-wasted state,* the therapy causes marked changes in fluid and electrolyte status and in levels of glucose, amino acids, minerals, and vitamins. Therefore, record daily intake and output accurately. Specify the volume and type of each fluid, and calculate the daily calorie intake. **INS**

• Monitor the results of routine laboratory tests, and report abnormal findings to the physician *to allow for appropriate changes in the parenteral nutrition solu-*

tion. Such tests typically include measurement of serum electrolyte, calcium, blood urea nitrogen, creatinine, and blood glucose levels at least three times weekly; serum magnesium and phosphorus levels twice weekly; liver function studies, complete blood count and differential, and serum albumin and transferrin levels weekly; and urine nitrogen balance and creatinine-height index studies weekly. A serum zinc level is obtained at the start of parenteral nutrition therapy. The physician may also order serum prealbumin, total lymphocyte count, amino acid levels, fatty acid-phospholipid fraction, skin testing, and expired gas analysis. (Also see "Total parenteral nutrition monitoring," page 177.)

• Physically assess the patient daily. If ordered, measure arm circumference and skinfold thickness over the triceps. Weigh him at the same time each morning after he voids; he should be weighed in similar clothing and on the same scale. Suspect fluid imbalance if he gains more than 1 lb (0.5 kg) daily.

• Change the dressing over the catheter according to your facility's policy or whenever the dressing becomes wet, soiled, or nonocclusive. Always use strict sterile technique. **INS** When performing dressing changes, watch for signs of phlebitis and catheter retraction from the vein. Measure the catheter length from the insertion site to the hub for verification.

• Change the tubing and filters every 24 hours or according to your facility's policy. **INS**

• Closely monitor the catheter site for swelling, *which may indicate infiltration.* Extravasation of parenteral nutrition solution can lead to tissue necrosis. (See *Correcting parenteral nutrition problems.*)

⬤ **CONTROVERSIAL ISSUE** *Most practice standards state that a specific line should be designated for parenteral nutrition and that line shouldn't be used for another purpose. Practice guidelines for some facilities may also require that a specific port be reserved for TPN.*

• Use caution when using the parenteral nutrition line for other functions. Don't use a single-lumen CV catheter to infuse blood or blood products, to give a bolus injection, to administer simultaneous I.V. solutions, to measure CV pressure, or to draw blood for laboratory tests.

• Provide regular mouth care. Also provide emotional support. Keep in mind that patients commonly as-

Correcting parenteral nutrition problems

This chart outlines common complications of parenteral nutrition along with their signs and symptoms and appropriate interventions.

Complications	Signs and symptoms	Interventions
Metabolic problems		
Hepatic dysfunction	Elevated serum aspartate aminotransferase, alkaline phosphatase, and bilirubin levels	Reduce total calorie and dextrose intake, making up lost calories by administering lipid emulsion. Change to cyclical infusion. Use specific hepatic formulations only if patient has encephalopathy.
Hypercapnia	Heightened oxygen consumption, increased carbon dioxide production, and measured respiratory quotient of 1 or greater	Reduce total calorie and dextrose intake and balance dextrose and fat calories.
Hyperglycemia	Fatigue, restlessness, confusion, anxiety, weakness, polyuria, dehydration, elevated serum glucose level and, in severe hyperglycemia, delirium or coma	Restrict dextrose intake by decreasing either infusion rate or dextrose concentration. Compensate for calorie loss by administering lipid emulsion. Begin insulin therapy.
Hyperosmolarity	Confusion, lethargy, seizures, hyperosmolar hyperglycemic nonketotic syndrome, hyperglycemia, dehydration, and glycosuria	Discontinue dextrose infusion. Administer insulin and half-normal saline solution with 10 to 20 mEq/L of potassium to rehydrate patient.
Hypocalcemia	Polyuria, dehydration, and elevated blood and urine glucose levels	Increase calcium supplements.
Hypoglycemia	Sweating, shaking, and irritability after infusion has stopped	Increase dextrose intake or decrease exogenous insulin intake.
Hypokalemia	Muscle weakness, paralysis, paresthesia, and arrhythmias	Increase potassium supplements.
Hypomagnesemia	Tingling around mouth, paresthesia in fingers, mental changes, and hyperreflexia	Increase magnesium supplements.
Hypophosphatemia	Irritability, weakness, paresthesia, coma, and respiratory arrest	Increase phosphate supplements.
Metabolic acidosis	Elevated serum chloride level and reduced serum bicarbonate level	Increase acetate and decrease chloride in parenteral nutrition solution.
Metabolic alkalosis	Reduced serum chloride level and elevated serum bicarbonate level	Decrease acetate and increase chloride in parenteral nutrition solution.
Zinc deficiency	Dermatitis, alopecia, apathy, depression, taste changes, confusion, poor wound healing, and diarrhea	Increase zinc supplements.

(continued)

Correcting parenteral nutrition problems *(continued)*

Complications	Signs and symptoms	Interventions
Mechanical problems		
Clotted I.V. catheter	Interrupted flow rate and resistance to flushing and blood withdrawal	Attempt to aspirate clot. If unsuccessful, instill a thrombolytic agent, such as alteplase, to clear catheter lumen, as ordered.
Cracked or broken tubing	Fluid leaking from tubing	Apply a padded hemostat above break *to prevent air from entering line.*
Dislodged catheter	Catheter out of vein	Apply pressure to site with a sterile gauze pad.
Too-rapid infusion	Nausea, headache, and lethargy	Adjust infusion rate and, if applicable, check infusion pump.
Other problems		
Air embolism	Apprehension, chest pain, tachycardia, hypotension, cyanosis, seizures, loss of consciousness, and cardiac arrest	Clamp catheter. Place patient in a steep, left lateral Trendelenburg position. Administer oxygen, as ordered. If cardiac arrest occurs, begin cardiopulmonary resuscitation. When catheter is removed, cover insertion site with dressing for 24 to 48 hours.
Extravasation	Swelling and pain around insertion site	Stop infusion. Assess patient for cardiopulmonary abnormalities; chest X-ray may be required.
Phlebitis	Pain, tenderness, redness, and warmth at insertion site	Apply gentle heat to area, and elevate insertion site, if possible.
Pneumothorax and hydrothorax	Dyspnea, chest pain, cyanosis, and decreased breath sounds	Assist with chest tube insertion and maintain chest tube suctioning, as ordered.
Septicemia	Red and swollen catheter site, chills, fever, and leukocytosis	Remove catheter and culture tip. Obtain blood culture if patient has fever. Give appropriate antibiotics.
Venous thrombosis	Erythema and edema at insertion site; ipsilateral swelling of arm, neck, face, and upper chest; pain at insertion site and along vein; malaise; fever; and tachycardia	Notify practitioner and remove catheter promptly. Administer heparin, if ordered. Venous flow studies may be ordered.

sociate eating with positive feelings and become disturbed when they can't eat.

● Teach the patient the potential adverse effects and complications of parenteral nutrition. Encourage the patient to inspect his mouth regularly for signs of parotitis, glossitis, and oral lesions. Tell him that he may have fewer bowel movements while receiving parenteral nutrition therapy. Encourage him to remain physically active *to help his body use the nutrients more fully.*

TEACHING *Patients who require prolonged or indefinite parenteral nutrition may be able to receive the therapy at home. Home parenteral nutrition reduces the need for long hospitalizations and allows the patient to resume many of his normal activities. Meet with a home care pa-*

tient before discharge to make sure he knows how to perform the administration procedure and how to handle complications.

Nursing diagnoses
- Imbalanced nutrition: Less than body requirements
- Risk for infection

Expected outcomes
The patient will:
- show no further evidence of weight loss
- tolerate oral, tube, or I.V. feeding without adverse effects
- maintain body temperature within normal limits
- maintain white blood cell and differential counts within normal limits.

Complications
- Catheter-related sepsis is the most serious complication of parenteral nutrition.
- Although rare, a malpositioned subclavian or jugular vein catheter may lead to thrombosis or sepsis.
- An air embolism, a potentially fatal complication, can occur during I.V. tubing changes if the tubing is inadvertently disconnected. It may also result from undetected hairline cracks in the tubing.
- Extravasation of parenteral nutrition solution can cause necrosis and then sloughing of the epidermis and dermis.

Documentation
Document the times of the dressing, filter, and solution changes; the condition of the catheter insertion site; your observations of the patient's condition; and complications and interventions. (See *Documenting TPN.*)

Supportive references
American Society for Parenteral and Enteral Nutrition. *Nutritional Support Nursing Core Curriculum,* 3rd ed. Columbus, Ohio: ASPEN, 1996.

"ASPEN Standards of Practice: Standards for Home Nutrition Support," *Nutrition in Clinical Practice* 14(3):151-62, June 1999.

Bliss, D.Z., and Dysart, M. "Using Needleless Intravenous Access Devices for Administering Total Parenteral Nutrition (TPN): Practice Update," *Nutrition in Clinical Practice* 14(6):299-303, December 1999.

> ### Documenting TPN
>
> If a patient is receiving total parenteral nutrition (TPN), be sure to record:
>
> - central line type and location
> - insertion site condition
> - volume and rate of the solution infused
> - your observations of any adverse reactions and your interventions
> - when you discontinue a central or peripheral I.V. line for TPN
> - date and time and the type of dressing applied after TPN was discontinued
> - administration site appearance.

Duerksen, D.R., et al. "Peripherally Inserted Central Catheters for Parenteral Nutrition: A Comparison of Centrally Inserted Catheters," *Journal of Parenteral and Enteral Nutrition* 23(2):85-90, March-April 1999.

"Standard 23. Expiration and Beyond-use Dates. Infusion Nursing Standards of Practice," *Journal of Infusion Nursing* 29(1S):S29, January-February 2006.

"Standard 32. Filters. Infusion Nursing Standards of Practice," *Journal of Infusion Nursing* 29(1S):S33-35, January-February 2006.

"Standard 69. Parenteral Nutrition. Infusion Nursing Standards of Practice," *Journal of Infusion Nursing* 29(1S):S75-76, January-February 2006.

Trissel, L.A., et al. "Compatibility of Medications with 3-in-1 Parenteral Nutrition Admixtures," *Journal of Parenteral and Enteral Nutrition* 23(2):67-74, March-April 1999.

Total parenteral nutrition monitoring

Total parenteral nutrition (TPN) requires careful monitoring. Because the typical patient is in a protein-wasting state, TPN therapy causes marked changes in fluid and electrolyte status and in glucose, amino acid, mineral, and vitamin levels. If the patient displays an adverse reaction or signs of complications, the TPN regimen can be changed as needed. **INS**

Assessment of the patient's nutritional status includes a physical examination, anthropometric measurements, biochemical determinations, and tests of cell-mediated immunity. Assessment of the patient's condition *to detect complications* requires recognition of the signs and symptoms of possible complications, understanding laboratory test results, and careful record keeping.

Because the TPN solution is high in glucose content, the infusion must start slowly *to allow the patient's pancreatic beta cells to adapt to it by increasing insulin output.* Within the first 3 to 5 days of TPN, the typical adult patient can tolerate 3 L of solution daily without adverse reactions. Lipid emulsions also require monitoring.

During TPN administration, the nurse should be especially observant of signs of metabolic and electrolyte disturbances and should also assess the catheter site daily for signs and symptoms of infection or other catheter-related problems. **INS**

Equipment

TPN solution and administration equipment• blood glucose meter• stethoscope• sphygmomanometer• watch with second hand• scale• input and output chart• time tape• additional equipment for nutritional assessment, as ordered

Preparation of equipment

● For information on preparing the infusion pump and TPN solution, see appropriate procedures in this section.
● Attach a time tape to the TPN container *to allow approximate measurement of fluid intake.*
● Make sure that each bag or bottle has a label listing the expiration date, glucose concentration, and total volume of solution. (If the bag or bottle is damaged and you don't have an immediate replacement, hang a bag of dextrose 10% in water until the new container is ready.)

Implementation

● Explain the procedure to the patient *to diminish his anxiety and encourage cooperation.* Instruct him to inform you if he experiences unusual sensations during the infusion. **INS** **PCP**
● Record the patient's vital signs every 4 hours, or more often if necessary, *because increased tempera-*ture is one of the earliest signs of catheter-related sepsis. **INS**
● Perform I.V. site care and dressing changes at least three times per week (once per week for transparent semipermeable dressings) or whenever the dressing becomes wet, soiled, or nonocclusive. Use strict sterile technique. **INS**
● Physically assess the patient daily. If ordered, measure arm circumference and skinfold thickness over the triceps.
● Weigh the patient at the same time each morning (after voiding), in similar clothing, and on the same scale. Compare these data with his fluid intake and output record. *Weight gain, particularly early in treatment, may indicate fluid overload* rather than increasing fat and protein stores. A patient shouldn't gain more than 3 lb (1.4 kg) per week; a gain of 1 lb (0.5 kg) per week is a reasonable goal in most cases. Suspect fluid imbalance if the patient gains more than 1 lb daily. Assess for peripheral and pulmonary edema.
● Monitor the patient for signs and symptoms of glucose metabolism disturbance, fluid and electrolyte imbalances, and nutritional aberrations. Remember that some patients may require supplemental insulin for the duration of TPN; the pharmacy usually adds insulin directly to the TPN solution. **INS**
● Monitor electrolyte and protein levels frequently — daily at first for electrolytes and twice per week for serum albumin. Later, as the patient's condition stabilizes, you won't need to monitor these values quite as closely. (Be aware that in a severely dehydrated patient, albumin levels may actually drop initially as treatment restores hydration.)
● Pay close attention to magnesium and calcium levels. If these electrolytes have been added to the TPN solution, the dosage may need adjusting *to maintain normal serum levels.* Assess the patient for signs and symptoms of magnesium and calcium imbalances. **ASPEN** **INS**
● Monitor serum glucose levels every 6 hours initially, then once per day, and stay alert for signs and symptoms of hyperglycemia, such as thirst and polyuria. Periodically confirm blood glucose meter readings with laboratory tests. **INS**
● Check renal function by monitoring blood urea nitrogen and creatinine levels — *increases can indicate excess amino acid intake.* Also assess nitrogen balance with 24-hour urine collection.

• Assess liver function by periodically monitoring liver enzyme, bilirubin, triglyceride, and cholesterol levels. *Abnormal values may indicate an intolerance or an excess of lipid emulsions or problems with metabolizing the protein or glucose in the TPN formula.*

• Change the I.V. administration set according to your facility's policy. Use sterile technique and coordinate the change with a solution change. Keep in mind that the tubing, injection caps, stopcocks, catheter, and even the patient's skin are potential sources of microbial contamination. The catheter hub, where most manipulations take place, is especially vulnerable. (The TPN formula itself, which is prepared under sterile conditions in the pharmacy, is rarely the source of infection.)

• Many facilities require changing I.V. administration sets every 24 hours, which is what most infection-control practitioners recommend for TPN infusions. However, some now wait 48 to 72 hours. *Because the risk of contamination is so high with TPN,* each facility should continuously evaluate protocols based on quality-control findings. **INS**

• Monitor the patient for signs of inflammation, infection, or sepsis, the most common complications of TPN. Microbial contamination of the venous access device is the usual cause. Watch for redness and drainage at the venous access site, and monitor the patient for fever and other signs and symptoms of sepsis. **INS**

• While weaning the patient from TPN, document his dietary intake and work with the nutritionist to determine the total calorie and protein intake. Also teach other health care staff caring for the patient the importance of recording food intake. Use percentages of food consumed ("ate 50% of a baked potato") instead of subjective descriptions ("had a good appetite") *to provide a more accurate account of patient intake.*

• Provide emotional support. Keep in mind that patients commonly associate eating with positive feelings and become disturbed when eating is prohibited.

• Provide frequent mouth care.

• Keep the patient active *to enable him to use nutrients more fully.*

• When discontinuing TPN, decrease the infusion rate slowly, depending on the patient's current glucose intake, *to minimize the risk of hyperinsulinemia and resulting hypoglycemia.* Weaning usually takes place over 24 to 48 hours but can be completed in 4 to 6 hours if the patient receives sufficient oral or I.V. carbohydrates. **ASPEN**

Special considerations

• Always maintain strict sterile technique when handling the equipment used to administer therapy. *Because the TPN solution serves as a medium for bacterial growth and the central venous (CV) line provides systemic access,* the patient risks infection and sepsis.

• When using a filter, position it as close to the access site as possible. Check the filter's porosity and pounds-per-square-inch (psi) capacity *to make sure it exceeds the number of psi exerted by the infusion pump.* **INS**

• Don't allow TPN solutions to hang for more than 24 hours. **INS**

• Be careful when using the TPN line for other functions. If using a single-lumen CV catheter, don't use the line to infuse blood or blood products, to give a bolus injection, to administer simultaneous I.V. solutions, to measure CV pressure, or to draw blood for laboratory tests. Never add medication to a TPN solution container. Also, avoid using a three-way stopcock, if possible, *because add-on devices increase the risk of infection.*

• When a patient is severely malnourished, starting TPN may spark "refeeding syndrome," which includes a rapid drop in potassium, magnesium, and phosphorus levels. *To avoid compromising cardiac function,* initiate feeding slowly and monitor the patient's blood values especially closely until they stabilize. **ASPEN**

Nursing diagnoses

• Risk for infection
• Risk for injury

Expected outcomes

The patient will:

• maintain temperature within normal limits
• maintain complete blood count and differential within normal limits
• have culture results that show no evidence of pathogens
• avoid complications associated with therapy.

Complications

Catheter-related, metabolic, and mechanical complications can occur during TPN administration.

Documentation

Record serial monitoring indexes on the appropriate flowchart *to determine the patient's progress and response.* Note abnormal, adverse, or altered responses.

Supportive references

"Standard 23. Expiration and Beyond-use Dates. Infusion Nursing Standards of Practice," *Journal of Infusion Nursing* 29(1S):S29, January-February 2006.

"Standard 29. Add-on Devices and Junction Securement. Infusion Nursing Standards of Practice," *Journal of Infusion Nursing* 29(1S):S32, January-February 2006.

"Standard 48. Administration Set Change. Infusion Nursing Standards of Practice," *Journal of Infusion Nursing* 29(1S):S48-51, January-February 2006.

"Standard 69. Parenteral Nutrition. Infusion Nursing Standards of Practice," *Journal of Infusion Nursing* 29(1S):S75-76, January-February 2006.

Transfusion reaction management

A transfusion reaction typically stems from a major antigen-antibody reaction and can result from a single or massive transfusion of blood or blood products. Although many reactions occur during transfusion or within 96 hours afterward, infectious diseases transmitted during a transfusion may go undetected until days, weeks, or months later, when signs and symptoms appear.

A transfusion reaction requires immediate recognition and prompt nursing action to prevent further complications and, possibly, death — particularly if the patient is unconscious or so heavily sedated that he can't report the common symptoms. (See *Managing transfusion reactions.*)

Equipment

Normal saline solution • I.V. administration set • sterile urine specimen container • needle, syringe, and tubes for blood samples • transfusion reaction report form • optional: oxygen, epinephrine, hypothermia blanket, leukocyte removal filter

Implementation

● As soon as you suspect an adverse reaction, stop the transfusion and start the saline infusion (using a new I.V. administration set) at a keep-vein-open rate *to maintain venous access.* Don't discard the blood bag or administration set. **AABB INS**
● Notify the physician.
● Monitor the patient's vital signs every 15 minutes or as indicated by the severity and type of reaction. **AABB INS**
● Compare the labels on all blood containers with corresponding patient identification forms *to verify that the transfusion was the correct blood or blood product.* **AABB INS**
● Notify the blood bank of a possible transfusion reaction and collect blood samples, as ordered. Immediately send the samples, all transfusion containers (even if empty), and the administration set to the blood bank. *The blood bank will test these materials to further evaluate the reaction.*
● Collect the first posttransfusion urine specimen, mark the collection slip "Possible transfusion reaction," and send it to the laboratory immediately. *The laboratory tests this urine specimen for the presence of hemoglobin, which indicates a hemolytic reaction.* **AABB INS**
● Closely monitor intake and output. Note evidence of oliguria or anuria *because hemoglobin deposition in the renal tubules can cause renal damage.* **Science**
● If prescribed, administer oxygen, epinephrine, or other drugs, and apply a hypothermia blanket *to reduce fever.*
● Make the patient as comfortable as possible, and provide reassurance as necessary.

Special considerations

● Treat all transfusion reactions as serious until proven otherwise. If the physician anticipates a transfusion reaction, such as one that may occur in a leukemia patient, he may order prophylactic treatment with antihistamines or antipyretics to precede blood administration.
● *To avoid a possible febrile reaction,* the physician may order the blood washed to remove as many leukocytes as possible, or a leukocyte removal filter may be used during the transfusion.

Nursing diagnoses

● Decreased cardiac output

(Text continues on page 184.)

Managing transfusion reactions

A patient receiving a transfusion of processed blood products risks certain complications, such as hemosiderosis and hypothermia, for example. This chart describes *endogenous reactions,* those caused by an antigen-antibody reaction in the recipient, and *exogenous reactions,* those caused by external factors in administered blood.

Reaction and causes	Signs and symptoms	Nursing interventions
Endogenous		
Allergic • Allergen in donor blood • Donor blood hypersensitive to certain drugs	• Anaphylaxis (chills, facial swelling, laryngeal edema, pruritus, urticaria, wheezing), fever, nausea and vomiting	• Administer antihistamines, as prescribed. • Monitor patient for anaphylactic reaction, and administer epinephrine and corticosteroids if indicated. *Prevention* • As prescribed, premedicate patient with diphenhydramine (Benadryl) before subsequent transfusion. • Observe patient closely for first 30 minutes of transfusion.
Bacterial contamination • Organisms that can survive cold, such as *Pseudomonas* or *Staphylococcus*	• Chills, fever, vomiting, abdominal cramping, diarrhea, shock, signs of renal failure	• Provide broad-spectrum antibiotics, corticosteroids, or epinephrine, as prescribed. *Prevention* • Maintain strict blood-storage control. • Change blood administration set and filter every 4 hours or after every two units. • Infuse each unit of blood over 2 to 4 hours; stop infusion if time span exceeds 4 hours. • Maintain sterile technique when administering blood products. • Inspect blood before transfusion for air, clots, and dark purple color.
Febrile • Bacterial lipopolysaccharides • Antileukocyte recipient antibodies directed against donor white blood cells	• Fever up to 104° F (40° C), chills, headache, facial flushing, palpitations, cough, chest tightness, increased pulse rate, flank pain	• Relieve symptoms with an antipyretic or antihistamine, as ordered. • If patient requires further transfusions, use frozen red blood cells (RBCs), add a special leukocyte removal filter to blood line, or premedicate him with acetaminophen, as ordered, before starting another transfusion. *Prevention* • Premedicate patient with an antipyretic, an antihistamine and, possibly, a steroid. • Use leukocyte-poor or washed RBCs. Use a leukocyte removal filter specific to blood component.

(continued)

Managing transfusion reactions *(continued)*

Reaction and causes	Signs and symptoms	Nursing interventions
Endogenous *(continued)*		
Hemolytic • ABO or Rh incompatibility • Intradonor incompatibility • Improper crossmatching • Improperly stored blood	• Chest pain, dyspnea, facial flushing, fever, chills, shaking, hypotension, flank pain, hemoglobinuria, oliguria, bloody oozing at infusion site or surgical incision site, burning sensation along vein receiving blood, shock, renal failure	• Monitor blood pressure. • Manage shock with I.V. fluids, oxygen, epinephrine, a diuretic, and a vasopressor, as ordered. • Obtain posttransfusion-reaction blood samples and urine specimens for analysis. • Observe for signs of hemorrhage resulting from disseminated intravascular coagulation. *Prevention* • Before the transfusion, check donor and recipient blood types to ensure blood compatibility. • Transfuse blood slowly for first 30 minutes of transfusion.
Plasma protein incompatibility • Immunoglobulin (Ig) A incompatibility	• Abdominal pain, diarrhea, dyspnea, chills, fever, flushing, hypotension	• Administer oxygen, fluids, epinephrine or, possibly, a steroid, as ordered. *Prevention* • Tranfuse only IgA-deficient blood or well-washed RBCs.
Exogenous		
Bleeding tendencies • Low platelet count in stored blood, causing thrombocytopenia	• Abnormal bleeding and oozing from a cut, a break in the skin surface or the gums; abnormal bruising and petechiae	• Administer platelets, fresh frozen plasma (FFP), or cryoprecipitate, as ordered. • Monitor platelet count. *Prevention* • Use only fresh blood (less than 7 days old) when possible.
Circulatory overload • May result from infusing whole blood too rapidly	• Increased plasma volume, back pain, chest tightness, chills, fever, dyspnea, flushed feeling, headache, hypertension, increased central venous and jugular vein pressure	• Monitor blood pressure. • Administer diuretics, as ordered. *Prevention* • Transfuse blood slowly. • Don't exceed two units in 4 hours; fewer for elderly patients, infants, or patients with cardiac conditions.
Elevated blood ammonia level • Increased ammonia level in stored donor blood	• Confusion, forgetfulness, lethargy	• Monitor ammonia level in blood. • Decrease amount of protein in patient's diet. • If indicated, give neomycin or laculose (Cholac). *Prevention* • Use only RBCs, FFP, or fresh blood, especially if patient has hepatic disease.

Managing transfusion reactions *(continued)*

Reaction and causes	Signs and symptoms	Nursing interventions
Exogenous *(continued)*		
Hemosiderosis ● Increased level of hemosiderin (iron-containing pigment) from RBC destruction, especially after many transfusions	● Iron plasma level exceeding 200 mg/dl	● Perform phlebotomy to remove excess iron. ***Prevention*** ● Administer blood only when absolutely necessary.
Hypocalcemia ● Citrate toxicity occurs when citrate-treated blood is infused rapidly (Citrate binds with calcium, causing a calcium deficiency, or normal citrate metabolism becomes impeded by hepatic disease.)	● Arrhythmias, hypotension, muscle cramps, nausea and vomiting, seizures, tingling in fingers	● Slow or stop transfusion, depending on patient's reaction. Expect a more severe reaction in hypothermic patients or patients with elevated potassium level. ***Prevention*** ● Infuse blood slowly.
Hypothermia ● Rapid infusion of large amounts of cold blood, which decreases body temperature	● Chills; shaking; hypotension; arrhythmias, especially bradycardia; cardiac arrest, if core temperature falls below 86° F (30° C)	● Stop transfusion. ● Warm patient with blankets. ● Obtain an electrocardiogram (ECG). ***Prevention*** ● Warm blood to 95° to 98° F (35° to 36.7° C) especially before massive transfusions.
Increased oxygen affinity for hemoglobin ● Decreased level of 2,3-diphosphoglycerate in stored blood, causing an increase in the oxygen's hemoglobin affinity (When this occurs, oxygen stays in the patient's bloodstream and isn't released into body tissues.)	● Depressed respiratory rate, especially in patients with chronic lung disease	● Monitor arterial blood gas levels, and provide respiratory support, as needed. ***Prevention*** ● Use only RBCs or fresh blood, if possible.
Potassium intoxication ● An abnormally high level of potassium in stored plasma caused by RBC hemolysis	● Diarrhea, intestinal colic, flaccidity, muscle twitching, oliguria, renal failure, bradycardia progressing to cardiac arrest, ECG changes with tall, peaked T waves	● Obtain an ECG. ● Administer sodium polystyrene sulfonate (Kayexalate) orally or by enema. ***Prevention*** ● Use fresh blood when administering massive transfusions.

- Deficient fluid volume
- Ineffective tissue perfusion: Cardiopulmonary

Expected outcomes

The patient will:
- maintain pulse rate not less than __ and not greater than ___; and blood pressure not less than ___ and not greater than ____
- not exhibit any arrhythmias
- maintain intake and output within normal range
- attain hemodynamic stability
- maintain heart and respiratory rates and pulse within normal range.

Documentation

Record the time and date of the transfusion reaction, the type and amount of infused blood or blood products, the clinical signs of the transfusion reaction in order of occurrence, the patient's vital signs, specimens sent to the laboratory for analysis, treatment given, and the patient's response to treatment. If required by policy, complete the transfusion reaction form.

Supportive references

American Association of Blood Banks. *Technical Manual*, 13th ed. Vengelen-Tyler, V., ed. Bethesda, Md.: AABB, 1999.

Cook, L.S. "Blood Transfusion Reactions Involving an Immune Response," *Journal of Intravenous Nursing* 20(1):5-14, January-February 1997.

Joint Commission on Accreditation of Healthcare Organizations. *Comprehensive Accreditation Manual for Home Care.* Oakbrook Terrace, Ill.: JCAHO, 2002. *www.jcaho.gov.*

Joint Commission on Accreditation of Healthcare Organizations. *Comprehensive Accreditation Manual for Hospitals.* Oakbrook Terrace, Ill.: JCAHO, 2002.

"Standard 14. Assessment and Monitoring. Infusion Nursing Standards of Practice," *Journal of Intravenous Nursing* 23(6S):S19-20, November-December 2000.

"Standard 48. Administration Set Change. Infusion Nursing Standards of Practice," *Journal of Infusion Nursing* 29(1S):S48-51, January-February 2006.

"Standard 70. Transfusion Therapy. Infusion Nursing Standards of Practice," *Journal of Infusion Nursing* 29(1S):S76-77, January-February 2006.

Weinstein, S.M. *Plumer's Principles and Practice of Intravenous Therapy,* 7th ed. Philadelphia: Lippincott Williams & Wilkins, 2001.

Vascular access ports

Surgically implanted under local anesthesia by a physician, a vascular access device consists of a silicone catheter attached to a reservoir, which is covered with a self-sealing silicone rubber septum. It's most commonly used for patients who require I.V. therapy for at least 6 months. The most common type of vascular access device is a vascular access port (VAP). (See *Understanding vascular access ports.*)

The VAP reservoir can be made of titanium (as with implanted infusion ports), stainless steel, or molded plastic. Type selected depends on the patient's needs.

Implanted in a pocket under the skin, the attached indwelling catheter tunnels through the subcutaneous tissue into a vein and the catheter is advanced *so that the catheter tip lies in a central vein* — for example, the subclavian vein. A VAP can also be used for arterial access or be implanted into the epidural space, peritoneum, or pericardial or pleural cavity.

Sterile technique must be maintained when accessing the VAP. Correct needle placement is verified by aspiration of blood and should be done before administering medications or I.V. solutions. The noncoring needle used to access the port should be changed every 7 days. Hemodynamic monitoring and venipuncture shouldn't be performed on the extremity containing the implanted device. **AABB** **INS**

Typically, VAPs deliver intermittent infusions. Most commonly used for chemotherapy, a VAP can also deliver I.V. fluids, medications, and blood. It can also be used to obtain blood samples.

VAPs offer several advantages, which include minimal activity restrictions, few steps for the patient to perform, and few dressing changes (except when used to maintain continuous infusions or intermittent infusion devices). Implanted devices are easier to maintain than external devices. For instance, they require heparinization only once after each use (or periodically if not in use). They also pose less risk of infection *because they have no exit site to serve as an entry for microorganisms.*

Because VAPs create only a slight protrusion under the skin, many patients find them easier to accept than external infusion devices. Because the device is implanted, however, it may be harder for the patient to manage, particularly if he'll be administering medication or fluids daily or frequently. And because accessing the device requires inserting a needle through subcutaneous tissue, patients who fear or dislike needle punctures may be uncomfortable using a VAP and may require a local anesthetic. In addition, implantation and removal of the device require surgery and hospitalization.

Implanted VAPs are contraindicated in patients who have been unable to tolerate other implanted devices and in those who may develop an allergic reaction.

Equipment

To implant a VAP

Noncoring needles of appropriate type and gauge (a noncoring needle has a deflected point, which slices the port's septum) • VAP • sterile gloves • mask • 2% chlorhexidine swabs • extension set tubing, if needed • local anesthetic (lidocaine without epinephrine) • ice pack • 10- and 20-ml syringes • normal saline and heparin flush solutions • I.V. solution • sterile dressings • luer-lock injection cap • clamp • adhesive skin closures • suture removal set

To administer a bolus injection

Extension set • 10-ml syringe filled with normal saline solution • clamp • syringe containing the prescribed medication • optional: sterile syringe filled with heparin flush solution

To administer a continuous infusion

Prescribed I.V. solution or drugs • I.V. administration set • filter, if ordered • extension set • clamp • 10-ml syringe filled with normal saline solution • adhesive tape • sterile 2″ × 2″ gauze pad • sterile tape • transparent semipermeable dressing

Some health care facilities use an implantable port access kit.

Preparation of equipment

● Confirm the size and type of the device and the insertion site with the physician.
● Attach the tubing to the solution container, prime the tubing with fluid, fill the syringes with saline or heparin flush solution, and prime the noncoring needle and extension set.

Understanding vascular access ports

Typically, a vascular access port (VAP) is used to deliver intermittent infusions of medication, chemotherapy, and blood products. Because the device is completely covered by the patient's skin, *the risk of extrinsic contamination is reduced.* Patients may prefer this type of central line because it doesn't alter the body image and requires less routine catheter care.

The VAP consists of a catheter connected to a small reservoir. A septum designed to withstand multiple punctures seals the reservoir.

To access the port, a special noncoring needle is inserted perpendicular to the reservoir.

Top-entry VAP

● All priming must be done using strict sterile technique, and all tubing must be free from air.
● After you've primed the tubing, recheck all connections for tightness. Make sure that all open ends are covered with sealed caps.

Implementation

● Wash your hands *to prevent the spread of microorganisms.* **CDC**

Assisting with implantation of a VAP

● Reinforce to the patient the practitioner's explanation of the procedure, its benefit to the patient, and what's expected of him during and after implantation. **PCP**

● Although the practitioner is responsible for obtaining consent for the procedure, make sure that the written document is signed, witnessed, and in the chart.

● Allay the patient's fears and answer questions about movement restrictions, cosmetic concerns, and-management regimens. **PCP**

● Check the patient's history for hypersensitivity to local anesthetics or iodine.

● The surgeon will surgically implant the VAP, probably using a local anesthetic (similar to insertion of a central venous [CV] catheter). Occasionally, a patient may receive a general anesthetic for VAP implantation.

● First, the surgeon makes a small incision and introduces the catheter, typically into the superior vena cava through the subclavian, jugular, or cephalic vein. After fluoroscopy verifies correct placement of the catheter tip, the physician creates a subcutaneous pocket over a bony prominence in the chest wall. Then he tunnels the catheter to the pocket. Next, he connects the catheter to the reservoir, places the reservoir in the pocket, and flushes it with heparin solution. Finally, he sutures the reservoir to the underlying fascia and closes the incision.

Preparing to access the port

● The VAP can be used immediately after placement, although some edema and tenderness may persist for about 72 hours. This makes the device initially difficult to palpate and slightly uncomfortable for the patient.

● Prepare to access the port, following the specific steps for top-entry ports.

● Confirm the patient's identity using two patient identifiers according to facility policy. **JCAHO**

● Using sterile technique, inspect the area around the port for signs of infection or skin breakdown. **INS**

● Place an ice pack over the area for several minutes *to alleviate possible discomfort from the needle puncture.* Alternatively, administer a local anesthetic after cleaning the area.

● Wash your hands thoroughly. Put on sterile gloves and a mask and wear them throughout the procedure. **CDC**

● Clean the area with an alcohol pad, starting at the center of the port and working outward with a firm, circular motion over a 4″ to 5″ (10- to 12.5-cm) diam-

eter. Repeat this procedure twice. Allow the site to dry, then clean the area with 2% chlorhexidine swabs in the same manner. Repeat this procedure twice. **INS**

● If your facility's policy calls for a local anesthetic, check the patient's record for possible allergies. As indicated, anesthetize the insertion site by injecting 0.1 ml of lidocaine (without epinephrine).

● Palpate the area over the port *to find its septum.*

● Anchor the port with your nondominant hand. Then using your dominant hand, aim the needle at the center of the device.

● Insert the needle perpendicular to the port septum. Push the needle through the skin and septum until you reach the bottom of the reservoir.

● Check needle placement by aspirating for blood return. **INS**

● If you can't obtain blood, remove the needle and repeat the procedure. *Inability to obtain blood may indicate sludge buildup (from medications) in the port reservoir.* If so, you may need to use a fibrinolytic agent to free the occlusion. Ask the patient to raise his arms and perform Valsalva's maneuver. If you still don't get a blood return, notify the physician; *a fibrin sleeve on the distal end of the catheter may be occluding the opening.* (See *Managing VAP problems.*) **INS**

● Flush the device with normal saline solution. If you detect swelling or if the patient reports pain at the site, remove the needle and notify the physician.

✓ **CLINICAL IMPACT** *A continuous infusion device may be more cost effective than manually flushing the VAP.*

Administering a bolus injection

● Attach the 10-ml syringe filled with saline solution to the end of the extension set and remove all the air. Now attach the extension set to the noncoring needle. Check for blood return. Then flush the port with normal saline solution, according to your facility's policy. **AABB** **INS**

● Clamp the extension set and remove the saline syringe.

● Connect the medication syringe to the extension set. Open the clamp and inject the drug, as ordered.

● Examine the skin surrounding the needle for signs of infiltration, such as swelling or tenderness. If you note these signs, stop the injection and intervene appropriately. **INS**

Managing VAP problems

This chart outlines common problems with vascular access ports (VAPs) along with possible causes and nursing interventions.

Problems and possible causes	Nursing interventions
Inability to flush the device or draw blood	
Catheter lodged against vessel wall	• Reposition patient. • Teach patient to change his position *to free catheter from vessel wall*. • Raise the arm that's on same side as catheter. • Roll patient to his opposite side. • Have patient cough, sit up, or take a deep breath. • Infuse 10 ml of normal saline solution into catheter. • Regain access to catheter or VAP using a new needle.
Clot formation	• Assess patency by trying to flush VAP while patient changes position. • Notify practitioner; obtain an order for fibrinolytic agent instillation. • Teach patient to recognize clot formation, to notify practitioner if it occurs, and to avoid forcibly flushing VAP.
Incorrect needle placement or needle not advanced through septum	• Regain access to device. • Teach home care patient to push down firmly on noncoring needle device in septum and to verify needle placement by aspirating for blood return.
Kinked catheter, catheter migration, or port rotation	• Notify practitioner immediately. • Tell patient to notify practitioner if he has trouble using VAP.
Kinked tubing or closed clamp	• Check tubing or clamp.
Inability to palpate the device	
Deeply implanted port	• Note portal chamber scar. • Use deep palpation technique. • Ask another nurse to try locating VAP. • Use a 1½″ or 2″ noncoring needle to access VAP.

• When the injection is complete, clamp the extension set and remove the medication syringe.

• Open the clamp and flush with 5 ml of normal saline solution after each drug injection *to minimize drug incompatibility reactions.* **INS**

• Flush with heparin solution according to your facility's policy.

Administering a continuous infusion

• Remove all air from the extension set by priming it with an attached syringe of normal saline solution.

Now attach the extension set to the noncoring needle. **INS**

• Flush the port system with normal saline solution. Clamp the extension set and remove the syringe.

• Connect the administration set, and secure the connections with sterile tape if necessary.

• Unclamp the extension set and begin the infusion.

• Affix the needle to the skin. Then apply a transparent semipermeable dressing. (See *Continuous infusion: Securing the needle,* page 188.)

• Examine the site carefully for infiltration. If the patient complains of stinging, burning, or pain at the

Continuous infusion: Securing the needle

When starting a continuous infusion, you must secure the right-angle, noncoring needle to the skin. If the needle hub isn't flush with the skin, place a folded sterile dressing under the hub, as shown. Then apply adhesive skin closures across it.

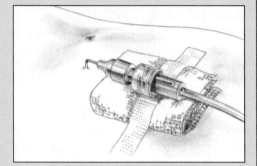

Secure the needle and tubing, using the chevron-taping technique.

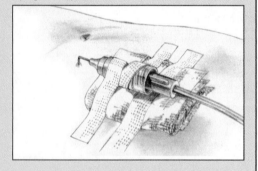

Apply a transparent semipermeable dressing over the entire site.

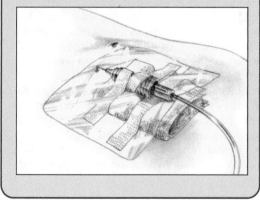

site, discontinue the infusion and intervene appropriately. **INS**

● When the solution container is empty, obtain a new I.V. solution container, as ordered.

● Flush with normal saline solution followed by heparin solution according to your facility's policy.

Special considerations

● After implantation, monitor the site for signs of hematoma and bleeding. Edema and tenderness may persist for up to 72 hours. The incision site requires routine postoperative care for 7 to 10 days. You'll also need to assess the implantation site for signs of infection, device rotation, or skin erosion. You don't need to apply a dressing to the wound site except during infusions or *to maintain an intermittent infusion device.*

● While the patient is hospitalized, a luer-lock injection cap may be attached to the end of the extension set to provide ready access for intermittent infusions. *Besides saving nursing time, a luer-lock cap reduces the discomfort of accessing the port and prolongs the life of the port septum by decreasing the number of needle punctures.*

● If the patient is receiving a continuous or prolonged infusion, change the dressing and needle every 7 days. You'll also need to change the tubing and solution, as you would for a long-term CV infusion. If the patient is receiving an intermittent infusion, flush the port periodically with heparin solution. When the VAP isn't being used, flush it every 4 weeks. During the course of therapy, you may have to clear a clotted VAP, as ordered. **INS**

● If clotting threatens to occlude the VAP, the physician may order a fibrinolytic agent to clear the catheter. *Because such agents increase the risk of bleeding,* fibrinolytic agents may be contraindicated in patients who have had surgery within the past 10 days; in those who have active internal bleeding, such as GI bleeding; and in those who have experienced central nervous system damage, such as infarction, hemorrhage, traumatic injury, surgery, or primary or metastatic disease, within the past 2 months.

● Besides performing routine care measures, you must be prepared to handle several common problems that may arise during an infusion with a VAP. These common problems include an inability to flush the VAP, withdraw blood from it, or palpate it.

TEACHING *If the patient is going home, he'll need thorough teaching about procedures as well as follow-up visits from a home care nurse to ensure safety and successful treatment. If he'll be accessing the port himself, explain that the most uncomfortable part of the procedure is the actual insertion of the needle into the skin.*

After the needle has penetrated the skin, the patient will feel mostly pressure. Eventually, the skin over the port will become desensitized from frequent needle punctures. Until then, the patient may want to use a topical anesthetic.

Stress the importance of pushing the needle into the port until the patient feels the needle bevel touch the back of the port. Many patients tend to stop short of the back of the port, leaving the needle bevel in the rubber septum.

Also stress the importance of monthly flushes when no more infusions are scheduled. If possible, instruct a family member in all aspects of care.

Nursing diagnoses
● Deficient knowledge (procedure and device)
● Risk for infection

Expected outcomes
The patient will:
● communicate the need to know more about the procedure and device
● state or demonstrate an understanding of what has been taught
● maintain temperature within normal limits
● maintain white blood cell and differential counts within normal limits
● have culture results that show no evidence of pathogens.

Complications
A patient who has a VAP faces risks similar to those associated with CV catheters. They include infection, thrombus formation, and occlusion. (See *Risks of VAP therapy,* page 190.)

Documentation
Record your assessment findings and interventions according to your facility's policy. Include the type, amount, rate, and duration of the infusion; appearance of the site; and adverse reactions and nursing interventions.

Also keep a record of all needle and dressing changes for continuous infusions; blood samples obtained, including the type and amount; and patient teaching topics covered. Finally, document the removal of the infusion needle, the status of the site, the use of the heparin flush, and any problems you found and resolved.

Supportive references

Brock-Cascanet, P.H. "Treating Occluded VADs in the Home Setting," *Infusion* 5(4):18-27, January 1999.

Davis, S.N., et al. "Activity and Dosage of Alteplase Dilution for Clearing Occlusions of Venous-Access Devices," *American Journal of Health System Pharmacy* 57(11):1039-45, June 2000.

Heath, J., and Jones, S. "Utilization of an Elastomeric Continuous Infusion Device to Maintain Catheter Patency," *Journal of Intravenous Nursing* 24(2):102-106, March-April 2001.

Kincaid, E.H. "'Blind' Placement of Long Term Central Venous Access Devices: Report of 589 Consecutive Procedures," *American Surgeon* 65:520-24, June 1999.

"Standard 40. Local Anesthesia. Infusion Nursing Standards of Practice," *Journal of Infusion Nursing* 29(1S):S41, January-February 2006.

"Standard 43. Catheter Stabilization. Infusion Nursing Standards of Practice," *Journal of Infusion Nursing* 29(1S):S44, January-February 2006.

"Standard 44. Dressings. Infusion Nursing Standards of Practice," *Journal of Infusion Nursing* 29(1S):S44-45, January-February 2006.

"Standard 45. Implanted Ports and Pumps. Infusion Nursing Standards of Practice," *Journal of Infusion Nursing* 29(1S):S45-46, January-February 2006.

"Standard 53. Phlebitis. Infusion Nursing Standards of Practice," *Journal of Infusion Nursing* 29(1S):S58-59, January-February 2006.

"Standard 54. Infiltration. Infusion Nursing Standards of Practice," *Journal of Infusion Nursing* 29(1S):S59-60, January-February 2006.

"Standard 55. Extravasation. Infusion Nursing Standards of Practice," *Journal of Infusion Nursing* 29(1S):S61-62, January-February 2006.

"Standard 60. Catheter Clearance. Infusion Nursing Standards of Practice," *Journal of Infusion Nursing* 29(1S):S65, January-February 2006.

Risks of VAP therapy

This chart shows possible complications of vascular access port (VAP) therapy and outlines signs and symptoms, possible causes, and nursing interventions.

Complication	Signs and symptoms	Possible causes	Nursing interventions
Extravasation	• Burning sensation or swelling in subcutaneous tissue	• Needle dislodged into subcutaneous tissue • Needle incorrectly placed in VAP • Needle position not confirmed; needle pulled out of septum • Rupture of catheter along tunnel route	• Stop infusion, but don't remove needle. • Notify practitioner; prepare to administer an antidote, if ordered. *Prevention* • Teach patient how to gain access to device, verify its placement, and secure needle before initiating an infusion.
Fibrin sheath formation	• Blocked port and catheter lumen • Inability to flush port or administer infusion • Possible swelling, tenderness, and erythema in neck, chest, and shoulder	• Adherence of platelets to catheter	• Notify practitioner; prepare to administer a thrombolytic agent. *Prevention* • Use port only to infuse fluids and medications; don't use it to obtain blood samples. • Administer only compatible substances through port.
Site infection or skin breakdown	• Erythema and warmth at port site • Oozing or purulent drainage at VAP site or pocket • Fever	• Infected incision or VAP pocket • Poor postoperative healing	• Assess site daily for redness; note drainage. • Notify practitioner. • Administer antibiotics, as prescribed. • Apply warm soaks for 20 minutes four times per day. *Prevention* • Teach patient to inspect for and report redness, swelling, drainage, or skin breakdown at port site.
Thrombosis	• Inability to flush port or administer infusion	• Frequent blood sampling • Infusion of packed red blood cells (RBCs)	• Notify practitioner; obtain an order to administer a fibrinolytic agent. *Prevention* • Flush VAP thoroughly right after obtaining a blood sample. • Administer packed RBCs as a piggyback with normal saline solution and use an infusion pump; flush with normal saline solution between units.

Volume-control sets

A volume-control set — an I.V. line with a graduated chamber — delivers precise amounts of fluid and shuts off when the fluid is exhausted, *preventing air from entering the I.V. line.* It may be used as a secondary line in adults for intermittent infusion of medication.

ALERT *A volume-control set is used as a primary line in children for continuous infusion of fluids or medication.*

Equipment

Volume-control set • I.V. pole (for setting up a primary I.V. line) • I.V. solution • 20G to 22G 1" needle or needle-free adapter • alcohol pads • medication in labeled syringe • tape • label

Although various models of volume-control sets are available, each one consists of a graduated fluid chamber (120 to 250 ml) with a spike and a filtered air line on top and administration tubing underneath. Floating-valve sets have a valve at the bottom that closes when the chamber empties; membrane-filter sets have a rigid filter at the bottom that, when wet, prevents the passage of air.

Preparation of equipment
● Ensure the sterility of all equipment and inspect it carefully *to ensure the absence of flaws.*
● Take the equipment to the patient's bedside.

Implementation
● Wash your hands, and explain the procedure to the patient. If an I.V. line is already in place, observe its insertion site for signs of infiltration and infection. **CDC** **PCP**
● Remove the volume-control set from its box, and close all the clamps.
● Remove the protective cap from the volume-control set spike, insert the spike into the I.V. solution container, and hang the container on the I.V. pole.
● Open the air vent clamp and close the upper slide clamp. Then open the lower clamp on the I.V. tubing, slide it upward until it's slightly below the drip chamber, and close the clamp (as shown below).

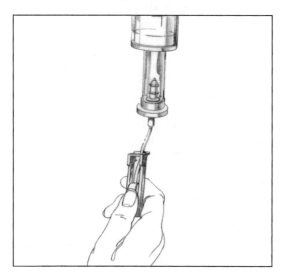

● If you're using a valve set, open the upper clamp until the fluid chamber fills with about 30 ml of solution. Then close the clamp and carefully squeeze the drip chamber until it's half full. **INS**
● If you're using a volume-control set with a membrane filter, open the upper clamp until the fluid chamber fills with about 30 ml of solution, and then close the clamp.
● Open the lower clamp and squeeze the drip chamber flat with two fingers of your opposite hand (as shown below). *If you squeeze the drip chamber with the lower clamp closed, you'll damage the membrane filter.*

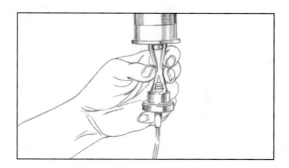

● Keeping the drip chamber flat, close the lower clamp. Now release the drip chamber so that it fills halfway.
● Open the lower clamp, prime the tubing, and close the clamp. To use the set as a primary line, insert the distal end of the tubing into the catheter or needle hub. To use the set as a secondary line, attach a needle to the adapter on the volume-control set. Wipe the Y-port of the primary tubing with an alcohol pad, and insert the needle. Then tape the connection. **AABB** **INS**
● If you're using a needle-free system, attach the distal end of the tubing to the Y-port of the primary tubing, following the manufacturer's instructions. **MFR**
● To add medication, wipe the injection port on the volume-control set with an alcohol pad, and inject the medication. Place a label on the chamber, indicating the drug, dose, and date. Don't write directly on the chamber *because the plastic absorbs ink.* **INS**
⚠ **ALERT** *Inadequate drug mixing can result in adverse effects. To avoid complications, never add medications to a hanging I.V. solution.*

✔ **CLINICAL IMPACT** *After adding medication to the administration set, a medication or solution should be infused or discarded within 24 hours. This expiration time may be extended beyond 24 hours if all of the following conditions are met:*
- *strict sterile technique is used during the initial infusion system setup*
- *a closed infusion administration system without injection ports or add-on devices is used*
- *no violation in the administration system is documented*
- *the prescribed medications and solutions are stable for the anticipated administration time.* **INS**
- Open the upper clamp, fill the fluid chamber with the prescribed amount of solution, and close the clamp. Gently rotate the chamber (as shown below) *to mix the medication.*

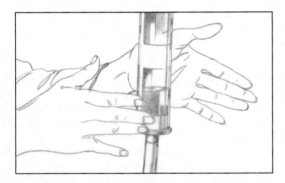

- Turn off the primary solution (if present) or lower the drip rate *to maintain an open line.*
- Open the lower clamp on the volume-control set, and adjust the drip rate as ordered. After completion of the infusion, open the upper clamp and let 10 ml of I.V. solution flow into the chamber and through the tubing *to flush them.*
- If you're using the volume-control set as a secondary I.V. line, close the lower clamp and reset the flow rate of the primary line. If you're using the set as a primary I.V. line, close the lower clamp, refill the chamber to the prescribed amount, and begin the infusion again.

Special considerations
- Always check compatibility of the medication and the I.V. solution. If you're using a membrane-filter

set, avoid administering suspensions, lipid emulsions, blood, or blood components through it.
- If you're using a floating-valve set, the diaphragm may stick after repeated use. If it does, close the air vent and upper clamp, invert the drip chamber, and squeeze it. If the diaphragm opens, reopen the clamp and continue to use the set.
- If the drip chamber of a floating-valve diaphragm set overfills, immediately close the upper clamp and air vent, invert the chamber, and squeeze the excess fluid from the drip chamber back into the graduated fluid chamber.

Nursing diagnoses
- Risk for imbalanced fluid volume

Expected outcomes
The patient will:
- maintain fluid intake and output at appropriate levels
- maintain vital signs within normal range.

Documentation
If you add a drug to the volume-control set, record the amount and type of medication, amount of fluid used to dilute it, and date and time of infusion.

Supportive references

Phillips, L.D. *Manual of I.V. Therapeutics,* 3rd ed. Philadelphia: F.A. Davis Co., 2001.

"Standard 15. Product Evaluation, Integrity, and Defect Reporting. Infusion Nursing Standards of Practice," *Journal of Infusion Nursing* 29(1S):S23, January-February 2006.

"Standard 48. Administration Set Change. Infusion Nursing Standards of Practice," *Journal of Infusion Nursing* 29(1S):S48-51, January-February 2006.

"Standard 68. Parenteral Medication and Solution Administration. Infusion Nursing Standards of Practice," *Journal of Infusion Nursing* 29(1S):S74-75, January-February 2006.

Weinstein, S.M. *Plumer's Principles and Practices of Intravenous Therapy,* 7th ed. Philadelphia: Lippincott Williams & Wilkins, 2001.

Cardiovascular care

Cardiovascular disorders affect millions of people every year and are, collectively, the leading cause of death in the United States. Because the care of patients with cardiovascular disorders is shared by practitioners of every type of nursing practice, cardiovascular care ranks as one of the most rapidly growing areas of nursing. Nurses face a constant challenge to keep up with new drugs and diagnostic tests as well as other innovative treatments.

The information presented in this chapter provides the latest evidence-based **EB** information from recent research and recommendations from various professional groups regarding care for this patient population. These groups include the American Heart Association **AHA** and its Advanced Cardiac Life Support **ACLS** guidelines, the American College of Cardiology **ACC**, the American Association of Critical-Care Nurses **AACN**, the Joint National Committee on Prevention, Detection, Evaluation, and Treatment of High Blood Pressure **JNC**, Emergency Nurse Association **ENA**, Joint Commission on Accreditation of Health Care Organizations **JCAHO**, and the Centers for Disease Control and Prevention **CDC**. Additional points are supported by the American Hospital Association's Patient Care Partnership **PCP** and fundamental tenets of science **Science**. Other points derive from specific manufacturers' recommendations **MFR** for the use of their equipment. You'll also learn about the kinds of equipment used in cardiac care and the best practices for various settings and situations.

Patient teaching

Nurses assume much of the responsibility for preparing patients physically and psychologically for hospitalization and ongoing care. They play a pivotal role in teaching patients and their families about disease prevention and lifestyle modification, tests and procedures, drugs and other treatments, and follow-up care. Patient and family teaching not only reduces stress but also improves patient compliance with prescribed therapy.

Monitoring

Cardiac and hemodynamic monitoring are vital aspects of cardiovascular care. Cardiac monitoring commonly involves either hardwire or telemetry systems that continually record the patient's cardiac activity. It's also useful to assess the patient's cardiac rhythm, gauge his response to drug therapy or diagnostic procedures, and provide opportunities for early intervention to prevent complications. Once only used in the critical care setting, cardiac monitoring is now utilized in high-risk obstetric care, general medical, pediatric, and transplantation departments.

Hemodynamic monitoring has become widely used since its inception in the 1970s. It uses invasive techniques to monitor the flow, pressure, and resistance of the cardiovascular system. Made with a pulmonary artery catheter, these measurements are used to guide therapy. Hemodynamic monitoring includes pulmonary artery pressure monitoring, right atrial pressure monitoring, pulmonary artery wedge pressure monitoring, cardiac output measurement, temporary pacing through the pulmonary artery catheter, and continuous evaluation of mixed venous oxygen saturation.

Treatment

In cardiovascular emergencies, nurses may perform or assist in lifesaving procedures, such as cardiopulmonary resuscitation, defibrillation, cardioversion, and temporary pacing. Carrying out these procedures requires in-depth knowledge of cardiovascular anatomy, physiology, and equipment as well as sound assessment and intervention techniques. Only nurses who are knowledgeable of the best practice regarding cardiovascular care can ensure the optimal outcome for their patients.

Ambulatory blood pressure monitoring

Ambulatory blood pressure monitoring (ABPM) allows measurement of blood pressure and cardiac activity over time without confining the patient to the health care facility. ABPM records the variations that occur in a patient's blood pressure during normal activity. Such monitoring more readily allows diagnosis of sustained hypertension and response to treatment than isolated blood pressure measurements taken in the physician's office.

The American Heart Association's *Seventh Report of the Joint National Committee* suggests that ABPM values are usually lower than physician office readings. Recent studies show that patients with a 24-hour ABPM greater than 135/85 mm Hg are two times more likely to have a cardiovascular event than those with a 24-hour ABPM less than 135/85 mm Hg, regardless of the blood pressure reading in the physician's office. **AHA** **JNC**

INNOVATIVE PRACTICE *ABPM can reduce health care costs by identifying patients who are normotensive but who would have been identified as having mild hypertension on the basis of office measurements alone. It can be used to rule out a diagnosis of sustained hypertension or determine a range in variability in labile hypertension, to monitor the effectiveness of therapy and evaluate drug-resistant hypertension, to determine diurnal blood pressure variations in patients with diabetes or autonomic insufficiency, and to evaluate blood pressure discrepancies. It's also useful in evaluating patients whose blood pressure measurements in the office are normal, but who have demonstrated progressive target organ injury. ABPM also can be used to avoid prescribing medication for patients who don't really need it.*

Equipment

Monitor (with new battery) that contains a cuff, microphone, and microprocessor that pumps the cuff and records measurements • carrying case with strap • 1″ adhesive tape • logbook or diary

Implementation

TEACHING *Explain the procedure to the patient and show him how to place the equip-*

ment into the carrying case and connect the neck strap.
- *Explain to the patient that he may need to wear a blood pressure cuff for 24 hours after activation of the monitor and tell him not to remove the cuff unless told to do so.*
- *Explain to the patient that he will have a carrying case with a strap to carry the 2-lb (0.9 kg) monitor.*
- *Tell the patient that he'll need to maintain an activity log during the 24-hour monitoring period. He should record the time, activities he performs, and any symptoms (such as headache, dizziness, light-headedness, palpitations, or chest pain) that occur.*
- *Explain to the patient the importance of maintaining his usual routine, including working, eating, sleeping, using the bathroom, and taking his medication.*
- *Suggest to the patient that he wear a watch to make keeping the log easier.*
- *Tell the patient that he'll need a follow-up appointment to review results 48 to 72 hours after removal of the monitor.*
- *Show the patient how to position the microphone over the brachial artery on the inner aspect of the nondominant arm, just above the elbow. Secure the microphone with tape. Then choose an appropriate-size blood pressure cuff.* **Science**
- *Explain that you will calibrate the monitor while the patient sits and then stands by measuring simultaneous blood pressure readings, using the ABPM unit and a mercury sphygmomanometer attached to the monitor with a T-tube device.* **JNC**
- *Show the patient how to use the tape to secure the microphone on the brachial area of his arm in case the microphone becomes loose.*
- *Tell the patient to keep the cuff arm still and free from extraneous noise when he feels the cuff inflating and deflating to ensure that measurements are accurate.*
- *Tell the patient to avoid activities — such as mowing the lawn, golfing, running, and playing tennis — that call for isometric use of the upper extremities to help avoid erroneous blood pressure measurements during such activities.*

Special considerations

● If the patient's skin is extremely oily, scaly, or diaphoretic, wash the electrode site with soap and water, then rub with a dry 4″ × 4″ gauze pad before applying the electrode.
● If the patient can't return to the office immediately after the monitoring period, show him how to remove the equipment and store the monitor, blood pressure cuff, and log.
● If the patient is wearing a patient-activated electrocardiogram, tell him that he can wear the monitor for up to 7 days. Tell him how to initiate the recording manually when symptoms occur.

Nursing diagnoses

● Health-seeking behaviors (blood pressure monitoring)

Expected outcomes

The patient will:
● demonstrate how to use ABPM
● state an understanding of the reason for monitoring
● state his blood pressure range
● express an interest in learning new behaviors to help reduce blood pressure.

Documentation

Document the indications for monitoring, noting the date and time the monitor was applied. Record the patient's medication regimen and blood pressure before monitoring. Be sure to include the patient's event log in the documentation. Document postprocedure results and actions taken.

Supportive references

American College of Physicians-American Society of Internal Medicine — Medical Specialty Society. "Diagnosing Syncope," June 1997.

Heaven, D.J., and Sutton, R. "Syncope," *Critical Care Medicine* 28(10 Suppl):N116-20, October 2000.

Institute for Clinical Systems Improvement. "Hypertension Diagnosis and Treatment," November 2000. *www.icsi.org/guide/HTN.pdf.*

O'Brien, E., et al. "Use and Interpretation of Ambulatory Blood Pressure Monitoring: Recommendations of the British Hypertension Society," *British Medical Journal* 320(7242):1128-34, April 2000.

"Seventh Report of the Joint National Committee on Prevention, Detection, Evaluation, and Treatment of High Blood Pressure," *Hypertension* 42:1206-52, 2003.

Yarows, S.A., et al. "Home Blood Pressure Monitoring," *Archives of Internal Medicine* 160(9):1251-57, May 2000.

Zimetbaum, P.J., and Josephson, M.E. "The Evolving Role of Ambulatory Arrhythmia Monitoring in General Clinical Practice," *Annals of Internal Medicine* 130(10):848-56, May 1999.

Zimetbaum, P.J., et al. "Diagnostic Yield and Optimal Duration of Continuous-Loop Event Monitoring for the Diagnosis of Palpitations: A Cost-Effective Analysis," *Annals of Internal Medicine* 128(11):890-95, June 1998.

Arterial pressure monitoring

Direct arterial pressure monitoring permits continuous measurement of systolic, diastolic, and mean pressures and allows arterial blood sampling. Because direct measurement reflects systemic vascular resistance in addition to blood flow, it's generally more accurate than indirect methods (such as palpation and auscultation of Korotkoff sounds or audible pulse), which are based on blood flow alone.

Direct monitoring is recommended when highly accurate or frequent blood pressure measurements are required; for example, in patients with low cardiac output and high systemic vascular resistance. It also should be used for patients who are receiving titrated doses of vasoactive drugs or need frequent blood sampling.

Indirect monitoring, which carries few associated risks, is commonly performed by applying pressure to an artery (such as by inflating a blood pressure cuff around the arm) to decrease blood flow. As pressure is released, flow resumes and can be palpated or auscultated. Korotkoff sounds presumably result from a combination of blood flow and arterial wall vibrations; with reduced flow, these vibrations may be less pronounced.

Equipment
Catheter insertion

Gloves ● sterile gown ● mask ● protective eyewear ● sterile gloves ● 16G to 20G catheter (type and length depend on the insertion site, the patient's height and weight, and other anticipated uses of the line) • pre-assembled preparation kit (if available) • sterile drapes • sheet protector • prepared pressure transducer system • ordered local anesthetic • sutures • syringe and needle (21G to 25G, 1″) • I.V. pole • tubing and medication labels • site care kit (containing sterile dressing and hypoallergenic tape) • arm board and soft wrist restraint (for a femoral site, an ankle restraint) • optional: shaving kit (for femoral artery insertion)

Blood sample collection
If an open system is in place: gloves • gown • mask • protective eyewear • sterile 4″ × 4″ gauze pads • sheet protector • 500-ml I.V. bag • 5- to 10-ml syringe for discard sample • syringes of appropriate size and number for ordered laboratory tests • laboratory request forms and labels • needleless device (depending on your facility's policy) • Vacutainers; if a closed system is in place: gloves • gown • mask • protective eyewear • syringes of appropriate size and number for ordered laboratory tests • laboratory request forms and labels • alcohol pads • blood transfer unit • Vacutainers

Arterial line tubing changes
Gloves • gown • mask • protective eyewear • sheet protector • preassembled arterial pressure tubing with a flush device and disposable pressure transducer • sterile gloves • 500-ml bag of I.V. flush solution (such as dextrose 5% in water or normal saline solution) • 500 or 1,000 units of heparin • syringe and needle (21G to 25G, 1″) • medication label • pressure bag • site care kit • tubing labels

Arterial catheter removal
Gloves • mask • gown • protective eyewear • two sterile 4″ × 4″ gauze pads • sheet protector • sterile suture removal set • dressing • hypoallergenic tape

Femoral line removal
Additional sterile 4″ × 4″ gauze pads • small sandbag (which you may wrap in a towel or place in a pillowcase) • adhesive bandage

Catheter-tip culture
Sterile scissors • sterile container

Preparation of equipment
● Before setting up and priming the monitoring system, wash your hands thoroughly. **CDC**

● Maintain asepsis by wearing personal protective equipment (PPE) throughout preparation. **CDC**
● Label all medications, medication containers, and other solutions on and off the sterile field. **JCAHO**
● When you've completed the equipment preparation, set the alarms on the bedside monitor according to your facility's policy.

Implementation
● Confirm the patient's identity using two patient identifiers according to facility policy **JCAHO**
● Explain the procedure, including the purpose of arterial pressure monitoring and the anticipated duration of catheter placement, to the patient and his family. Make sure that the patient signs a consent form. If he can't sign, ask a responsible family member to give written consent. **PCP**
● Check the patient's history for an allergy or a hypersensitivity to iodine, heparin, latex, or the ordered local anesthetic.
● Maintain asepsis by wearing PPE throughout all procedures described here. **CDC**
● Position the patient for easy access to the catheter insertion site. Place a sheet protector under the site.
● If the catheter will be inserted into the radial artery, perform Allen's test *to assess collateral circulation in the hand*. (See "Arterial puncture," page 22.) **Science**

Inserting an arterial catheter
● Using a preassembled preparation kit, the physician prepares and anesthetizes the insertion site. He covers the surrounding area with sterile drapes. The catheter is then inserted into the artery and attached to the fluid-filled pressure tubing.
● While the physician holds the catheter in place, activate the fast-flush release *to flush blood from the catheter*. After each fast-flush operation, observe the drip chamber *to verify that the continuous flush rate is as desired*. A waveform should appear on the bedside monitor.
● The physician may suture the catheter in place, or you may secure it with hypoallergenic tape. Cover the insertion site with a dressing, as specified by your facility's policy.
● Immobilize the insertion site. With a radial or brachial site, use an arm board and soft wrist restraint (if the patient's condition so requires). With a femoral site, assess the need for an ankle restraint; maintain the patient on bed rest, with the head of the

bed raised no more than 30 degrees, *to prevent the catheter from kinking.* Level the zeroing stopcock of the transducer with the phlebostatic axis, and then zero the system to atmospheric pressure. **EB**
● Activate monitor alarms, as appropriate.

Obtaining a blood sample from an open system
● Assemble the equipment, taking care not to contaminate the dead-end cap, stopcock, and syringes. Deactivate or temporarily silence the monitor alarms, if this is permitted by your facility's policy.
● Locate the stopcock nearest the patient. Open a sterile 4" × 4" gauze pad. Remove the dead-end cap from the stopcock and place it on the gauze pad.
● Insert the syringe for the discard sample into the stopcock. (This sample is discarded because it's diluted with flush solution.) Follow your facility's policy on how much discard blood to collect. Usually, you'll withdraw 5 to 10 ml through a 5- or 10-ml syringe.
● Turn the stopcock off to the flush solution. Slowly retract the syringe to withdraw the discard sample. If you feel resistance, reposition the affected extremity and check the insertion site for obvious problems such as catheter kinking. After correcting the problem, resume blood withdrawal. Then turn the stopcock halfway back to the open position *to close the system in all directions.* **Science**
● Remove the discard syringe and dispose of the blood in the syringe, observing universal precautions. (See "Standard precautions," page 105.) **CDC**
● Place the syringe for the laboratory sample in the stopcock, turn the stopcock off to the flush solution, and slowly withdraw the required amount of blood. For each additional sample required, repeat this procedure. If the physician has ordered coagulation tests, obtain blood for this sample from the final syringe *to prevent dilution from the flush device.*
● After you've obtained blood for the final sample, turn the stopcock off to the syringe and remove the syringe. Activate the fast-flush release *to clear the tubing.* Then turn off the stopcock to the patient, and repeat the fast flush *to clear the stopcock port.*
● Turn the stopcock off to the stopcock port, and replace the dead-end cap. Reactivate the monitor alarms. Attach the needleless device to the filled syringes, and transfer the blood samples to the appropriate Vacutainers, labeling them according to your facility's policy. Send all samples to the laboratory with appropriate documentation.
● Check the monitor for return of the arterial waveform and pressure reading. (See *Understanding the arterial waveform,* page 198.)

Obtaining a blood sample from a closed system
● Confirm the patient's identity using two patient identifiers according to facility policy. **JCAHO**
● Assemble the equipment, maintaining aseptic technique. Locate the closed-system reservoir and blood sampling site. Deactivate or temporarily silence monitor alarms, if this is permitted by your facility's policy.
● Clean the sampling site with an alcohol pad.
● Holding the reservoir upright, grasp the flexures and slowly fill the reservoir with blood over 3 to 5 seconds. (*This blood serves as discard blood.*) If you feel resistance, reposition the affected extremity, and check the catheter site for obvious problems such as kinking. Then resume blood withdrawal.
● Turn the one-way valve off to the reservoir by turning the handle perpendicular to the tubing. Using a syringe with an attached cannula, insert the cannula into the sampling site. (Make sure that the plunger is depressed to the bottom of the syringe barrel.) Slowly fill the syringe. Then grasp the cannula near the sampling site, and remove the syringe and cannula as one unit. Repeat the procedure, as needed, to fill the required number of syringes. If the physician has ordered coagulation tests, obtain blood for those tests from the final syringe *to prevent dilution from the flush solution.*
● After filling the syringes, turn the one-way valve to its original position, parallel to the tubing. Now smoothly and evenly push down on the plunger until the flexures lock in place in the fully closed position and all fluid has been reinfused. The fluid should be reinfused over a 3- to 5-second period. Then activate the fast-flush release to clear blood from the tubing and reservoir.
● Clean the sampling site with an alcohol pad. Reactivate the monitor alarms. Using the blood transfer unit, transfer blood samples to the appropriate Vacutainers, labeling them according to your facility's policy. Send all samples to the laboratory with appropriate documentation.

Understanding the arterial waveform

Normal arterial blood pressure produces a characteristic waveform, representing ventricular systole and diastole. The waveform has five distinct components: the anacrotic limb, systolic peak, dicrotic limb, dicrotic notch, and end diastole.

The *anacrotic limb* marks the waveform's initial upstroke, which results as blood is rapidly ejected from the ventricle through the open aortic valve into the aorta. The rapid ejection causes a sharp rise in arterial pressure, which appears as the waveform's highest point. This is called the *systolic peak.*

As blood continues into the peripheral vessels, arterial pressure falls, and the waveform begins a downward trend. This part is called the *dicrotic limb.* Arterial pressure usually will continue to fall until pressure in the ventricle is less than pressure in the aortic root. When this occurs, the aortic valve closes. This event appears as a small notch (the *dicrotic notch*) on the waveform's downside.

When the aortic valve closes, diastole begins, progressing until the aortic root pressure gradually descends to its lowest point. On the waveform, this is known as *end diastole.*

Normal arterial waveform

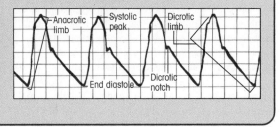

Changing arterial line tubing

● Confirm the patient's identity using two patient identifiers according to facility policy. **JCAHO**
● Wash your hands and follow standard precautions. **CDC** (See "Standard precautions," 105.) Assemble the new pressure monitoring system.
● Consult your facility's policy and procedure manual to determine how much tubing length to change.
● Inflate the pressure bag to 300 mm Hg, check it for air leaks, and then release the pressure.
● Prepare the I.V. flush solution and prime the pressure tubing and transducer system. At this time, add medication and tubing labels. Apply 300 mm Hg of pressure to the system. Then hang the I.V. bag on a pole. **EB**
● Place the sheet protector under the affected extremity. Remove the dressing from the catheter insertion site, taking care not to dislodge the catheter or cause vessel trauma. Deactivate or temporarily silence the monitor alarms, if this is permitted by your facility's policy.
● Turn off the flow clamp of the tubing segment to be changed. Disconnect the tubing from the catheter hub, taking care not to dislodge the catheter. Immediately insert new tubing into the catheter hub. Secure the tubing, and then activate the fast-flush release to clear it.

● Reactivate the monitor alarms. Apply an appropriate dressing.
● Level the zeroing stopcock of the transducer with the phlebostatic axis, and zero the system to atmospheric pressure. **EB**

Removing an arterial line

● Consult your facility's policy to determine whether you're permitted to perform this procedure.
● Confirm the patient's identity using two patient identifiers according to facility policy. **JCAHO**
● Explain the procedure to the patient. **PCP**
● Assemble all equipment. Wash your hands. Observe standard precautions, including wearing PPE, for this procedure. **CDC**
● Record the patient's systolic, diastolic, and mean blood pressures. If a manual, indirect blood pressure hasn't been assessed recently, obtain one now *to establish a new baseline.* **AACN**
● Turn off the monitor alarms, and then turn off the flow clamp to the flush solution.
● Carefully remove the dressing over the insertion site. Remove any sutures, using the suture removal kit, and then carefully check *to ensure that all sutures have been removed.*

● Withdraw the catheter using a gentle, steady motion. Keep the catheter parallel to the artery during withdrawal *to reduce the risk of traumatic injury.*

● Allow a small amount of blood out following the catheter removal and before applying pressure to the site. This will ensure that any clot adhered to the catheter is removed with the catheter.

● Apply pressure to the site with a sterile 4″ × 4″ gauze pad. Maintain pressure for at least 10 minutes (longer if bleeding or oozing persists). Apply additional pressure to a femoral site, or if the patient has coagulopathy or is receiving anticoagulants. **Science**

● Cover the site with an appropriate dressing and secure the dressing with tape. If stipulated by facility policy, make a pressure dressing for a femoral site by folding in half four sterile 4″ × 4″ gauze pads, and apply the dressing. Cover the dressing with a tight adhesive bandage, and then cover the bandage with a sandbag, if ordered. Maintain the patient on bed rest for 4 to 6 hours or as ordered.

● If the physician has ordered a culture of the catheter tip (to diagnose a suspected infection), gently place the catheter tip on a 4″ × 4″ sterile gauze pad. When the bleeding is under control, hold the catheter over the sterile container. Using sterile scissors, cut the tip so it falls into the sterile container. Label the specimen and send it to the laboratory.

● Observe the site for bleeding. Assess circulation in the extremity distal to the site by evaluating color, pulses, and sensation. Repeat this assessment every 15 minutes for the first hour, every 30 minutes for the next hour, and then hourly for the next 2 hours, or as ordered. **AACN**

Special considerations

● Observing the pressure waveform on the monitor can enhance arterial pressure assessment. An abnormal waveform may reflect an arrhythmia (such as atrial fibrillation) or other cardiovascular problems, such as aortic stenosis, aortic insufficiency, pulsus alternans, or pulsus paradoxus. (See *Recognizing abnormal waveforms,* page 200.)

● Change the pressure tubing every 2 to 3 days, according to your facility's policy. Change the dressing at the catheter site at intervals specified by facility policy. Regularly assess the site for signs of infection, such as redness and swelling. Notify the physician immediately if you note any such signs.

● Be aware that erroneous pressure readings may result from a clotted or positional catheter, loose connections, extra stopcocks or extension tubing, inadvertent entry of air into the system, or improper calibration, leveling, or zeroing of the monitoring system. If the catheter lumen clots, the flush system may be improperly pressurized. Regularly assess the amount of flush solution in the I.V. bag, and maintain 300 mm Hg of pressure in the pressure bag.

Nursing diagnoses

● Decreased cardiac output

Expected outcomes

The patient will:
● maintain an adequate cardiac output
● exhibit no arrhythmias
● maintain a blood pressure and pulse rate within normal limits.

Complications

● Direct arterial pressure monitoring can cause such complications as arterial bleeding, infection, air embolism, arterial spasm, or thrombosis.

Documentation

Document the date of system setup *so that all caregivers will know when to change the components.* Document the dynamic response or square wave test every 8 to 12 hours *to verify the accuracy of the waveform and readings.* (See *Square wave test,* page 201.) Document systolic, diastolic, and mean pressure readings as well. Record circulation in the extremity distal to the site by assessing color, pulses, and sensation. Carefully document the amount of flush solution infused *to avoid hypervolemia and volume overload and to ensure accurate assessment of the patient's fluid status.*

Make sure that the patient's position is documented when each blood pressure reading is obtained. *This is important for determining trends.*

Supportive references

Imperial-Perez, F., and McRae, M. "Protocols for Practice: Applying Research at the Bedside. Arterial Pressure Monitoring," *Critical Care Nurse* 19(2):105-107, April 1999.

(Text continues on page 202.)

Recognizing abnormal waveforms

Understanding a normal arterial waveform is relatively straightforward, but an abnormal waveform is more difficult to decipher. Abnormal patterns and markings, however, may provide important diagnostic clues to the patient's cardiovascular status, or they may simply signal trouble in the monitor. Use this chart to help you recognize and resolve waveform abnormalities.

Abnormality	Possible causes	Nursing interventions
Alternating high and low waves in a regular pattern	Ventricular bigeminy Cardiac tamponade	● Check the patient's electrocardiogram to confirm ventricular bigeminy. The tracing should reflect premature ventricular contractions every second beat. ● Assess the patient for signs of tamponade.
Flattened waveform	Overdamped waveform Hypotensive patient	● Check the dynamic response or square wave test. An overdampened waveform should be suspected if a slurred upstroke occurs at the beginning of the wave and after the initial downstroke if there's a loss of oscillations. Check for kinks or obstructions in the line or tubing. Clear the line of air or blood. Repeat the square wave test to verify optimal waveform. ● If the square wave test indicates an optimal waveform, assess and treat the patient for hypotension.
Slightly rounded waveform with consistent variations in systolic height	Patient on ventilator with positive end-expiratory pressure	● Check the patient's systolic blood pressure regularly. The difference between the highest and lowest systolic pressure reading should be less than 10 mm Hg. If the difference exceeds that amount, suspect pulsus paradoxus, possibly from cardiac tamponade.
Slow upstroke	Aortic stenosis	● Check the patient's heart sounds for signs of aortic stenosis. Also, notify the physician, who will document suspected aortic stenosis in his notes.
Diminished amplitude on inspiration	Pulsus paradoxus, possibly from cardiac tamponade, constrictive pericarditis, or lung disease	● Note systolic pressure during inspiration and expiration. If inspiratory pressure is at least 10 mm Hg less than expiratory pressure, call the physician. ● If you're also monitoring pulmonary artery pressure, observe for a diastolic plateau. This occurs when the mean central venous pressure (right atrial pressure), mean pulmonary artery pressure, and mean pulmonary artery wedge pressure are within 5 mm Hg of one another.

CLINICAL IMPACT

Square wave test

When using a pressure monitoring system, you must ensure and document the system's accuracy. Along with leveling and zeroing the system to atmospheric pressure at the phlebostatic axis and interpreting waveforms, you can ensure accuracy by performing the square wave test (or dynamic response test). To perform the test:

● Activate the fast-flush device for 1 second, and then release. Obtain a graphic printout.
● Observe for the desired response: the pressure wave rises rapidly, squares off, and is followed by a series of oscillations. (See illustration below.)
● Know that these oscillations should have an initial downstroke, which extends below the baseline and just 1 to 2 oscillations after the initial downstroke. Usually, but not always, the first upstroke is about one-third the height of the initial downstroke.
● Be aware that the intervals between oscillations should be no more than 0.04 to 0.08 second (1 to 2 small boxes).

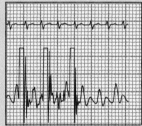

Underdamped square wave

If you observe extra oscillations after the initial downstroke or more than 0.08 second between oscillations, the waveform is underdamped. (See illustration at top of next column.) This can cause falsely high pressure readings and artifact in the waveforms. It can be corrected by:
● removing excess tubing or extra stopcocks from the system
● inserting a damping device (available from pressure tubing companies)
● dampening the wave by inserting a small air bubble at the transducer stopcock.

Repeat the square wave test, read the pressure waveform, and then remove the small air bubble.

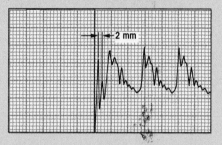

Overdamped square wave

If you observe a slurred upstroke at the beginning of the square wave and a loss of oscillations after the initial downstroke, the waveform is overdamped. (See illustration below.) This can cause falsely low pressure readings, and you can lose the sharpness of waveform peaks and the dicrotic notch. It can be corrected by:
● clearing the line of any blood or air
● checking to make sure there are no kinks or obstructions in the line
● ensuring that you're using short, low-compliance tubing.

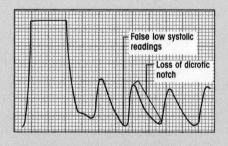

Adapted with permission from Quaal, S.J. "Improving the Accuracy of Pulmonary Artery Catheter Measurements," *Journal of Cardiovascular Nursing* 15(2):71-82, January 2001. © 2001 Aspen Publishers.

Kaye, J., et al. "Patency of Radial Arterial Catheters," *American Journal of Critical Care* 10(2):104-11, March 2001.

Keeling, A.W., et al. "Reducing Time in Bed After Percutaneous Transluminal Coronary Angioplasty (TIBS III)," *American Journal of Critical Care* 9(3):185-87, May 2000.

Lynn-McHale Wiegand, D.J., and Carlson, K.K. *AACN Procedure Manual for Critical Care*, 5th ed. Philadelphia: W.B. Saunders Co., 2005. **EB**

Rice, W.P., et al. "A Comparison of Hydrostatic Leveling Methods in Invasive Pressure Monitoring," *Critical Care Nurse* 20(6):21-30, December 2000.

Task Force of the American College of Critical Care Medicine, Society of Critical Medicine. "Guidelines for Intensive Care Unit Admission, Triage, and Discharge," *Critical Care Medicine* 27(3):633-38, March 1999.

Task Force of the American College of Critical Care Medicine, Society of Critical Medicine. "Practice Parameters for Hemodynamic Support of Sepsis in Adult Patients: 2004 Update," *Critical Care Medicine* 32(9):1928-48, September 2004.

Automated external defibrillation

Automated external defibrillators (AEDs) are commonly used to meet the need for early defibrillation, which is generally considered the most effective treatment for ventricular fibrillation (VF). Some health care facilities now require an AED in every noncritical care unit. Their use is common in such public places as shopping malls, sports stadiums, and airplanes. Instruction in using the AED is required as part of basic life support (BLS) and advanced cardiac life support (ACLS) training.

✔ **CLINICAL IMPACT** *Studies have shown that established Public Access to Defibrillation programs (laypersons who are trained to use an AED) have a survival of 41% to 74% from sudden cardiac arrest with ventricular fibrillation when cardiopulmonary resuscitation (CPR) is initiated immediately and defibrillation occurs within 3 to 5 minutes.* **AHA**

The 2005 American Heart Association guidelines for CPR and emergency cardiovascular care recommend the integration of CPR with the use of an AED. The guidelines recommend that:

● early defibrillation is appropriate. Compression before defibrillation may be considered when emergency medical service (EMS) arrival is greater than 4 to 5 minutes.

● one shock followed by immediate CPR, beginning with chest compressions, should be used. The rhythm should be checked after 5 cycles of CPR, or 2 minutes. The three-shock sequence is no longer recommended by the AHA.

● if more than one rescuer is present, one rescuer should start CPR while the other prepares the AED.

● AEDs can be used in children ages 1 to 8. For this age-group, an AED with a pediatric dose attenuator system should be used, if available.

● health care providers should be trained, equipped, and retrained to perform defibrillation. **AHA**

AEDs provide early defibrillation — even when no health care provider is present. The AED interprets the victim's cardiac rhythm and gives the operator step-by-step directions on how to proceed if defibrillation is indicated. Most AEDs have a "quick-look" feature that allows visualization of the rhythm with the paddles before electrodes are connected.

The AED is equipped with a microcomputer that senses and analyzes a patient's heart rhythm at the push of a button. Then it audibly or visually prompts you to deliver a shock. AED models all have the same basic function but offer different options. For example, all AEDs communicate directions by messages on a display screen, give voice commands, or both. Some AEDs simultaneously display a patient's heart rhythm.

All devices record your interactions with the patient during defibrillation, either on a cassette tape or in a solid-state memory module. Some AEDs have an integral printer for immediate event documentation. Facility policy determines who's responsible for reviewing all AED interactions; the patient's physician always has that option. Local and state regulations govern who's responsible for collecting AED case data for reporting purposes.

There are two types of defibrillators: one with monophasic waveforms and the other with biphasic waveforms. Monophasic waveform defibrillators were introduced first and many are still used today. When using this type of defibrillator, the initial shock should be set at 360 joules with second and subsequent shocks set at 360 joules. **AHA**

Biphasic waveforms are used in most AEDs and manual defibrillators. When using this type of defibrillator, an energy setting of 150 to 200 joules should be used for the first shock and the same, or higher, setting for second and subsequent shocks. The optimal energy level for a biphasic waveform defibrillator hasn't been determined. The optimal dose for each device that has proven most effective in eliminating VF should be noted on the defibrillator. **AHA**

Equipment

AED • two prepackaged electrodes

Implementation

- Upon discovering that the patient is unresponsive to your questions, pulseless, and apneic, follow BLS and ACLS protocols. Ask a colleague to bring the AED into the patient's room and set it up before the code team arrives.
- Open the foil packets containing the two electrode pads. Attach the white electrode cable connector to one pad and the red electrode cable connector to the other. The electrode pads aren't site specific.
- Expose the patient's chest. Remove the plastic backing film from the electrode pads, and place the electrode pad attached to the white cable connector on the right upper portion of the patient's chest, just beneath his clavicle.
- Place the pad attached to the red cable connector to the left of the heart's apex. To help remember where to place the pads, think, "White — right, red — ribs." (Placement for both electrode pads is the same as for manual defibrillation or cardioversion.)
- Firmly press the AED's ON button and wait while the machine performs a brief self-test. Most AEDs signal readiness by a computerized voice that says, "Stand clear" or by emitting a series of loud beeps. (If the AED were malfunctioning, it would convey the message, "Do not use the AED. Remove and continue CPR.") Remember to report AED malfunctions in accordance with your facility's policy.
- Now the machine is ready to analyze the patient's heart rhythm. Ask everyone to stand clear, and press the ANALYZE button when the machine prompts you to do so. Be careful not to touch or move the patient while the AED is in analysis mode. (If you get the message, "Check electrodes," make sure that the electrodes are correctly placed and the patient cable is se-

curely attached; then press the ANALYZE button again.)

- In 15 to 30 seconds, the AED will analyze the patient's rhythm. When he needs a shock, the AED will display a "Stand clear" message and emit a beep that changes into a steady tone as it's charging.
- When the AED is fully charged and ready to deliver a shock, it will prompt you to press the SHOCK button. (Some fully automatic AED models automatically deliver a shock within 15 seconds after analyzing the patient's rhythm. If a shock wasn't needed, the AED would display, "No shock indicated," and prompt you, "Check patient.")
- Make sure that no one is touching the patient or his bed, and call out, "Stand clear." Then press the shock button on the AED. Most AEDs are ready to deliver a shock within 15 seconds.
- After the first shock, continue CPR, beginning with chest compression until 5 cycles or about 2 minutes of CPR have been provided. Don't delay compressions to recheck rhythm or pulse. After 5 cycles of CPR, the AED should analyze the rhythm and deliver another shock, if indicated. **AHA**
- If a nonshockable rhythm is detected, the AED should instruct you to resume CPR. Then continue the algorithm sequence until the code team leader arrives.
- After the code, remove and transcribe the AED's computer memory module or tape, or prompt the AED to print a rhythm strip with code data. Follow your facility's policy for analyzing and storing code data.

Special considerations

- Defibrillators vary from one manufacturer to the next, so familiarize yourself with your facility's equipment. **MFR**
- Defibrillator operation should be checked at least every 8 hours and after each use.

Nursing diagnoses

- Decreased cardiac output
- Ineffective tissue perfusion: Cardiopulmonary

Expected outcomes

The patient will:
- exhibit no arrhythmias
- maintain a blood pressure and pulse rate within normal limits

• maintain an adequate cardiac output.

Complications
• Defibrillation can cause accidental electric shock to those providing care.
• Use of an insufficient amount of conduction medium can lead to skin burns.

Documentation
After using an AED, give a synopsis to the code team leader. Remember to report:
• the patient's name, age, medical history, and chief complaint
• the time you found the patient in cardiac arrest
• when you started CPR
• when you applied the AED
• how many shocks the patient received
• when the patient regained a pulse at any point
• what postarrest care was given, if any
• physical assessment findings.

Later, be sure to document the code on the appropriate form.

Supportive references
American Heart Association. "2005 AHA Guidelines for Cardiopulmonary Resuscitation and Emergency Cardiovascular Care. International Consensus on Science," *Circulation* 112(22 Suppl):IV-1-IV-211, November 2005.

American Heart Association. "Highlights of the 2005 AHA Guidelines for CPR and ECC," *Currents in ECC* 16(4):1-27, Winter 2005-2006.

Hazinsk, M., et al. "Lay Rescuer Automated External Defibrillator ("Public Access Defibrillation") Programs," *Circulation* 111(24):3336-40, June 2005.

Balloon valvuloplasty

Although the treatment of choice for valvular heart disease is surgery, balloon valvuloplasty is an alternative to valve replacement in patients with critical stenoses. This technique enlarges the orifice of a heart valve that has been narrowed by a congenital defect, calcification, rheumatic fever, or aging. It evolved from percutaneous transluminal coronary angioplasty and uses the same balloon-tipped catheters for dilatation.

Balloon valvuloplasty was first performed successfully on pediatric patients, then on elderly patients who have stenotic valves complicated by other med-

ical problems such as chronic obstructive pulmonary disease. It's indicated for patients who face a high risk from surgery and for those who refuse surgery.

ALERT *Balloon valvuloplasty has proved to be more tolerable than surgery for elderly patients, especially those older than age 80.*

This procedure is done in the cardiac catheterization laboratory under local anesthesia. The physician inserts a balloon-tipped catheter through the patient's femoral vein or artery, threads it into the heart, and repeatedly inflates it against the leaflets of the diseased valve. This increases the size of the orifice, improving valvular function and helping prevent complications from decreased cardiac output. (See *How balloon valvuloplasty works.*)

The nurse's role includes teaching the patient and his family about valvuloplasty and monitoring the patient for potential complications.

Equipment
Povidone-iodine solution • local anesthetic • valvuloplasty or balloon-tipped catheter • I.V. solution and tubing • electrocardiogram (ECG) monitor and electrodes • pulmonary artery (PA) catheter • contrast medium • oxygen • nasal cannula • sedative • emergency medications • shaving supplies or depilatory cream • heparin for injection • introducer kit for balloon catheter • sterile gown, gloves, mask, cap, and drapes • sterile marker • sterile labels • 5-lb (2.3-kg) sandbag • optional: nitroglycerin

Implementation PCP
TEACHING *Reinforce the physician's explanation of balloon valvuloplasty, including its risks and alternatives, to the patient and his family.*

Reassure the patient that although he'll be awake during the procedure, he'll receive a sedative and a local anesthetic beforehand.

Teach the patient what to expect. For example, inform him that his groin area will be shaved and cleaned with an antiseptic; he'll feel a brief, stinging sensation when the local anesthetic is injected; and he may feel pressure as the catheter moves along the vessel. Describe the warm, flushed feeling he's likely to experience from injection of the contrast medium.

Tell him that the procedure may last up to 4 hours and that he may feel discomfort from lying on a hard table for that long.

Before balloon valvuloplasty

- Make sure that the patient has no allergies to shell-fish, iodine, or contrast media and that he or a family member has signed a consent form. **EB**
- Withhold food and fluids (except for medications) for at least 6 hours before valvuloplasty or as ordered (usually after midnight the night before the procedure).
- Ensure that the results of routine laboratory studies and blood typing and crossmatching are available.
- Insert an I.V. line *to provide access for medications.*
- Take baseline peripheral pulses in all extremities.
- Shave the insertion sites or use a depilatory cream, and then clean the sites with povidone-iodine solution.
- Give the patient a sedative, as ordered.
- Have the patient void.
- When the patient arrives at the cardiac catheterization laboratory, apply ECG electrodes and ensure I.V. line patency.

During balloon valvuloplasty

- Administer oxygen by nasal cannula.
- The physician will put on a sterile gown, gloves, mask, and cap and open the sterile supplies. A member of the team will label all medications, medication containers, and other solutions on and off the sterile field. **JCAHO**
- The physician prepares and anesthetizes the catheter insertion site (usually at the femoral artery). He may insert a PA catheter if one isn't in place.
- He then inserts a large guide catheter into the site and threads a valvuloplasty or balloon-tipped catheter up into the heart.
- The physician injects a contrast medium *to visualize the heart valves and assess the stenosis.* He also injects heparin to prevent the catheter from clotting.
- Using low pressure, he inflates the balloon on the valvuloplasty catheter for a short time, usually 12 to 30 seconds, gradually increasing the time and pressure. If the stenosis isn't reduced, a larger balloon may be used.
- After completion of valvuloplasty, a series of angiograms are taken *to evaluate the effectiveness of the treatment.*
- The physician sutures the guide catheter in place. He'll remove it after the effects of the heparin have worn off.

How balloon valvuloplasty works

In balloon valvuloplasty, the physician inserts a balloon-tipped catheter through the femoral vein or artery and threads it into the heart. After locating the stenotic valve, he inflates the balloon, increasing the size of the valve opening.

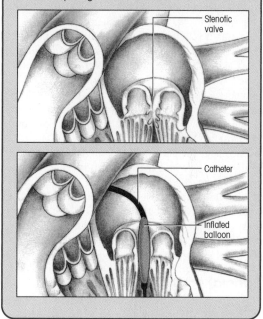

After balloon valvuloplasty

- When the patient returns to the unit, he may be receiving I.V. heparin or nitroglycerin. He may also have a sandbag on the insertion site *to prevent hematoma formation.*
- Monitor ECG rhythm and arterial pressures. **AACN** **AHA**
- Monitor the insertion site frequently for signs of hemorrhage *because exsanguination can occur rapidly.* **AACN** **AHA**
- *To prevent excessive hip flexion and migration of the catheter,* keep the affected leg straight and elevate the head of the bed no more than 15 degrees. If necessary, use a soft restraint.
- Monitor the patient's vital signs every 15 minutes for the first hour, every 30 minutes for the next 2 hours, and then hourly for the next 5 hours. If his vi-

tal signs are unstable, notify the practitioner and continue to check them every 5 minutes. **AACN** **AHA**

● When you take the patient's vital signs, assess peripheral pulses distal to the catheter insertion site as well as the color, sensation, temperature, and capillary refill time of the affected extremity. **AACN** **AHA**

● Assess the catheter site for hematoma, ecchymosis, and hemorrhage. If a hematoma expands, mark the site and alert the physician.

● Auscultate regularly for murmurs, which may indicate worsening valvular insufficiency. Notify the physician if you detect a new or worsening murmur.

● *To help the kidneys excrete the contrast medium,* provide I.V. fluids at a rate of at least 100 ml/hour. Assess the patient for signs of fluid overload, such as jugular vein distention, atrial and ventricular gallops, dyspnea, pulmonary congestion, tachycardia, hypertension, and hypoxemia. Monitor his intake and output closely. **Science**

● Encourage the patient to perform deep-breathing exercises *to prevent atelectasis.* This is especially important in an elderly patient. **Science**

● After the guide catheter is removed (usually 6 to 12 hours after valvuloplasty), apply direct pressure for at least 10 minutes and monitor the site frequently.

● Note the patient's tolerance of the procedure and his condition afterward.

Special considerations

● Assess the patient's vital signs constantly during the procedure, especially if it's an aortic valvuloplasty. During balloon inflation, the aortic outflow tract is completely obstructed, causing blood pressure to fall dangerously low. Ventricular ectopy is also common during balloon positioning and inflation. Start treatment for ectopy when symptoms develop or when ventricular tachycardia is sustained. Carefully assess the patient's respiratory status — changes in rate and pattern can be the first sign of a complication such as an embolism.

● Assess pedal pulses with a Doppler stethoscope. They'll be difficult to detect, especially if the catheter sheath remains in place. Assess for complications: embolism, hemorrhage, chest pain, and cardiac tamponade. Using heparin and a large-bore catheter can lead to arterial hemorrhage. This complication can be reversed with protamine sulfate when the sheath is removed, or the sheath can be left in place and removed 6 to 8 hours after heparin is discontinued.

Chest pain can result from blood flow obstruction during aortic valvuloplasty, so assess for symptoms of myocardial ischemia. Also stay alert for symptoms of cardiac tamponade (decreased or absent peripheral pulses, pale or cyanotic skin, hypotension, and paradoxical pulse), which requires emergency surgery.

Nursing diagnoses

● Decreased cardiac output

Expected outcomes

The patient will:
● exhibit no arrhythmias
● maintain a blood pressure and pulse rate within normal limits
● express comfort after activity.

Complications

● Severe complications, such as myocardial infarction or calcium emboli (embolization of debris released from the calcified valve), are rare.

● Other complications include bleeding or hematoma at the insertion site, arrhythmias, circulatory disorders distal to the insertion site, guide wire perforation of the ventricle leading to tamponade, disruption of the valve ring, restenosis of the valve, and valvular insufficiency, which can contribute to heart failure and reduced cardiac output.

● Infection and an allergic reaction to the contrast medium can also occur.

Documentation

Document complications and interventions.

Supportive references

Buchwald, A.B., et al. "Efficacy of Balloon Valvuloplasty in Patients with Critical Aortic Stenosis and Cardiogenic Shock — The Role of Shock Duration," *Clinical Cardiology* 24(3):214-18, March 2001.

Tarka, E.A., et al. "Hemodynamic Effects of Long-Term Outcome of Percutaneous Balloon Valvuloplasty in Patients with Mitral Stenosis and Atrial Fibrillation," *Clinical Cardiology* 23:673-77, September 2000.

Tong, A.D. "Pulmonic Stenosis and Balloon Valvuloplasty," Congenital Heart Information Network, May 2001. *www.tchin.org.*

Turi, Z.G. "Balloon Valvuloplasty: Mitral Valve," in Yusuf, S., ed. *Evidence-Based Cardiology.* London: BMJ Publishing Group, 1998. **EB**

Webb, J.G. "Percutaneous aortic valve implantation retrograde from the femoral artery," *Circulation* 113 (6):842-50, February 2006.

Cardiac monitoring

In the 1960s, mortality rates for myocardial infarction fell due to two major factors: the recognition of arrhythmias as a cause of death and the development of external defibrillation as an effective mode of therapy. These discoveries led to the creation of coronary care units, the birth of a new nursing specialty, and the use of continuous electrocardiography (ECG) monitoring for patients with cardiovascular diseases or disorders.

Because it allows for continuous observation of the heart's electrical activity, cardiac monitoring is commonly used for patients with conduction disturbances and patients at risk for arrhythmias or myocardial ischemia.

Like other forms of ECG, cardiac monitoring uses electrodes placed on the patient's chest to transmit electrical signals that are converted into a tracing of cardiac rhythm on an oscilloscope.

Two types of monitoring may be performed: hardwire or telemetry. In *hardwire monitoring*, the patient is connected to a monitor at the bedside. The rhythm display appears at the bedside, but it may also be transmitted to a console or central station at a remote location. *Telemetry* uses a small transmitter connected to the ambulatory patient to send electrical signals to another location, where they're displayed on a monitor screen. Battery powered and portable, telemetry allows the patient to be mobile and safe from the potential risk of electrical leakage and accidental shock that may occur with hardwire monitoring. Telemetry is especially useful for monitoring arrhythmias that occur during sleep, rest, exercise, or stressful situations. However, unlike hardwire monitoring, telemetry can monitor only heart rate and rhythm.

Regardless of the type, most cardiac monitors can recognize, store, and display the patient's heart rate and rhythm, produce a printed record of the rhythm, and sound an alarm if the patient's rate, rhythm, or cardiac waveforms change. For example, ST-segment monitoring helps detect myocardial ischemia, electrolyte imbalance, coronary artery spasm, and hypoxic events. The ST segment represents early ventricular repolarization, and changes in this waveform component reflect alterations in myocardial oxygenation. Any monitoring lead that views an ischemic heart region will reveal ST-segment changes. The monitor's software establishes a template of the patient's normal QRST pattern from the selected leads; then the monitor displays ST-segment changes. Some monitors display such changes continuously, others only on command. (See *Lead selection*.)

Lead selection

Your patient's clinical condition determines the leads you'll monitor. *Note:* If the monitor can detect arrhythmias, know which leads perform this function. Even if you don't continuously monitor these leads, periodically check the quality of their waveforms because the arrhythmia detection algorithm will fail without adequate waveforms.

Clinical concern	Lead
Bundle branch block	V_1 or V_6
Ischemia based on the area of infarction or site of percutaneous coronary intervention	
Anterior	V_3, V_4
Septal	V_1, V_2
Lateral	I, aV_L, V_5, V_6
Inferior	II, III, aV_F
Right ventricle	V_{4R}
Junctional rhythm with retrograde P waves	II
Optimal view of atrial activity	I, II, or Lewis lead (positive and negative electrodes at the 2nd and 4th intercostal spaces at the right sternal border)
Ventricular ectopy, wide complex tachycardia	V_1 (may use V_6 along with V_1)
Ventricular pacing	V_1 or II

Equipment

Cardiac monitor • leadwires • patient cable • disposable pregelled electrodes (number of electrodes varies from three to five, depending on the patient's needs) • alcohol pads • 4″ × 4″ gauze pads • optional: shaving supplies and washcloth

Telemetry monitoring

Transmitter • transmitter pouch • telemetry battery pack, leads, and electrodes

Preparation of equipment

● Plug the cardiac monitor into an electrical outlet and turn it on to warm up the unit while you prepare the equipment and patient.
● Insert the cable into the appropriate socket in the monitor.
● Connect the leadwires to the cable. In some systems, the leadwires are permanently secured to the cable. Each leadwire should indicate the attachment location: right arm (RA), left arm (LA), right leg (RL), left leg (LL), and chest (C). This should appear on the leadwire — if it's permanently connected — or at the connection of the leadwires and cable to the patient.
● Connect an electrode to each of the leadwires, carefully checking that each leadwire is in its correct outlet.

Telemetry monitoring

● Insert a new battery into the transmitter. Be sure to match the poles on the battery with the polar markings on the transmitter case.
● If the leadwires aren't permanently affixed to the telemetry unit, attach them securely. If they must be attached individually, be sure to connect each one to the correct outlet.

Implementation

● Confirm the patient's identity using two patient identifiers according to facility policy. **JCAHO**
● Explain the procedure to the patient, provide privacy, and ask him to expose his chest.
● Wash your hands. **CDC**
● Determine electrode positions on the patient's chest, based on the system and lead you're using. (See *Positioning monitoring leads.*)

● If the leadwires and patient cable aren't permanently attached, verify that the electrode placement corresponds to the label on the patient cable.
● If necessary, shave an area about 4″ (10 cm) in diameter around each electrode site. **EB** Clean the area with soap and water and dry it completely *to remove skin secretions that may interfere with electrode function.* Gently abrade the dried area by rubbing it briskly until it reddens *to remove dead skin cells and to promote better electrical contact with living cells.* (Some electrodes have a small, rough patch for abrading the skin; otherwise, use a dry washcloth or gauze pad.)
● Remove the backing from the pregelled electrode. Check the gel for moistness. If the gel is dry, discard it and replace it with a fresh electrode.
● Apply the electrode to the site and press firmly *to ensure a tight seal.* Repeat with the remaining electrodes.
● When all the electrodes are in place, check for a tracing on the cardiac monitor. Assess the quality of the ECG. (See *Identifying cardiac monitor problems,* pages 211 and 212.)
● To verify that each beat is being detected by the monitor, compare the digital heart rate display with your count of the patient's heart rate.
● If necessary, use the gain control to adjust the size of the rhythm tracing, and use the position control to adjust the waveform position on the recording paper.
● Set the upper and lower limits of the heart rate alarm, based on your facility's policy. Turn the alarm on.

Telemetry monitoring

● Wash your hands. **CDC** Explain the procedure to the patient and provide privacy. **PCP**
● Expose the patient's chest, and select the lead arrangement. Remove the backing from one of the gelled electrodes. Check the gel for moistness. If it's dry, discard the electrode and obtain a new one.
● Apply the electrode to the appropriate site by pressing the electrode against the skin. Press your fingers in a circular motion around the electrode *to fix the gel and stabilize the electrode.* Repeat for each electrode.
● Attach an electrode to the end of each leadwire.
● Place the transmitter in the pouch. Tie the pouch strings around the patient's neck and waist, making

(Text continues on page 212.)

Positioning monitoring leads

This chart shows the correct electrode positions for some of the monitoring leads you'll use most often. For each lead, you'll see electrode placement for a five-leadwire system, a three-leadwire system, and a telemetry system that consists of positive, negative, and ground leads.

In the three- and five-lead hardwire systems, the electrode positions for one lead may be identical to the electrode positions for another lead. In this case, you simply change the lead selector switch to the setting that corre-sponds to the lead you want. In some cases, you'll need to reposition the electrodes.

Many monitoring systems now obtain and store wave-forms in several leads simultaneously, allowing the nurse or physician to review and record the same event in different leads.

The illustrations below use these abbreviations: RA, right arm; LA, left arm; RL, right leg; LL, left leg; C, chest; and G, ground.

Five-leadwire system	Three-leadwire system	Telemetry system

Lead I

Lead II

Lead III

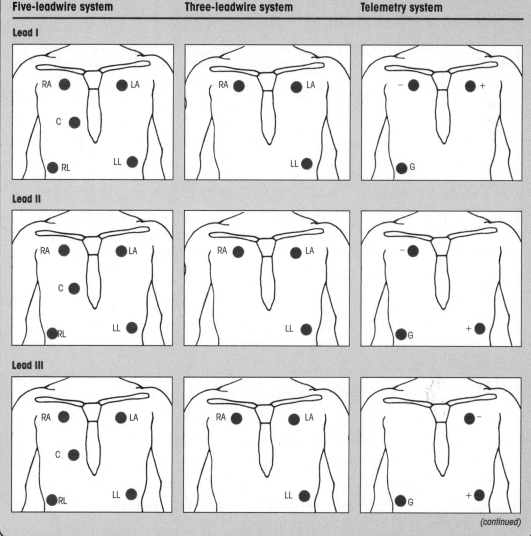

(continued)

Positioning monitoring leads *(continued)*

Five-leadwire system	Three-leadwire system	Telemetry system

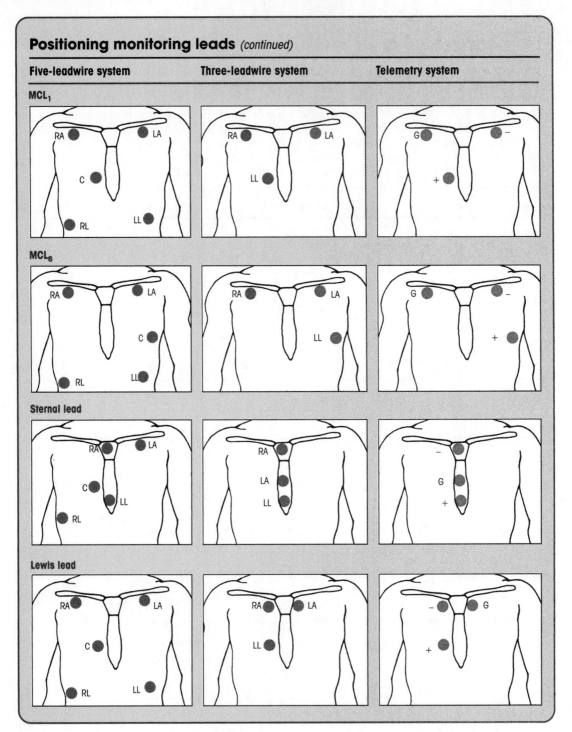

MCL₁

MCL₆

Sternal lead

Lewis lead

Identifying cardiac monitor problems

Problem	Possible causes	Solutions
False-high-rate alarm	• Monitor interpreting large T waves as QRS complexes, which doubles the rate • Skeletal muscle activity	• Reposition electrodes to lead where QRS complexes are taller than T waves. Decrease gain if necessary. • Place electrodes away from major muscle masses.
False-low-rate alarm	• Shift in electrical axis from patient movement, making QRS complexes too small to register • Low QRS amplitude • Poor contact between electrode and skin	• Reapply electrodes. Set gain so height of complex is greater than 1 mV. • Increase gain. • Reapply electrodes.
Low amplitude	• Gain dial set too low • Poor contact between skin and electrodes; dried gel; broken or loose leadwires; poor connection between patient and monitor; malfunctioning monitor; physiologic loss of QRS amplitude	• Increase gain. • Check connections on all leadwires and monitoring cable. Replace electrodes as necessary.
Wandering baseline 	• Poor position or contact between electrodes and skin • Thoracic movement with respirations	• Reposition or replace electrodes. • Reposition electrodes.
Artifact (waveform interference) 	• Patient having seizures, chills, or anxiety • Patient movement • Electrodes applied improperly • Static electricity • Electrical short circuit in leadwires or cable • Interference from decreased room humidity	• Notify physician and treat patient as ordered. Keep patient warm and reassure him. • Help patient relax. • Check electrodes and reapply, if necessary. • Make sure cables don't have exposed connectors. • Change patient's static-causing gown or pajamas. • Replace broken equipment. Use stress loops when applying leadwires. • Regulate humidity to 40%.
Broken leadwires or cable	• Stress loops not used on leadwires • Cables and leadwires cleaned with alcohol or acetone, causing brittleness	• Replace leadwires and retape them, using stress loops. • Clean cable and leadwires with soapy water. *Don't allow cable ends to become wet.* • Replace cable as necessary.

(continued)

Identifying cardiac monitor problems (continued)

Problem	Possible causes	Solutions
60-cycle interference (fuzzy baseline)	• Electrical interference from other equipment in room • Patient's bed improperly grounded	• Attach all electrical equipment to common ground. • Check plugs to make sure prongs aren't loose. • Attach bed ground to room's common ground.
Skin excoriation under electrode	• Patient allergic to electrode adhesive • Electrode on skin too long	• Remove electrodes and apply nonallergenic electrodes and nonallergenic tape. • Remove electrode, clean site, and reapply electrode at new site.

sure that the pouch fits comfortably. Place the transmitter in the patient's gown or bathrobe pocket.
• Check the patient's waveform for clarity, position, and size. Adjust the gain and baseline, as needed. (If necessary, ask the patient to remain resting or sitting in his room while you locate his telemetry monitor at the central station.)
• To obtain a rhythm strip, press the RECORD key at the central station. Label the strip with the patient's name, room number, date, and time. Also identify the rhythm. Place the rhythm strip in the appropriate location in the patient's chart.

Special considerations
• Make sure that all electrical equipment and outlets are grounded *to avoid electric shock and interference (artifacts)*. Also make sure that the patient is clean and dry *to prevent electric shock*.
• Avoid opening the electrode packages until just before using them *to prevent the gel from drying out*.
• Avoid placing the electrodes on bony prominences, hairy areas, areas where defibrillator pads will be placed, or areas for chest compression.
• If the patient's skin is exceptionally oily, scaly, or diaphoretic, rub the electrode site with a dry 4″ × 4″ gauze pad before applying the electrode *to help reduce interference in the tracing*.
• Assess skin integrity, and reposition the electrodes every 24 hours or as necessary. **Science**
• If the patient is being monitored by telemetry, show him how the transmitter works. If applicable, show him the button that produces a recording of his

ECG or signal at the central station. Teach him how to push the button whenever he has symptoms. *Depending on the monitoring system, this records an event and causes the central console to print a rhythm strip*. Stress that the patient shouldn't remove the unit.

Nursing diagnoses
• Decreased cardiac output
• Fear

Expected outcomes
The patient will:
• exhibit no arrhythmias
• have skin that remains warm and dry
• carry out activities of daily living without his heart rate exceeding or dropping below the expected limits
• state an understanding of the procedure
• express comfort with the procedure (cardiac monitoring).

Documentation
Record in your notes the date and time that monitoring begins and the monitoring lead used. Document a rhythm strip at least every 8 hours and with any changes in the patient's condition (or as stated by your facility's policy). Label the rhythm strip with the patient's name and room number, the date, and the time, lead recorded, and rhythm interpretation.

Other methods for measuring cardiac output

Cardiac output (CO) can be measured continuously by using a specialized pulmonary artery catheter. The catheter intermittently heats blood adjacent to the catheter and senses a change in blood temperature at the catheter tip using a fast-response thermistor. This method requires no manual injections, and values are taken, averaged, and updated automatically every several minutes.

In the Fick method of measuring, especially useful in detecting low CO levels, the blood's oxygen content is measured before and after it passes through the lungs. First, blood is removed from the pulmonary and the brachial arteries and analyzed for oxygen content. Then, a spirometer measures oxygen consumption — the amount of air entering the lungs each minute. Next, CO is calculated using this formula:

$$\text{CO (L/minute)} = \frac{\text{oxygen consumption (ml/minute)}}{\text{arterial oxygen content} - \text{venous oxygen content (ml/minute)}}$$

In the dye dilution test, a known volume and concentration of dye is injected into the pulmonary artery and measured by simultaneously sampling the amount of dye in the brachial artery. To calculate CO, these values are entered into a formula or plotted into a time and dilution-concentration curve. A computer, similar to the one used for the thermodilution test, performs the computation. Dye dilution measurements are particularly helpful in detecting intracardiac shunts and valvular regurgitation.

Supportive references

American Heart Association. "Practice Standards for Electrocardiographic Monitoring in Hospital Settings," *Circulation* 110:2721-46, 2004.

Bickwermert, M. "This Lead, That Lead, What Lead? Lead Placement: Basics Reviewed and Revisited." Presented at National Teaching Institute, American Association of Critical-Care Nurses, 1999. **EB**

Chambrin, M.C., et al. "Multicentric Study of Monitoring Alarms in the Adult Intensive Care Unit (ICU): A Descriptive Analysis," *Intensive Care Medicine* 25(12): 1360-66, December 1999.

Lynn-McHale Wiegand, D.J., and Carlson, K.K. *AACN Procedure Manual for Critical Care,* 5th ed. Philadelphia: W.B. Saunders Co., 2005.

Martin, N., and Hendrickson, P. "Telemetry Monitoring in Acute and Critical Care," *Critical Care Nursing Clinics of North America* 11(1):77-85, March 1999.

Schull, M.J., and Redelmeier, D.A. "Continuous Electrocardiographic Monitoring and Cardiac Arrest Outcomes in 8,932 Telemetry Ward Patients," *Academic Emergency Medicine* 7(6):647-52, June 2000.

Cardiac output measurement

Cardiac output (CO) — the amount of blood pumped by the heart per minute — helps evaluate cardiac function. Each ventricle has a CO of 4 to 6 L/minute. The most widely used method of calculating this measurement is the bolus thermodilution technique. This technique is based on the previously popular indicator-dilution technique. Performed at the patient's bedside, the thermodilution technique is the most practical method for evaluating the cardiac status of critically ill patients and those suspected of having cardiac disease. Other methods include continuous measurement using thermodilution, the Fick method, and the dye dilution test. (See *Other methods for measuring cardiac output*.)

To measure CO, a quantity of solution colder than the patient's blood is injected into the right atrium via a port on a pulmonary artery (PA) catheter. This indicator solution mixes with the blood as it travels through the right ventricle into the pulmonary artery, and a thermistor on the catheter registers the change in temperature of the flowing blood. A computer then plots the temperature change over time as a curve and calculates flow based on the area under the curve. (See *Cardiac output curves,* page 214.)

Cardiac output curves

The illustrations below show cardiac output (CO) curves produced at the bedside using a pulmonary artery catheter (thermodilution method). Patients with a high CO have a curve with a small area beneath it, whereas patients with a low CO have a large area beneath the curve. Patients with uneven injection have an uneven upstroke on the curve. Presence of artifact commonly represents incorrect CO measurement.

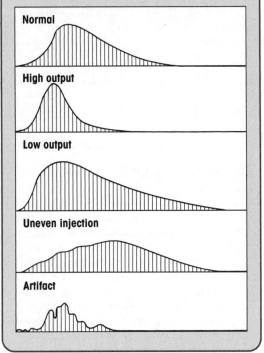

Normal

High output

Low output

Uneven injection

Artifact

◆ **CONTROVERSIAL ISSUE** *Iced or room-temperature injectant may be used. The choice should be based on your facility's policy as well as the patient's status. The accuracy of the bolus thermodilution technique depends on the computer being able to differentiate the temperature change caused by the injectant in the pulmonary artery and the temperature changes in the pulmonary artery. Because iced injectant is colder than room-temperature injectant, it provides a stronger signal to be detected.*

Typically, however, room-temperature injectant is more convenient and provides equally accurate measurements. Iced injectant may be more accurate in patients with high or low CO, in patients with hypothermia, or when smaller volumes of injectant must be used (3 to 5 ml), as in patients with volume restrictions or in children.

Equipment
Thermodilution method

Thermodilution PA catheter in position • output computer and cables (or a module for the bedside cardiac monitor) • closed or open injectant delivery system • 10-ml syringe • 500-ml bag of dextrose 5% in water or normal saline solution • crushed ice and water (if iced injectant is used)

The newer bedside cardiac monitors measure CO continuously, using either an invasive or a noninvasive method. If your bedside monitor doesn't have this capability, you'll need a freestanding CO computer.

Preparation of equipment

● Wash your hands thoroughly, and assemble the equipment at the patient's bedside. **CDC**
● Insert the closed injectant system tubing into the 500-ml bag of I.V. solution.
● Connect the 10-ml syringe to the system tubing and prime the tubing with I.V. solution until there's no air. Then clamp the tubing.
● The steps that follow differ, depending on the temperature of the injectant.

Room-temperature injectant closed delivery system

● Confirm the patient's identity using two patient identifiers according to facility policy. **JCAHO**
● After clamping the tubing, connect the primed system to the stopcock of the proximal injectant lumen of the PA catheter.
● Connect the temperature probe from the CO computer to the closed injectant system's flow-through housing device.
● Connect the CO computer cable to the thermistor connector on the PA catheter and verify the blood temperature reading.
● Turn on the computer and enter the correct computation constant, as provided by the catheter's manu-

facturer. **MFR** The constant is determined by the volume and temperature of the injectant as well as the size and type of catheter.

ALERT *With children, you'll need to adjust the computation constant to reflect a smaller volume and catheter size.*

Iced injectant closed delivery system

- Confirm the patient's identity using two patient identifiers according to facility policy. **JCAHO**
- After clamping the tubing, place the coiled segment into the Styrofoam container and add crushed ice and water to cover the entire coil.
- Let the solution cool for 15 to 20 minutes.
- The rest of the steps are the same as those for the room-temperature injectant closed delivery system.

Implementation

TEACHING *Make sure that the patient is in a comfortable position. Tell him not to move during the procedure because movement can cause an error in measurement.*

Explain to the patient that the procedure will help determine how well his heart is pumping and that he'll feel no discomfort.

Room-temperature injectant closed delivery system

- Verify the presence of a PA waveform on the cardiac monitor.
- Unclamp the I.V. tubing and withdraw exactly 10 ml of solution. Reclamp the tubing. **AACN**
- Turn the stopcock at the catheter injectant hub *to open a fluid path between the injectant lumen of the PA catheter and the syringe.*
- Press the START button on the CO computer or wait for the "Inject" message to flash.
- Inject the solution smoothly within 4 seconds, making sure that it doesn't leak at the connectors.
- If available, analyze the contour of the thermodilution washout curve on a strip chart recorder for a rapid upstroke and a gradual, smooth return to baseline. **AACN**
- Repeat these steps until three values are within 10% to 15% of the median value. Compute the average, and record the patient's CO. **AACN**

- Return the stopcock to its original position, and make sure that the injectant delivery system tubing is clamped.
- Verify the presence of a PA waveform on the cardiac monitor.
- Discontinue CO measurements when the patient is hemodynamically stable and weaned from his vasoactive and inotropic medications. You can leave the PA catheter inserted for pressure measurements.
- Disconnect and discard the injectant delivery system and the I.V. bag. Cover exposed stopcocks with air-occlusive caps.
- Monitor the patient for signs or symptoms of inadequate perfusion, including restlessness, fatigue, changes in level of consciousness, decreased capillary refill time, diminished peripheral pulses, oliguria, and pale, cool skin.

Iced injectant closed delivery system

- Unclamp the I.V. tubing and withdraw 5 ml of solution into the syringe.

ALERT *When using an iced injectant closed delivery system on a child, use 3 ml or less of solution.*

- Inject the solution to flow past the temperature sensor while observing the injectant temperature that registers on the computer. Verify that the injectant temperature is between 43° and 54° F (6.1° and 12.2° C).
- Verify the presence of a PA waveform on the cardiac monitor.
- Withdraw exactly 10 ml of cooled solution before reclamping the tubing. **AACN**
- Turn the stopcock at the catheter injectant hub to open a fluid path between the injectant lumen of the PA catheter and the syringe.
- Press the START button on the CO computer or wait for the "Inject" message to flash.
- Inject the solution smoothly within 4 seconds, making sure that it doesn't leak at the connectors.
- If available, analyze the contour of the thermodilution washout curve on a strip chart recorder for a rapid upstroke and a gradual, smooth return to baseline. **AACN**
- Wait 1 minute between injections, and repeat the procedure until three values are within 10% to 15% of the median value. Compute the average, and record the patient's CO.

- Return the stopcock to its original position, and make sure that the injectant delivery system tubing is clamped.
- Verify the presence of a PA waveform on the cardiac monitor.

Special considerations

- The normal range for CO is 4 to 8 L/minute. The adequacy of a patient's CO is better assessed by calculating his cardiac index (CI), adjusted for his body size.
- To calculate the patient's CI, divide his CO by his body surface area (BSA), a function of height and weight. For example, a CO of 4 L/minute might be adequate for a 65″, 120-lb (165-cm, 54-kg) patient (normally a BSA of 1.59 and a CI of 2.5) but would be inadequate for a 74″, 230-lb (188-cm, 104-kg) patient (normally a BSA of 2.26 and a CI of 1.8). The normal CI for adults ranges from 2.5 to 4.2 L/minute/m²; for pregnant women, 3.5 to 6.5 L/minute/m².

ALERT *Normal CI for infants and children is 3.5 to 4 L/minute/m². Normal CI for elderly adults is 2 to 2.5 L/minute/m².*

- Add the fluid volume injected for CO determinations to the patient's total intake. Injectant delivery of 30 ml/hour will contribute 720 ml to the patient's 24-hour intake.
- After CO measurement, make sure that the clamp on the injectant bag is secured *to prevent inadvertent delivery of the injectant to the patient.*

CLINICAL IMPACT *There are limitations to the use of the thermodilution method. It can't be used in a patient with a large intracardiac shunt, in whom a PA catheter may pose a danger. Thermodilution is also contraindicated in a patient with a ventricular septal defect because of improper mixing of the thermal indicator with blood, and also can't be used if a patient has tricuspid regurgitation due to blood regurgitation, prolonging the mixing time and movement of the thermal indicator. Due to these limitations, other noninvasive techniques, such as Doppler CO determination, are being developed. The Doppler method uses a transducer placed on the suprasternal notch and aims an ultrasound beam toward the aortic root to measure blood velocity. It's currently still in the evalua-tive phase, but if it's successful, it will greatly reduce the hazards of CO determination via an invasive line.*

Nursing diagnoses

- Decreased cardiac output

Expected outcomes

The patient will:
- have a diminished workload of his heart
- exhibit no arrhythmias
- maintain a blood pressure and pulse rate within normal limits.

Documentation

Document the patient's CO, CI, and other hemodynamic values and vital signs at the time of measurement. Note his position during measurement and other unusual occurrences, such as bradycardia or neurologic changes.

Supportive references

American Society of Anesthesiologists. "Practice Guidelines for Pulmonary Artery Catheterization. An Updated Report by the American Society of Anesthesiologists Task Force on Pulmonary Artery Catheterization," 2003. *www.asahq.org/practice/pulm/pulm_artery.html.*

Bridges, E.J. "Monitoring Pulmonary Artery Pressures: Just the Facts," *Critical Care Nurse* 20(6):59-80, December 2000.

Daily, E.K. "Hemodynamic Waveform Analysis," *Journal of Cardiovascular Nursing* 15(2):6-22, January 2001.

Druding, M.C. "Integrating Hemodynamic Monitoring and Physical Assessment," *Dimensions of Critical Care Nursing* 19(4):25-30, July-August 2000.

Gawlinski, A. "Measuring Cardiac Output: Intermittent Bolus Thermodilution Method," *Critical Care Nurse* 24(5):74-78, October 2004.

Keckeisen, M. "Monitoring Pulmonary Artery Pressure," *Critical Care Nurse* 19(6):88-91, December 1999.

Lynn-McHale Wiegand, D.J., and Carlson, K.K. *AACN Procedure Manual for Critical Care,* 5th ed. Philadelphia: W.B. Saunders Co., 2005.

Ott, K., et al. "New Technologies in the Assessment of Hemodynamic Parameters," *Journal of Cardiovascular Nursing* 15(2):41-55, January 2001.

Quaal, S.J. "Improving the Accuracy of Pulmonary Artery Catheter Measurements," *Journal of Cardiovascular Nursing* 15(2):71-82, January 2001.

Rice, W.P., et al. "A Comparison of Hydrostatic Leveling Methods in Invasive Pressure Monitoring," *Critical Care Nurse* 20(6):20-30, December 2000.

Savino, J.S., et al. "Cardiac Surgery in the Adult," in *Cardiac Anesthesia.* Cohn, L.H., and Edmunds, L.H., eds. New York: McGraw-Hill Book Co., 2003.

Cardiopulmonary resuscitation

Cardiopulmonary resuscitation (CPR) seeks to restore and maintain the patient's respiration and circulation after his heartbeat and breathing have stopped. Basic life support (BLS) procedures should be performed according to the 2005 American Heart Association (AHA) guidelines. CPR is a BLS procedure performed on victims of cardiac arrest. Another BLS procedure is clearing an obstructed airway.

CLINICAL IMPACT *Recent research has contributed to several changes in the AHA guidelines for BLS for health care providers. Some of these changes include:*

A lone rescuer should activate the emergency medical service (EMS), get an automated external defibrillator (AED), and return to the victim to perform CPR. This sequence should be tailored to take into account the cause of the arrest. If the victim has a sudden collapse and the cause is likely cardiac, the above sequence should be followed. If the victim has hypoxic arrest, the lone health care provider should do 5 cycles of CPR before activating EMS and retrieving an AED.

For an infant or a child, the lone rescuer should perform CPR first for 5 cycles and then activate EMS. As written above, the sequence should be tailored to the most likely cause of the arrest.

Rescue breaths should be delivered over 1 second and should be sufficient to produce a visible chest rise. In the past, rescuers were taught to give breaths over 1 to 2 seconds. It's been found that hyperventilation can be harmful.

The compression to ventilation ratio has changed. The new rates are 30:2 for infants, children, and adults for one-person CPR; for two-person CPR, 15:2 for infants and children and 30:2 for adults.

CONTROVERSIAL ISSUE *The AHA has made several changes to adult BLS guidelines for lay rescuers. One major change is that they no longer are taught to use a jaw thrust to open the airway of injured victims. The head tilt-chin lift should be used for all victims because the jaw thrust is difficult to perform.*

Another change is that lay rescuers are now taught to give 2 rescue breaths and immediately begin 30 chest compressions without stopping to check for a pulse. The AHA found that lay rescuers can't reliably check for a pulse within 10 seconds or accurately assess other signs of circulation. **AHA**

Most adults in sudden cardiac arrest develop ventricular fibrillation and require defibrillation; CPR alone doesn't improve their chances of survival. Early activation of EMS, CPR, delivery of a shock with a defibrillator, and early advanced cardiac life support (ACLS) all contribute to an improved chance for survival.

Equipment

CPR requires no special equipment except a hard surface on which to place the patient.

Implementation **AHA**

● See the *AHA BLS algorithm*, page 218, and follow the step-by-step instructions for CPR for the health care provider as described here.

One-person rescue
● If you're the sole rescuer, expect to call for help to open the patient's airway; check for breathing, and assess for circulation before beginning compressions.

Opening the airway **AHA**
● Assess the victim to determine if he's unconscious (as shown at top of page 219). Gently shake his shoulders and shout, "Are you okay?" This helps to ensure that you don't start CPR on a person who's conscious. Check whether he has an injury, particularly to the head or neck. If you suspect a head or neck injury, move him as little as possible to reduce the risk of paralysis.

BLS algorithm AHA

The American Heart Association (AHA) has issued this algorithm for adult basic life support (BLS) for the health care provider. The boxes bordered with dotted lines indicate actions or steps that are performed by the health care provider, not the lay rescuer.

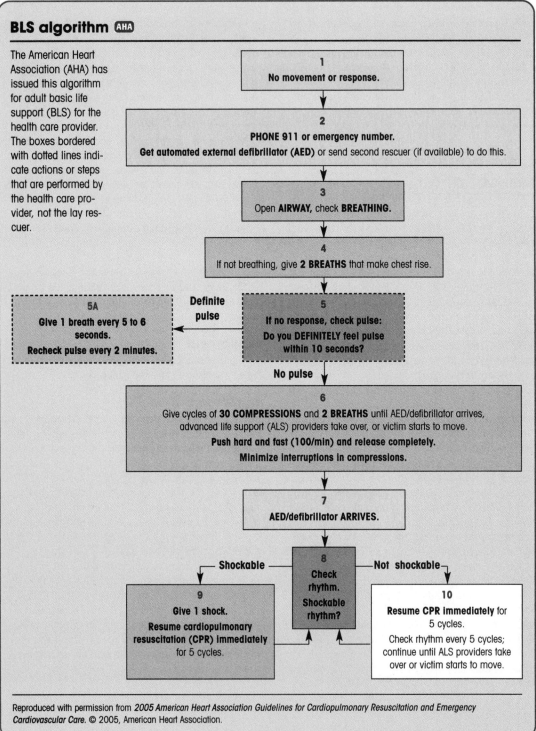

1
No movement or response.

2
PHONE 911 or emergency number.
Get automated external defibrillator (AED) or send second rescuer (if available) to do this.

3
Open AIRWAY, check BREATHING.

4
If not breathing, give 2 BREATHS that make chest rise.

5
If no response, check pulse:
Do you DEFINITELY feel pulse within 10 seconds?

Definite pulse →

5A
Give 1 breath every 5 to 6 seconds.
Recheck pulse every 2 minutes.

No pulse ↓

6
Give cycles of 30 COMPRESSIONS and 2 BREATHS until AED/defibrillator arrives, advanced life support (ALS) providers take over, or victim starts to move.
Push hard and fast (100/min) and release completely.
Minimize interruptions in compressions.

7
AED/defibrillator ARRIVES.

8
Check rhythm. Shockable rhythm?

— Shockable —

— Not shockable —

9
Give 1 shock.
Resume cardiopulmonary resuscitation (CPR) immediately for 5 cycles.

10
Resume CPR immediately for 5 cycles.
Check rhythm every 5 cycles; continue until ALS providers take over or victim starts to move.

Reproduced with permission from *2005 American Heart Association Guidelines for Cardiopulmonary Resuscitation and Emergency Cardiovascular Care.* © 2005, American Heart Association.

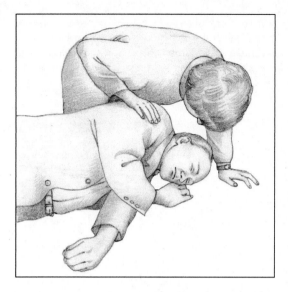

● Call out for help. Send someone to contact EMS or call a code, and get the AED. Place the victim in a supine position on a hard, flat surface. When moving him, roll his head and torso as a unit. Avoid twisting or pulling his neck, shoulders, or hips (as shown below).

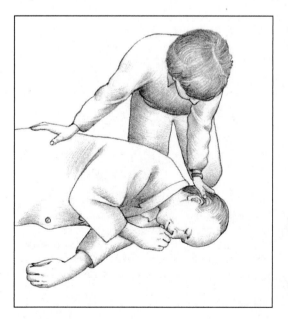

● Kneel near his shoulders. This position will give you easy access to his head and chest (as shown below).

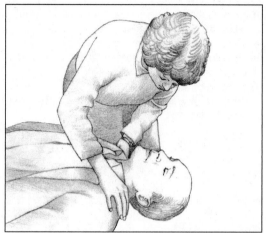

● In many cases, the muscles controlling the victim's tongue will be relaxed, causing the tongue to obstruct the airway. If the victim doesn't appear to have a neck injury, use the head-tilt, chin-lift maneuver *to open his airway.* To accomplish this, first place your hand that's closer to the victim's head on his forehead. Then apply firm pressure. The pressure should be firm enough to tilt the victim's head back. Next place the fingertips of your other hand under the bony part of his lower jaw near the chin. Now lift the victim's chin. At the same time, keep his mouth partially open (as shown below).

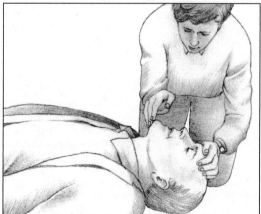

● Avoid placing your fingertips on the soft tissue under the victim's chin because this maneuver may inadvertently obstruct the airway you're trying to open.
● If you suspect a neck injury, use the jaw thrust maneuver without head extension instead of the head-tilt, chin-lift maneuver. Kneel at the victim's head with your elbows on the ground. Rest your thumbs on his lower jaw near the corners of the mouth, pointing your thumbs toward his feet. Then place your fingertips around the lower jaw. To open the airway, lift the lower jaw with your fingertips (as shown below).

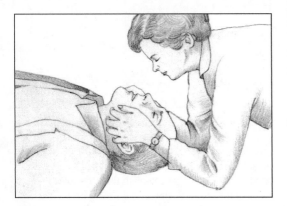

Checking for breathing AHA

● While maintaining the open airway, look, listen, and feel for breathing. Place your ear over the victim's mouth and nose. Now, listen for the sound of air moving, and note whether his chest rises and falls. You may also feel airflow on your cheek. If he starts to breathe, keep the airway open and continue checking his breathing until help arrives (as shown below).

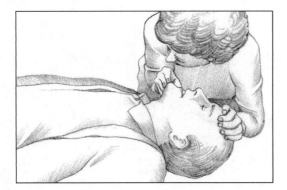

● If you don't detect adequate breathing within 10 seconds after opening his airway, begin rescue breathing. Pinch his nostrils shut with the thumb and index finger of the hand you've had on his forehead (as shown below).

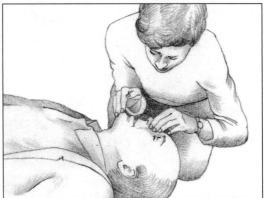

● Take a regular (not deep) breath and place your mouth over the victim's mouth, creating a tight seal (as shown below). Give 2 breaths, each over 1 second. Each ventilation should have enough volume to produce a visible chest rise.

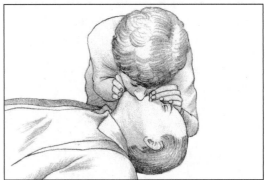

● If the first ventilation isn't successful, reposition the victim's head and try again. If you're still not successful, he may have a foreign-body airway obstruction. Check for loose dentures. If dentures or other objects are blocking the airway, clear the airway.

Assessing circulation

● Keep one hand on the victim's forehead so his airway remains open. With your other hand, palpate the carotid artery that's closer to you. To do this, place your index and middle fingers in the groove between the trachea and the sternocleidomastoid muscle. Palpate for 10 seconds (as shown below).

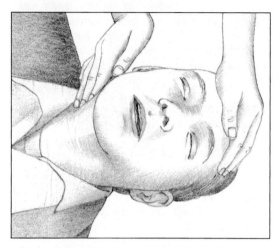

● If you detect a pulse, don't begin chest compressions. Instead, perform rescue breathing by giving the victim 10 to 12 ventilations per minute (or one every 5 to 6 seconds). Each breath should be given over 1 second and cause a visible chest rise. After 2 minutes, recheck his pulse but spend only 10 seconds doing so.
● If there's no pulse, start giving chest compressions. Make sure that your knees are apart for a wide base of support. Using the hand closer to his feet, locate the lower margin of the rib cage (as shown below). Then move your fingertips along the margin to the notch where the ribs meet the sternum.

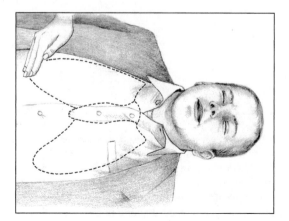

● Place your middle finger on the notch and your index finger next to your middle finger. The long axis of the heel of your hand will be aligned with the long axis of the sternum (as shown below) in the center of the chest between the nipples.

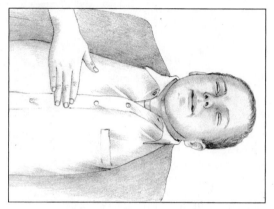

● Put the heel of your other hand on the sternum, next to the index finger. The long axis of the heel of your hand will be aligned with the long axis of the sternum (as shown below).

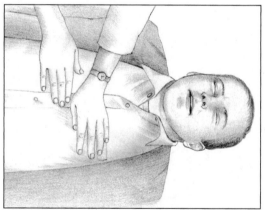

● Take the first hand off the notch and put it on top of the hand on the sternum. Make sure that you have one hand directly on top of the other and your fingers aren't on his chest (as shown at top of next page). This position will keep the force of the compression on the sternum and reduce the risk of a rib fracture, lung puncture, or liver laceration.

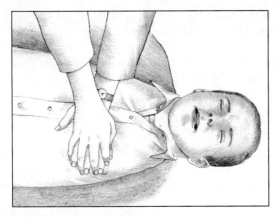

● With your elbows locked, arms straight, and your shoulders directly over your hands (as shown below), you're ready to give chest compressions. Using the weight of your upper body, compress the victim's sternum 1½″ to 2″ (4 to 5 cm), delivering the pressure through the heels of your hands. After each compression, release the pressure and allow the chest to return to its normal position so that the heart can fill with blood. Don't change your hand position during compressions — you might injure the victim.

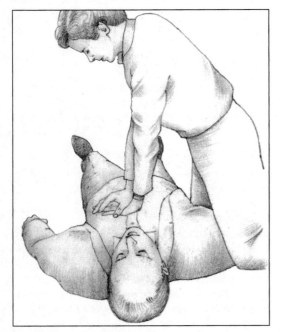

● Give 30 chest compressions at a rate of approximately 100 per minute. Push hard and fast. Open the airway and give 2 ventilations. Then find the proper hand position again and deliver 30 more compressions. Continue chest compressions until EMS arrives or another rescuer arrives with the AED. Health care providers should interrupt chest compressions as infrequently as possible. Interruptions should last no longer than 10 seconds except for special interventions, such as use of the AED or insertion of an airway.

Two-person rescue AHA

If another rescuer arrives while you're giving CPR, follow these steps:

● If the EMS team hasn't arrived, tell the second rescuer to repeat the call for help. If he's not a health care professional, ask him to stand by. Then, after about 2 minutes or 5 cycles of compressions and ventilations, you should switch. The switch should occur in less than 5 seconds.

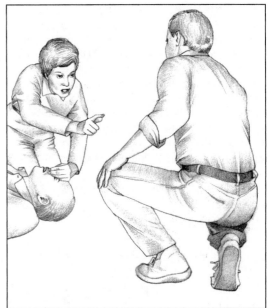

● If the rescuer is another health care professional, the two of you can perform two-person CPR. He should start assisting after you've finished 5 cycles of 30 compressions, 2 ventilations, and a pulse check.
● The second rescuer should get into place opposite you. While you're checking for a pulse, he should be

finding the proper hand placement for delivering chest compressions (as shown below).

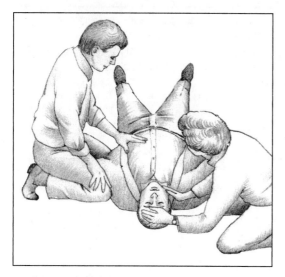

● If you don't detect a pulse, say, "No pulse, continue CPR," and give 2 ventilations. Then the second rescuer should begin delivering compressions at a rate of 100 per minute (as shown below). Compressions and ventilations should be administered at a ratio of 30 compressions to 2 ventilations. The compressor (at this point, the second rescuer) should count out loud so the ventilator can anticipate when to give ventilations. To ensure that the ventilations are effective, they should cause a visible chest rise.

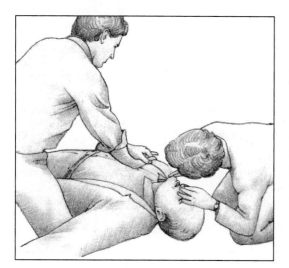

● The compressor role should switch after 5 cycles of compressions and ventilations. The switch should occur in less than 5 seconds.
● As shown below, both of you should continue giving CPR until an AED or defibrillator arrives, the ACLS providers take over, or the victim starts to move.

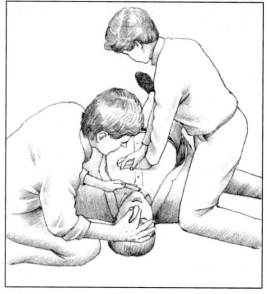

Special considerations
● Some health care providers may hesitate to give mouth-to-mouth rescue breathing. For this reason, the AHA recommends that all health care professionals learn how to use disposable airway equipment.

Nursing diagnoses
● Decreased cardiac output
● Ineffective breathing pattern

Expected outcomes
The patient will:
● maintain a blood pressure and pulse rate within normal limits
● maintain an adequate cardiac output
● resume independent ventilation
● have arterial blood gas levels return to baseline.

Potential hazards of CPR

Cardiopulmonary resuscitation (CPR) can cause various complications, including injury to bones and vital organs. This chart describes the causes of CPR hazards and lists preventive steps.

Hazard	Causes	Assessment findings	Preventive measures
Sternum and rib fractures	• Osteoporosis • Malnutrition • Improper hand placement	• Paradoxical chest movement • Chest pain or tenderness that increases with inspiration • Crepitus • Palpation of movable bony fragments over the sternum • On palpation, sternum feels unattached to surrounding ribs	*While performing CPR* • Don't rest your hands or fingers on the patient's ribs. • Interlock your fingers. • Keep your bottom hand in contact with the chest, but release pressure after each compression. • Compress the sternum at the recommended depth for the patient's age.
Pneumothorax, hemothorax, or both	• Lung puncture from fractured rib	• Chest pain and dyspnea • Decreased or absent breath sounds over the affected lung • Tracheal deviation from midline • Hypotension • Hyperresonance to percussion over the affected area along with shoulder pain	• Follow the measures listed for sternum and rib fractures.
Injury to the heart and great vessels (pericardial tamponade, atrial or ventricular rupture, vessel laceration, cardiac contusion, punctures of the heart chambers)	• Improperly performed chest compressions • Transvenous or transthoracic pacing attempts • Central line placement during resuscitation • Intracardiac drug administration	• Jugular vein distention • Muffled heart sounds • Pulsus paradoxus • Narrowed pulse pressure • Electrical alternans (decreased electrical amplitude of every other QRS complex) • Adventitious heart sounds • Hypotension • Electrocardiogram changes (arrhythmias, ST-segment elevation, T-wave inversion, and marked decrease in QRS voltage)	• Perform chest compressions properly.
Organ laceration (primarily liver and spleen)	• Forceful compression • Sharp edge of a fractured rib or xiphoid process	• Persistent right upper quadrant tenderness (liver injury) • Persistent left upper quadrant tenderness (splenic injury) • Increasing abdominal girth	• Follow the measures listed for sternum and rib fractures.
Aspiration of stomach contents	• Gastric distention and an elevated diaphragm from high ventilatory pressures	• Fever, hypoxia, and dyspnea • Auscultation of wheezes and crackles • Increased white blood cell count • Changes in color and odor of lung secretions	• Intubate early. • Insert a nasogastric tube and apply suction if gastric distention is marked.

Complications

● CPR can cause certain complications — especially if the compressor doesn't place his hands properly on the sternum. These complications include fractured ribs, a lacerated liver, and punctured lungs.
● Gastric distention, a common complication, results from giving too much air during ventilation. (See *Potential hazards of CPR.*)

Documentation

Whenever you perform CPR, document why you initiated it, whether the victim suffered from cardiac or respiratory arrest, when you found the victim and started CPR, and how long the victim received CPR. Note his response and any complications. Also include interventions taken to correct complications.

If the victim also received ACLS, document which interventions were performed, who performed them, when they were performed, and what equipment was used.

Supportive references

American Association for Respiratory Care. "Clinical Practice Guideline. Resuscitation and Defibrillation in the Health Care Setting — 2004 Revision and Update," *Respiratory Care* 89(9):1085-99, September 2004.

American Heart Association. "2005 AHA Guidelines for Cardiopulmonary Resuscitation and Emergency Cardiovascular Care: International Consensus on Science," *Circulation* 112(22 Suppl):IV-1-IV-221, November 2005.

American Heart Association "Highlights of the 2005 AHA Guideline for CPR and ECC," *Currents* 16(4):1-27, Winter 2005-2006.

Cardioversion, synchronized

Used to treat tachyarrhythmias, cardioversion delivers an electric charge to the myocardium at the peak of the R wave. This causes immediate depolarization, interrupting reentry circuits and allowing the sinoatrial node to resume control. Synchronizing the electric charge with the R wave ensures that the current won't be delivered on the vulnerable T wave and thus disrupt repolarization.

Synchronized cardioversion is the treatment of choice for arrhythmias that don't respond to vagal massage or drug therapy, such as unstable supraventricular tachycardia, unstable atrial fibrillation, unstable atrial flutter, and unstable monomorphic ventricular tachycardia.

Cardioversion should be performed according to the 2005 American Heart Association (AHA) guidelines and should be preceded by assessing the patient's cardiac and metabolic status. This assessment should include electrolyte values, particularly potassium values, which should be in the normal range, and knowledge of renal function (creatinine level), which guides the dosage of adjunctive medications. The serum digoxin level should be in the nontoxic range. When possible, the patient should be in optimal functional status at the time of the procedure. Arterial blood gas (ABG) analysis may be relevant in the patient with chronic lung disease. Written informed consent should be obtained from the patient after appropriate discussion of the procedure. The procedure should be carried out in an area where a general anesthetic or sedative agent can be administered and, if necessary, cardiopulmonary resuscitation measures can be conducted. **AHA**

Cardioversion may be an elective or urgent procedure, depending on how well the patient tolerates the arrhythmia. For example, if the patient is hemodynamically unstable, he would require urgent cardioversion. Remember that when preparing for cardioversion, the patient's condition can deteriorate quickly, necessitating immediate defibrillation.

CLINICAL IMPACT *The 2005 AHA guidelines for the treatment of symptomatic (unstable) tachycardias recommend immediate synchronized cardioversion. If the patient is stable, a 12-lead electrocardiogram (ECG) is done to further classify the tachycardia. Unstable signs include altered mental status, shock or hypotension, and ongoing chest pain.* **AHA**

Equipment

Cardioverter-defibrillator ● conductive gel pads ● anterior, posterior, or transverse paddles ● ECG monitor with recorder ● sedative ● oxygen therapy equipment ● airway ● handheld resuscitation bag ● emergency pacing equipment ● emergency cardiac medications ● automatic blood pressure cuff (if available) ● pulse oximeter (if available)

Implementation

- Explain the procedure to the patient, and make sure that he has signed a consent form. **PCP**
- Check the patient's recent serum potassium and magnesium levels and ABG results. Also check recent digoxin levels. Although the patient taking digoxin may undergo cardioversion, he tends to require lower energy levels to convert. If the patient takes digoxin, withhold the dose on the day of the procedure.
- If possible, withhold all food and fluids for 6 to 12 hours before the procedure.
- Obtain a 12-lead ECG to serve as a baseline.
- Check to see if the physician has ordered administration of any cardiac drugs before the procedure. Also verify that the patient has a patent I.V. site in case drug administration becomes necessary.
- Connect the patient to a pulse oximeter and automatic blood pressure cuff, if available.
- Consider administering oxygen for 5 to 10 minutes before cardioversion *to promote myocardial oxygenation*. If the patient wears dentures, evaluate whether they support his airway or may cause an airway obstruction. If they may cause an obstruction, remove them. **Science**
- Place the patient in the supine position and assess his vital signs, level of consciousness (LOC), cardiac rhythm, and peripheral pulses.
- Remove an oxygen delivery device just before cardioversion *to avoid possible combustion*.
- Have epinephrine (Adrenalin), lidocaine (Xylocain), and atropine at the patient's bedside.
- Make sure that the resuscitation bag is at the patient's bedside.
- Administer a sedative, as ordered. The patient should be heavily sedated but still able to breathe adequately.
- Carefully monitor the patient's blood pressure and respiratory rate until he recovers.
- Press the POWER button to turn on the defibrillator. Next, push the SYNC button *to synchronize the machine with the patient's QRS complexes*. Make sure that the SYNC button flashes with each of the patient's QRS complexes. You should also see a bright green flag flash on the monitor.
- Turn the ENERGY SELECT dial to the ordered amount of energy. Advanced cardiac life support (ACLS) protocols call for an initial shock of 50 to 100 joules for a patient with unstable supraventricular tachycardia, 100 to 200 joules for a patient with atrial fibrillation, 100 to 200 joules for a patient with atrial fibrillation,

50 to 100 joules for a patient with atrial flutter, and 100 joules for a patient who has monomorphic ventricular tachycardia with a pulse. If there's no response with the first shock, the health care provider should increase the joules in a step-wise manner. **ACLS**

- Remove the paddles from the machine, and prepare them as you would if you were defibrillating the patient. Place the conductive gel pads or paddles in the same positions as you would to defibrillate.
- Make sure that everyone stands away from the bed, and then push the discharge buttons. Hold the paddles in place and wait for the energy to be discharged — the machine has to synchronize the discharge with the QRS complex.
- Check the waveform on the monitor. If the arrhythmia fails to convert, repeat the procedure two or three more times at 3-minute intervals. Gradually increase the energy level with each additional countershock.
- After cardioversion, frequently assess the patient's LOC and respiratory status, including airway patency, respiratory rate and depth, and the need for supplemental oxygen. *Because the patient will be heavily sedated, he may require airway support.*
- Record a postcardioversion 12-lead ECG, and monitor the patient's ECG rhythm for 2 hours. Check the patient's chest for electrical burns.

Special considerations

- If the patient is attached to a bedside or telemetry monitor, disconnect the unit before cardioversion. *The electric current it generates could damage the equipment.*
- Remove any patches with metallic backings such as nitroglycerin patches. This backing may cause arcing during cardioversion.
- Be aware that improper synchronization may result if the patient's ECG tracing contains artifact-like spikes, such as peaked T waves or bundle-branch blocks when the R′ wave may be taller than the R wave.
- Although the electric shock of cardioversion won't usually damage an implanted pacemaker, avoid placing the paddles directly over the pacemaker.
- Reset the synchronization mode after each cardioversion because many defibrillators automatically default back to the synchronized mode.

Nursing diagnoses
- Decreased cardiac output
- Fear

Expected outcomes
The patient will:
- exhibit no arrhythmias
- maintain a blood pressure and pulse rate within normal limits
- state an understanding of the procedure.

Complications
- Common complications following cardioversion include transient, harmless arrhythmias, such as atrial, ventricular, and junctional premature beats.
- Serious ventricular arrhythmias, such as ventricular fibrillation, may also occur. However, this type of arrhythmia is more likely to result from high amounts of electrical energy, digoxin toxicity, severe heart disease, electrolyte imbalance, or improper synchronization with the R wave.

Documentation
Document the procedure, including the voltage delivered with each attempt, rhythm strips before and after the procedure, and how the patient tolerated the procedure.

Supportive references
American Heart Association. "2005 AHA Guidelines for Cardiopulmonary Resuscitation and Emergency Cardiovascular Care: International Consensus on Science," *Circulation* 112(22 Suppl):IV-1-IV-211, November 2005.

Central venous pressure monitoring

In central venous pressure (CVP) monitoring, a catheter is inserted through a vein and advanced until its tip lies in or near the right atrium. Because no major valves lie at the junction of the vena cava and right atrium, pressure at end diastole reflects back to the catheter.

CVP monitoring provides information about the body's blood volume or fluid status and right ventricular function. The central venous (CV) line also pro-

---

Converting cm H$_2$O to mm Hg

Central venous pressure (CVP) may be measured in centimeters of water (cm H$_2$O) or millimeters of mercury (mm Hg), with 1 mm Hg = 1.36 cm H$_2$O. However, it's recorded in mm Hg. To convert a reading in cm H$_2$O to a reading in mm Hg, use this equation:

$$\frac{CVP \text{ in cm } H_2O}{1.36} = CVP \text{ in mm Hg}$$

---

vides access to a large vessel for rapid, high-volume fluid administration and allows for rapid dilution of medications and frequent blood withdrawal for laboratory samples.

CVP can be monitored *intermittently* or *continuously*. According to the American Association of Critical-Care Nurses (AACN) guidelines, there are three methods for measuring pressure in the right atrium: using a water manometer attached to a CV catheter, using the proximal lumen of a pulmonary artery (PA) catheter, or using a line placed directly into the right atrium and attached to a transducer system. CVP is recorded in millimeters of mercury (mm Hg). When measured by a water manometer, CVP is reported in centimeters of water (cm H$_2$O). (See *Converting cm H$_2$O to mm Hg*.)

Normal CVP ranges from 5 to 10 cm H$_2$O. Any condition that alters venous return, circulating blood volume, or cardiac performance may affect CVP. If circulating volume increases (such as with enhanced venous return to the heart), CVP rises. If circulating volume decreases (such as with reduced venous return), CVP drops.

Equipment
Intermittent CVP monitoring
Disposable CVP manometer set • leveling device (such as a rod from a reusable CVP pole holder or a carpenter's level or rule) • additional stopcock (to attach the CVP manometer to the catheter) • extension tubing (if needed) • I.V. pole • I.V. solution • I.V. drip chamber and tubing

Continuous CVP monitoring

Pressure monitoring kit with disposable pressure transducer • leveling device • bedside pressure module • continuous I.V. flush solution • pressure bag

Withdrawal of blood samples through CV line

Appropriate number of syringes for the ordered tests • 5- or 10-ml syringe for the discard sample (Syringe size depends on the tests ordered.)

Use of intermittent CV line

Syringe with normal saline solution • syringe with heparin flush solution

Removal of CV catheter

Sterile gloves • suture removal set • sterile gauze pads • povidone-iodine ointment • dressing • tape

Implementation

● Gather the necessary equipment. Explain the procedure to the patient *to reduce his anxiety.*
● Assist the practitioner as he inserts the CV catheter. (The procedure is similar to that used for PA pressure monitoring, except that the catheter is advanced only as far as the superior vena cava.)

Intermittent CVP readings with water manometer

● Confirm the patient's identity using two patient identifiers according to facility policy. **JCAHO**
● With the CV line in place, position the patient flat. Align the base of the manometer with the previously determined zero reference point by using a leveling device. Because CVP reflects right atrial pressure, you must align the right atrium (the zero reference point) with the zero mark on the manometer. To find the right atrium, locate the fourth intercostal space at the midaxillary line. This is the phlebostatic axis. Mark the appropriate place on the patient's chest *so that all subsequent recordings will be made using the same location.* **AACN**
● If the patient can't tolerate a flat position, place him in semi-Fowler's position. Use the same degree of elevation for all subsequent measurements.
● Attach the water manometer to an I.V. pole or place it next to the patient's chest. Make sure that the zero reference point is level with the right atrium. (See *Measuring CVP with a water manometer.*)

● Verify that the water manometer is connected to the I.V. tubing. Typically, markings on the manometer range from –2 to 38 cm H_2O. However, the manufacturer's markings may differ, so be sure to read the directions before setting up the manometer and obtaining readings. **MFR**
● Turn the stopcock off to the patient, and slowly fill the manometer with I.V. solution until the fluid level is 10 to 20 cm H_2O higher than the patient's expected CVP value. Don't overfill the tube *because fluid that spills over the top can become a source of contamination.* **AACN**
● Turn the stopcock off to the I.V. solution and open to the patient. The fluid level in the manometer will drop. When the fluid level comes to rest, it will fluctuate slightly with respirations. Expect it to drop during inspiration and to rise during expiration.
● Record CVP at the end of expiration, when intrathoracic pressure has a negligible effect. Depending on the type of water manometer used, note the value either at the bottom of the meniscus or at the midline of the small floating ball. **AACN**
● After you've obtained the CVP value, turn the stopcock to resume the I.V. infusion. Adjust the I.V. drip rate as required.
● Place the patient in a comfortable position.

Continuous CVP readings with water manometer

● Make sure that the stopcock is turned so that the I.V. solution port, CVP column port, and patient port are open. Be aware that with this stopcock position, infusion of the I.V. solution increases CVP. Therefore, expect higher readings than those taken with the stopcock turned off to the I.V. solution. If the I.V. solution infuses at a constant rate, CVP will change as the patient's condition changes, although the initial reading will be higher.
● Assess the patient closely for changes.

Continuous CVP readings with pressure monitoring system

● Make sure that the CV line or the proximal lumen of a PA catheter is attached to the system. (If the patient has a CV line with multiple lumens, one lumen may be dedicated to continuous CVP monitoring and the other lumens used for fluid administration.) **AACN**

Measuring CVP with a water manometer

To ensure accurate central venous pressure (CVP) readings, make sure that the manometer base is aligned with the patient's right atrium (the zero reference point). The manometer set usually contains a leveling rod to allow you to determine this quickly.

After adjusting the manometer's position, examine the typical three-way stopcock (as shown at right). By turning it to any position shown, you can control the direction of fluid flow. Four-way stopcocks are also available.

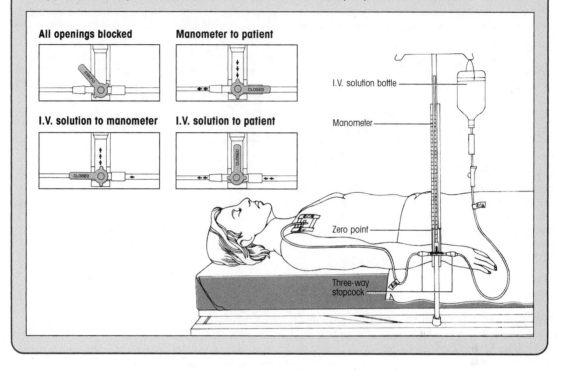

All openings blocked

Manometer to patient

I.V. solution to manometer

I.V. solution to patient

I.V. solution bottle

Manometer

Zero point

Three-way stopcock

● Set up a pressure transducer system. Connect pressure tubing from the CVP catheter hub to the transducer. Then connect the flush solution container to a flush device.

● To obtain values, position the patient flat. If he can't tolerate this position, use semi-Fowler's position. Locate the level of the right atrium by identifying the phlebostatic axis. Zero the transducer, leveling the transducer air-fluid interface stopcock with the right atrium. Read the CVP value from the digital display on the monitor, and note the waveform. Make sure that the patient is still when the reading is taken *to prevent artifact*. Be sure to use this position for all subsequent readings.

● Perform and document the dynamic response or square wave test every 8 to 12 hours to verify the optimal waveform. **AACN**

CV line removal

● You may assist the physician in removing a CV line. (In some states, a nurse is permitted to remove the catheter with a physician's order or when acting under facility policy and protocol.)

● If the head of the bed is elevated, minimize the risk of air embolism during catheter removal—for instance, place the patient in Trendelenburg's position if the line was inserted using a superior approach. If he can't tolerate this, position him flat. **AACN**

● Turn the patient's head to the side opposite the catheter insertion site. Remove the dressing and ex-

pose the insertion site. If sutures are in place, remove them carefully.
● Turn the I.V. solution off.
● Put on sterile gloves. **CDC**
● Pull the catheter out in a slow, smooth motion and then apply pressure to the insertion site.
● Clean the insertion site, apply povidone-iodine ointment, and cover it with a sterile gauze dressing, as ordered. Remove gloves, and wash your hands.
● Assess the patient for signs of respiratory distress, *which may indicate an air embolism.*

Special considerations

● As ordered, arrange for daily chest X-rays *to check catheter placement.*
● Care for the insertion site according to your facility's policy. Typically, you'll change the dressing every 24 to 48 hours.
● Be sure to wash your hands before performing dressing changes and to use aseptic technique and sterile gloves when re-dressing the site. When removing the old dressing, observe for signs of infection, such as redness, and note if the patient complains of tenderness. Apply ointment if directed by your facility's policy, and then cover the site with a sterile gauze dressing or a clear occlusive dressing.
● After the initial CVP reading, reevaluate readings frequently *to establish a baseline for the patient.* Authorities recommend obtaining readings at 15-, 30-, and 60-minute intervals to establish a baseline. If the patient's CVP fluctuates by more than 2 cm H_2O, suspect a change in his clinical status and report this finding to the physician.
● Change the I.V. solution every 24 hours and the I.V. tubing every 48 hours, according to your facility's policy. Expect the physician to change the catheter every 72 hours. Label the I.V. solution, tubing, and dressing with the date, time, and your initials.

Nursing diagnoses

● Risk for infection

Expected outcomes

The patient will:
● maintain vital signs and laboratory values within normal limits
● remain free from infection.

Complications

● Complications of CVP monitoring include pneumothorax (which typically occurs upon catheter insertion), sepsis, thrombus, vessel or adjacent organ puncture, and air embolism.

Documentation

Document all dressing, tubing, and solution changes. Document the patient's tolerance of the procedure, the date and time of catheter removal, and the type of dressing applied. Note the condition of the catheter insertion site and whether a culture specimen was collected. Note any complications and actions taken.

Supportive references

Bridges, E.J. "Monitoring Pulmonary Artery Pressures: Just the Facts," *Critical Care Nurse* 20(6):59-80, December 2000.

Daily, E.K. "Hemodynamic Waveform Analysis," *Journal of Cardiovascular Nursing* 15(2):6-22, January 2001.

Druding, M.C. "Integrating Hemodynamic Monitoring and Physical Assessment," *Dimensions of Critical Care Nursing* 19(4):25-30, July-August 2000.

Keckeisen, M. "Monitoring Pulmonary Artery Pressure," *Critical Care Nurse* 19(6):88-91, December 1999.

Lynn-McHale Wiegand, D.J., and Carlson, K.K. *AACN Procedure Manual for Critical Care*, 5th ed. Philadelphia: W.B. Saunders Co., 2005.

Quaal, S.J. "Improving the Accuracy of Pulmonary Artery Catheter Measurements," *Journal of Cardiovascular Nursing* 15(2):71-82, January 2001.

Rice, W.P., et al. "A Comparison of Hydrostatic Leveling Methods in Invasive Pressure Monitoring," *Critical Care Nurse* 20(6):21-30, December 2000.

Code management

The goals of any code are to restore the patient's spontaneous heartbeat and respirations and also to prevent hypoxic damage to the brain and other vital organs. Fulfilling these goals requires a team approach. Ideally, the team should consist of health care workers trained in advanced cardiac life support (ACLS), although nurses trained in basic life support (BLS) may also be a part of the team. Sponsored by the American Heart Association (AHA), the ACLS course incorporates BLS skills with advanced resuscitation techniques. BLS and ACLS procedures and protocols should be performed according to the 2005 AHA guidelines.

In most health care facilities, ACLS-trained nurses provide the first resuscitative efforts to cardiac arrest patients, commonly administering cardiac medications and performing defibrillation before the physician's arrival. Because ventricular fibrillation (VF) usually precedes sudden cardiac arrest, initial resuscitative efforts focus on rapid recognition of arrhythmias and, when indicated, defibrillation. If monitoring equipment isn't available, you should simply perform BLS measures. Of course, the scope of your responsibilities in any situation depends on your facility's policies and procedures and your state's nurse practice act.

A code may be called for patients with absent pulse, apnea, VF, ventricular tachycardia, and asystole. Some facilities allow family members to be present during a code; check your facility's policy regarding this issue.

CONTROVERSIAL ISSUE *The Emergency Nurses Association (ENA) has adopted a position statement regarding family presence during resuscitation. The ENA states that the family is the patient's major support system and that being with their loved one during resuscitation helps to meet the family's and the patient's needs. In addition, allowing family members to be present during a code facilitates the grieving process by, "bringing a sense of reality to the treatment efforts and the patient's clinical status." Family presence during pediatric resuscitation is recommended in the 2005 AHA pediatric resuscitation guidelines.* **AHA** **ENA**

The 2005 AHA guidelines for cardiopulmonary resuscitation (CPR) and emergency cardiovascular care stress the importance of good BLS care as the foundation of ACLS. Basic CPR and early defibrillation are of primary importance because they can significantly increase the patient's chances of survival. Drug therapy is the second priority. Recommended priorities include:
- starting CPR
- attempting defibrillation
- establishing I.V. access
- considering drug therapy
- inserting an advanced airway.

The 2005 AHA guidelines also stress that compressions shouldn't be interrupted unless a shock is being delivered or a rhythm check is being performed.

Health care providers shouldn't attempt to check for a pulse after a shock is delivered, but the pulse check should occur after 5 cycles of CPR, if a rhythm is detected.

Equipment

Oral, nasal, and endotracheal (ET) airways • one-way valve masks • oxygen source • oxygen flowmeter • intubation supplies • handheld resuscitation bag • suction supplies • nasogastric (NG) tube • goggles, masks, and gloves • cardiac arrest board • peripheral I.V. supplies, including 14G and 18G peripheral I.V. catheters • central I.V. supplies, including an 18G thin-wall catheter, a 6-cm needle catheter, and a 16G 15- to 20-cm catheter • I.V. administration sets (including microdrip and minidrip) • I.V. fluids, including dextrose 5% in water (D_5W), normal saline solution, and lactated Ringer's solution • electrocardiogram (ECG) monitor and leads • cardioverter-defibrillator • conductive medium • cardiac drugs, including adenosine (Adenocard), amiodarone (Cordarone), atropine, calcium chloride, dobutamine (Dobutrex), dopamine (Intropin), epinephrine (Adrenaline), isoproterenol (Isuprel), lidocaine (Xylocaine), procainamide (Pronestyl), and vasopressin (Pitressin) • optional: transthoracic pacemaker, percutaneous transvenous pacer, cricothyrotomy kit, and end-tidal carbon dioxide detector

Preparation of equipment

- Because effective emergency care depends on reliable and accessible equipment, the equipment as well as the personnel must be ready for a code at any time. (See *Organizing your crash cart,* page 232.)
- You also should be familiar with the cardiac drugs you may have to administer. (See *Common emergency cardiac drugs,* pages 233 and 234)
- Always be aware of the patient's code status as defined by the physician's orders, the patient's advance directive, and the family's wishes. If the physician has ordered, "no code," make sure that the physician has written and signed the order. If possible, have the patient or a responsible family member co-sign the order. **PCP**
- For some patients, you may need to consider whether the family wishes to be present during a code. If they want to be present and if a nurse or clergyman can remain with them, consider allowing them to remain during the code.

INNOVATIVE
PRACTICE

Organizing your crash cart

When responding to a code, you can't waste time searching the drawers of your crash cart for the equipment you need. One way to make sure that you know the precise location of everything is to follow the ABCD plan to an organized crash cart. Label the crash cart drawers with the letters A, B, C, and D, and fill them as follows.

A: Airway control drawer
This drawer should contain all of the equipment necessary for maintaining a patient's airway. It should include oral, nasal, and endotracheal (ET) airways; an intubation tray containing a laryngoscope and blades; an extra laryngoscope; lidocaine ointment; tape; a 10-ml syringe to inflate the ET balloon; extra batteries and lightbulbs; and suction devices.

B: Breathing drawer
This drawer should contain all of the equipment needed to support the patient's ventilation and oxygenation. Oxygenation is maintained with nasal cannulas, face masks, and Venturi masks. Ventilation is supported by maintaining gastric compression with nasogastric tubes.

C: Circulation drawer
In this drawer, place anything needed to start a central or peripheral I.V. line, such as catheters, tubing, start kits, pump tubing, and 250-ml or 500-ml bags of I.V. solutions (dextrose 5% in water and normal saline solution).

D: Drug drawer
This drawer should contain all medications needed for advanced cardiac life support.

Implementation
- If you're the first to arrive at the site of a code, call for help and instruct another person to retrieve the emergency equipment. Then assess the patient's level of consciousness (LOC), airway, breathing, and circulation, and begin CPR. Use a pocket mask, if available, to ventilate the patient.
- When the emergency equipment arrives, have the second BLS provider place the cardiac arrest board under the patient and then assist with two-rescuer CPR. Meanwhile, have the nurse assigned to the patient relate the patient's medical history and describe the events leading to cardiac arrest.
- A third person, either a nurse certified in BLS or a respiratory therapist, will then attach the handheld resuscitation bag to the oxygen source and begin to ventilate the patient with 100% oxygen.
- When the ACLS-trained nurse arrives, she'll expose the patient's chest and apply defibrillator pads. She'll then apply the paddles to the patient's chest to obtain a "quick look" at the patient's cardiac rhythm. If the patient is in VF, ACLS protocol calls for defibrillation as soon as possible with 120 to 200 joules. Then, resume CPR immediately. A rhythm check isn't done at this time. It's done after 5 cycles of CPR and if a rhythm is detected, perform a pulse check. The ACLS-trained nurse will act as code leader until the physician arrives.
- If not already in place, apply ECG electrodes and attach the patient to the defibrillator's cardiac monitor. Avoid placing electrodes on bony prominences or hairy areas. Also avoid the areas where the defibrillator pads will be placed and where chest compressions will be given.
- After 5 cycles of CPR, the patient's rhythm will be checked and, if necessary, another shock will be given at the same or higher dose, and then continue CPR while the defibrillator is charging. After another 5 cycles of CPR, the patient's rhythm will be checked and another shock will be given at the same or higher dose, if necessary.
- As CPR and defibrillation is occurring, you or an ACLS-trained nurse will then start two peripheral I.V. lines with large-bore I.V. catheters. Be sure to use only a large vein, such as the antecubital vein, *to allow for rapid fluid administration and to prevent drug extravasation.*
- As soon as the I.V. catheter is in place, begin an infusion of normal saline solution or lactated Ringer's solution *to help prevent circulatory collapse.* D_5W continues to be acceptable, but the latest ACLS guidelines encourage the use of normal saline solution or lactated Ringer's solution *because D_5W can produce hyperglycemic effects during cardiac arrest.*

Common emergency cardiac drugs

You may be called on to administer several cardiac drugs during a code. This chart lists the most common emergency cardiac drugs, along with their actions, indications, and dosages.

Drug	Actions	Indications	Typical adult dosage
adenosine (Adenocard)	• Slows conduction through atrioventricular (AV) node; may interrupt reentry through AV node • Shortens duration of atrial action potential during supraventricular tachycardia	• Supraventricular tachycardia, including those associated with accessory bypass tracts	• 6 mg I.V. push over 1 to 3 seconds initially; may be increased to 12 mg if conversion has not occurred within 2 minutes; may repeat 12 mg in 1 to 2 minutes if needed. Each dose should be followed by a 20-ml saline flush. • *Caution:* Slower-than-recommended administration decreases drug's effectiveness.
amiodarone (Cordarone)	• Thought to prolong refractory period and action potential, duration	• Supraventricular tachycardia • Persistent ventricular tachycardia (VT) or ventricular fibrillation (VF)	• For wide complex tachycardia, 150 mg over 10 minutes, followed by 1 mg/minute infusion for 6 hours, then 0.5 mg/minute. • For cardiac arrest, 300 mg I.V. push or I.O.; repeat 150 mg I.V. push in 3 to 5 minutes. Dilute in 20 to 30 ml D_5W. Maximum dose 2.2 g I.V./24 hour.
atropine	• Accelerates AV conduction and heart rate by blocking vagal nerve	• Symptomatic bradycardia • Asystole • Pulseless electrical activity (PEA) (slow rate)	• 0.5 mg I.V. push (for asystole or PEA, 1 mg); repeated every 3 to 5 minutes until heart rate 60 beats/minute up to 3 mg total.
dobutamine (Dobutrex)	• Increases myocardial contractility without raising oxygen demand	• Heart failure • Cardiogenic shock	• 2 to 20 mcg/kg/minute by continuous I.V. infusion. Titrate so that heart rate isn't greater than 10% of baseline.
dopamine (Intropin)	• Produces inotropic effect, increasing cardiac output, blood pressure, and renal perfusion	• Hypotension (except when caused by hypovolemia)	• Continuous I.V. infusion at 2 to 20 mcg/kg/minute *Note:* Always dilute and give I.V. drip, never I.V. push. Titrate to patient response. • *Caution:* Don't administer in same I.V. line with alkaline solution.
epinephrine (Adrenalin)	• Increases heart rate, peripheral resistance, and blood flow to heart (enhancing myocardial and cerebral oxygenation) • Strengthens myocardial contractility • Increases coronary perfusion pressure during cardiopulmonary resuscitation	• VF • Pulseless VT • Pulseless electrical activity • Asystole • Hypotension (secondary agent) • Symptomatic bradycardia	• 10 ml of 1:10,000 solution (1 mg) I.V. push or I.O. initially; may be repeated every 3 to 5 minutes, as needed. After each dose, flush 20 ml of I.V. fluid if administered peripherally. • 2 to 2½ times the I.V. dose, endotracheally if no I.V. line is available. (*Note:* 1:1,000 solution contains 1 mg/ml, so it must be diluted in 9 ml of normal saline solution to provide 1 mg/10 ml.) • For hypotension, 1 mg/500 ml of D_5W by continuous infusion, starting at 1 mcg/min and titrated to desired effect (2 to 10 mcg/minute). • *Caution:* Don't administer in same I.V. line with alkaline solutions. • Many reports have shown that doses of 10 mg I.V. or more are needed to achieve resuscitation. *(continued)*

Common emergency cardiac drugs *(continued)*

Drug	Actions	Indications	Typical adult dosage
isoproterenol (Isuprel)	• Enhances automaticity and accelerates conduction • Increases heart rate and cardiac contractility, but exacerbates ischemia and arrhythmias in patients with ischemic heart disease	• Indicated only for temporary control of severe bradycardia unresponsive to atropine (while awaiting pacemaker insertion) • Torsades de pointes	• Continuous I.V. infusion at 2 to 10 mcg/minute titrated p.r.n. to obtain an adequate heart rate. Monitor heart rate and blood pressure carefully. Doses that increase heart rate to greater than 130 beats/minute may induce ventricular arrhythmias.
lidocaine (Xylocaine)	• Depresses automaticity and conduction of ectopic impulses in ventricles, especially in ischemic tissue • Raises fibrillation threshold, especially in an ischemic heart	• Cardiac arrest from VF or VT	• 1 to 1.5 mg/kg (usually 50 to 75 mg) I.V. push or I.O. initially; may be followed by 0.5 to 0.75 mg/kg bolus dose every 5 to 10 minutes up to total of 3 mg/kg. • Continuous I.V. infusion of 2 g/500 ml of D_5W at (1 to 4 mg/minute) to prevent recurrence of lethal arrhythmias; reduced by 50% after 24 hour.
magnesium sulfate	• Mechanism of action is unclear but drug may help in cardiac arrest associated with refractory VT or VF	• Cardiac arrest associated with refractory VT • Torsades de pointes • Ventricular arrhythmias due to digoxin toxicity	• For cardiac arrest associated with torsades de pointes, 1 to 2 g I.V. in 10 ml of D_5W over 5 to 20 minutes. • For torsades de pointes without cardiac arrest, 1 to 2 g in 50 to 100 ml of D_5W over 5 to 60 minutes; follow with 0.5 to 1 g/hour I.V.
procainamide (Pronestyl)	• Depresses automaticity and conduction • Prolongs refraction in atria and ventricles	• Suppresses PVCs • VT • Supraventricular arrhythmias	• 20 mg/minute I.V. infusion up to total of 17 mg/kg, followed by maintenance dose of 1 to 4 mg/minute by I.V. infusion. Administration is limited by the need for slow infusion.
vasopressin (Pitressin)	• Causes peripheral vasoconstriction	• Refractory VF • Pulseless VT • VF	• 40 units I.V. or I.O. as a single dose, one time only.
verapamil (Isoptin)	• Slows conduction through AV node • Causes vasodilation • Produces negative inotropic effect on heart, depressing myocardial contractility	• Paroxysmal supraventricular tachycardia with narrow QRS complex and rate control in atrial fibrillation	• 2.5 to 5 mg I.V. push over 2 minutes initially (over 3 minutes in older adult). Repeat dose of 5 to 10 mg every 15 to 30 minutes, if needed. Total dose 20 mg. Monitor electrocardiogram and blood pressure.

• While one nurse starts the I.V. lines, the other nurse will set up portable or wall suction equipment and suction the patient's oral secretions, as necessary, *to maintain an open airway.*
• The ACLS-trained nurse will then prepare and administer emergency cardiac drugs, as needed. (See *ACLS pulseless arrest algorithm,* pages 236 and 237.)

Keep in mind that drugs administered through a central line reach the myocardium more quickly than those administered through a peripheral line.
• The ACLS pulseless arrest algorithm shows the timing of drug administration and shock administration. Drug doses should be given immediately after a rhythm check.

- If the patient doesn't have an accessible I.V. line, you may administer medications, such as epinephrine, lidocaine, vasopressin, and atropine through an ET tube. To do so, dilute the drugs in 10 ml of normal saline solution or sterile water and then instill them into the patient's ET tube. Afterward, ventilate the patient manually *to improve absorption by distributing the drug throughout the bronchial tree.*
- The ACLS-trained nurse will also prepare for and assist with ET intubation or other advanced airway. Compression interruption should be minimized during advanced airway placement.
- Suction the patient as needed. After the patient has been intubated, the health care provider should use clinical assessment and confirmation devices to check ET tube placement. Assessment includes visualizing chest expansion, auscultation of equal breath sounds, and auscultation of no breath sounds over the epigastrium. Devices used to check tube placement include exhaled carbon dioxide detectors and esophageal detectors. When the tube is correctly positioned, tape it securely. *To serve as a reference,* mark the point on the tube level with the patient's lips.
- Meanwhile, other members of the code team should keep a written record of the events. Other duties include prompting participants about when to perform certain activities (such as when to check a pulse or take vital signs), overseeing the effectiveness of CPR, and keeping track of the time between therapies. Each team member should know what each participant's role is *to prevent duplicating effort.* Finally, someone from the team should make sure that the primary nurse's other patients are reassigned to another nurse.
- If the family is at the facility during the code, have someone, such as a clergy member or social worker, remain with them. Keep the family informed of the patient's status.
- If the family isn't at the facility, contact them as soon as possible. Encourage them not to drive to the facility, but offer to call someone who can give them a ride.

Special considerations
- When the patient's condition has stabilized, assess his LOC, breath sounds, heart sounds, peripheral perfusion, bowel sounds, and urine output. Take his vital signs every 15 minutes, and monitor his cardiac rhythm continuously.
- Make sure that the patient receives an adequate supply of oxygen, whether through a mask or ventilator.
- Check the infusion rates of all I.V. fluids, and use infusion pumps to deliver vasoactive drugs. *To evaluate the effectiveness of fluid therapy,* insert an indwelling catheter if the patient doesn't already have one.
- Also insert an NG tube *to relieve or prevent gastric distention.*
- If appropriate, reassure the patient and explain what's happening. Allow the patient's family to visit as soon as possible. If the patient dies, notify the family and allow them to see the patient as soon as possible.
- *To make sure that your code team performs optimally,* schedule a time to review the code.

Nursing diagnoses
- Compromised family coping
- Decreased cardiac output

Expected outcomes
The patient (and his family) will:
- express their concerns and fears
- have restored heart rhythm
- maintain a blood pressure and pulse rate within normal limits.

Complications
- Even when performed correctly, CPR can cause fractured ribs, liver laceration, lung puncture, and gastric distention.
- Defibrillation can cause electric shock, and emergency intubation can result in esophageal or tracheal laceration, subcutaneous emphysema, or accidental right mainstem bronchus intubation.
- Decreased or absent breath sounds on the left side of the chest and normal breath sounds on the right may signal accidental right mainstem bronchus intubation.

Documentation
During the code, document the events in as much detail as possible. Note whether the arrest was witnessed or unwitnessed, the time of the arrest, the

(Text continues on page 238.)

ACLS pulseless arrest algorithm ⓐcⓛs ⓐⓗⓐ

This American Heart Association algorithm outlines the steps an advanced cardiac life support (ACLS)-certified nurse should take to treat rhythms that produce cardiac arrest, such as ventricular fibrillation (VF), rapid ventricular tachycardia (VT), pulseless electrical activity, and asystole. If you aren't ACLS-certified, the algorithm will help you know what to expect in such an emergency.

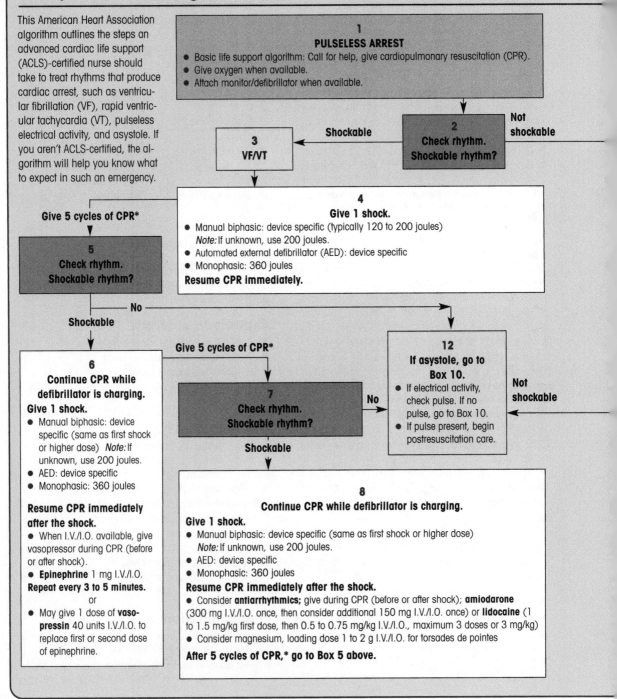

1
PULSELESS ARREST
- Basic life support algorithm: Call for help, give cardiopulmonary resuscitation (CPR).
- Give oxygen when available.
- Attach monitor/defibrillator when available.

2
Check rhythm.
Shockable rhythm?

Shockable → Not shockable

3
VF/VT

4
Give 1 shock.
- Manual biphasic: device specific (typically 120 to 200 joules)
  Note: If unknown, use 200 joules.
- Automated external defibrillator (AED): device specific
- Monophasic: 360 joules
Resume CPR immediately.

Give 5 cycles of CPR*

5
Check rhythm.
Shockable rhythm?

No

Shockable

6
Continue CPR while defibrillator is charging.
Give 1 shock.
- Manual biphasic: device specific (same as first shock or higher dose) *Note:* If unknown, use 200 joules.
- AED: device specific
- Monophasic: 360 joules

Resume CPR immediately after the shock.
- When I.V./I.O. available, give vasopressor during CPR (before or after shock).
- **Epinephrine** 1 mg I.V./I.O. **Repeat every 3 to 5 minutes.**
  or
- May give 1 dose of **vasopressin** 40 units I.V./I.O. to replace first or second dose of epinephrine.

Give 5 cycles of CPR*

7
Check rhythm.
Shockable rhythm?

No

Shockable

12
If asystole, go to Box 10.
- If electrical activity, check pulse. If no pulse, go to Box 10.
- If pulse present, begin postresuscitation care.

Not shockable

8
Continue CPR while defibrillator is charging.
Give 1 shock.
- Manual biphasic: device specific (same as first shock or higher dose)
  Note: If unknown, use 200 joules.
- AED: device specific
- Monophasic: 360 joules
Resume CPR immediately after the shock.
- Consider **antiarrhythmics;** give during CPR (before or after shock); **amiodarone** (300 mg I.V./I.O. once, then consider additional 150 mg I.V./I.O. once) or **lidocaine** (1 to 1.5 mg/kg first dose, then 0.5 to 0.75 mg/kg I.V./I.O., maximum 3 doses or 3 mg/kg)
- Consider magnesium, loading dose 1 to 2 g I.V./I.O. for torsades de pointes
After 5 cycles of CPR,* go to Box 5 above.

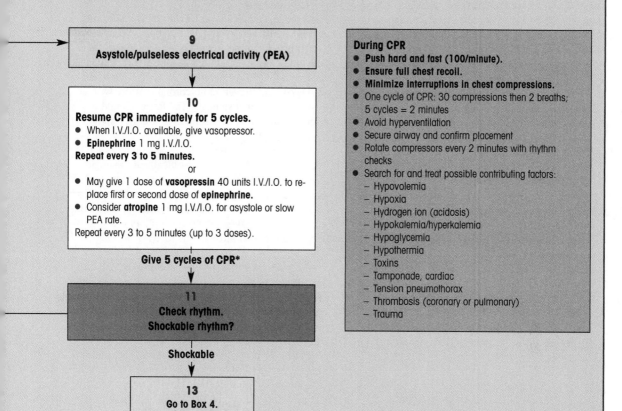

9
Asystole/pulseless electrical activity (PEA)

10
Resume CPR immediately for 5 cycles.
- When I.V./I.O. available, give vasopressor.
- **Epinephrine** 1 mg I.V./I.O.
Repeat every 3 to 5 minutes.

or

- May give 1 dose of **vasopressin** 40 units I.V./I.O. to re-place first or second dose of **epinephrine.**
- Consider **atropine** 1 mg I.V./I.O. for asystole or slow PEA rate.
Repeat every 3 to 5 minutes (up to 3 doses).

Give 5 cycles of CPR*

11
Check rhythm.
Shockable rhythm?

Shockable

13
Go to Box 4.

During CPR
- **Push hard and fast (100/minute).**
- **Ensure full chest recoil.**
- **Minimize interruptions in chest compressions.**
- One cycle of CPR: 30 compressions then 2 breaths; 5 cycles = 2 minutes
- Avoid hyperventilation
- Secure airway and confirm placement
- Rotate compressors every 2 minutes with rhythm checks
- Search for and treat possible contributing factors:
  – Hypovolemia
  – Hypoxia
  – Hydrogen ion (acidosis)
  – Hypokalemia/hyperkalemia
  – Hypoglycemia
  – Hypothermia
  – Toxins
  – Tamponade, cardiac
  – Tension pneumothorax
  – Thrombosis (coronary or pulmonary)
  – Trauma

*After an advanced airway is placed, rescuers no longer deliver "cycles" of CPR. Give continuous chest compressions without pauses for breaths. Give 8 to 10 breaths/minute. Check rhythm every 2 minutes.

time CPR was begun, the time the ACLS-trained nurse arrived, and the total resuscitation time. Also document the number of defibrillations, the times they were performed, the joule level, the patient's cardiac rhythm before and after the defibrillation, and whether the patient had a pulse.

Document all drug therapy, including dosages, routes of administration, and the patient's response. You'll also want to record all procedures, such as peripheral and central line insertion, pacemaker insertion, and ET tube insertion, with the time performed and the patient's tolerance of the procedure. Also keep track of all arterial blood gas values.

Record whether the patient is transferred to another unit or facility along with his condition at the time of transfer and whether or not his family was notified. Finally, document complications and the measures taken to correct them. When your documentation is complete, have the physician and ACLS nurse review and then sign the document.

Supportive references

American Heart Association. "2005 AHA Guidelines for Cardiopulmonary Resuscitation and Emergency Cardiovascular Care: International Consensus on Science," *Circulation* 112(22 Suppl):IV-1-IV-211, November 2005.

American Heart Association. "Highlights of the 2005 American Heart Association Guidelines for CPR and ECC," *Currents* 16(4):1-27, Winter 2005-2006.

Emergency Nurses Association. "Emergency Nurses Association Position Statement: Family Presence at the Bedside During Invasive Procedures and/or Resuscitation," July 2001. *www.ena.org/publications/index.htm.*

Martinez, J.A., and Weiss, L.D. "Medical and Legal Implications of Cardiac Arrest Protocols," Annual Meeting of the American Association of Critical-Care Nurses. Orlando, Fla., October 2000. *www.aacn.org/aacn/conteduc.nsf.*

Coronary angioplasty

A nonsurgical approach to opening coronary vessels narrowed by arteriosclerosis, percutaneous transluminal coronary angioplasty (PTCA) uses a balloon-tipped catheter that's inserted into a narrowed coronary artery. This procedure, performed in the cardiac catheterization laboratory under local anesthesia, relieves pain due to angina and myocardial ischemia.

The current techniques of PTCA allow patients (with favorable anatomy) to have either single- or multivessel PTCA at low risk and with a high likelihood of initial success. For this reason, the new recommendations by the American College of Cardiology (ACC), the American Heart Association (AHA), and the Society for Cardiovascular Angiography and Interventions are largely based upon the patient's clinical condition, specific coronary lesion morphology and anatomy, left ventricular (LV) function, and associated medical conditions. Less emphasis is placed on how many lesions or vessels require PTCA. The ideal candidate for PTCA has single- or double-vessel disease excluding the left main coronary artery with at least 50% proximal stenosis. The lesion should be discrete, uncalcified, concentric, and not located near a bifurcation.

Cardiac catheterization usually accompanies PTCA to assess the stenosis and the efficacy of the angioplasty. Catheterization is used as a visual tool to direct the balloon-tipped catheter through the vessel's area of stenosis. As the balloon is inflated, the plaque is compressed against the vessel wall, allowing coronary blood to flow more freely. (See *Performing PTCA.*)

Your responsibilities include teaching the patient and his family about the procedure and assessing the patient for complications afterward.

PTCA provides an alternative for patients who are poor surgical risks because of chronic medical problems. It's also useful for patients who have total coronary occlusion, unstable angina, and plaque buildup in several areas and for those with poor LV function.

Newer procedures, such as brachytherapy and drug-eluting stents, show promise in preventing or treating restenosis. (See *Preventing restenosis.*)

Equipment

Povidone-iodine solution • local anesthetic • I.V. solution and tubing • electrocardiogram (ECG) monitor and electrodes • oxygen • nasal cannula • shaving supplies or depilatory cream • sedative • pulmonary artery (PA) catheter • contrast medium • emergency medications • heparin for injection • 5-lb (2.3-kg) sandbag • introducer kit for PTCA catheter • sterile gown, gloves, and drapes • sterile marker • sterile labels • optional: nitroglycerin, soft restraints

Performing PTCA

Percutaneous transluminal coronary angioplasty (PTCA) is a procedure that opens an occluded coronary artery without opening the chest. It's performed in the cardiac catheterization laboratory after coronary angiography confirms the presence and location of the occlusion. After the occlusion is located, the physician threads a guide catheter through the patient's femoral artery and into the coronary artery under fluoroscopic guidance (as shown below).

When the guide catheter's position at the occlusion site is confirmed by angiography, the physician carefully introduces a double-lumen balloon that's smaller than the catheter lumen. He then directs the balloon through the lesion, where a marked pressure gradient will be obvious. The physician alternately inflates (as shown below) and deflates the balloon until an angiogram verifies successful arterial dilation and the pressure gradient has decreased.

Top-entry vascular access port (VAP)

Side-entry VAP

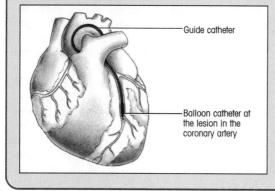

Guide catheter

Balloon catheter at the lesion in the coronary artery

Flattened plaque

Inflated balloon

Preventing restenosis

Restenosis is the recurrence of a coronary artery blockage at the site of treatment. Restenosis is a major drawback in treating coronary artery disease with angioplasty or stents. One option for patients who have developed restenosis in previously implanted stents is brachytherapy or coronary artery radiation.

Most restenosis is caused by thrombosis or blood clotting at the site of treatment. Anti-clotting drugs such as clopidogrel (Plavix) can partially prevent this type of restenosis. However, some restenosis at the site of treatment is due to actual tissue growth of endothelial cells that normally line the blood vessels. Radiation therapy or brachytherapy can be used to target these areas and treat restenosis even after stent placement.

Brachytherapy is delivered by insertion of a new type of catheter designed to apply the radiation to a localized area. The catheter is passed into the coronary arteries

and across the target area. Once the target area is "bracketed" by the catheter, the radiation is applied. Brachytherapy seems to reduce the rate of restenosis within stents by approximately 30% to 50%.

While radiation for in-stent restenosis is a promising approach, there are drawbacks to this therapy and it doesn't always work. More important than treating the restenosis is to prevent it from happening. The most promising option appears to be the insertion of drug-eluting stents coated with a medication such as sirolimus (Rapamune). A large scale randomized double-blind study showed sustained reduction in the incidence of re-blockage by more than 90%. In 2003, this product received Food and Drug Administration approval, making it the first combination drug device intended to help reduce restenosis of a treated coronary artery. **EB1**

Implementation

TEACHING *Explain the procedure to the patient and his family to reduce the patient's fear and promote cooperation.* **PCP**

Inform the patient that the procedure lasts 1 to 4 hours and that he may feel some discomfort from lying on a hard table for that long. **PCP**

Tell the patient that a catheter will be inserted into an artery or a vein in his groin and that he may feel pressure as the catheter moves along the vessel.

Reassure the patient that although he'll be awake during the procedure, he'll be given a sedative. Explain that the physician or nurse may ask him how he's feeling and that he should tell them if he experiences angina.

Explain that the physician will inject a contrast medium to outline the lesion's location. Warn the patient that he may feel a hot, flushing sensation or transient nausea during the injection.

Before coronary angioplasty

● Check the patient's history for allergies; if he has had allergic reactions to shellfish, iodine, or contrast media, notify the physician. **EB2**

● Give 650 mg of aspirin the evening before the procedure, as ordered, *to prevent platelet aggregation.* **Science**

● Make sure that the patient signs a consent form. **PCP**

● Restrict food and fluids for at least 6 hours before the procedure or as ordered.

● Make sure that the results of coagulation studies, complete blood count, serum electrolyte studies, and blood typing and crossmatching are available. **ACC** **AHA**

● Insert an I.V. line *in case emergency medications are needed.*

● Shave hair from the insertion site (groin or brachial area), or use a depilatory cream. Then clean the area with povidone-iodine solution.

● Give the patient a sedative, as ordered.

● Take baseline peripheral pulses in all extremities.

During coronary angioplasty

● When the patient arrives at the cardiac catheterization laboratory, apply ECG electrodes and ensure I.V. line patency.

● Administer oxygen through a nasal cannula.

● The physician puts on a sterile gown and gloves. Open the sterile supplies. Label all medications, medication containers, and other solutions on and off the sterile field. **CDC** **JCAHO**

● The physician prepares and drapes the site and injects a local anesthetic. If the patient doesn't have a PA catheter in place, the physician may insert one now.

● The physician inserts a large guide catheter into the artery and sutures it in place. Then he threads an angioplasty catheter through the guide catheter. An angioplasty catheter is thinner and longer and has a balloon at its tip. Using a thin, flexible guide wire, he then threads the catheter up through the aorta and into the coronary artery to the area of stenosis.

● The physician injects a contrast medium through the angioplasty catheter and into the obstructed coronary artery *to outline the lesion's location and help assess the blockage.* He also injects heparin, *to prevent the catheter from clotting,* and intracoronary nitroglycerin, *to dilate coronary vessels and prevent spasm, if needed.*

● The physician inflates the catheter's balloon for a gradually increasing amount of time and pressure. The expanding balloon compresses the atherosclerotic plaque against the arterial wall, expanding the arterial lumen. Because balloon inflation deprives the myocardium distal to the inflation area of blood, the patient may experience angina at this time. If balloon inflation fails to decrease the stenosis, a larger balloon may be used.

● After angioplasty, serial angiograms help determine the effectiveness of treatment.

● The physician removes the angioplasty catheter while leaving the guide catheter in place, in case the procedure needs to be repeated because of vessel occlusion. The guide catheter is usually removed 8 to 24 hours after the procedure.

After coronary angioplasty

● When the patient returns to the unit, he may be receiving I.V. heparin or nitroglycerin. If he's bleeding at the catheter insertion site, he may also have a sandbag on it *to prevent hematoma.* **AHA**

● Assess the patient's vital signs every 15 minutes for the first hour and then every 30 minutes for 4 hours, unless his condition warrants more frequent checking. **AACN** **AHA**

● Assess peripheral pulses distal to the catheter insertion site as well as the color, sensation, temperature, and capillary refill of the affected extremity.

● Monitor ECG rhythm and arterial pressures.

ALERT *Because coronary spasm may occur during or after PTCA, monitor the ECG for ST- and T-wave changes, and take the patient's vital signs frequently. Coronary artery dissection may occur with no early symptoms, but it can cause restenosis of the vessel. Stay alert for symptoms of ischemia, which requires emergency coronary revascularization.*

● Instruct the patient to remain in bed for 8 hours and to keep the affected extremity straight; if he's restless and moving his extremities, apply soft restraints, if necessary. Elevate the head of the bed 15 to 30 degrees.

● Assess the catheter site for hematoma, ecchymosis, and hemorrhage. If an area of expanding hematoma appears, mark the site and alert the physician. If bleeding occurs, locate the artery and apply manual pressure, and then notify the physician. **AACN** **AHA**

● Administer I.V. fluids as ordered — usually 100 ml/hour — *to promote excretion of the contrast medium.* Be sure to assess for signs of fluid overload (jugular vein distention, atrial and ventricular gallops, dyspnea, pulmonary congestion, tachycardia, hypertension, and hypoxemia). **Science**

● After the physician removes the catheter, apply direct pressure for at least 10 minutes and monitor the site frequently.

Special considerations
● PTCA is contraindicated in left main coronary artery disease, especially when the patient is a poor surgical risk; in patients with variant angina or critical valvular disease; and in patients with vessels occluded at the aortic wall orifice.

Nursing diagnoses
● Ineffective tissue perfusion: Cardiopulmonary

Expected outcomes
The patient will:
● maintain hemodynamic stability
● exhibit peripheral pulses that remain present and strong.

Complications
● The most common complication is prolonged angina.
● Other complications include coronary artery perforation, balloon rupture, reocclusion (necessitating a

coronary artery bypass graft), myocardial infarction, pericardial tamponade, hematoma, hemorrhage, reperfusion arrhythmias, and closure of the vessel.
● Vascular stents may be inserted to prevent vessel closure. (See *Vascular stents.*)

Vascular stents

Acute vessel closure and late restenosis are two serious complications of percutaneous transluminal coronary angioplasty (PTCA). To prevent these problems, physicians are performing a new procedure called stenting. The balloon-expandable stent consists of a stainless steel tube, the walls of which have a rectangular design. When the stent expands, each rectangle stretches to a diamond shape. The expanded stent supports the artery and helps prevent restenosis.

The stent is used in patients at risk for abrupt clotting after PTCA. Stents may also be inserted after failed PTCA to keep the patient stable until he can undergo coronary artery bypass surgery, or a stent may be used as an alternative to surgery.

For insertion, the stent is put on a standard balloon angioplasty catheter and positioned over a guide wire. Fluoroscopy verifies correct placement, and then the stent is expanded and the catheter is removed (as shown).

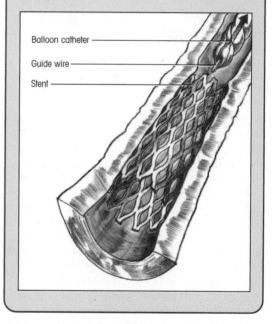

Balloon catheter

Guide wire

Stent

Documentation

Note the patient's tolerance of the procedure and his condition after it, including his vital signs and the condition of the extremity distal to the insertion site. Document any complications and interventions.

Supportive references

American College of Cardiology, American Heart Association, Society for Cardiovascular Angiography and Interventions. "2005 Guideline Update for Percutaneous Coronary Intervention." *www.americanheart.org/*

McCabe, P.J., et al. "Evaluation of Nursing Care after Diagnostic Coronary Angiography," *American Journal of Critical Care* 10(5):330-40, September 2001. **EB2**

Morice, M., et al. "Sirolimus- vs. Paclitaxel-eluding Stents in de Novo Coronary Artery Lesions: The REALITY Trial: A Randomized Controlled Trial," *JAMA* 295(8): 895-904, February 2006. **EB1**

Schickel, S.I., et al. "Achieving Femoral Artery Hemostasis after Cardiac Catheterization: A Comparison of Methods," *American Journal of Critical Care* 8(6): 406-409, November 1999.

Defibrillation

The 2005 American Heart Association (AHA) guidelines identify defibrillation as the standard treatment for ventricular fibrillation (VF), after cardiopulmonary resuscitation (CPR). CPR prolongs VF and prolongs the time that defibrillation can occur. CPR alone isn't likely to correct VF; therefore, early defibrillation is critical. Defibrillation involves using electrode paddles to direct an electric current through the patient's heart. The current causes the myocardium to depolarize, which in turn encourages the sinoatrial node to resume control of the heart's electrical activity. Successful defibrillation depends on the appropriate selection of energy to generate sufficient flow through the heart to achieve defibrillation while minimizing injury to the heart. Modern defibrillators deliver current in waveforms, and are available in monophasic and biphasic models. Defibrillators with monophasic waveforms deliver current in one direction. Few monophasic waveform defibrillators are being manufactured, but some are still in use. Biphasic waveforms deliver current that flows in a positive direction for a specific duration and then reverses and flows in a negative direction for the remaining time of electrical discharge. Lower energy shocks are required and have been shown to be as effective as the higher energy shocks used with monophasic waveform defibrillators in terminating VF.

Because VF leads to death if not corrected, the success of defibrillation depends on early recognition and quick treatment of this arrhythmia. In addition to treating VF, defibrillation may also be used to treat ventricular tachycardia that doesn't produce a pulse.

Patients with a history of VF may be candidates for an implantable cardioverter-defibrillator, a sophisticated device that automatically discharges an electric current when it senses a ventricular tachyarrhythmia. (See *Understanding the ICD.*)

Equipment

Defibrillator • external paddles • internal paddles (sterilized for cardiac surgery) • conductive medium pads • electrocardiogram (ECG) monitor with recorder • oxygen therapy equipment • handheld resuscitation bag • airway equipment • emergency pacing equipment • emergency cardiac medications

Implementation

● Assess the patient *to determine the lack of a pulse.* Call for help and perform CPR until the defibrillator and emergency equipment arrive. **AHA**

● Refer to the sequence for defibrillation as described under "Code management," page 230, and "Automated external defibrillation," page 202.

● If defibrillation restores a normal rhythm, check the patient's central and peripheral pulses and obtain a blood pressure reading, heart rate, and respiratory rate. Assess the patient's level of consciousness, cardiac rhythm, breath sounds, skin color, and urine output. Obtain baseline arterial blood gas levels and a 12-lead ECG. Provide supplemental oxygen, ventilation, and medications, as needed. Check the patient's chest for electrical burns and treat them, as ordered, with corticosteroids or lanolin-based creams.

● Prepare the defibrillator for immediate reuse.

Special considerations

● When applying conductive pads, make sure to place them 1″ (2.5 cm) away from any implantable device the patient may have.

● Defibrillators vary from one manufacturer to the next, so familiarize yourself with your facility's

equipment. **MFR** Defibrillator operation should be checked at least every 8 hours and after each use.
● Defibrillation can be affected by several factors, including paddle size and placement, condition of the patient's myocardium, duration of the arrhythmia, chest resistance, and the number of countershocks.

Nursing diagnoses
● Decreased cardiac output

Expected outcomes
The patient will:
● exhibit no arrhythmias
● maintain a blood pressure and pulse rate within normal limits.

Complications
● Defibrillation can cause accidental electric shock to those providing care.
● Use of an insufficient amount of conductive medium can lead to skin burns.

Documentation
Document the procedure, including the patient's ECG rhythm before and after defibrillation; the number of times defibrillation was performed; the voltage used with each attempt; whether a pulse returned; the dosage, route, and time of drug administration; whether CPR was used; how the airway was maintained; and the patient's outcome.

Supportive references
American Heart Association. "2005 AHA Guidelines for Cardiopulmonary Resuscitation and Emergency Cardiovascular Care: International Consensus on Science," *Circulation* 112(22 Suppl):IV-1-IV-211, November 2005.
American Heart Association. "Highlights of the 2005 American Heart Association Guidelines for CPR and ECC," *Currents* 16(4):1-27, Winter 2005-2006.

Electrocardiography

Electrocardiography (ECG), a display of the electric currents generated by the heart, is one of the most valuable and frequently used diagnostic tools. These impulses move through the heart's conduction system, creating electric currents that can be monitored on the body's surface. Electrodes attached to the skin

---

Understanding the ICD

The implantable cardioverter-defibrillator (ICD) has a programmable pulse generator and lead system that monitors the heart's activity, detects ventricular bradyarrhythmias and tachyarrhythmias, and responds to each with different interventions. These interventions include antitachycardia pacing, cardioversion, defibrillation, and bradycardia pacing.

ICDs can be programmed to pace the atrium and the ventricle. Implantation is similar to that of a permanent pacemaker. The cardiologist positions the lead or leads in the endocardium of the right ventricle (and the right atrium if both chambers require pacing) and then connects the other end to a generator that's implanted in the right or left upper chest near the collarbone. Newer ICDs can also be placed to provide biventricular pacing.

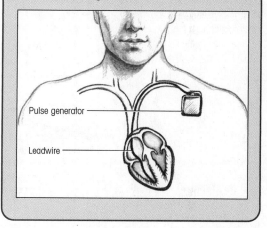

Pulse generator

Leadwire

---

can detect these electric currents and transmit them to an instrument that produces a record (the ECG) of cardiac activity.

ECG can be used to identify myocardial ischemia and infarction, rhythm and conduction disturbances, chamber enlargement, valve function, and the effects of electrolytes and drugs on the heart.

To determine which patients would benefit from an ECG, the American Heart Association (AHA) and the American College of Cardiology (ACC) have set guidelines for ECG use. These guidelines classify patients into three groups: patients with known cardiovascular disease or dysfunction; patients who are suspected of having, or who are at increased risk for

Reviewing ECG waveforms and components

An electrocardiogram (ECG) waveform has three basic components: P wave, QRS complex, and T wave. These elements can be further divided into the PR interval, J point, ST segment, U wave, and QT interval.

P wave and PR interval

The P wave represents atrial depolarization. The PR interval represents the time it takes an impulse to travel from the atria through the atrioventricular nodes and bundle of His. The PR interval measures from the beginning of the P wave to the beginning of the QRS complex.

QRS complex

The QRS complex represents ventricular depolarization (the time it takes for the impulse to travel through the bundle branches to the Purkinje fibers). The Q wave appears as the first negative deflection in the QRS complex; the R wave, as the first positive deflection. The S wave appears as the second negative deflection or the first negative deflection after the R wave.

J point and ST segment

Marking the end of the QRS complex, the J point also indicates the beginning of the ST segment. The ST segment represents part of ventricular repolarization.

T wave and U wave

Usually following the same deflection pattern as the P wave, the T wave represents ventricular repolarization. The U wave follows the T wave, but isn't always seen.

QT interval

The QT interval represents ventricular depolarization and repolarization. It extends from the beginning of the QRS complex to the end of the T wave.

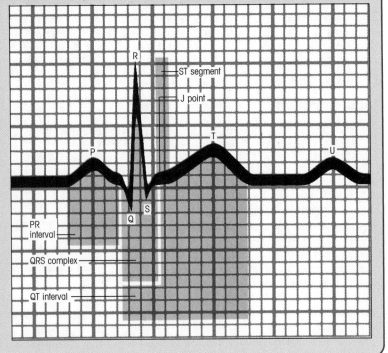

developing, cardiovascular disease or dysfunction; and patients with no apparent or suspected heart disease or dysfunction. **AHA**

The standard 12-lead ECG uses a series of electrodes placed on the extremities and the chest wall to assess the heart from 12 different views (leads). The 12 leads consist of three standard bipolar limb leads (designated leads I, II, and III), three unipolar augmented leads (leads aV_R, aV_L, and aV_F), and six unipolar precordial leads (leads V_1 to V_6). The limb leads and augmented leads show the heart from the frontal plane. The precordial leads show the heart from the horizontal plane.

The ECG device measures and averages the differences among the electrical potential of the electrode sites for each lead and graphs them over time. This creates the standard ECG complex, called P-QRS-T. The P wave represents atrial depolarization; the QRS complex, ventricular depolarization; and the T wave, ventricular repolarization. (See *Reviewing ECG waveforms and components*.)

Variations of the standard ECG include stress ECG and ambulatory ECG. (See "Holter monitoring," page 252.) Stress ECG monitors heart rate, blood pressure, and ECG waveforms as the patient walks on a treadmill or pedals a stationary bicycle. For patients unable to perform exercises, pharmacologic agents, such as adenosine (Adenocard) or dobutamine (Dobutrex), can be used to produce the same cardiovascular stress as exercise to allow for testing. For ambulatory ECG, the patient wears a portable Holter monitor to record heart activity continually over 24 hours.

Today, ECG is typically accomplished using a multichannel method. All electrodes are attached to the patient at once, and the machine prints a simultaneous view of all leads.

Equipment

ECG machine • recording paper • disposable pregelled electrodes • 4" × 4" gauze pads • optional: shaving supplies, marking pen

Preparation of equipment

• Place the ECG machine close to the patient's bed, and plug the cord into the wall outlet.
• If the patient is already connected to a cardiac monitor, remove the electrodes to accommodate the precordial leads and to minimize electrical interference on the ECG tracing.
• Keep the patient away from electrical fixtures and power cords.

Implementation

• Confirm the patient's identity using two patient identifiers according to facility policy. **JCAHO**
• As you set up the machine to record a 12-lead ECG, explain the procedure to the patient. Tell him that the test records the heart's electrical activity and that it may be repeated at certain intervals. Emphasize that no electrical current will enter his body. Also, tell him that the test typically takes about 5 minutes. **PCP**
• Have the patient lie supine in the center of the bed with his arms at his sides. You may raise the head of the bed *to promote comfort*. Expose his arms and legs, and cover him appropriately. His arms and legs

should be relaxed *to minimize muscle trembling, which can cause electrical interference.* **AHA**
• If the bed is too narrow, place the patient's hands under his buttocks *to prevent muscle tension.* Also use this technique if the patient is shivering or trembling. Make sure that his feet aren't touching the bed board.
• Select flat, fleshy areas to place the electrodes. Avoid muscular and bony areas. If the patient has an amputated limb, choose a site on the stump. **AHA**
• If an area is excessively hairy, shave it. Clean excess oil or other substances from the skin *to enhance electrode contact.*
• Peel off the contact paper of the disposable electrodes and apply them directly to the prepared site, as recommended by the manufacturer's instructions. **MFR** *To guarantee the best connection to the leadwire,* position disposable electrodes on the patient's legs with the lead connection pointing superiorly. **AHA**
• Connect the limb leadwires to the electrodes. Make sure that the metal parts of the electrodes are clean and bright. *Dirty or corroded electrodes prevent a good electrical connection.*
• You'll see that the tip of each leadwire is lettered and color-coded for easy identification. The white or RA leadwire goes to the right arm; the green or RL leadwire, to the right leg; the red or LL leadwire, to the left leg; the black or LA leadwire, to the left arm; and the brown or V_1 to V_6 leadwire, to the chest.
• Expose the patient's chest. Put a disposable electrode at each electrode position. (See *Positioning chest electrodes,* page 246.) If the patient is a woman, be sure to place the chest electrodes below the breast tissue. In a large-breasted woman, you may need to displace the breast tissue laterally.
• Check to see that the paper speed selector is set to the standard 25 mm/second and that the machine is set to standard voltage. The machine will record a normal standardization mark — a square that's the height of two large squares or 10 small squares on the recording paper. Then, if necessary, enter the appropriate patient identification data. **AHA**
• If a part of the waveform extends beyond the paper when you record the ECG, adjust the normal standardization to half-standardization. Note this adjustment on the ECG strip *because this will need to be considered in interpreting the results.*

Positioning chest electrodes

To ensure accurate test results, position chest electrodes as follows:

V_1—Fourth intercostal space at right border of sternum

V_2—Fourth intercostal space at left border of sternum

V_3—Halfway between leads V_2 and V_4

V_4—Fifth intercostal space at midclavicular line

V_5—Fifth intercostal space at anterior axillary line (halfway between leads V_4 and V_6)

V_6—Fifth intercostal space at midaxillary line, level with lead V_4.

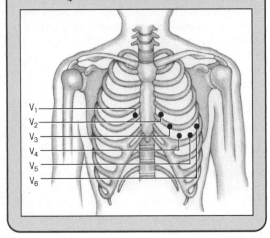

● Now you're ready to begin the recording. Ask the patient to relax and breathe normally. Tell him to lie still and not to talk when you record his ECG. Then press the AUTO button. Observe the tracing quality. The machine will record all 12 leads automatically, recording three consecutive leads simultaneously. Some machines have a display screen so you can preview waveforms before the machine records them on paper.

● When the machine finishes recording the 12-lead ECG, remove the electrodes and clean the patient's skin. After disconnecting the leadwires from the electrodes, dispose of or clean the electrodes, as indicated.

● If serial ECGs are expected, consider marking the electrode positions on the patient's skin. Consistent lead placement enhances the comparison of serial ECGs and eliminates inaccuracy due to lead placement.

Special considerations

● Small areas of hair on the patient's chest or extremities may be shaved, but this usually isn't necessary.

● If the patient's skin is exceptionally oily, scaly, or diaphoretic, rub the electrode site with a dry 4″ × 4″ gauze pad before applying the electrode *to help reduce interference in the tracing.* During the procedure, ask the patient to breathe normally. If his respirations distort the recording, ask him to hold his breath briefly *to reduce baseline wander in the tracing.*

● If the patient has a pacemaker, you can perform an ECG with or without a magnet, according to the physician's orders. Be sure to note the presence of a pacemaker and the use of the magnet (to turn off the pacemaker's sensing function) on the strip.

Nursing diagnoses

● Deficient knowledge (procedure)

Expected outcomes

The patient will:

● state an understanding of the need for an ECG

● ask questions when new information warrants clarification.

Documentation

Label the ECG recording with the patient's name, room number, and facility identification number. Document in your notes the test's date and time and significant responses by the patient as well. Record the date, time, patient's name, and room number on the ECG itself. Note appropriate clinical information on the ECG.

Supportive references

Lynn-McHale Wiegand, D.J., and Carlson, K.K. *AACN Procedure Manual for Critical Care,* 5th ed. Philadelphia: W.B. Saunders Co., 2005.

Schlant, R.C., et al. "Guidelines for Electrocardiography," *Journal of the American College of Cardiology* 19(3): 473-81, March 1992.

Electrocardiography, posterior-chest lead

Evidence-based research has proven that a 12-lead electrocardiogram (ECG) has limited sensitivity in detecting posterior myocardial infarction (MI) because of a limited view through the lung and muscle barriers. Because of the heart's posterior surface, changes associated with myocardial damage aren't apparent on a standard 12-lead ECG. The major findings of these studies have shown that the addition of posterior leads V_7, V_8, and V_9 to the 12-lead ECG increases the sensitivity and specificity of identifying a posterior wall MI and may provide clues to posterior wall infarction so that appropriate treatment can begin.

CONTROVERSIAL ISSUE *A study has found that the widely used criterion of 1 mm for ischemia is inadequate to detect elevation in the ST segment in the posterior leads during left coronary occlusion. This study used a measurement of 0.5 mm, exceeding the normal ST-segment variation of 0.2 mm. Results from this study indicated that approximately half of the subjects had ST elevation ranging from 0.5 to 1.0 mm in the posterior leads during left coronary occlusion. This finding suggests that posterior leads provide additional diagnostic value to the standard 12-lead ECG when a modified ischemic criterion of 0.5 mm is applied.* **EB**

Usually, the posterior lead ECG is performed with a standard ECG and only involves recording the additional posterior leads. ST-segment elevation of 1 mm or more in at least two posterior leads (leads V_7, V_8, and V_9) indicates a posterior wall MI.

Equipment

Multichannel or single-channel ECG machine with recording paper • disposable pregelled electrodes • 4″ × 4″ gauze pads • optional: shaving supplies, moist cloth

Implementation

● Confirm the patient's identity using two patient identifiers according to facility policy. **JCAHO**
● Prepare the electrode sites according to the manufacturer's instructions. **MFR** *To ensure good skin contact*, shave the site if the patient has considerable back hair.

● These leads are placed opposite the anterior leads, V_4, V_5, and V_6, on the left side of the patient's back, following the same horizontal line. Begin by attaching a disposable electrode to the lead V_7 position on the left posterior midaxillary line at the same horizontal level as lead V_6 at the fifth intercostal space. Then attach the V_4 leadwire to the V_7 electrode. **EB**
● Next, attach a disposable electrode to the patient's back at the lead V_8 position on the left midscapular line at the same horizontal level as lead V_6 at the fifth intercostal space, and attach the V_5 leadwire to this electrode. **EB**
● Finally, attach a disposable electrode to the patient's back at the lead V_9 position, just left of the spinal column at the same horizontal level as lead V_6 at the fifth intercostal space. Then, attach the V_6 leadwire to the V_9 electrode. (See *Placing electrodes for posterior ECG*, page 248.) **EB**
● If you're using a single-channel ECG machine, put electrode gel at the locations for leads V_7, V_8, and V_9. Then connect the brown leadwire to the V_7 electrode.
● Turn on the machine and make sure that the paper speed is set at 25 mm/second. If necessary, standardize the machine. Press AUTO and the machine will record.
● If you're using a single-channel ECG machine, turn the selector knob to "V" to record the V_7 lead. Then stop the machine. Reposition the electrode to the V_8 position and record that lead. Repeat the procedure for the V_9 position.
● When the ECG is complete, remove the electrodes and clean the patient's skin with a gauze pad or moist cloth. If you think you may need more than one posterior lead ECG, mark the electrode sites on his skin *to permit accurate comparison for future tracings*.

Special considerations

● The number of leads may vary according to the cardiologist's preference. (If right posterior leads are requested, position the patient on his left side. These leads, known as V_{7R}, V_{8R}, and V_{9R}, are located at the same landmarks on the right side of the patient's back.)
● Some ECG machines won't operate unless you connect all leadwires. In that case, you may need to connect the limb leadwires and the leadwires for V_1, V_2, and V_3.

Placing electrodes for posterior ECG

To ensure an accurate electrocardiogram (ECG) reading, make sure that the posterior leads V_7, V_8, and V_9 are placed at the same level horizontally as the V_6 lead at the fifth intercostal space. Place lead V_7 at the posterior axillary line, lead V_9 at the paraspinal line, and lead V_8 halfway between leads V_7 and V_9.

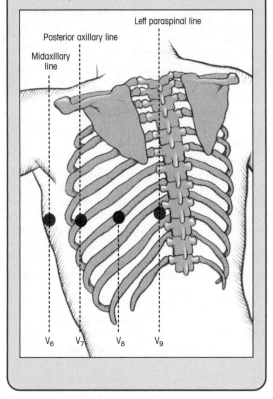

Left paraspinal line

Posterior axillary line

Midaxillary line

V_6 V_7 V_8 V_9

Nursing diagnoses

● Deficient knowledge (procedure)

Expected outcomes

The patient will:
● state an understanding of the need for a posterior ECG
● ask questions when new information warrants clarification.

Documentation

Document the procedure in your nurses' notes. Make sure that the patient's name, age, room number, time, date, and physician's name are clearly written on the ECG along with the relabeled lead tracings. Document any patient teaching you may have performed as well as the patient's tolerance of the procedure.

Supportive references

Khaw, K., et al. "Improved Detection of Posterior Myocardial Wall Ischemia with the 15-Lead Electrocardiogram," *American Heart Journal* 138(5 Part I):934-40, November 1999.

Wung, S-F., and Drew, B.J. "New Electrocardiographic Criteria for Posterior Wall Acute Myocardial Ischemia Validated by a Percutaneous Transluminal Coronary Angioplasty Model of Acute Myocardial Infarction," *American Journal of Cardiology* 87(8):970-74, April 2001. **EB**

Electrocardiography, right-chest lead

Unlike a standard 12-lead electrocardiogram (ECG), which is used primarily to evaluate left ventricular function, a right-chest lead ECG reflects right ventricular function and provides clues to damage or dysfunction in this chamber.

Right ventricular infarction should be suspected in patients with acute inferior wall myocardial infarction (MI). Damage to the right ventricle occurs approximately 25% to 50% of patients who have had an inferior wall MI. For those patients with suspected right ventricular involvement, a right-chest lead ECG should be performed.

Early identification of a right ventricular MI is essential because this type of MI is associated with significant morbidity and mortality. ST-segment elevation of 1 mm or more in the right precordial lead V_{4R} indicates a right ventricular MI.

Treatment for right ventricular infarction differs from treatment of other types of MI. Instead of judiciously hydrating a patient to prevent heart failure, the patient with right ventricular infarction requires administration of I.V. fluids to maintain adequate filling pressures on the right side of the heart. This helps the right ventricle eject an adequate volume of blood at a sufficient pressure and supports left ventricular filling. **AHA**

If a right-chest lead ECG isn't routinely performed at your facility, consider the need for this test in a patient with an inferior wall MI who shows signs of poor left ventricular output and clear lung sounds on auscultation.

Equipment

Multichannel ECG machine • paper • pregelled disposable electrodes • 4″ × 4″ gauze pads

Implementation

• Confirm the patient's identity using two patient identifiers according to facility policy. **JCAHO**
• Take the equipment to the patient's bedside, and explain the procedure to him. Inform him that the physician has ordered a right-chest lead ECG, a procedure that involves placing electrodes on his wrist, ankles, and chest. Reassure him that the test is painless and takes only a few minutes, during which he'll need to lie quietly on his back.
• Make sure that the paper speed is set at 25 mm/second and amplitude at 1 mV/10 mm.
• Place the patient in a supine position or, if he has difficulty lying flat, in semi-Fowler's position. Provide privacy, and expose his arms, chest, and legs. (Cover a female patient's chest with a drape until you apply the chest leads.)
• Examine the patient's wrists and ankles for the best areas to place the electrodes. Choose flat and fleshy (not bony or muscular) hairless areas such as the inner aspects of the wrist and ankles. Clean the sites with gauze pads *to promote good skin contact.* **AHA**
• Connect the leadwires to the electrodes. The leadwires are color-coded and lettered. Place the white or right arm (RA) wire on the right arm; the black or left arm (LA) wire on the left arm; the green or right leg (RL) wire on the right leg; and the red or left leg (LL) wire on the left leg.
• Then examine the patient's chest *to locate the correct sites for chest lead placement* (as shown at top of next column). If the patient is a woman, you'll place the electrodes under the breast tissue.

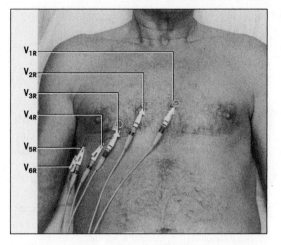

• Use your fingers to feel between the patient's ribs (the intercostal spaces). Start at the second intercostal space on the left (the notch felt at the top of the sternum, where the manubrium joins the body of the sternum). Count down two spaces to the fourth intercostal space. Then apply a disposable electrode to the site and attach leadwire V_{1R} to that electrode. **AHA**
• Move your fingers across the sternum to the fourth intercostal space on the right side of the sternum. Apply a disposable electrode to that site and attach lead V_{2R}. **AHA**
• Move your finger down to the fifth intercostal space and over to the midclavicular line. Place a disposable electrode here and attach lead V_{4R}. Apply a disposable electrode midway on this line from V_{2R} and attach lead V_{3R}. **AHA**
• Move your finger horizontally from lead V_{4R} to the right midaxillary line. Apply a disposable electrode to this site and attach lead V_{6R}. **AHA**
• Move your fingers along the same horizontal line to the midpoint between lead V_{4R} and V_{6R}. This is the right anterior midaxillary line. Apply a disposable electrode to this site and attach lead V_{5R}. **AHA**
• Turn on the ECG machine. Ask the patient to breathe normally but not to talk during the recording *so that muscle movement won't distort the tracing.* Enter appropriate patient information required by the machine you're using. If necessary, standardize the machine. This will cause a square tracing of 10 mm (two large squares) to appear on the ECG paper when the machine is set for 1 mV (1 mV = 10 mm).

• Press the AUTO key. The ECG machine will record all 12 leads automatically. Check your facility's policy for the number of readings to obtain. (Some facilities require at least two ECGs so that one copy can be sent out for interpretation while the other remains at the bedside.)

• When you're finished recording the ECG, turn off the machine. Clearly label the ECG with the patient's name, date, and time. Also label the tracing as, "right chest ECG" to distinguish it from a standard 12-lead ECG. Make sure that the leads are correctly labeled: V_{1R} through V_{6R}. Remove the electrodes and help the patient get comfortable.

• If serial right-chest lead ECGs are anticipated, consider marking the electrode sites on the patient's skin to facilitate consistent lead placement.

Special considerations

• For best results, place the electrodes symmetrically on the limbs. If the patient's wrist or ankle is covered by a dressing or if the patient is an amputee, choose an area that's available on both sides.

Nursing diagnoses

• Deficient knowledge (procedure)

Expected outcomes

The patient will:
• state an understanding of the need for the procedure
• ask appropriate questions.

Documentation

Document the procedure in the nurses' notes, and document the patient's tolerance to the procedure. Place a copy of the tracing in the patient's chart.

Supportive references

Haji, S.A., and Movahed, A. "Right Ventricular Infarction — Diagnosis and Treatment," *Clinical Cardiology* 23(7):473-82, July 2000.

Horan, L.G., and Flowers, N.D. "Right Ventricular Infarction: Specific Requirements of Management," *American Family Physician* 60(6):1727-34, October 1999.

Kosuge, M., et al. "Implications of the Absence of ST-Segment Elevation in Lead V_{4R} in Patients Who Have Inferior Wall Acute Myocardial Infarction with Right

Ventricular Involvement," *Clinical Cardiology* 24(3):225-30, March 2001.

Electrocardiography, signal-averaged

Signal-averaged electrocardiography (ECG) primarily helps to identify patients at risk for sustained ventricular tachycardia (VT). Because this cardiac arrhythmia can be a precursor of sudden death after a myocardial infarction (MI) or with other cardiac abnormalities, the results of signal-averaged ECG can allow appropriate preventive measures.

Using a computer-based ECG, signal averaging detects low-amplitude signals or late electrical potentials, which reflect slow conduction or disorganized ventricular activity occurring as depolarization, proceeding through healthy myocardial bundles separated by fibrotic tissue from other bundles, or passing through abnormal or infarcted regions of the ventricles. The signal-averaged ECG is developed by recording the noise-free surface ECG in three specialized leads for several hundred beats. (See *Placing electrodes for signal-averaged ECG.*) Signal averaging enhances signals that would otherwise be missed because of increased amplitude and sensitivity to ventricular activity. For instance, on the standard 12-lead ECG, "noise" created by muscle tissue, electronic artifacts, and electrodes masks late potentials, which have a low amplitude. This procedure is used to evaluate the risk of sustained VT in patients with malignant VT, those recovering from an MI, with unexplained syncope, with nonischemic dilated cardiomyopathy, following surgical treatment of an arrhythmia, or with nonsustained VT.

The American College of Cardiology (ACC) has recommended the signal-averaged ECG only for evaluation of patients recovering from an MI or those with ischemic heart disease or unexplained syncope. Emerging research indicates other potential beneficial applications of this technology, including:

• identifying the risk of sustained ventricular arrhythmias in nonischemic cardiomyopathy and hypertrophic obstructive cardiomyopathy

• evaluating the success of surgical treatment for sustained VT

• assessing the efficacy of antiarrhythmic medications

- assessing successful restoration of coronary artery blood flow
- detecting acute rejection in heart transplantation
- identifying sinus node dysfunction. **ACC** **EB**

Equipment

Signal-averaged ECG machine • signal-averaged computer • record of patient's surface ECG for 200 to 300 QRS complexes • three bipolar electrodes or leads • shaving supplies

Implementation

- Confirm the patient's identity using two patient identifiers according to facility policy. **JCAHO**
- Inform the patient that this procedure will take 10 to 30 minutes and will help the physician determine the risk of a certain type of arrhythmia. If appropriate, mention that it may be done along with other tests, such as echocardiography, Holter monitoring, and a stress test. **PCP**
- Ensure a quiet environment with no interruption during the test.
- Place the patient in the supine position, and tell him to lie as still as possible. Tell him he shouldn't speak and should breathe normally during the procedure.
- If the patient has hair on his chest, shave the area, wash the area with soap and water, and dry it before placing the electrodes on it.
- Place the leads in the X, Y, and Z positions.
- The ECG machine gathers input from these leads and amplifies, filters, and samples the signals. The computer collects and stores data for analysis. The crucial values are those showing QRS complex duration, duration of the portion of the QRS complex with an amplitude under 40 ?V, and the root mean square voltage of the last 40 msec.

Special considerations

- *Because muscle movements may cause a false-positive result,* patients who are restless or in respiratory distress are poor candidates for signal-averaged ECG. Proper electrode placement and skin preparation are essential to this procedure.
- Results indicating low-amplitude signals include a QRS complex duration greater than 110 msec; a duration of more than 40 msec for the amplitude portion under 40 µV; and a root mean square voltage of less than 25 µV during the last 40 msec of the QRS com-

plex. However, all three factors need not be present to consider the result positive or negative. The final interpretation hinges on individual patient factors.

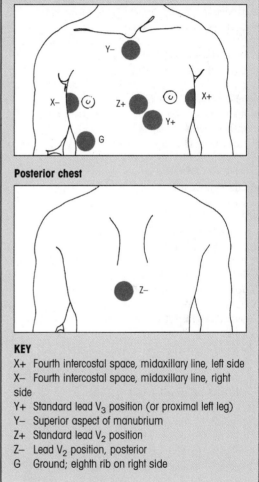

Placing electrodes for signal-averaged ECG

To prepare the patient for signal-averaged electrocardiography (ECG), place the electrodes in the X, Y, and Z orthogonal positions (as shown below). These positions bisect one another to provide a three-dimensional, composite view of ventricular activation.

Anterior chest

Posterior chest

KEY
X+ Fourth intercostal space, midaxillary line, left side
X– Fourth intercostal space, midaxillary line, right side
Y+ Standard lead V_3 position (or proximal left leg)
Y– Superior aspect of manubrium
Z+ Standard lead V_2 position
Z– Lead V_2 position, posterior
G Ground; eighth rib on right side

- Results of signal-averaged ECG help the physician determine whether the patient is a candidate for invasive procedures, such as electrophysiologic testing or angiography.
- Keep in mind that the significance of signal-averaged ECG results in patients with bundle-branch heart block is unknown *because myocardial activation doesn't follow the usual sequence in these patients.*

Nursing diagnoses
- Anxiety
- Decreased cardiac output

Expected outcomes
The patient will:
- cope with diagnosis of an MI without demonstrating severe signs of anxiety
- maintain a blood pressure and pulse rate within normal limits
- exhibit no arrhythmias.

Complications
- Usually none

Documentation
Document the time of the procedure, why the procedure was done, and how the patient tolerated it.

Supportive references

"ACC Expert Consensus Document — Signal-Averaged Electrocardiography," *Journal of the American College of Cardiology* 27(1):238-49, January 1996. **EB**

Fauchier, L., et al. "Long-Term Prognostic Value of Time Domain Analysis of Signal-Averaged Electrocardiography in Idiopathic Dilated Cardiomyopathy," *American Journal of Cardiology* 85(5):618-23, March 2000.

Gant, R.H., et al. "The Expanding Role of Signal-Averaged Electrocardiography," *Critical Care Nurse* 19(5):61-67, October 1999.

Goedel-Meinen, L., et al. "Prognostic Value of an Abnormal Signal-Averaged Electrocardiogram in Patients with Nonischemic Dilated Cardiomyopathy," *American Journal of Cardiology* 87(6):809-12, March 2001.

Yamada, T., et al. "Identification of Sinus Node Dysfunction by Use of P-wave Signal-Averaged Electrocardiograms in Paroxysmal Atrial Fibrillation: A Prospective Study," *American Heart Journal* 142(2):286-93, August 2001.

Holter monitoring

Holter monitoring (also called *continuous electrocardiograph monitoring*) allows for the measurement of blood pressure and cardiac activity over time without confining the patient to a facility. Holter monitoring records variations in electrocardiogram (ECG) waveforms during normal activity.

Indications for Holter monitoring include evaluating the status of a patient recuperating from a myocardial infarction who has left ventricular dysfunction, to evaluate arrhythmias in a patient with heart failure or idiopathic cardiomyopathy, to assess pacemaker function and assist in optimal programming, to evaluate cardiac signs and symptoms (syncope), to evaluate the type and frequency of cardiac arrhythmias, to assess antiarrhythmic drug therapy, and to determine the relationship among cardiac events, the patient's symptoms, and associated cardiac symptoms. **ACC**

Monitoring can be over a 24-hour period, or the ECG rhythm may be recorded intermittently when the patient experiences symptoms and then triggers the device. Such intermittent monitoring may occur over 7 to 30 days, and the data may be periodically transmitted to the physician's office over the telephone.

Equipment
Holter unit with new battery • cable wires • disposable pregelled electrodes • carrying case with strap • 4″ × 4″ gauze pad • soap and water • logbook or diary • optional: clippers

Implementation
- Ask the patient if he's allergic to electrode gel. **PCP**
- Place equipment into the carrying case and connect the neck strap.

> **TEACHING** *Explain to the patient that his cardiac activity will be monitored for 24 hours before the monitor is removed. Tell him that he'll feel no pain from the procedure but that the tape and monitor may cause mild discomfort.* **ACC**

Explain to the patient that he may need to wear a microprocessor for 24 hours after activation of the monitor, and tell him not to remove the microprocessor or electrodes unless told to do so. Explain that he'll have a carrying case with a strap to carry the 2-lb (0.9-kg) monitor. **ACC**

Tell the patient that he'll need to maintain an activity log during the 24-hour monitoring period. He should record the time, activities he performs, and any symptoms (such as headache, dizziness, light-headedness, palpitations, or chest pain) that occur. **ACC**

Explain to the patient the importance of maintaining his usual routine, including working, eating, sleeping, using the bathroom, and taking his medication.

Encourage the patient to wear loose-fitting clothes, with tops that open in the front. Suggest that he wear a watch to make keeping the log easier.

Tell the patient that he can sponge bathe but shouldn't get the equipment wet.

Tell the patient he'll need a follow-up appointment to review results 48 to 72 hours after removing the monitor.

● As appropriate, tell the patient that you need to clip the hairs on his chest so that you can place the electrodes properly. After clipping, wash the areas with soap and water to remove body oils.
● Connect the wires to the electrodes and to the monitor.
● Apply each electrode to the patient's chest by removing the paper backing, securing the edges of the electrode, and then pressing the center to ensure proper contact.
● Show the patient how to reattach loosened electrodes by depressing the center; tell him to return to the office if an electrode becomes fully dislodged.
● Tell the patient to avoid magnets, metal detectors, high-voltage areas, and electric blankets, which may cause artifacts or interfere with monitoring. **EB**

Special considerations
● If the patient's skin is extremely oily, scaly, or diaphoretic, wash the patient's chest with water, and then rub with a dry 4″ × 4″ gauze pad before applying the electrodes.
● If the patient can't return to the office immediately after the monitoring period, show him how to remove the equipment and store the monitor and log.
● If the patient is wearing a patient-activated ECG, tell him that he can wear the monitor for up to 7 days. Tell him how to initiate the recording manually when symptoms occur.

Nursing diagnoses
● Deficient knowledge (procedure)

Expected outcomes
The patient will:
● state an understanding of the need for a Holter monitor
● ask appropriate questions.

Documentation
Include in your documentation the indications for monitoring and the date the monitor was placed. Document the duration the monitor was worn and the results. Be sure to include the patient's log in your documentation. Also include the ECG strip taken before the monitor was placed. Record any medications the patient is taking.

Supportive references
American College of Cardiology and American Heart Association. "ACC/AHA Clinical Competence Statement on Electrocardiography and Ambulatory Electrocardiograph," *Circulation* 104:3169-78, December 2001.

"American College of Cardiology Position Statement— Ambulatory Blood Pressure Monitoring," *Journal of the American College of Cardiology* 23(16):1511-13, May 1994.

American College of Physicians-American Society of Internal Medicine (ACP-ASIM)—Medical Specialty Society, "Diagnosing Syncope," June 1997.

Heaven, D.J., and Sutton, R. "Syncope," *Critical Care Medicine* 28(10 Suppl):N116-20, October 2000.

Institute for Clinical Systems Improvement (ICSI). "Hypertension Diagnosis and Treatment," November 2000. *www.icsi.org.guidelst.htm*.

O'Brien, E., et al. "Use and Interpretation of Ambulatory Blood Pressure Monitoring: Recommendations of the British Hypertension Society," *British Medical Journal* 320(7242):1128-34, April 2000.

"Seventh Report of the Joint National Committee on Prevention, Detection, Evaluation, and Treatment of High Blood Pressure," *Hypertension* 42:1206-52, December 2003.

Yarows, S.A., et al. "Home Blood Pressure Monitoring," *Archives of Internal Medicine* 160(19):1251-57, May 2000. **EB**

Zimetbaum, P.J., and Josephson, M.E. "The Evolving Role of Ambulatory Arrhythmia Monitoring in General

How the intra-aortic balloon pump works

Made of polyurethane, the intra-aortic balloon is attached to an external pump console by means of a large-lumen catheter. The illustrations here show the direction of blood flow when the pump inflates and deflates the balloon.

Balloon inflation
The balloon inflates as the aortic valve closes and diastole begins. Diastole increases perfusion to the coronary arteries.

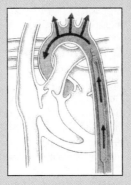

Balloon deflation
The balloon deflates before ventricular ejection, when the aortic valve opens. This permits ejection of blood from the left ventricle against a lowered resistance. As a result, aortic end-diastolic pressure and afterload decrease and cardiac output rises.

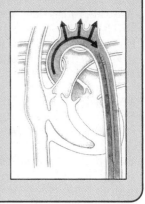

Clinical Practice," *Annals of Internal Medicine* 130(10): 848-56, May 1999.

Zimetbaum, P.J., et al. "Diagnostic Yield and Optimal Duration of Continuous-Loop Event Monitoring for the Diagnosis of Palpitations," *Annals of Internal Medicine* 128(11):890-95, June 1998.

Intra-aortic balloon counterpulsation

Providing temporary support for the heart's left ventricle, intra-aortic balloon counterpulsation (IABC) mechanically displaces blood within the aorta by means of an intra-aortic balloon attached to an external pump console. The balloon is usually inserted through the common femoral artery and positioned with its tip just distal to the left subclavian artery. (See *How the intra-aortic balloon pump works*, and *Interpreting intra-aortic balloon waveforms*.) It monitors myocardial perfusion and the effects of drugs on myocardial function and perfusion. When used correctly, IABC improves two key aspects of myocardial physiology: It increases the supply of oxygen-rich blood to the myocardium, and it decreases myocardial oxygen demand.

IABC is recommended for patients with a wide range of low-cardiac-output disorders or cardiac instability, including refractory angina, ventricular arrhythmias associated with ischemia, and pump failure caused by cardiogenic shock, intraoperative myocardial infarction (MI), or low cardiac output after bypass surgery. IABC is also indicated for patients with low cardiac output secondary to acute mechanical defects after an MI, such as ventricular septal defect, papillary muscle rupture, and left ventricular aneurysm.

Perioperatively, the technique is used to support and stabilize patients with a suspected high-grade lesion who are undergoing such procedures as angioplasty, thrombolytic therapy, cardiac surgery, and cardiac catheterization.

IABC is contraindicated in patients with severe aortic regurgitation, aortic aneurysm, or severe peripheral vascular disease.

Equipment

IABC console and balloon catheters • insertion kit • Dacron graft (for surgically inserted balloon) • electrocardiogram (ECG) monitor and electrodes • sedative • pain medication • pulmonary artery (PA) catheter setup • temporary pacemaker setup • 18G angiography needle • sterile drape • sterile gloves • gown • mask •

Interpreting intra-aortic balloon waveforms

During intra-aortic balloon counterpulsation, you can use electrocardiogram and arterial pressure waveforms to determine whether the balloon pump is functioning properly.

Normal inflation-deflation timing

Balloon inflation occurs after aortic valve closure; deflation, during isovolumetric contraction, just before the aortic valve opens. In a properly timed waveform, like the one shown at right, the inflation point lies at or slightly above the dicrotic notch. Inflation and deflation cause a sharp V shape. Peak diastolic pressure exceeds peak systolic pressure; peak systolic pressure exceeds assisted peak systolic pressure.

Early inflation

With early inflation, the inflation point lies before the dicrotic notch. Early inflation dangerously increases myocardial stress and decreases cardiac output.

Early deflation

With early deflation, a U shape appears and peak systolic pressure is less than or equal to assisted peak systolic pressure. This won't decrease afterload or myocardial oxygen consumption.

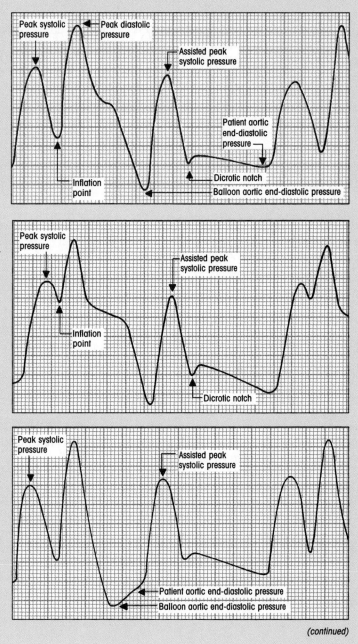

(continued)

Interpreting intra-aortic balloon waveforms *(continued)*

Late inflation

With late inflation, the dicrotic notch precedes the inflation point, and the notch and the inflation point create a W shape. This can lead to a reduction in peak diastolic pressure, coronary and systemic perfusion augmentation time, and augmented coronary perfusion pressure.

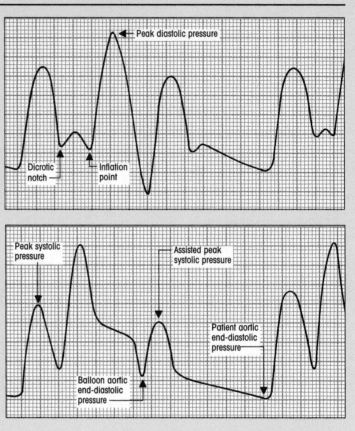

Peak diastolic pressure

Dicrotic notch

Inflation point

Late deflation

With late deflation, peak systolic pressure exceeds assisted peak systolic pressure. This threatens the patient by increasing afterload, myocardial oxygen consumption, cardiac workload, and preload. It occurs when the balloon has been inflated for too long.

Peak systolic pressure

Assisted peak systolic pressure

Patient aortic end-diastolic pressure

Balloon aortic end-diastolic pressure

---

sutures • povidone-iodine swabs • suction setup • oxygen setup and ventilator, if necessary • defibrillator and emergency medications • fluoroscope • indwelling catheter • urinometer • arterial blood gas (ABG) analysis kits and tubes for laboratory studies • povidone-iodine swabs • dressing materials • 4″ × 4″ gauze pads • shaving supplies • I.V. heparin

Preparation of equipment

● Depending on your facility's policy, you or a perfusionist must balance the pressure transducer in the external pump console and calibrate the oscilloscope monitor to ensure accuracy.

Implementation

TEACHING *Explain to the patient that the physician will place a special balloon catheter in his aorta to help his heart pump more easily. Briefly explain the insertion procedure, and mention that the catheter will be connected to a large console next to his bed. Tell him that the balloon will temporarily reduce his heart's workload to promote rapid healing of the ventricular muscle. Let him know that it will be removed after his heart can resume an adequate workload.* **PCP**

Preparing for intra-aortic balloon insertion

● Make sure that the patient or a family member understands and signs a consent form. Verify that the form is attached to the patient's chart.

● Obtain the patient's baseline vital signs, including PA pressure. (A PA line should already be in place.) Attach the patient to an ECG machine for continuous monitoring. Apply chest electrodes in a standard lead II position — or in whatever position that produces the largest R wave *because the R wave triggers balloon inflation and deflation.* Obtain a baseline ECG rhythm strip. **AACN** **ACC**

● Attach another set of ECG electrodes to the patient unless the ECG pattern is being transmitted from the patient's bedside monitor to the balloon pump monitor through a phone cable. Administer oxygen as ordered and as necessary.

● Make sure that the patient has an arterial line, a PA line, and a peripheral I.V. line in place. *The arterial line is used for withdrawing blood samples, monitoring blood pressure, and assessing the timing and effectiveness of therapy. The PA line allows measurement of PA pressure, aspiration of blood samples, and cardiac output studies.* Increased pulmonary artery wedge pressure (PAWP) indicates increased myocardial workload and ineffective balloon pumping. Cardiac output studies are usually performed with and without the balloon *to check the patient's progress.* The central lumen of the intra-aortic balloon, used to monitor central aortic pressure, produces an augmented pressure waveform that allows you to check for proper timing of the inflation-deflation cycle and demonstrates the effects of counterpulsation, elevated diastolic pressure, and reduced end-diastolic and systolic pressures. **AACN** **ACC**

● Insert an indwelling urinary catheter with a urinometer *so you can measure the patient's urine output and assess his fluid balance and renal function. To reduce the risk of infection,* shave or clip hair bilaterally from the lower abdomen to the lower thigh, including the pubic area. **AACN**

● Observe and record the patient's peripheral leg pulse, and document sensation, movement, color, and temperature of the legs.

● Administer a sedative, as ordered. Shave the insertion site if needed.

● Have the defibrillator, suction setup, temporary pacemaker setup, and emergency medications readily available in case the patient develops complications during insertion such as an arrhythmia. **AACN** **ACC**

● Before the physician inserts the balloon, he puts on sterile gloves, gown, and mask. He cleans the site with povidone-iodine solution, and drapes the area using a sterile drape.

Inserting the intra-aortic balloon percutaneously

● The physician may insert the balloon percutaneously through the femoral artery into the descending thoracic aorta, using a modified Seldinger technique. First, he accesses the vessel with an 18G angiography needle and removes the inner stylet.

● The physician passes the guide wire through the needle and removes the needle. Next, he passes an introducer (dilator and sheath assembly) over the guide wire into the vessel until 1″ (2.5 cm) remains above the insertion site. He then removes the inner dilator, leaving the introducer sheath and guide wire in place.

● After passing the balloon over the guide wire into the introducer sheath, the physician advances the catheter into position, 3/8″ to 3/4″ (1 to 2 cm) distal to the left subclavian artery, under fluoroscopic guidance.

● The physician attaches the balloon to the control system to initiate counterpulsation. The balloon catheter then unfurls.

Inserting the intra-aortic balloon surgically

● If the physician chooses not to insert the catheter percutaneously, he usually inserts it through a femoral arteriotomy.

● After making an incision and isolating the femoral artery, the physician attaches a Dacron graft to a small opening in the arterial wall.

● He then passes the catheter through this graft. With fluoroscopic guidance, as needed, he advances the catheter up the descending thoracic aorta and positions the catheter tip between the left subclavian artery and the renal arteries.

● The physician sews the Dacron graft around the catheter at the insertion point and connects the other end of the catheter to the pump console. (See *Surgical insertion sites for an intra-aortic balloon,* page 258.)

● If the balloon can't be inserted through the femoral artery, the physician inserts it in an antegrade direc-

Surgical insertion sites for an intra-aortic balloon

If an intra-aortic balloon can't be inserted percutaneously, the physician will insert it surgically, using a femoral or transthoracic approach.

Femoral approach

Insertion through the femoral artery requires a cutdown and an arteriotomy. The physician passes the balloon through a Dacron graft that has been sewn to the artery.

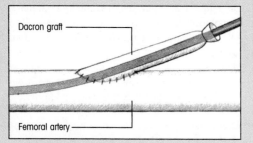

Dacron graft

Femoral artery

Transthoracic approach

If femoral insertion is unsuccessful, the physician may use a transthoracic approach. He inserts the balloon in an antegrade direction through the subclavian artery and then positions it in the descending thoracic aorta.

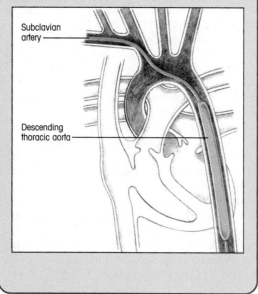

Subclavian artery

Descending thoracic aorta

tion through the anterior wall of the ascending aorta. He positions it $^3/_8''$ to $^3/_4''$ beyond the left subclavian artery and brings the catheter out through the chest wall.

Monitoring the patient after balloon insertion

ALERT *If the control system malfunctions or becomes inoperable, don't let the balloon catheter remain dormant for more than 30 minutes. Get another control system and attach it to the balloon, and then resume pumping. In the meantime, inflate the balloon manually, using a 60-cc syringe and room air a minimum of once every 5 minutes, to prevent thrombus formation in the catheter.*

● The physician will clean the insertion site with povidone-iodine swabs and apply a sterile dressing.
● Obtain a chest X-ray *to verify correct balloon placement.*
● Assess and record pedal and posterior tibial pulses as well as color, sensation, and temperature in the affected limb every 15 minutes for 1 hour and then hourly. Notify the physician immediately if you detect circulatory changes *because it may be necessary to remove the balloon.* **AACN** **ACC**
● Observe and record the patient's baseline arm pulses, arm sensation and movement, and arm color and temperature every 15 minutes for 1 hour after balloon insertion and then every 2 hours while the balloon is in place. *Loss of left arm pulses may indicate upward balloon displacement.* Notify the physician of any changes.
● Monitor the patient's urine output every hour. Note baseline blood urea nitrogen (BUN) and serum creatinine levels, and monitor these levels daily. *Changes in urine output and BUN and serum creatinine levels may signal reduced renal perfusion from downward balloon displacement.* **AACN**
● Auscultate and record bowel sounds every 4 hours. Check for abdominal distention and tenderness as well as changes in the patient's elimination patterns.
● Measure the patient's temperature every 1 to 4 hours. If it's elevated, obtain blood samples for a culture, send them to the laboratory immediately, and notify the physician. Culture any drainage at the insertion site.
● Monitor the patient's hematologic status. Observe for bleeding gums, blood in urine or stools, petechiae,

and bleeding at the insertion site. Monitor his platelet count, hemoglobin level, and hematocrit daily. Expect to administer blood products *to maintain hematocrit at 30%*. If the platelet count drops, expect to administer platelets.

● If the patient is heparinized, monitor partial thromboplastin time (PTT) every 6 hours while the I.V. heparin dose is adjusted *to maintain PTT at 1.5 to 2 times the normal value* and then every 12 to 24 hours while the balloon remains in place. **AACN** **ACC**

● Measure PA pressure and PAWP every 1 to 2 hours, as ordered. A rising PAWP reflects preload, signaling increased ventricular pressure and workload; notify the physician if this occurs. Some patients require I.V. nitroprusside (Nipride) during IABC *to reduce preload and afterload.*

● Obtain samples for ABG analysis, as ordered.

● Monitor serum electrolyte levels — especially sodium and potassium — *to assess the patient's fluid and electrolyte balance and help prevent arrhythmias.* **AACN**

● Watch for signs and symptoms of a dissecting aortic aneurysm: a blood pressure differential between the left and right arms, elevated blood pressure, syncope, pallor, diaphoresis, dyspnea, a throbbing abdominal mass, a reduced red blood cell count with an elevated white blood cell count, and pain in the chest, abdomen, or back. *Notify the physician immediately if you note any of these findings.* **AACN** **Science**

Weaning the patient from IABC

● Assess the cardiac index, systemic blood pressure, and PAWP *to help the physician evaluate the patient's readiness for weaning* — usually about 24 hours after balloon insertion. The patient's hemodynamic status should be stable on minimal doses of inotropic agents, such as dopamine (Intropin) or dobutamine (Dobutrex). **AACN**

● To begin weaning, gradually decrease the frequency of balloon augmentation to 1:2 and 1:4, as ordered. Although your facility has its own weaning protocol, be aware that assist frequency is usually maintained for 1 hour or longer. If the patient's hemodynamic indices remain stable during this time, weaning may continue.

● Avoid leaving the patient on a low augmentation setting for more than 1 to 2 hours *to prevent embolus formation.* **ACC**

● Assess the patient's tolerance of weaning. Signs and symptoms of poor tolerance include confusion and disorientation, urine output below 30 ml/hour, cold and clammy skin, chest pain, arrhythmias, ischemic ECG changes, and an elevated PAWP. If the patient develops any of these problems, notify the physician at once.

Removing the intra-aortic balloon

● The balloon is removed when the patient's hemodynamic status remains stable after the frequency of balloon augmentation is decreased. The control system is turned off and the connective tubing is disconnected from the catheter *to ensure balloon deflation.*

● The physician withdraws the balloon until the proximal end of the catheter contacts the distal end of the introducer sheath.

● The physician then applies pressure below the puncture site and removes the balloon and introducer sheath as a unit, allowing a few seconds of free bleeding *to prevent thrombus formation.*

● *To promote distal bleedback,* the physician applies pressure above the puncture site.

● Apply direct pressure to the site for 30 minutes or until bleeding stops. (In some facilities, this is the physician's responsibility.)

● If the balloon was inserted surgically, the physician will close the Dacron graft and suture the insertion site. The cardiologist usually removes a percutaneous catheter.

● After balloon removal, provide wound care according to your facility's policy. Record the patient's pedal and posterior tibial pulses and the color, temperature, and sensation of the affected limb. Enforce bed rest, as appropriate (usually for 24 hours).

Special considerations

● Before using the IABC control system, make sure that you know what the alarms and messages mean and how to respond to them.

⚠ **ALERT** *Alarms and messages require an immediate response.*

● Change the dressing at the balloon insertion site every 24 hours or as needed, using strict sterile technique. Don't let povidone-iodine solution come in contact with the catheter. **AACN**

● Make sure that the head of the bed is elevated no more than 30 degrees.

● Watch for pump interruptions, which may result from loose ECG electrodes or leadwires, static or 60-cycle interference, catheter kinking, or improper body alignment.

● Make sure the PTT is within normal limits before the balloon is removed *to prevent hemorrhage at the insertion site*.

Nursing diagnoses

● Decreased cardiac output

Expected outcomes

The patient will:
● exhibit positive pedal pulses
● exhibit no pedal edema
● have skin that's warm and dry.

Complications

● IABC may cause numerous complications. The most common, arterial embolism, stems from clot formation on the balloon surface.

● Other potential complications include extension or rupture of an aortic aneurysm, balloon rupture, femoral or iliac artery perforation, femoral artery occlusion, and sepsis.

● Bleeding at the insertion site may become aggravated by pump-induced thrombocytopenia caused by platelet aggregation around the balloon.

Documentation

Document all aspects of patient assessment and management, including the patient's response to therapy. If you're responsible for the IABC device, document all routine checks, problems, and troubleshooting measures. If a technician is responsible for the IABC device, record only when and why the technician was notified as well as the result of his actions on the patient, if any. Also document teaching given to the patient, his family, or his close friends as well as their responses.

Supportive references

Lynn-McHale Wiegand, D.J., and Carlson, K.K. *AACN Procedure Manual for Critical Care*, 5th ed. Philadelphia: W.B. Saunders Co., 2005.

Pacemaker (permanent) insertion and care

Designed to operate for 3 to 20 years, a permanent pacemaker is a self-contained device that the surgeon implants in a pocket beneath the patient's skin. This is usually done in the operating room or cardiac catheterization laboratory. Nursing responsibilities involve monitoring the electrocardiogram (ECG) and maintaining sterile technique.

Today, permanent pacemakers function in the demand mode, allowing the patient's heart to beat on its own but preventing it from falling below a preset rate. Pacing electrodes can be placed in the atria, ventricles, or both (atrioventricular sequential, dual chamber). (See *Understanding pacemaker codes*.) The most common pacing codes are VVI for single-chamber pacing and DDD for dual-chamber pacing. To keep the patient healthy and active, newer-generation pacemakers are specially designed to increase the heart rate with exercise. (See *Pacemaker innovations*.)

Candidates for permanent pacemakers include patients with myocardial infarction and persistent bradyarrhythmia and patients with complete heart block or slow ventricular rates stemming from congenital or degenerative heart disease or cardiac surgery. Patients who suffer from Stokes-Adams syndrome as well as those with Wolff-Parkinson-White or sick sinus syndrome may also benefit from permanent pacemaker implantation. **AHA**

CLINICAL IMPACT *Much research has been done regarding the application of permanent pacemakers in patients other than those with symptomatic bradycardia. Permanent pacemakers are also being used in patients with hypertrophic obstructive cardiomyopathy, dilated cardiomyopathy, atrial fibrillation, neurocardiogenic syndrome, and long-QT syndrome. Biventricular pacing has been shown to be an effective way of maximizing heart function in patients with heart failure who have intraventricular conductor defects. This has been shown to reduce hospitalization and improve symptoms in patients with heart failure.*

Equipment

Sphygmomanometer ● stethoscope ● ECG monitor and strip-chart recorder ● sterile dressing tray ● povidone-iodine ointment ● shaving supplies ● sterile gauze dressing ● hypoallergenic tape ● sedatives ● alcohol pads • emergency resuscitation equipment • sterile gown and mask • optional: I.V. line for emergency medications

Implementation

● Explain the procedure to the patient. Provide and review literature from the manufacturer or the American Heart Association (AHA) so he can learn about the pacemaker and how it works. Emphasize that the pacemaker merely augments his natural heart rate.
● Make sure that the patient or a responsible family member signs a consent form, and ask the patient if he's allergic to anesthetics or iodine.

Before pacemaker insertion

● For pacemaker insertion, shave the patient's chest from the axilla to the midline and from the clavicle to the nipple line on the side selected by the physician.
● Establish an I.V. line at a keep-vein-open rate *so that you can administer emergency drugs if the patient experiences a ventricular arrhythmia.*
● Obtain the patient's baseline vital signs and a baseline ECG. **AHA**
● Provide sedation, as ordered.

During pacemaker insertion

● If you'll be present to monitor arrhythmias during the procedure, put on a gown and mask.
● Connect the ECG monitor to the patient, and run a baseline rhythm strip. Make sure that the machine has enough paper to run additional rhythm strips during the procedure.
● In *transvenous* placement, the physician, guided by a fluoroscope, passes the electrode catheter through the cephalic or external jugular vein and positions it in the right ventricle. He attaches the catheter to the pulse generator, inserts this into the chest wall, and sutures it closed, leaving a small outlet for a drainage tube.

After pacemaker insertion

● Monitor the patient's ECG to check for arrhythmias and to ensure correct pacemaker functioning. **AACN**
● Monitor the I.V. flow rate; the I.V. line is usually kept in place for 24 to 48 hours postoperatively to allow for possible emergency treatment of arrhythmias.
● Check the dressing for signs of bleeding and infection (swelling, redness, or exudate). Prophylactic antibiotics may be ordered for up to 7 days after implantation. **AACN**

Understanding pacemaker codes

A permanent pacemaker's 5-letter code simply refers to how it's programmed. Typically, only the first three letters are used.

First letter
A = atrium
V = ventricle
D = dual (both chambers)
O = not applicable

Second letter
A = atrium
V = ventricle
D = dual (both chambers)
O = not applicable

Third letter
I = inhibited
T = triggered
D = dual (inhibited and triggered)
O = not applicable

Fourth letter
P = Basic functions programmable
M = Multiprogrammable parameters
C = Communication functions
R = Rate responsive

Fifth letter
P = Pacing ability
S = Shock
D = Dual ability to shock and pace
O = None

● Change the dressing and apply povidone-iodine ointment at least once every 24 to 48 hours, or according to the physician's orders and your facility's policy. If the dressing becomes soiled or if the site is exposed to air, change the dressing immediately, regardless of when you last changed it. **AACN**
● Check the patient's vital signs and level of consciousness (LOC) every 15 minutes for the first hour,

---

Pacemaker innovations

Traditional pacemakers use one or two leads to sense and pace the right atrium (RA), right ventricle (RV), or both, to maintain a good heart rate and keep the atrium and ventricle working together. Biventricular pacemakers have three leads rather than two: one to pace the right atrium, one to pace the right ventricle, and one to pace the left ventricle. Both ventricles are paced at the same time, causing them to contract simultaneously, increasing cardiac output.

TEACHING

Teaching about permanent pacemakers

If your patient is going home with a permanent pacemaker, be sure to teach him about daily care, safety and activity guidelines, and other precautions as described here.

Daily care
- Clean your pacemaker site gently with soap and water when you take a shower or bath. Leave the incision exposed to the air.
- Inspect your skin around the incision. A slight bulge is normal, but call your physician if you feel discomfort or notice swelling, redness, a discharge, or other problems.
- Check your pulse for 1 minute as your nurse or physician showed you — on the side of your neck, inside your elbow, or on the thumb side of your wrist. Your pulse rate should be the same as your pacemaker rate or faster. Contact your physician if you think your heart is beating too fast or too slow.
- Take your medications, including those for pain, as prescribed. Even with a pacemaker, you still need the medication your physician ordered.

Safety and activity
- Keep your pacemaker instruction booklet handy, and carry your pacemaker identification card at all times. This card has your pacemaker model number and other information needed by health care personnel who treat you.
- You can resume most of your usual activities when you feel comfortable doing so, but don't drive until the physician gives you permission. Also avoid heavy lifting and stretching exercises for at least 4 weeks or as directed by your physician.
- Try to use both arms equally to prevent stiffness. Check with your physician before you golf, swim, play tennis, or perform other strenuous activities.

Electromagnetic interference
- Today's pacemakers are designed and insulated to eliminate most electrical interference. You can safely operate common household electrical devices, including microwaves, razors, and sewing machines. And you can ride in or operate a motor vehicle without it affecting your pacemaker.
- Take care to avoid direct contact with large running motors, high-powered CB radios and other similar equipment, welding machinery, and radar devices.
- If your pacemaker activates the metal detector in an airport, show your pacemaker identification card to the security official.
- Because the metal in your pacemaker makes you ineligible for certain diagnostic studies, such as magnetic resonance imaging, be sure to inform your physicians, dentist, and other health care providers that you have a pacemaker.

Special precautions
- If you feel light-headed or dizzy when you're near electrical equipment, moving away from the device should restore normal pacemaker function. Ask your physician about particular electrical devices.
- Notify your physician if you experience signs of pacemaker failure, such as palpitations, a fast heart rate, a slow heart rate (5 to 10 beats less than the pacemaker's setting), dizziness, fainting, shortness of breath, swollen ankles or feet, anxiety, forgetfulness, or confusion.

Checkups
- Be sure to schedule and keep regular appointments with your physician.
- If your physician checks your pacemaker status by telephone, keep your transmission schedule and instructions in a handy place.

---

every hour for the next 4 hours, every 4 hours for the next 48 hours, and then once per shift.

ALERT *Confused, elderly patients with second-degree heart block won't show immediate improvement in their LOC.*

Special considerations
- If the patient wears a hearing aid, the pacemaker battery is placed on the opposite side accordingly.
- Provide the patient with an identification card that lists the pacemaker type and manufacturer, serial

number, pacemaker rate setting, date implanted, and the physician's name. (See *Teaching about permanent pacemakers.*)
● Watch for signs of pacemaker malfunction.

Nursing diagnoses
● Deficient knowledge (procedure)

Expected outcomes
The patient (and his family) will:
● state an understanding of the need for the procedure
● state an understanding of discharge instructions and the signs and symptoms to watch for at home.

Complications
● Insertion of a permanent pacemaker places the patient at risk for certain complications, such as infection, lead displacement, a perforated ventricle, cardiac tamponade, or a lead fracture and disconnection.

ALERT *Watch for signs and symptoms of a perforated ventricle, with resultant cardiac tamponade: persistent hiccups, distant heart sounds, pulsus paradoxus, hypotension with narrow pulse pressure, increased venous pressure, cyanosis, jugular vein distention, decreased urine output, restlessness, or complaints of fullness in the chest. If the patient develops any of these, notify the physician immediately.*

Documentation
Document the type of pacemaker used, the serial number and the manufacturer's name, the pacing rate, the date of implantation, and the physician's name. Note whether the pacemaker successfully treated the patient's arrhythmia and the condition of the incision site.

Supportive references
American College of Cardiology and the American Heart Association. "2002 Guideline Update for Implantation of Cardiac Pacemakers and Anti-arrhythmia Devices." *www.americanheart.org.*
American College of Cardiology and the American Heart Association. "ACC/AHA/NASPE 2002 Guideline Update for Implantation of Cardiac Pacemakers and Antiarrhythmia Devices: Summary Article," *Circulation* 106:2145-61, October 2002.
Clark, A. "Troubleshooting Cardiac Pacemaker Problems," 2000. *www.nursingceu.com.*
Gould, P.A., et al. "Biventricular Pacing in Heart Failure: A Review," *Expert Review of Cardiovascular Therapy* 4(1):97-109, January 2006.
Obias-Manno, D. "Unconventional Applications in Pacemaker therapy," *AACN Clinical Issues* 12(1):127-39, February 2001.

Pacemaker (temporary) insertion and care

Usually inserted in an emergency, a temporary pacemaker consists of an external, battery-powered pulse generator and a lead or electrode system. The temporary pacemaker used may be one of four types: transcutaneous, transvenous, transthoracic, and epicardial.

In a life-threatening situation, a transcutaneous pacemaker is the best choice. (See *Indications for transcutaneous pacing,* page 264.) This device works by sending an electrical impulse from the pulse generator to the patient's heart by way of two electrodes, which are placed on the front and back of the patient's chest. Transcutaneous pacing is quick and effective, but it's used only until the physician can institute transvenous pacing.

CONTROVERSIAL ISSUE *According to the American Heart Association (AHA), the use of transcutaneous pacing for pulseless electrical activity (PEA) or asystole has been disappointing. Several studies have examined whether transcutaneous pacing has any benefit for PEA by speeding up the rate of the electrical activity or any benefit for postshock asystole that's only seconds old. Results have proven that transcutaneous pacing has been ineffective for both of these conditions.* **AHA**

Transcutaneous pacing is recommended by the 2005 AHA guidelines for cardiopulmonary resuscitation (CPR) and emergency cardiovascular care for symptomatic bradycardia when a pulse is present. If transcutaneous pacing doesn't correct the problem, transvenous pacing is indicated. Transvenous pacing involves threading an electrode catheter through a vein into the patient's right atrium or right ventricle. The electrode then attaches to an external pulse generator. As a result, the pulse generator can provide an

Indications for transcutaneous pacing

The American Heart Association recommends transcutaneous pacing for these indications:

Class I
- Symptomatic bradycardia with hemodynamic instability unresponsive to atropine
- High degree block (Mobitz type II second-degree block or third-degree atrioventricular block)

Class IIa
- Bradycardia with an escape rhythm unresponsive to drug therapy
- Cardiac arrest with profound bradycardia, or pulseless electrical activity due to drug overdose, acidosis, or electrolyte abnormalities

Class IIb
Supraventricular or ventricular tachycardia refractory to drug therapy or cardioversion
   Note: Overdrive pacing should be used for these patients.

electrical stimulus directly to the endocardium. This is the most common type of pacemaker.

Clinical indications include the management of bradycardia, tachyarrhythmias, and other conduction system disturbances. The purpose of temporary transvenous pacemaker insertion is to maintain circulatory integrity by providing for standby pacing should sudden complete heart block ensue, to increase the heart rate during periods of symptomatic bradycardia, and occasionally to control sustained supraventricular or ventricular tachycardia. **AHA**

As an elective surgical procedure or as an emergency measure during CPR, a physician may choose to insert a *transthoracic pacemaker.* To insert this type of pacemaker, the physician performs a procedure similar to pericardiocentesis, in which he uses a cardiac needle to pass an electrode through the chest wall and into the right ventricle. This procedure carries a significant risk of coronary artery laceration and cardiac tamponade.

During cardiac surgery, the surgeon may insert electrodes through the epicardium of the right ventricle and, if he wants to institute atrioventricular sequential pacing, the right atrium. From there, the electrodes pass through the chest wall, where they remain available if temporary pacing becomes necessary. This is called *epicardial pacing.*

Besides helping to correct conduction disturbances, a temporary pacemaker may help diagnose conduction abnormalities. For example, during a cardiac catheterization or electrophysiology study, the physician may use a temporary pacemaker to localize conduction defects. In the process, he may also learn whether the patient is at risk for developing an arrhythmia.

Among the contraindications to pacemaker therapy are electromechanical dissociation and ventricular fibrillation.

Equipment
Transcutaneous pacing
Transcutaneous pacing generator • transcutaneous pacing electrodes • cardiac monitor

Transvenous pacing
All equipment listed for other types of temporary pacing • bridging cable • percutaneous introducer tray or venous cutdown tray • sterile gowns • linen-saver pad • antimicrobial soap • alcohol pads • 1% lidocaine • 5-ml syringe • fluoroscopy equipment, if necessary • fenestrated drape • prepackaged cutdown tray (for antecubital vein placement only) • sutures • receptacle for infectious waste

Transthoracic pacing
All equipment listed for temporary pacemakers • transthoracic or cardiac needle

Epicardial pacing
All equipment listed for temporary pacemakers • atrial epicardial wires • ventricular epicardial wires • sterile rubber finger cot • sterile dressing materials (if the wires won't be connected to a pulse generator)

Other types of temporary pacing
Temporary pacemaker generator with new battery • guide wire or introducer • electrode catheter • sterile gloves • sterile dressings • adhesive tape • antiseptic solution • sterile marker • sterile labels • nonconduct-

ing tape or rubber surgical glove • emergency cardiac drugs • intubation equipment • defibrillator • cardiac monitor with strip-chart recorder • equipment to start a peripheral I.V. line, if appropriate • I.V. fluids • sedative • optional: elastic bandage or gauze strips, restraints

Implementation

● If applicable, explain the procedure to the patient.

Transcutaneous pacing

● If necessary, clip the hair over the areas of electrode placement. However, don't shave the area. If you nick the skin, the current from the pulse generator could cause discomfort and the nicks could become irritated or infected after the electrodes are applied.

● Attach monitoring electrodes to the patient in the lead I, II, or III position. Do this even if the patient is already on telemetry monitoring because you'll need to connect the electrodes to the pacemaker. If you select the lead II position, adjust the LL (left leg) electrode placement to accommodate the anterior pacing electrode and the patient's anatomy. **AACN**

● Plug the patient cable into the electrocardiogram (ECG) input connection on the front of the pacing generator. Set the selector switch to the MONITOR ON position.

● You should see the ECG waveform on the monitor. Adjust the R-wave beeper volume to a suitable level and activate the alarm by pressing the ALARM ON button. Set the alarm for 10 to 20 beats lower and 20 to 30 beats higher than the intrinsic rate.

● Press the START/STOP button for a printout of the waveform.

● Now you're ready to apply the two pacing electrodes. First, make sure that the patient's skin is clean and dry to ensure good skin contact.

● Pull off the protective strip from the posterior electrode (marked BACK) and apply the electrode on the left side of the back, just below the scapula and to the left of the spine.

● The anterior pacing electrode (marked FRONT) has two protective strips — one covering the jellied area and one covering the outer rim. Expose the jellied area and apply it to the skin in the anterior position — to the left side of the precordium in the usual lead V_2 to V_5 position. Move this electrode around to get the best waveform. Then expose the electrode's

outer rim and firmly press it to the skin. (See *Proper electrode placement for a temporary pacemaker,* page 266.) **AACN**

● Now you're ready to pace the heart. After making sure that the energy output in milliamperes (mA) is on 0, connect the electrode cable to the monitor output cable.

● Check the waveform, looking for a tall QRS complex in lead II.

● Next, turn the selector switch to PACER ON. Tell the patient that he may feel a thumping or twitching sensation. Reassure him that you'll give him medication if he can't tolerate the discomfort.

● Now set the rate dial to 10 to 20 beats higher than the patient's intrinsic rhythm. Look for pacer artifact or spikes, which will appear as you increase the rate. If the patient doesn't have an intrinsic rhythm, set the rate at 60. **AACN**

● Slowly increase the amount of energy delivered to the heart by adjusting the OUTPUT mA dial. Do this until capture is achieved — you'll see a pacer spike followed by a widened QRS complex that resembles a premature ventricular contraction (PVC). This is the pacing threshold. To ensure consistent capture, increase output by 10%, but don't go higher because you could cause the patient needless discomfort.

● With full capture, the patient's heart rate should be approximately the same as the pacemaker rate set on the machine. The usual pacing threshold is 40 to 80 mA.

Transvenous pacing

● Check the patient's history for hypersensitivity to local anesthetics. Then, attach the cardiac monitor to the patient and obtain a baseline assessment, including the patient's vital signs, skin color, level of consciousness (LOC), heart rate and rhythm, and emotional state. Next, insert a peripheral I.V. line if the patient doesn't already have one. Then begin an I.V. infusion of dextrose 5% in water at a keep-vein-open rate.

● Insert a new battery into the external pacemaker generator and then test it to make sure that it has a strong charge. Connect the bridging cable to the generator, and align the positive and negative poles. *This cable allows slack between the electrode catheter and the generator, reducing the risk of accidental catheter displacement.*

Proper electrode placement for a temporary pacemaker

Place the pacing electrodes for a noninvasive temporary pacemaker at heart level on the patient's chest and back, with the heart lying between them. This placement ensures that the electrical stimulus will travel to the heart in the shortest distance.

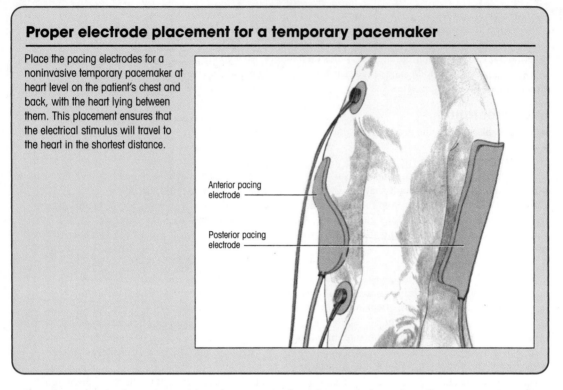

Anterior pacing electrode

Posterior pacing electrode

● Place the patient in the supine position. If necessary, clip the hair around the insertion site. Next, open the supply tray while maintaining a sterile field. Label all medications, medication containers, and other solutions on and off the sterile field. **JCAHO** Using sterile technique, clean the insertion site with antimicrobial soap and then wipe the area with antiseptic solution. Cover the insertion site with a fenestrated drape. *Because fluoroscopy may be used during the placement of leadwires,* put on a protective apron. **AACN**

● Provide the physician with the local anesthetic.

● After anesthetizing the insertion site, the physician will puncture the brachial, femoral, subclavian, or jugular vein. Then he'll insert a guide wire or an introducer and advance the electrode catheter.

● As the catheter advances, watch the cardiac monitor. When the electrode catheter reaches the right atrium, you'll notice large P waves and small QRS complexes. Then, as the catheter reaches the right ventricle, the P waves will become smaller while the QRS complexes enlarge. When the catheter touches the right ventricular endocardium, expect to see elevated ST segments, PVCs, or both.

● When in the right ventricle, the electrode catheter will send an impulse to the myocardium, causing depolarization. If the patient needs atrial pacing, either alone or with ventricular pacing, the physician may place an electrode in the right atrium.

● Meanwhile, continuously monitor the patient's cardiac status and treat arrhythmias, as appropriate. Also assess the patient for jaw pain and earache; *these symptoms indicate that the electrode catheter has missed the superior vena cava and has moved into the neck instead.*

● When the electrode catheter is in place, attach the catheter leads to the bridging cable, lining up the positive and negative poles.

● Check the battery's charge by pressing the BATTERY TEST button.

● Set the pacemaker as ordered.

● The physician will then suture the catheter to the insertion site. Afterward, put on sterile gloves and apply a sterile dressing to the site. Label the dressing with the date and time of application.

Transthoracic pacing

● Clean the skin to the left of the xiphoid process with povidone-iodine solution. Work quickly *because CPR must be interrupted for the procedure.*

● After interrupting CPR, the physician will insert a transthoracic needle through the patient's chest wall to the left of the xiphoid process into the right ventricle. He'll then follow the needle with the electrode catheter.

● Connect the electrode catheter to the generator, lining up the positive and negative poles. Watch the cardiac monitor for signs of ventricular pacing and capture.

● After the physician sutures the electrode catheter into place, use sterile technique to apply a sterile 4″ × 4″ gauze dressing to the site. Tape the dressing securely, and label it with the date and time of application.

● Check the patient's peripheral pulses and vital signs *to assess cardiac output.* If you can't palpate a pulse, continue performing CPR.

● If the patient has a palpable pulse, assess the patient's vital signs, ECG, and LOC.

Epicardial pacing

● During your preoperative teaching, inform the patient that epicardial pacemaker wires may be placed during cardiac surgery.

● During cardiac surgery, the physician will hook epicardial wires into the epicardium just before the end of the surgery. Depending on the patient's condition, the physician may insert either atrial or ventricular wires, or both.

● If indicated, connect the electrode catheter to the generator, lining up the positive and negative poles. Set the pacemaker as ordered.

● If the wires won't be connected to an external pulse generator, place them in a sterile rubber finger cot. Then cover the wires and the insertion site with a sterile, occlusive dressing. *This will help protect the patient from microshock and infection.*

Special considerations

● Take care to prevent microshock. This includes warning the patient not to use electrical equipment that isn't grounded, such as telephones, electric shavers, televisions, or lamps.

● Other safety measures include placing a plastic cover supplied by the manufacturer over the pacemaker controls *to avoid an accidental setting change.* Also, insulate the pacemaker by covering all exposed metal parts, such as electrode connections and pacemaker terminals, with nonconducting tape, or place the pacing unit in a dry, rubber surgical glove. If the patient is disoriented or uncooperative, use restraints *to prevent accidental removal of pacemaker wires.* If the patient needs emergency defibrillation, make sure that the pacemaker can withstand the procedure. If you're unsure, disconnect the pulse generator *to avoid damage.*

● When using a transcutaneous pacemaker, don't place the electrodes over a bony area *because bone conducts current poorly.* With a female patient, place the anterior electrode under her breast but not over her diaphragm. If the physician inserts the electrode through the brachial or femoral vein, immobilize the patient's arm or leg *to avoid putting stress on the pacing wires.*

● After insertion of a temporary pacemaker, assess the patient's vital signs, skin color, LOC, and peripheral pulses *to determine the effectiveness of the paced rhythm.* Perform a 12-lead ECG to serve as a baseline, and then perform additional ECGs daily or with clinical changes. Also, if possible, obtain a rhythm strip before, during, and after pacemaker placement; any time that pacemaker settings are changed; and whenever the patient receives treatment because of a complication due to the pacemaker. **AACN**

● Continuously monitor the ECG tracing, noting capture, sensing, rate, intrinsic beats, and competition of paced and intrinsic rhythms. If the pacemaker is sensing correctly, the sense indicator on the pulse generator should flash with each beat. (See *Handling pacemaker malfunction,* pages 268 and 269.)

● Record the date and time of pacemaker insertion, the type of pacemaker, the reason for insertion, and the patient's response. Note the pacemaker settings. Document any complications and the interventions taken.

● If the patient has epicardial pacing wires in place, clean the insertion site with povidone-iodine solution and change the dressing daily. At the same time, monitor the site for signs of infection. Always keep the pulse generator nearby in case pacing becomes necessary.

Nursing diagnoses

● Decreased cardiac output

Handling pacemaker malfunction

Occasionally, a temporary pacemaker may fail to function appropriately. When this occurs, you need to take immediate action to correct the problem. Here you'll learn which steps to take when your patient's pacemaker fails to pace, capture, or sense intrinsic beats.

Failure to pace

This happens when the pacemaker either doesn't fire or fires too often. The pulse generator may not be working properly, or it may not be conducting the impulse to the patient.

Nursing interventions

● If the pacing or sensing indicator flashes, check the connections to the cable and the position of the pacing electrode in the patient by X-ray. The cable may have come loose, or the electrode may have been dislodged, pulled out, or broken.
● If the pulse generator is turned on but the indicators still aren't flashing, change the battery. If that doesn't help, use a different pulse generator.
● Check the settings if the pacemaker is firing too rapidly. If they're correct, or if altering them (according to your

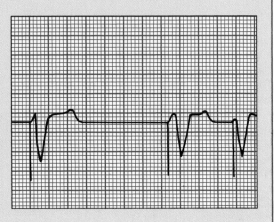

facility's policy or the physician's order) doesn't help, change the pulse generator.

Failure to capture

Here, you see pacemaker spikes but the heart isn't responding. This may be caused by changes in the pacing threshold from ischemia, an electrolyte imbalance (high or low potassium or magnesium levels), acidosis, an adverse reaction to a medication, a perforated ventricle, fibrosis, or the electrode position.

Nursing interventions

● If the patient's condition has changed, notify the physician and ask him for new settings.
● If pacemaker settings are altered by the patient or others, return them to their correct positions. Then make sure that the face of the pacemaker is covered with a plastic shield. Also, tell the patient or others not to touch the dials.
● If the heart isn't responding, try any or all of these suggestions: Carefully check all connections; increase the milliamperes slowly (according to your facility's policy or the physician's order); turn the patient on his left side, then on his right (if turning him to the left didn't

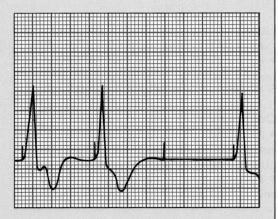

help); reverse the cable in the pulse generator so the positive electrode wire is in the negative terminal and the negative electrode wire is in the positive terminal; or schedule an anteroposterior or lateral chest X-ray to determine the electrode position.

Handling pacemaker malfunction *(continued)*

Failure to sense intrinsic beats

This could cause ventricular tachycardia or ventricular fibrillation if the pacemaker fires on the vulnerable T wave. This could be caused by the pacemaker sensing an external stimulus as a QRS complex, which could lead to asystole, or by the pacemaker not being sensitive enough, which means it could fire anywhere within the cardiac cycle.

Nursing interventions

● If the pacing is undersensing, turn the sensitivity control completely to the right. If it's oversensing, turn it slightly to the left.
● If the pacemaker isn't functioning correctly, change the battery or the pulse generator.
● Remove items in the room causing electromechanical interference (razors, radios, cautery devices). Check the ground wires on the bed and other equipment for obvious damage. Unplug each piece and see if the interference stops. When you locate the cause, notify the staff engineer and ask him to check it.

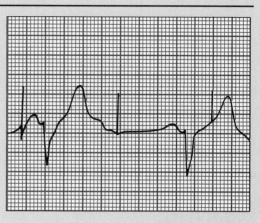

● If the pacemaker is still firing on the T wave and all else has failed, turn off the pacemaker. Make sure that atropine is available in case the patient's heart rate drops. Be prepared to call a code and start cardiopulmonary resuscitation, if necessary.

Expected outcomes

The patient will:
● maintain a blood pressure and pulse rate within normal limits
● maintain an adequate cardiac output.

Complications

● Complications associated with pacemaker therapy include microshock, equipment failure, and competitive or fatal arrhythmias.
● Transcutaneous pacemakers may also cause skin breakdown and muscle pain and twitching when the pacemaker fires.
● Transvenous pacemakers may cause such complications as pneumothorax or hemothorax, cardiac perforation and tamponade, diaphragmatic stimulation, pulmonary embolism, thrombophlebitis, and infection.
● If the physician threads the electrode through the antecubital or femoral vein, venous spasm, thrombophlebitis, or lead displacement may result.
● Complications of transthoracic pacemakers include pneumothorax, cardiac tamponade, emboli, sepsis,

lacerations of the myocardium or coronary artery, and perforations of a cardiac chamber.
● Epicardial pacemakers carry a risk of infection, cardiac arrest, and diaphragmatic stimulation.

Documentation

Record the reason for pacing, the time it started, and the locations of the electrodes. For a transvenous or transthoracic pacemaker, note the date, time, and reason for the temporary pacemaker.

For any temporary pacemaker, record the pacemaker settings. Note the patient's response to the procedure, along with any complications and the interventions taken. If possible, obtain rhythm strips before, during, and after pacemaker placement and whenever pacemaker settings are changed or when the patient receives treatment for a complication caused by the pacemaker. As you monitor the patient, record his response to temporary pacing and note changes in his condition.

Supportive references

American Association for Respiratory Care. "Resuscitation and Defibrillation in the Health Care Setting — 2004 Revision and Update," *Respiratory Care* 49(9):1085-99, September 2004. *www.rcjournal.com/ online_resources/cpgs/rachcpg.html.*

American Heart Association. "2005 AHA Guidelines for Cardiopulmonary Resuscitation and Emergency Cardiovascular Care: International Consensus on Science." *Circulation* 112(22 Suppl):IV-1-IV-211, November 2005.

Pulmonary artery pressure and pulmonary artery wedge pressure monitoring

Continuous pulmonary artery pressure (PAP) and intermittent pulmonary artery wedge pressure (PAWP) measurements provide important information about left ventricular function and preload. You can use this information not only for monitoring but also for aiding diagnosis, refining your assessment, guiding interventions, and projecting patient outcomes.

Nearly all acutely ill patients are candidates for PAP monitoring — especially those who are hemodynamically unstable, who need fluid management or continuous cardiopulmonary assessment, or who are receiving multiple or frequently administered cardioactive drugs. There are several clinical conditions in which the use of a pulmonary artery (PA) catheter is generally recommended. These include:

● the assessment of intravascular volume, particularly in patients with severe pulmonary edema, heart failure, or oliguric renal failure
● as a guide for therapy in severe refractory shock or multiorgan failure
● as a guide for therapy to maximize oxygen delivery to tissues in some selected patients. **ACC**

Two physicians, Swan and Ganz, invented the original PAP monitoring catheter, which has two lumens. The device still bears their name (Swan-Ganz catheter) but is commonly called a PA catheter. Current versions have up to six lumens, allowing more hemodynamic information to be gathered. Besides distal and proximal lumens used to measure pressures, a PA catheter has a balloon inflation lumen that inflates the balloon for PAWP measurement and a thermistor connector lumen that allows cardiac output measurement. Some catheters also have a pacemaker wire lumen that provides a port for pacemaker electrodes and measures continuous mixed venous oxygen saturation. (See *PA catheters: Basic to complex.*)

CLINICAL IMPACT *New capabilities have been added to some PA catheters, dramatically enhancing the available hemodynamic data. These include continuous cardiac output, mixed venous oxyhemoglobin, and right ventricular ejection fraction. Other new technologies could potentially replace PA monitoring. These include exhaled carbon dioxide and esophageal Doppler. Further research is needed to define their optimal clinical use.*

Fluoroscopy usually isn't required during catheter insertion because the catheter is flow directed, following venous blood flow from the right heart chambers into the pulmonary artery. Also, the pulmonary artery, right atrium, and right ventricle produce characteristic pressures and waveforms that can be observed on the monitor to help track catheter-tip location. Marks on the catheter shaft, with 10-cm graduations, assist tracking by showing how far the catheter is inserted.

The PA catheter is inserted into the heart's right side with the distal tip lying in the pulmonary artery. Left-sided pressures can be assessed indirectly.

No specific contraindications for PAP monitoring exist. However, some patients undergoing it require special precautions. These include elderly patients with pulmonary hypertension, those with left bundle-branch block, and those for whom a systemic infection would be life threatening.

Equipment

Balloon-tipped, flow-directed PA catheter ● prepared pressure transducer system ● I.V. solutions ● sterile gloves ● alcohol pads ● medication-added label ● monitor and monitor cable ● I.V. pole with transducer mount ● emergency resuscitation equipment ● electrocardiogram (ECG) monitor ● ECG electrodes ● arm board (for antecubital insertion) ● lead aprons (if fluoroscopy is necessary) ● sterile marker ● sterile labels ● sutures ● sterile 4″ × 4″ gauze pads or other dry, occlusive dressing material ● prepackaged introducer kit ● optional: dextrose 5% in water, shaving materials (for femoral insertion site), small sterile basin, sterile water

PA catheters: Basic to complex

Depending on the intended use, a pulmonary artery (PA) catheter may be simple or complex. The basic PA catheter has a distal and proximal lumen, a thermistor, and a balloon inflation gate valve. The distal lumen, which exits in the pulmonary artery, monitors PA pressure. Its hub usually is marked "P distal" or is color-coded yellow. The proximal lumen exits in the right atrium or vena cava, depending on the size of the patient's heart. It monitors right atrial pressure and can be used as the injected solution lumen for cardiac output determination and for infusing solutions. The proximal lumen hub usually is marked "Proximal" or is color-coded blue.

The thermistor, located about 1 ½" (4 cm) from the distal tip, measures temperature (aiding core temperature evaluation) and allows cardiac output measurement. The thermistor connector attaches to a cardiac output connector cable and then to a cardiac output monitor. Typically, it's red.

The balloon inflation gate valve is used for inflating the balloon tip with air. A stopcock connection, typically color-coded red, may be used.

Additional lumens

Some PA catheters have additional lumens used to obtain other hemodynamic data or permit certain interventions. For instance, a proximal infusion port, which exits in the right atrium or vena cava, allows additional fluid administration. A right ventricular lumen, exiting in the right ventricle, allows fluid administration, right ventricular pressure measurement, or use of a temporary ventricular pacing lead.

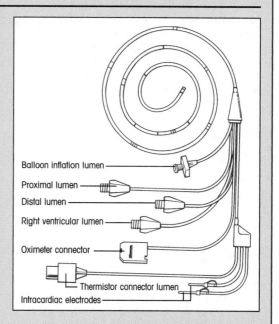

Balloon inflation lumen
Proximal lumen
Distal lumen
Right ventricular lumen
Oximeter connector
Thermistor connector lumen
Intracardiac electrodes

Some catheters have additional right atrial and right ventricular lumens for atrioventricular pacing. A right ventricular ejection fraction test-response thermistor, with PA and right ventricular sensing electrodes, allows volumetric and ejection fraction measurements. Fiber-optic filaments, such as those used in pulse oximetry, exit into the pulmonary artery and permit measurement of continuous mixed venous oxygen saturation.

If a prepackaged introducer kit is unavailable, obtain the following: introducer (one size larger than the catheter) • sterile tray containing instruments for procedure • masks • sterile gowns, gloves, and drapes • povidone-iodine ointment and solution • sutures • two 10-ml syringes • local anesthetic (1% to 2% lidocaine) • one 5-ml syringe • 25G ½" needle • 1" and 3" tape

Preparation of equipment

● To obtain reliable pressure values and clear waveforms, the pressure monitoring system and bedside monitor must be properly calibrated and zeroed.

● Make sure that the monitor has the correct pressure modules, and then calibrate it according to the manufacturer's instructions. **MFR**

● Turn the monitor on before gathering the equipment to give it time to warm up. Be sure to check the operations manual for the monitor you're using; some older monitors may need 20 minutes to warm up.

● Prepare the pressure monitoring system according to your facility's policy. Your facility's guidelines also may specify whether to mount the transducer on the I.V. pole or tape it to the patient and whether to add heparin to the flush solution.

- To manage complications from catheter insertion, be sure to have emergency resuscitation equipment on hand (defibrillator, oxygen, and supplies for intubation and emergency drug administration).
- Prepare a sterile field for insertion of the introducer and catheter. Label all medications, medication containers, and other solutions on and off the sterile field. **JCAHO** A bedside tray, placed on the same side as the insertion site for easier access, may be sufficient.

Implementation

- Confirm the patient's identity using two patient identifiers according to facility policy. **JCAHO**
- Check the patient's chart for heparin sensitivity, which contraindicates adding heparin to the flush solution. If the patient is alert, explain the procedure to him to reduce his anxiety. Mention that the catheter will monitor pressures from the pulmonary artery and heart. Reassure him that the catheter poses little danger and rarely causes pain. Tell him that if pain occurs at the introducer insertion site, the physician will order an analgesic or a sedative. **PCP**
- Be sure to tell the patient and his family not to be alarmed if they see the pressure waveform on the monitor "move around." Explain that the cause usually is artifact.

Positioning the patient for catheter placement

- Position the patient at the proper height and angle. If the physician will use a superior approach for percutaneous insertion (most commonly using the internal jugular or subclavian vein), place the patient flat or in a slight Trendelenburg position. Remove the patient's pillow to help engorge the vessel and prevent air embolism. Turn his head to the side opposite the insertion site.
- If the physician will use an inferior approach to access a femoral vein, position the patient flat. Be aware that with this approach, certain catheters are harder to insert and may require more manipulations.

Preparing the catheter

- Maintain aseptic technique and use standard precautions throughout catheter preparation and insertion. **CDC**
- Wash your hands. Clean the insertion site with povidone-iodine solution and drape it. **CDC**

- Put on a mask. Help the physician put on a sterile mask, gown, and gloves. **CDC**
- Open the outer packaging of the catheter, revealing the inner sterile wrapping. Using aseptic technique, the physician opens the inner wrapping and picks up the catheter. Take the catheter lumen hubs as he hands them to you.
- *To remove air from the catheter and verify its patency,* flush the catheter. In the more common flushing method, you connect the I.V. solutions aseptically to the appropriate pressure lines, and then flush them before insertion. *This method makes pressure waveforms easier to identify on the monitor during insertion.* **AACN**
- Alternatively, you may flush the lumens with sterile I.V. solution from sterile syringes attached to the lumens. Leave the filled syringes on during insertion.
- If the system has multiple pressure lines (such as a distal line to monitor PAP and a proximal line to monitor right atrial pressure), make sure that the distal PA lumen hub is attached to the pressure line that will be observed on the monitor. *Inadvertently attaching the distal PA line to the proximal lumen hub will prevent the proper waveform from appearing during insertion.* **AACN**
- Observe the diastolic values carefully during insertion. Make sure that the scale is appropriate for lower pressures. A scale of 0 to 25 mm Hg or 0 to 50 mm Hg (more common) is preferred. (With a higher scale, such as 0 to 100 or 0 to 250 mm Hg, waveforms appear too small and the location of the catheter tip will be hard to identify.) **AACN**
- *To verify balloon integrity,* the physician inflates it with air (usually 1.5 cc) before handing you the lumens to attach to the pressure monitoring system. He then observes the balloon for symmetry. He also may submerge it in a small, sterile basin filled with sterile water and observe it for bubbles, which indicate a leak.

Inserting the catheter

- Assist the physician as he inserts the introducer to access the vessel. He may perform a cutdown or (more commonly) insert the catheter percutaneously, as in a modified Seldinger technique.
- After the introducer is placed and the catheter lumens are flushed, the physician inserts the catheter through the introducer. In the internal jugular or subclavian approach, he inserts the catheter into the end of the introducer sheath with the balloon deflated, di-

Normal PA waveforms

During pulmonary artery (PA) catheter insertion, the monitor shows various waveforms as the catheter advances through the heart chambers.

Right atrium

When the catheter tip enters the right atrium, the first heart chamber on its route, a waveform like the one shown at right appears on the monitor. Note the two small upright waves. The a waves represent left atrial contraction; the v waves, increased pressure or volume in the left atrium during left ventricular systole.

Right ventricle

As the catheter tip reaches the right ventricle, you'll see a waveform with sharp systolic upstrokes and lower diastolic dips.

Pulmonary artery

The catheter then floats into the pulmonary artery, causing a waveform like the one shown at right. Note that the upstroke is smoother than on the right ventricular waveform. The dicrotic notch indicates pulmonic valve closure.

PAWP

Floating into a distal branch of the pulmonary artery, the balloon wedges where the vessel becomes too narrow for it to pass. The monitor now shows a pulmonary artery wedge pressure (PAWP) waveform, with two small uprises from left atrial systole and diastole. The balloon is then deflated and the catheter is left in the pulmonary artery. Observe for the return of the normal PA waveform.

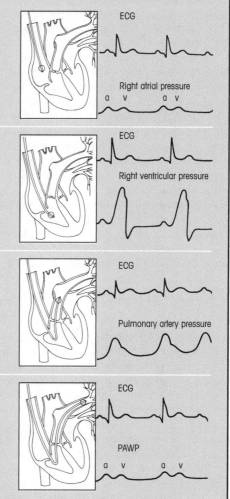

recting the curl of the catheter toward the patient's midline.

● As insertion begins, observe the bedside monitor for waveform variations. (See *Normal PA waveforms*.)
● When the catheter exits the end of the introducer sheath and reaches the junction of the superior vena cava and right atrium (at the 15- to 20-cm mark on the catheter shaft), the monitor shows oscillations that correspond to the patient's respirations. The balloon is then inflated with the recommended volume of air *to allow normal blood flow and aid catheter insertion.*

● Using a gentle, smooth motion, the physician advances the catheter through the heart chambers, moving rapidly to the pulmonary artery *because prolonged manipulation here may reduce catheter stiffness.*

● When the mark on the catheter shaft reaches 15 to 20 cm, the catheter enters the right atrium. The waveform shows two small, upright waves; pressure is low (from 2 to 4 mm Hg). Read pressure values in the mean mode *because systolic and diastolic values are similar.*

● The physician advances the catheter into the right ventricle, working quickly to minimize irritation. The waveform now shows sharp systolic upstrokes and lower diastolic dips. Depending on the size of the patient's heart, the catheter should reach the 30- to 35-cm mark. (The smaller the heart, the less catheter length will be needed to reach the right ventricle.) Record systolic and diastolic pressures. Systolic pressure normally ranges from 15 to 25 mm Hg; diastolic pressure, from 0 to 8 mm Hg.

● As the catheter floats into the pulmonary artery, note that the upstroke from right ventricular systole is smoother, and systolic pressure is nearly the same as right ventricular systolic pressure. Record systolic, diastolic, and mean pressures (typically ranging from 8 to 15 mm Hg). A dicrotic notch on the diastolic portion of the waveform indicates pulmonic valve closure. **AACN**

Wedging the catheter **AACN**

● To obtain a wedge tracing, the physician lets the inflated balloon float downstream with venous blood flow to a smaller, more distal branch of the pulmonary artery. Here, the catheter lodges, or wedges, causing occlusion of right ventricular and PA diastolic pressures. The tracing resembles the right atrial tracing because the catheter tip is recording left atrial pressure. The waveform shows two small uprises. Record PAWP in the mean mode (usually 6 to 12 mm Hg).

● A PAWP waveform, or wedge tracing, appears when the catheter has been inserted 45 to 50 cm. (In a large heart, a longer catheter length — up to 55 cm — typically is required. However, a catheter should never be inserted more than 60 cm.) Usually, 30 to 45 seconds elapse from the time the physician inserts the introducer until the wedge tracing appears.

● The physician deflates the balloon, and the catheter drifts out of the wedge position and into the pulmonary artery, its normal resting place.

● If the appropriate waveforms don't appear at the expected times during catheter insertion, the catheter may be coiled in the right atrium and ventricle. To correct this problem, deflate the balloon. To do this, unlock the gate valve or turn the stopcock to the ON position and then detach the syringe from the balloon inflation port. Back pressure in the pulmonary artery causes the balloon to deflate on its own. (Active air withdrawal may compromise balloon integrity.) *To verify balloon deflation,* observe the monitor for return of the PAP tracing.

● Typically, the physician orders a portable chest X-ray *to confirm catheter position.*

● Apply a sterile occlusive dressing to the insertion site.

● The Centers for Disease Control and Prevention (CDC) recommends changing the dressing whenever it's moist or every 24 to 48 hours, re-dressing the site according to your facility's policy, changing the catheter every 72 hours, changing the pressure tubing every 48 hours, and changing the flush solution every 24 hours. However, these recommendations were issued in 1982. Since then, some health care facilities have maintained closed-pressure monitoring systems for longer than the recommended times with no increase in infection rates. Nonetheless, before departing from CDC recommendations, determine your facility's policy. **CDC**

Obtaining intermittent PAP values

● After inserting the catheter and recording initial pressure readings, record subsequent PAP values and monitor waveforms. These values will be used to calculate other important hemodynamic indices. *To ensure accurate values,* make sure that the transducer is properly leveled and zeroed.

● Perform a dynamic response measurement or square wave test and document it every 8 to 12 hours to assess and validate optimal waveforms. (See *Square wave test,* page 201.) **AACN**

● If possible, obtain PAP values at end expiration (when the patient completely exhales). *At this time, intrathoracic pressure approaches atmospheric pressure and has the least effect on PAP.* If you obtain a reading during other phases of the respiratory cycle, respiratory interference may occur. For instance, during inspiration, when intrathoracic pressure drops, PAP may be falsely low because the negative pressure is transmitted to the catheter. During expiration, when intrathoracic pressure rises, PAP may be falsely high.

● For patients with a rapid respiratory rate and subsequent variations, you may have trouble identifying end expiration. The monitor displays an average of the digital readings obtained over time as well as those readings obtained during a full respiratory cycle. If possible, obtain a printout. Use the averaged values obtained through the full respiratory cycle. *To analyze trends accurately,* be sure to record values at consistent times during the respiratory cycle.

Taking a PAWP reading AACN

● PAWP is recorded by inflating the balloon and letting it float in a distal artery. Some facilities allow only physicians or specially trained nurses to take a PAWP reading because of the risk of PA rupture — a rare but life-threatening complication. If your facility permits you to perform this procedure, do so with extreme caution and make sure that you're thoroughly familiar with intracardiac waveform interpretation.

● To begin, verify that the transducer is properly leveled and zeroed. Detach the syringe from the balloon inflation hub. Draw 1.5 cc of air into the syringe, and then reattach the syringe to the hub. Watching the monitor, inject the air through the hub slowly and smoothly. When you see a wedge tracing on the monitor, immediately stop inflating the balloon. Never inflate the balloon beyond the volume needed to obtain a wedge tracing.

● Take the pressure reading at end expiration. Note the amount of air needed to change the PA tracing to a wedge tracing (normally, 1.25 to 1.5 cc). If the wedge tracing appeared with an injection of less than 1.25 cc, suspect that the catheter has migrated into a more distal branch and requires repositioning. If the balloon is in a more distal branch, the tracings may move up the oscilloscope, indicating that the catheter tip is recording balloon pressure rather than PAWP. This may lead to PA rupture.

Removing the catheter

● To assist the physician, inspect the chest X-ray for signs of catheter kinking or knotting. (In some states, you may be permitted to remove a PA catheter yourself under your facility's policy.)

● Obtain the patient's baseline vital signs and note the ECG pattern. AACN

● Explain the procedure to the patient. Place the head of the bed flat, unless ordered otherwise. If the catheter was inserted using a superior approach, turn the patient's head to the side opposite the insertion site. Gently remove the dressing.

● Remove any sutures securing the catheter, unless the introducer is left in place.

● Turn all stopcocks off to the patient. (You may turn stopcocks on to the distal port if you wish to observe waveforms. However, use caution because this may cause an air embolism.)

● Put on sterile gloves. After verifying that the balloon is deflated, withdraw the catheter slowly and smoothly. If you feel resistance, stop immediately, stay with the patient, and notify the physician at once. AACN CDC

● Watch the ECG monitor for arrhythmias.

● If the introducer was removed, apply pressure to the site, and check it frequently for signs of bleeding. Dress the site again, as necessary. If the introducer is left in place, observe the diaphragm for blood backflow, *which verifies the integrity of the hemostasis valve.* AACN

● Return all equipment to the appropriate location. You may turn off the bedside pressure modules but leave the ECG module on.

● Reassure the patient and his family that he'll be observed closely. Make sure that he understands that the catheter was removed because his condition has improved and he no longer needs it.

Special considerations

● Advise the patient to use caution when moving about in bed *to avoid dislodging the catheter.*

● Never leave the balloon inflated *because this may cause pulmonary infarction.* To determine if the balloon is inflated, check the monitor for a wedge tracing, which indicates inflation. (A PA tracing confirms balloon deflation.)

● Never inflate the balloon with more than the recommended air volume (specified on the catheter shaft) *because this may cause loss of elasticity or balloon rupture.* With appropriate inflation volume, the balloon floats easily through the heart chambers and rests in the main branch of the pulmonary artery, producing accurate waveforms. If the patient has a suspected left-to-right shunt, use carbon dioxide to

inflate the balloon, as ordered, *because it diffuses more quickly than air*. Never inflate the balloon with fluids *because they may not be able to be retrieved from inside the balloon, preventing deflation.*
- Be aware that the catheter may slip back into the right ventricle. *Because the tip may irritate the ventricle*, check the monitor for a right ventricular waveform to detect this problem promptly.
- *To minimize valvular trauma*, make sure that the balloon is deflated whenever the catheter is withdrawn from the pulmonary artery to the right ventricle or from the right ventricle to the right atrium.
- Perform and document the dynamic response or square wave test every 8 to 12 hours to validate the optimal waveform.

Nursing diagnoses
- Ineffective tissue perfusion: Cardiopulmonary

Expected outcomes
The patient will:
- maintain hemodynamic stability
- exhibit no arrhythmias.

Complications
- Complications of PA catheter insertion include PA perforation, pulmonary infarction, catheter knotting, local or systemic infection, cardiac arrhythmias, and heparin-induced thrombocytopenia.

Documentation
Document the date and time of catheter insertion, the physician who performed the procedure, the catheter insertion site, pressure waveforms and values for the various heart chambers, balloon inflation volume required to obtain a wedge tracing, any arrhythmias occurring during or after the procedure, type of flush solution used and its heparin concentration (if any), type of dressing applied, and the patient's tolerance of the procedure. Remember to initial and date the dressing.

After catheter removal, document the patient's tolerance of the removal procedure, and note any problems encountered during removal.

Supportive references
American Society of Anesthesiologists. "Practice Guidelines for Pulmonary Artery Catheterization: An Updated Report by the American Society of Anes-

thesiologists Task Force," *Anesthesiology* 99(4):988-1014, October 2003.

Bridges, E.J. "Monitoring Pulmonary Artery Pressures: Just the Facts," *Critical Care Nurse* 20(6):59-80, December 2000.

Daily, E.K. "Hemodynamic Waveform Analysis," *Journal of Cardiovascular Nursing* 15(2):6-22, 87-88, January 2001.

Druding, M.C. "Integrating Hemodynamic Monitoring and Physical Assessment," *Dimensions of Critical Care Nursing* 19(4):25-30, July-August 2000.

Keckeisen, M. "Monitoring Pulmonary Artery Pressure," *Critical Care Nurse* 19(6):88-91, December 1999.

Lynn-McHale Wiegand, D.J., and Carlson, K.K. *AACN Procedure Manual for Critical Care,* 5th ed. Philadelphia: W.B. Saunders Co., 2005.

Ott, K., et al. "New Technologies in the Assessment of Hemodynamic Parameters," *Journal of Cardiovascular Nursing* 15(2):41-55, January 2001.

Quaal, S.J. "Improving the Accuracy of Pulmonary Artery Catheter Measurements," *Journal of Cardiovascular Nursing* 15(2):71-82, January 2001.

Rice, W.P., et al. "A Comparison of Hydrostatic Leveling Methods in Invasive Pressure Monitoring," *Critical Care Nurse* 20(6):20, 22-30, December 2000.

Vagal maneuvers

When a patient suffers sinus, atrial, or junctional tachyarrhythmias, vagal maneuvers — Valsalva's maneuver and carotid sinus massage — can slow his heart rate. These maneuvers work by stimulating nerve endings, which respond as they would to an increase in blood pressure. They send this message to the brain stem, which in turn stimulates the autonomic nervous system to increase vagal tone and decrease the heart rate.

According to the American Heart Association (AHA), vagal maneuvers and adenosine (Adenocard) should be the initial treatment for stable reentry supraventricular tachycardia (SVT). It has been found that vagal maneuvers alone will correct SVT 20% to 25% of the time. **AHA**

In Valsalva's maneuver, the patient holds his breath and bears down, raising his intrathoracic pressure. When this pressure increase is transmitted to the heart and great vessels, venous return, stroke volume, and systolic blood pressure decrease. Within seconds, the baroreceptors respond to these changes by increasing the heart rate and causing peripheral vaso-constriction.

When the patient exhales at the end of the maneuver, his blood pressure rises to its previous level. This increase, combined with the peripheral vasoconstriction caused by bearing down, stimulates the vagus nerve, decreasing the heart rate.

ALERT *Valsalva's maneuver is contraindicated in patients with increased intracranial pressure. It shouldn't be taught to patients who aren't alert or cooperative.*

In carotid sinus massage, manual pressure applied to the left or right carotid sinus slows the heart rate. This method is used to diagnose and treat tachyarrhythmias.

The patient's response to carotid sinus massage depends on the type of arrhythmia. If he has sinus tachycardia, his heart rate will slow gradually during the procedure and speed up again after it. If he has atrial tachycardia, the arrhythmia may stop and the heart rate may remain slow because the procedure increases atrioventricular (AV) block. With atrial fibrillation or flutter, the ventricular rate may not change; AV block may even worsen. With paroxysmal atrial tachycardia, reversion to sinus rhythm occurs only 20% of the time. Nonparoxysmal tachycardia and ventricular tachycardia won't respond.

Vagal maneuvers are contraindicated in patients with severe coronary artery disease (CAD), acute myocardial infarction, or hypovolemia. Carotid sinus massage is contraindicated in patients with cardiac glycoside toxicity or cerebrovascular disease and in patients who have had carotid surgery.

Although usually performed by a physician, vagal maneuvers may also be done by a specially prepared nurse under a physician's supervision.

CONTROVERSIAL ISSUE *Because older patients commonly have undiagnosed atherosclerosis and carotid bruits aren't always present even with significant atherosclerosis, most experts avoid carotid sinus massage in elderly and late middle-age patients. In these patients, experts agree that Valsalva's maneuver should be used.*

Equipment

Crash cart with emergency medications and airway equipment • electrocardiogram (ECG) monitor and electrodes • I.V. catheter and tubing • tourniquet • dex-trose 5% in water (D$_5$W) • optional: shaving supplies, cardiotonic drugs

Implementation

- Confirm the patient's identity using two patient identifiers according to facility policy. **JCAHO**
- Explain the procedure to the patient *to ease his fears and promote cooperation.* Ask him to let you know if he feels light-headed.
- Place the patient in a supine position. Insert an I.V. line, if necessary. Then administer D$_5$W at a keep-vein-open rate, as ordered. *This line will be used if emergency drugs become necessary.*
- Prepare the patient's skin, shaving it if necessary, and attach ECG electrodes. Adjust the size of the ECG complexes on the monitor *so that you can see the arrhythmia clearly.*

Valsalva's maneuver

- Ask the patient to take a deep breath and bear down, as if he were trying to defecate. If he doesn't feel light-headed or dizzy and if no new arrhythmias occur, have him hold his breath and bear down for 10 seconds. **AHA**
- If he does feel dizzy or light-headed or if you see a new arrhythmia on the monitor — asystole for more than 6 seconds, frequent premature ventricular contractions (PVCs), or ventricular tachycardia or ventricular fibrillation — allow him to exhale and stop bearing down.
- After 10 seconds, ask him to exhale and breathe quietly. If the maneuver was successful, the monitor will show his heart rate slowing before he exhales.

Carotid sinus massage

- Begin by obtaining a rhythm strip, using the lead that shows the strongest P waves.
- Auscultate both carotid sinuses. If you detect bruits, inform the physician and don't perform carotid sinus massage. If you don't detect bruits, proceed as ordered. (See *Performing carotid sinus massage,* page 278.)
- Monitor the ECG throughout the procedure. Stop massaging when the ventricular rate slows sufficiently to permit diagnosis of the rhythm. Or stop as soon as any evidence of a rhythm change appears. Have the crash cart handy to give emergency treatment if a dangerous arrhythmia occurs. **AHA**

Performing carotid sinus massage

Before applying manual pressure to the patient's right carotid sinus, locate the bifurcation of the carotid artery on the right side of the neck. Turn the patient's head slightly to the left and hyperextend the neck. This brings the carotid artery closer to the skin and moves the sternocleidomastoid muscle away from the carotid artery.

Then, using a circular motion, gently massage the right carotid sinus between your fingers and the transverse processes of the spine for 3 to 5 seconds. Don't massage for more than 5 seconds *to avoid risking life-threatening complications.*

Internal carotid artery
External carotid sinus
Carotid body
Vagus nerve
Right common carotid artery
Left common carotid artery
Right subclavian artery
Cardiac plexus
Left subclavian artery

● If the procedure has no effect within 5 seconds, stop massaging the right carotid sinus and begin to massage the left. If this also fails, administer cardiotonic drugs, as ordered.

Special considerations
● Remember that a brief period of asystole — from 3 to 6 seconds — and several PVCs may precede conversion to normal sinus rhythm.
● If the vagal maneuver succeeded in slowing the patient's heart rate and converting the arrhythmia, continue monitoring him for several hours.

Nursing diagnoses
● Fear
● Ineffective tissue perfusion: Cardiopulmonary

Expected outcomes
The patient will:
● state an understanding of the procedure
● exhibit no physical signs and symptoms of fear
● maintain a blood pressure and pulse rate within normal limits
● exhibit no arrhythmias.

Complications
● Use caution when performing carotid sinus massage on elderly patients, patients receiving cardiac glycosides, and patients with heart block, hypertension, CAD, diabetes mellitus, or hyperkalemia. The procedure may cause arterial pressure to plummet in these patients, although it usually rises quickly afterward.

ALERT *Elderly patients with heart disease are especially susceptible to the adverse effects of vagal maneuvers.*

● Vagal maneuvers can occasionally cause bradycardia or complete heart block, so monitor the patient's cardiac rhythm closely. (See *Adverse effects of vagal maneuvers.*)

Documentation

Record the date and time of the procedure, who performed it, and why it was necessary. Note the patient's response, any complications, and the interventions taken. If possible, obtain a rhythm strip before, during, and after the procedure.

Supportive references

American Heart Association. "2005 AHA Guidelines for Cardiopulmonary Resuscitation and Emergency Cardiovascular Care: International Consensus on Science," *Circulation* 112(22 Suppl):IV-1-IV-211, November 2005.

Gilbert, C.J. "Common Supraventricular Tachycardias: Mechanisms and Management," *AACN Clinical Issues* 12(1):100-13, February 2001.

Mastering ACLS, 2nd ed. Philadelphia: Lippincott Williams & Wilkins, 2006.

Ventricular assist device

A temporary life-sustaining treatment for a failing heart, the ventricular assist device (VAD) diverts systemic blood flow from a diseased ventricle into an implanted or a paracorporeal pump. It maintains cardiac output, reduces ventricular work, and allows the myocardium to rest and contractility to improve. Although used most commonly to assist the left ventricle, this device may also assist the right ventricle or both ventricles. (See *VAD: Help for the failing heart,* page 280.)

Candidates for VADs include patients with massive myocardial infarction, irreversible cardiomyopathy, ventricular arrhythmias, acute myocarditis, an inability to be weaned from cardiopulmonary bypass, valvular disease, bacterial endocarditis, or heart transplant rejection. VADs also may be used in patients awaiting heart transplantation.

Indications for VAD therapy include bridge to transplant, bridge to recovery, and destination therapy.

Adverse effects of vagal maneuvers

Valsalva's maneuver and carotid sinus massage are useful for slowing the heart rate. However, they can cause complications, some of which are life-threatening.

Valsalva's maneuver

Valsalva's maneuver can cause bradycardia, accompanied by a decrease in cardiac output, possibly leading to syncope. The bradycardia will usually pass quickly, but if it doesn't or if it advances to complete heart block or asystole, begin basic life support (BLS) followed — if necessary — by advanced cardiac life support (ACLS).

Valsalva's maneuver can mobilize venous thrombi and cause bleeding. Monitor the patient for signs and symptoms of vascular occlusion, including neurologic changes, chest discomfort, and dyspnea. Report such problems at once, and prepare the patient for diagnostic testing or transfer him to the intensive care unit (ICU), as ordered.

Carotid sinus massage

Because carotid sinus massage can cause ventricular fibrillation, ventricular tachycardia, and standstill as well as worsening atrioventricular block that leads to junctional or ventricular escape rhythms, you'll need to monitor the patient's electrocardiogram (ECG) closely. If his ECG indicates complete heart block or asystole, start BLS at once, followed by ACLS. If emergency medications don't convert the complete heart block, the patient may need a temporary pacemaker.

Carotid sinus massage can cause cerebral damage from inadequate tissue perfusion, especially in elderly patients. It can also cause a stroke, either from decreased perfusion caused by total carotid artery blockage or from migrating endothelial plaque loosened by carotid sinus compression. Watch the patient carefully during and after the procedure for changes in his neurologic status. If you note any, tell the physician at once and prepare the patient for further diagnostic tests or transfer him to the ICU, as ordered.

VAD: Help for the failing heart

The ventricular assist device (VAD) functions somewhat like an artificial heart. The major difference is that the VAD assists the heart, whereas the artificial heart replaces it. The VAD is designed to aid one or both ventricles. The pumping chambers themselves may be implanted in the patient or may be external, depending on the VAD system.

A VAD with an implanted pump receives power through the skin either through a percutaneous lead or through a belt of electrical transformer coils (worn externally as a portable battery pack). It can also operate off an implanted, rechargeable battery for up to 1 hour at a time, depending on the VAD system.

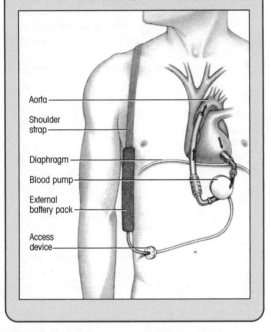

Aorta

Shoulder strap

Diaphragm

Blood pump

External battery pack

Access device

Destination therapy supports patients with VAD therapy until the end of their life, as an alternate to heart transplant for end-stage heart failure. Potential future indications for VADs may include permanent support for a failing heart.

Equipment

The VAD is inserted in the operating room. The equipment depends on the VAD system being used.

Implementation

● Before surgery, explain to the patient that food and fluid intake must be restricted and that you'll continuously monitor his cardiac function (using an electrocardiogram, a pulmonary artery [PA] catheter, and an arterial line). Offer the patient reassurance. Before sending him to the operating room, make sure that he has signed a consent form. **PCP**

● If time permits, shave the patient's chest and scrub it with an antiseptic solution.

● When the patient returns from surgery, administer analgesics, as ordered.

● Frequently monitor the patient's vital signs, intake, and output.

● Keep VAD exit sites immobile. The patient should be encouraged to rehabilitate as soon as clinically stable. **AACN**

● Monitor PA pressures. If you've been prepared to adjust the pump, maintain cardiac output at about 5 to 8 L/minute, central venous pressure at about 8 to 16 mm Hg, pulmonary artery wedge pressure at about 10 to 20 mm Hg, mean arterial pressure at greater than 60 mm Hg, and left atrial pressure at about 4 to 12 mm Hg. **AACN**

● Assess the patient who has a left VAD for signs and symptoms of right-sided heart failure.

● Monitor the patient for signs and symptoms of poor perfusion and ineffective pumping, including arrhythmias, hypotension, slow capillary refill, cool skin, oliguria or anuria, confusion, anxiety, and restlessness.

● Administer heparin as ordered and depending on the recommendation of the VAD system being used *to prevent clotting in the pump head and thrombus formation.* Check for bleeding, especially at the operative sites. Monitor laboratory studies, as ordered, especially complete blood count and coagulation studies. Follow your facility's anticoagulation protocol *because thromboembolism is a risk for the duration of VAD use.* **AACN**

● Assess the patient's incisions and the cannula insertion sites for signs of infection. Monitor the patient's white blood cell count and differential daily, and take rectal or core temperatures every 4 hours in the postoperative period. Maintain stability of all device exit sites *to promote tissue healing and decrease the risk of infection.*

● Change the dressing over the cannula sites daily or according to your facility's policy.

● Provide supportive care, including range-of-motion exercises and mouth and skin care.

● If VAD support is to be maintained for a prolonged period, follow your facility's protocol for assessments, dressings, and patient mobility as the patient's condition progresses.

● If the patient is going home with the device, give explicit discharge instructions based on the VAD system used.

Special considerations

● If the patient with an acute indication for a VAD fails to show improved ventricular function in a few days, the patient may need a transplant. If so, provide psychological support for the patient and his family as they endure evaluation or referral to a transplant center. You may also initiate the transplant process by contacting the appropriate agency.

● The psychological effects of the VAD can produce stress in the patient, his family, and his close friends. If appropriate, refer them to other support personnel.

● Understand that the patient with a VAD as a bridge to transplant may have a prolonged wait for heart transplantation. Maintaining or improving the patient's physical conditioning during this wait will improve posttransplant recovery and outcome.

Nursing diagnoses

● Compromised family coping
● Ineffective tissue perfusion: Cardiopulmonary

Expected outcomes

The patient (and his family) will:
● express their concerns about coping with patient's illness
● contact appropriate support sources
● remain oriented to person, place, and time
● exhibit no signs of poor perfusion
● maintain hemodynamic stability.

Complications

● The VAD carries a high risk of complications, including damaged blood cells, which can increase the likelihood of thrombus formation and subsequent pulmonary embolism or stroke.
● Other risks include infection and device failure.

Documentation

Note the patient's condition following insertion of the VAD. Document any pump adjustments as well as any complications and interventions according to your facility's policy.

Supportive references

Holmes, E.C. "Outpatient Management of Long-Term Assist Devices." *Cardiology Clinics* 21:93-99, February 2003.

Loh, E. "Maximizing Management of Patients with Decompensated Heart Failure," *Clinical Cardiology* 23(III Suppl):III, 1-5, March 2000.

Piccione, W. "Left Ventricular Assist Device Implantation: Short and Long-Term Surgical Complications," *Journal of Heart and Lung Transplantation* 19(8 Suppl):S89-94, August 2000.

Stevenson, L.W., et al. "Mechanical Cardiac Support 2000: Current Applications and Future Trial Design, June 2000, Bethesda, Maryland," *Journal of the American College of Cardiology* 37(1):340-70, January 2001.

Williams, M.R., and Oz, M.C. "Indications and Patient Selection for Mechanical Ventricular Assistance," *Annals of Thoracic Surgery* 71:586-91, March 2001.

6

Respiratory care

Respiratory diseases may be acute or chronic and may develop as a primary disorder or result from a cardiac condition. These conditions affect millions of people worldwide — no matter where you work, you're sure to encounter patients with respiratory conditions.

Caring for a patient with a respiratory condition will challenge your nursing skills. Not only is the patient's oxygenation compromised, but he may develop other problems, such as ineffective airway clearance and gas exchange, altered cardiac output, altered fluid volume, impaired thermoregulation, and decreased mobility. He may be anxious, cope ineffectively, and have an impaired ability to communicate. In addition, his nutritional status may be compromised. For such a patient, you'll need to develop an individual care plan to make sure that he achieves optimum gas exchange and physical function.

To meet your care goals, you need to have a working knowledge of the many therapies available to respiratory patients. Although many health care facilities have staff members who specialize in respiratory procedures, you still need to keep your knowledge up to date so you'll know and understand the rationales behind the patient's treatment and be able to perform or assist with procedures if necessary, recognize complications, and detect the need for additional therapy.

The information presented in this chapter will give you the most recent research in the form of evidence-based **EB** discoveries from the National Institutes of Health **NIH** and the Association for Healthcare Research and Quality **AHRQ**. Included are guidelines drawn up by professional groups, such as the American Association for Respiratory Care **AARC**, the American Association of Critical-Care Nurses **AACN**, the Society of Critical Care Medicine **SCCM**, the American Heart Association **AHA**, the American Lung Association **ALA**, the American Hospital Association's Patient Care Partnership **PCP**, and the Child Health

Corporation of America's Cooperative Pulse Oximetry FORUM **FORUM**. Some of the best practices in the chapter are grounded in fundamental principles of science **Science**. You'll also find recommendations from the Centers for Disease Control and Prevention **CDC** and the Joint Commission for Accreditation of Healthcare Organizations **JCAHO** so that you can give the best care to your patient. For points related to the equipment, manufacturers **MFR** may recommend specific guidelines.

Chest physiotherapy

Chest physiotherapy includes postural drainage, chest percussion and vibration, and coughing and deep-breathing exercises. Together, these techniques mobilize and eliminate secretions, reexpand lung tissue, and promote efficient use of respiratory muscles. Of critical importance to the bedridden patient, chest physiotherapy helps prevent or treat atelectasis and also may help prevent pneumonia — two respiratory complications that can seriously impede recovery. (See *Reducing health care-associated infections.*)

Postural drainage, or sequential repositioning of the patient, encourages peripheral pulmonary secretions to empty by gravity into the major bronchi or trachea when performed in conjunction with percussion and vibration. Secretions usually drain best with the patient positioned so that the bronchi are perpendicular to the floor. Lower and middle lobe bronchi usually empty best with the patient in the head-down position; upper lobe bronchi, in the head-up position. (See *Postural drainage positions,* pages 284 and 285.)

Percussing the chest with cupped hands mechanically dislodges thick, tenacious secretions from the bronchial walls. Vibration can be used with percussion, or as an alternative to it, in a patient who's frail, in pain, or recovering from thoracic surgery or trauma.

Candidates for chest physiotherapy include patients who expectorate large amounts of sputum (if sputum production is less than 25 ml/day, chest physiotherapy isn't needed), such as those with bronchiectasis and cystic fibrosis. The procedure hasn't proved effective in treating patients with status asthmaticus, lobar pneumonia, or acute exacerbations of chronic bronchitis when the patient has scant secretions and is being mechanically ventilated. Chest physiotherapy has little value for treating patients with stable, chronic bronchitis.

In critical care patients, including those on mechanical ventilation, postural drainage therapy (PDT) should be performed from every 4 to 6 hours, as indicated. The PDT order should be reevaluated at least every 48 hours, based on assessments from individual treatments.

In spontaneously breathing patients, PDT frequency should be determined by assessing the patient's response to therapy. Acute care patient orders should be reevaluated, based on patient response to therapy, at least every 72 hours or with a change in the patient's status. **AARC**

Contraindications for chest physiotherapy include active pulmonary bleeding with hemoptysis and the immediate posthemorrhage stage, fractured ribs or an unstable chest wall, lung contusions, pulmonary tuberculosis, untreated pneumothorax, acute asthma or bronchospasm, lung abscess or tumor, bony metastasis, head injury, recent myocardial infarction, and vomiting or immediately after eating. **AARC**

Equipment

Stethoscope • pillows • tilt or postural drainage table (if available) or adjustable hospital bed • emesis basin • facial tissues • suction equipment as needed • equipment for oral care • trash bag • optional: sterile specimen container, mechanical ventilator, supplemental oxygen

Preparation of equipment

● Gather the equipment at the patient's bedside.
● Set up suction equipment, if needed, and test its function.

Implementation

● Confirm the patient's identity using two patient identifiers according to facility policy. **JCAHO**

(Text continues on page 286.)

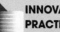

INNOVATIVE PRACTICE

Reducing health care-associated infections **EB**

Health care-associated infections (HAIs) most commonly attack the respiratory system, and complications from HAIs are a significant cause of patient deaths in hospitals. Patients on mechanical ventilators may have up to a 20-fold increase in the risk of hospital-acquired pneumonia. Western Medical Center, Tenet California Healthcare System, reduced HAIs in tracheal intubation using a multidisciplinary team approach.

Western Medical Center had a pneumonia rate of 10% to 15% in the intensive care unit (ICU), which was greater than the National Nosocomial Infections Surveillance System pooled mean. To reduce this rate, a multidisciplinary team was created to study the problem of reducing hospital-acquired pneumonia in high-risk ICU patients and implementing changes in nursing practice in the care of intubated patients admitted to the ICU.

Patients were evaluated using a Patient Identification for Rotational Therapy tool and those who were identified as high risk were placed on kinetic therapy within 48 hours. This therapy consists of rotation at a minimum of 40 degrees to either side for a minimum of 18 hours per day. High-risk patients also received nutritional therapy within 48 hours. Patients with long-term ventilator therapy received a tracheostomy and had a percutaneous endoscopic gastrostomy tube placed by day 7.

Patients were monitored using the Patient Identification for Rotational Therapy tool and specific quality indicators three times per week. Staff also received reinforcement in such areas as hand hygiene, suctioning, assessment skills, and modes of transmission.

The program resulted in a 43% decrease in hospital-acquired pneumonia in patients in the ICU. None of the patients placed on rotational therapy developed pneumonia. Of the patients receiving rotational therapy for pneumonia, 75% showed improvement within 48 hours. The length of time on a ventilator was reduced by 20% and length of stay in the ICU was decreased by 1 day.

Postural drainage positions

The following illustrations show the various postural drainage positions and the areas of the lungs affected by each.

Lower lobes: Posterior basal segments

Elevate the foot of the bed 30 degrees. Have the patient lie prone with his head lowered. Position pillows under his chest and abdomen. Percuss his lower ribs on both sides of his spine.

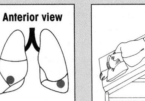

Posterior view

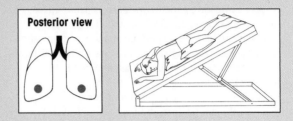

Lower lobes: Lateral basal segments

Elevate the foot of the bed 30 degrees. Instruct the patient to lie on his abdomen with his head lowered and his upper leg flexed over a pillow for support. Then have him rotate a quarter turn upward. Percuss his lower ribs on the uppermost portion of his lateral chest wall.

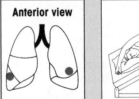

Anterior view

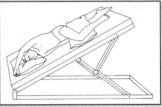

Lower lobes: Anterior basal segments

Elevate the foot of the bed 30 degrees. Instruct the patient to lie on his side with his head lowered. Then place pillows as shown. Percuss with a slightly cupped hand over his lower ribs just beneath the axilla. If an acutely ill patient has trouble breathing in this position, adjust the bed to an angle he can tolerate. Then begin percussion.

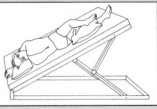

Anterior view

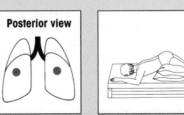

Lower lobes: Superior segments

With the bed flat, have the patient lie on his abdomen. Place two pillows under his hips. Percuss on both sides of his spine at the lower tips of his scapulae.

Posterior view

Right middle lobe: Medial and lateral segments

Elevate the foot of the bed 15 degrees. Have the patient lie on his left side with his head down and his knees flexed. Then have him rotate a quarter turn backward. Place a pillow beneath him. Percuss with your hand moderately cupped over the right nipple. For a woman, cup your hand so that its heel is under the armpit and your fingers extend forward beneath the breast.

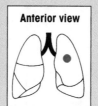

Anterior view

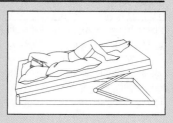

Left upper lobe: Superior and inferior segments, lingular portion

Elevate the foot of the bed 15 degrees. Have the patient lie on his right side with his head down and knees flexed. Then have him rotate a quarter turn backward. Place a pillow behind him, from shoulders to hips. Percuss with your hand moderately cupped over his left nipple. For a woman, cup your hand so that its heel is beneath the armpit and your fingers extend forward beneath the breast.

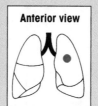

Anterior view

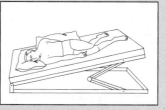

Upper lobes: Anterior segments

Make sure that the bed is flat. Have the patient lie on his back with a pillow folded under his knees. Then have him rotate slightly away from the side being drained. Percuss between his clavicle and nipple.

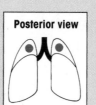

Anterior view

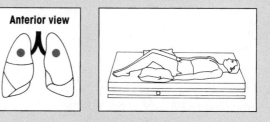

Upper lobes: Apical segments

Keep the bed flat. Have the patient lean back at a 30-degree angle against you and a pillow. Percuss with a cupped hand between his clavicles and the top of each scapula.

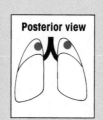

Posterior view

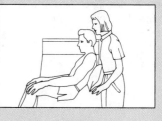

Upper lobes: Posterior segments

Keep the bed flat. Have the patient lean over a pillow at a 30-degree angle. Percuss and clap his upper back on each side.

Posterior view

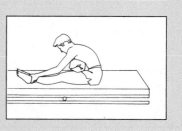

Performing percussion and vibration

To perform percussion, instruct the patient to breathe slowly and deeply, using the diaphragm, *to promote relaxation.* Hold your hands in a cupped shape, with fingers flexed and thumbs pressed tightly against your index fingers. Percuss each segment for 1 to 2 minutes by alternating your hands against the patient in a rhythmic manner. Listen for a hollow sound on percussion *to verify correct performance of the technique.*

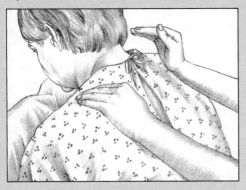

To perform vibration, ask the patient to inhale deeply and then exhale slowly through pursed lips. During exhalation, firmly press your fingers and the palms of your hands against the chest wall. Tense the muscles of your arms and shoulders in an isometric contraction *to send fine vibrations through the chest wall.* Vibrate during five exhalations over each chest segment.

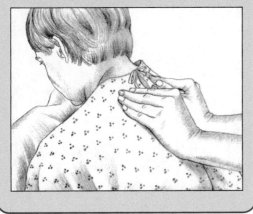

- Explain the procedure to the patient, provide privacy, and wash your hands. **CDC** **PCP**
- Auscultate the patient's lungs *to determine baseline respiratory status.*
- Position the patient as ordered. In generalized disease, drainage usually begins with the lower lobes, continues with the middle lobes, and ends with the upper lobes. In localized disease, drainage begins with the affected lobes and then proceeds to the other lobes *to avoid spreading the disease to uninvolved areas.*

TEACHING *Instruct the patient to remain in each position for 3 to 15 minutes. During this time, perform percussion and vibration as ordered. (See* Performing percussion and vibration.*)* **AARC**

- After PDT, percussion, or vibration, instruct the patient to cough *to remove loosened secretions.* First, tell him to inhale deeply through his nose and then exhale in three short huffs. Then have him inhale deeply again and cough through a slightly open mouth. Three consecutive coughs are highly effective. An effective cough sounds deep, low, and hollow; an ineffective one, high-pitched. Have the patient perform exercises for about 1 minute and then have him rest for 2 minutes. Gradually progress to a 10-minute exercise period four times daily. **Science**
- Provide oral hygiene *because secretions may have a foul taste or a stale odor.*
- Auscultate the patient's lungs *to evaluate the effectiveness of therapy.*

Special considerations

- For optimal effectiveness and safety, modify chest physiotherapy according to the patient's condition. For example, initiate or increase the flow of supplemental oxygen, if indicated. Also, suction the patient who has an ineffective cough reflex. If the patient tires quickly during therapy, shorten the sessions *because fatigue leads to shallow respirations and increased hypoxia.*
- Maintain adequate hydration in the patient receiving chest physiotherapy *to prevent mucus dehydration and promote easier mobilization.* Avoid performing postural drainage immediately before or within $1\frac{1}{2}$ hours after meals *to avoid nausea and aspiration of food or vomitus.*
- *Because chest percussion can induce bronchospasm,* any adjunct treatment (for example, intermittent

positive-pressure breathing or aerosol or nebulizer therapy) should precede chest physiotherapy.
● Refrain from percussing over the spine, liver, kidneys, or spleen *to avoid injury to the spine or internal organs*. Also, avoid performing percussion on bare skin or the female patient's breasts. Percuss over soft clothing (but not over buttons, snaps, or zippers), or place a thin towel over the chest wall. Remember to remove jewelry that might scratch or bruise the patient.

TEACHING *Explain coughing and deep-breathing exercises preoperatively so that the patient can practice them when he's pain-free and better able to concentrate. Postoperatively, splint the patient's incision using your hands or, if possible, teach the patient to splint it himself to minimize pain during coughing.*

Nursing diagnoses
● Impaired gas exchange
● Ineffective airway clearance
● Ineffective breathing pattern

Expected outcomes
The patient will:
● maintain adequate ventilation and normal oxygen levels
● express comfort during air exchange
● expectorate sputum
● have absent adventitious breath sounds (may worsen following therapy and then clear as secretions are cleared)
● maintain a patent airway
● breathe deeply and cough to remove secretions
● have a normal chest X-ray.

Complications
● During PDT in head-down positions, pressure on the diaphragm by abdominal contents can impair respiratory excursion and lead to hypoxia or orthostatic hypotension. The head-down position also may lead to increased intracranial pressure, which precludes the use of chest physiotherapy in a patient with acute neurologic impairment.
● Vigorous percussion or vibration can cause rib fracture, especially in the patient with osteoporosis.
● In a patient with emphysema who has blebs, coughing could lead to pneumothorax.

Documentation
Record the frequency, date, and time of chest physiotherapy; positions for postural drainage and length of time each is maintained; chest segments percussed or vibrated; the color, amount, odor, and viscosity of secretions produced and presence of any blood; any complications and interventions taken, and the patient's tolerance of treatment.

Supportive references
American Association for Respiratory Care. "AARC Clinical Practice Guideline: Directed Cough," *Respiratory Care* 38(5):495-99, May 1993.
American Association for Respiratory Care. "AARC Clinical Practice Guideline: Postural Drainage Therapy," *Respiratory Care* 36(12):1418-426, December 1991.
McCool, F.D., and Rosen, M.J. "Non-pharmacologic Airway Clearance Therapies: ACCP Evidence-based Clinical Practice Guidelines," *Chest* 129(1 Suppl): 250S-595, January 2006.
McKay, C. "Reducing Nosocomial Pneumonia in Critical Care," American Association of Critical-Care Nurses. *www.aacn.org*. Search word: McKay. **EB**
Vines, D.L., et al. "Current Respiratory Care, Part 1: Oxygen Therapy, Oximetry, Bronchial Hygiene," *Journal of Critical Illness* 15(9):507-10, 513-15, September 2000.

Cricothyrotomy

When endotracheal intubation or a tracheotomy can't be performed quickly to establish an airway, an emergency cricothyrotomy may be necessary. Performed rarely, this procedure involves puncturing the trachea through the cricothyroid membrane.

Usually, your role will be to assist a physician with this procedure. However, if a physician isn't available and the patient is likely to die before he can be intubated, you may have to perform the procedure yourself if you've been trained to do so. Ideally, cricothyrotomy is performed using sterile technique but, in an emergency, this may not be possible.

Equipment
Have one person stay with the patient while another collects the necessary equipment.

Performing an emergency cricothyrotomy

To perform an emergency cricothyrotomy, first put on sterile gloves and clean the patient's neck with a sterile gauze pad soaked in povidone-iodine solution. To reduce the risk of contamination, use a circular motion, working outward from the incision site.

● Locate the precise insertion site by sliding your thumb and fingers down to the thyroid gland. You'll know you've located its outer borders when the space between your fingers and thumb widens.

● Move your finger across the center of the gland, over the anterior edge of the cricoid ring.

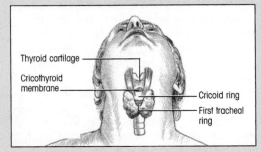

Thyroid cartilage
Cricothyroid membrane
Cricoid ring
First tracheal ring

Using a scalpel

● Make a horizontal incision, less than ½" (1.3 cm) long, in the cricothyroid membrane just above the cricoid ring.

● Insert a dilator to prevent tissue from closing around the incision. If a dilator isn't available, insert the handle of the scalpel and rotate it 90 degrees (as shown below).

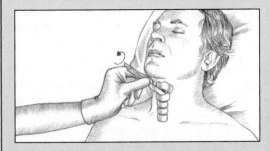

● If a small tracheostomy tube (#6 or smaller) is available, insert it into the opening and secure it *to help maintain a patent airway.* If a tracheostomy tube isn't available, tape the dilator or scalpel handle in place until a tracheostomy tube is available.

● If the patient can breathe spontaneously, attach a humidified oxygen source to the tracheostomy tube with a T tube; if he can't, attach a handheld resuscitation bag. You'll need to inflate the cuff of the tracheostomy tube with a syringe *to provide positive-pressure ventilation.*

● Auscultate bilaterally for breath sounds, and take the patient's vital signs.

● Dispose of the gloves properly and wash your hands. **CDC**

Using a needle

● Attach a 10-ml syringe to a 14G (or larger) through-the-needle or over-the-needle catheter. Then insert the catheter into the cricothyroid membrane just above the cricoid ring.

● Direct the catheter downward at a 45-degree angle, as shown below, to the trachea *to avoid damaging the vocal cords.* Maintain negative pressure by pulling back the syringe plunger as you advance the catheter. You'll know the catheter has entered the trachea when air enters the syringe.

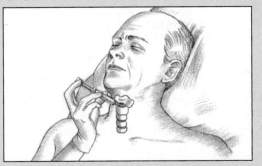

● When the catheter reaches the trachea, advance it and remove the needle and syringe. Tape the catheter in place.

● Attach the catheter hub to one end of the I.V. extension tubing. At the other end, attach a hand-operated release valve or a pressure-regulating adjustment valve. Connect the entire assembly to an oxygen source.

● Press the release valve to introduce oxygen into the trachea and inflate the lungs. When you can see that they're inflated, release the valve to allow passive exhalation. Adjust the pressure-regulating valve to the minimum pressure needed for adequate lung inflation.

● Auscultate bilaterally for breath sounds, and take the patient's vital signs.

● Dispose of the gloves properly and wash your hands. **CDC**

Scalpel or needle cricothyrotomy

Sterile gloves • povidone-iodine solution • sterile 4″ × 4″ gauze pads • dilator • tape • oxygen source

Scalpel cricothyrotomy

Scalpel • tracheostomy tube (#6 or smaller, if available) • handheld resuscitation bag or T tube and wide-bore oxygen tubing

Needle cricothyrotomy

14G (or larger) through-the-needle or over-the-needle catheter • 10-ml syringe • I.V. extension tubing • hand-operated release valve or pressure-regulating adjustment valve

Implementation

● Hyperextend the patient's neck to expose the area of the incision site.
● Have someone hold the patient's head in the correct position while you perform the procedure. (See *Performing an emergency cricothyrotomy.*)

Special considerations

● Immediately after the procedure, check for bleeding at the insertion site, subcutaneous emphysema or inadequate ventilation, and tracheal or vocal cord damage.

ALERT *Scalpel cricothyrotomy isn't recommended for children younger than age 12 because it could damage the cricoid cartilage, the only circumferential support to the upper trachea.*

Nursing diagnoses

● Impaired spontaneous ventilation

Expected outcomes

The patient will:
● maintain normal arterial blood gas levels
● maintain a respiratory rate within 5 breaths/minute of baseline.

Complications

● Hemorrhage, perforation of the thyroid or esophagus, and subcutaneous or mediastinal emphysema may occur from this procedure.
● Infection also may occur several days after the procedure.

Documentation

Document the date, time, and circumstances necessitating the procedure and the patient's vital signs. Note whether the patient initiated spontaneous respirations after the procedure. Record how much and by what method oxygen was delivered. If any procedures were performed after the airway was established — endotracheal intubation, for example — note them.

Supportive references

American Association for Respiratory Care. "AARC Clinical Practice Guideline: Management of Airway Emergencies," *Respiratory Care* 40(7):749-60, July 1995.

Blanda, M. "The Difficult Airway: Tools and Techniques for Acute Management," *Journal of Critical Illness* 15(7):358-60, 369-73, July 2000.

Rich, J.M., et al. "The SLAM Emergency Airway Flow Chart: A New Guide for Advanced Airway Practitioners," *AANA Journal* 72(6):431-39, December 2004.

Endotracheal intubation

Endotracheal (ET) intubation involves the oral or nasal insertion of a flexible tube through the larynx into the trachea for the purpose of controlling the airway and mechanically ventilating the patient. Performed by a physician, anesthetist, respiratory therapist, or nurse educated in the procedure, ET intubation usually occurs in emergencies, such as cardiopulmonary arrest, or in diseases such as epiglottiditis. However, intubation also may occur under more controlled circumstances such as just before surgery. In such instances, ET intubation requires patient teaching and preparation.

The 2005 International Consensus Conference on Cardiopulmonary Resuscitation and Emergency Cardiovascular Care Science provides recommendations on the skill level needed to intubate, methods of confirming ET tube placement, and alternatives to intubation.

The guidelines recommend that only health care workers with adequate training and experience or frequent retraining should perform ET intubation. If a health care worker isn't authorized to perform ET intubation, alternative measures, such as a laryngeal mask airway or an esophageal-tracheal Combitube, may be used. These alternatives are less likely to cause aspiration than the use of a bag-mask. **AHA**

Advantages of ET intubation include establishing and maintaining a patent airway, protecting against aspiration by sealing off the trachea from the digestive tract, permitting removal of tracheobronchial secretions in the patient who can't cough effectively, and providing a route for mechanical ventilation. Disadvantages include bypassing normal respiratory defenses against infection, reducing cough effectiveness, and preventing the patient from communicating.

Oral ET intubation is contraindicated in patients with acute cervical spinal injury and degenerative spinal disorders, while nasal intubation is contraindicated in patients with apnea, bleeding disorders, chronic sinusitis, or nasal obstructions.

Equipment

Two ET tubes (one spare) in appropriate size • 10-ml syringe • stethoscope • gloves • lighted laryngoscope with a handle and blades of various sizes, curved and straight • sedative • local anesthetic spray • mucosal vasoconstricting agent (for nasal intubation) • overbed or other table • water-soluble lubricant • adhesive or other strong tape or Velcro tube holder (see *Securing an ET tube*) • compound benzoin tincture • oral airway or bite block (for oral intubation) • suction equipment • handheld resuscitation bag with sterile swivel adapter • humidified oxygen source • optional: prepackaged intubation tray, sterile gauze pad, stylet, Magill forceps, sterile water, sterile basin

Preparation of equipment

● Gather the individual supplies, or use a prepackaged intubation tray that typically contains most of the necessary supplies.
● Select an ET tube of the appropriate size — typically, 2.5 to 5.5 mm, uncuffed, for children and 6 to 10 mm, cuffed, for adults. The typical size of an oral tube is 7.5 mm for women and 9 mm for men. Select a slightly smaller tube for nasal intubation.
● Check the light in the laryngoscope by snapping the appropriate-size blade into place; if the bulb doesn't light, replace the batteries or the laryngoscope, whichever is quicker.
● Using sterile technique, open the package containing the ET tube and, if desired, open the other supplies on an overbed table.

● Pour the sterile water into the sterile basin. Then, *to ease insertion,* lubricate the first 1″ (2.5 cm) of the distal end of the ET tube with the water-soluble lubricant, using aseptic technique. Do this by squeezing the lubricant directly onto the tube. Use only water-soluble lubricant *because it can be absorbed by mucous membranes.*
● Attach the syringe to the port on the tube's exterior pilot cuff.
● Slowly inflate the cuff, observing for uniform inflation. If desired, submerge the tube in the sterile water and watch for air bubbles. Use the syringe to deflate the cuff.
● A stylet may be used in oral intubation *to stiffen the tube.* Lubricate the entire stylet. Insert the stylet into the tube so that its distal tip lies about ½″ (1.3 cm) inside the distal end of the tube. Make sure that the stylet doesn't protrude from the tube *to avoid vocal cord trauma.*
● Prepare the humidified oxygen source and the suction equipment for immediate use.
● If the patient is in bed, remove the headboard *to provide easier access.*

Implementation

● Administer sedatives, as ordered, to induce amnesia or analgesia, and help calm and relax the conscious patient. Remove dentures and bridgework, if present. **Science**
● Administer oxygen until the ET tube is inserted *to prevent hypoxia.*
● Place the patient supine in the sniffing position *so that his mouth, pharynx, and trachea are extended.* For a blind intubation, place the patient's head and neck in a neutral position.
● Put on gloves. **CDC**
● For oral intubation, spray a local anesthetic, such as lidocaine (Xylocaine), deep into the posterior pharynx *to diminish the gag reflex and reduce patient discomfort.* For nasal intubation, spray a local anesthetic and a mucosal vasoconstrictor into the nasal passages *to anesthetize the nasal turbinates and reduce the chance of bleeding.*
● If necessary, suction the patient's pharynx just before ET tube insertion *to improve visualization of the patient's pharynx and vocal cords.*
● Time each intubation attempt, limiting attempts to less than 30 seconds *to prevent hypoxia.*

Securing an ET tube

Before securing an endotracheal (ET) tube, make sure that the patient's face is clean, dry, and free from beard stubble. If possible, suction his mouth and dry the ET tube just before taping. Check the reference mark on the tube to ensure correct placement. After securing, always check for bilateral breath sounds to ensure that the ET tube hasn't been displaced by manipulation. To secure the tube, use one of the methods described here.

Method 1
- Cut one piece of 1″ cloth adhesive tape long enough to wrap around the patient's head and overlap in front, and then cut an 8″ (20.3-cm) piece of tape and center it on the longer piece, sticky sides together.
- Cut a 5″ (12.7-cm) slit in each end of the longer tape (as shown).

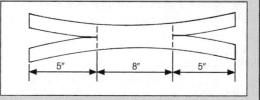

- Apply benzoin tincture to the patient's cheeks, under his nose, and under the lower lip. (Don't spray benzoin directly on the patient's face; the vapors can be irritating if inhaled and can harm the eyes.)
- Place the top half of one end of the tape under the patient's nose and wrap the lower half around the ET tube. Place the lower half of the other end of the tape along his lower lip and wrap the top half around the tube.

Method 2
- ET tube holders are available that can help secure an ET tube.
- Made of hard plastic or of softer material, the tube holder secures the ET tube in place. The tube holder is available in adult and pediatric sizes. Some models come with bite blocks attached.
- Place the strap around the patient's neck and secure it around the tube with Velcro fasteners (as shown).
- Because each model is different, check the manufacturer's guidelines for correct placement and care. **MFR**

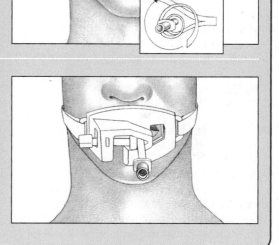

Intubation with direct visualization
- Stand at the head of the patient's bed. Using your right hand, hold the patient's mouth open by crossing your index finger over your thumb, placing your thumb on the patient's upper teeth and your index finger on his lower teeth. *This technique provides greater leverage.*

- Grasp the laryngoscope handle in your left hand, and gently slide the blade into the right side of the patient's mouth. Center the blade, and push the patient's tongue to the left. Hold the patient's lower lip away from his teeth *to prevent the lip from being traumatized.*

● Advance the blade to expose the epiglottis. When using a straight blade, insert the tip under the epiglottis; when using a curved blade, insert the tip between the base of the tongue and the epiglottis.

● Lift the laryngoscope handle upward and away from your body at a 45-degree angle *to reveal the vocal cords*. Avoid pivoting the laryngoscope against the patient's teeth *to avoid damaging them*.

● If desired, have an assistant apply pressure to the cricoid ring *to occlude the esophagus and minimize gastric regurgitation*. **EB**

● When performing oral intubation, insert the ET tube into the right side of the patient's mouth. When performing nasotracheal intubation, insert the ET tube through the nostril and into the pharynx. Then use Magill forceps to guide the tube through the vocal cords.

● Guide the tube into the vertical openings of the larynx between the vocal cords, being careful not to mistake the horizontal opening of the esophagus for the larynx. If the vocal cords are closed because of a spasm, wait a few seconds for them to relax, and then gently guide the tube past them *to avoid traumatic injury*.

● Advance the tube until the cuff disappears beyond the vocal cords. Avoid advancing the tube further *to avoid occluding a major bronchus or precipitate lung collapse*.

● Holding the ET tube in place, quickly remove the stylet, if present.

Blind nasotracheal intubation

● Pass the ET tube along the floor of the nasal cavity. If necessary, use gentle force to pass the tube through the nasopharynx and into the pharynx.

● Listen and feel for air movement through the tube as it's advanced *to ensure that the tube is properly placed in the airway*.

● Slip the ET tube between the vocal cords when the patient inhales *because the vocal cords separate on inhalation*.

● When the tube is past the vocal cords, the breath sounds should become louder. If at any time during tube advancement breath sounds disappear, withdraw the tube until they reappear.

After intubation

● Inflate the tube's cuff with 5 to 10 cc of air, until you feel resistance. When the patient is mechanically ventilated, you'll use the minimal-leak technique or the minimal occlusive volume technique to establish correct inflation of the cuff. (For instructions, see "Tracheal cuff pressure measurement," page 350.)

● Remove the laryngoscope. If the patient was intubated orally, insert an oral airway or bite block *to prevent the patient from obstructing airflow or puncturing the tube with his teeth*.

● Confirm ET tube placement by listening for bilateral breath sounds, observing chest expansion, and using techniques, such as capnography or capnometry.

● The 2005 guidelines recommend confirming ET tube placement using techniques other than physical examination, such as esophageal detector devices, qualitative end-tidal carbon dioxide indicators, and capnographic and capnometric devices. Be aware that devices that rely on exhaled carbon dioxide may not be accurate in patients in cardiac arrest *because of reduced lung perfusion* and in patients with large amounts of dead space in the lungs such as a patient with a large pulmonary embolus. Other methods that complement nonphysical examination techniques include observing for bilateral chest expansion, auscultating for bilateral breath sounds, absence of abdominal sounds, feeling for warm exhalations, and observing for condensation in the ET tube.

● If you determine that the tube isn't in the trachea, immediately deflate the cuff and remove the tube. After reoxygenating the patient to prevent hypoxia, repeat insertion using a sterile tube *to prevent contamination of the trachea*. **CDC**

● Auscultate bilaterally *to exclude the possibility of endobronchial intubation*. If you fail to hear breath sounds on both sides of the chest, you may have inserted the tube into one of the mainstem bronchi (usually the right one *because of its wider angle at the bifurcation*); such insertion occludes the other bronchus and lungs and results in atelectasis on the obstructed side. The tube also may be resting on the carina, resulting in dry secretions that obstruct both bronchi. (The patient's coughing and fighting the ventilator will alert you to the problem.) To correct these situations, deflate the cuff, withdraw the tube 1 to 2 mm, auscultate for bilateral breath sounds, and reinflate the cuff.

● When you've confirmed correct ET tube placement, administer oxygen or initiate mechanical ventilation, and suction, if indicated.

● To secure tube position, apply compound benzoin tincture to each cheek and let it dry. Tape the tube firmly with adhesive or another strong tape or use a Velcro tube holder.

● Inflate the cuff with the minimal-leak or minimal occlusive volume technique. For the minimal-leak technique, attach a 10-ml syringe to the port on the tube's exterior pilot cuff, and place a stethoscope on the side of the patient's neck. Inject small amounts of air with each breath until you hear no leak. Then aspirate 0.1 cc of air from the cuff *to create a minimal air leak.* Record the amount of air needed to inflate the cuff. For the minimal occlusive volume technique, follow the first two steps of the minimal-leak technique, but place the stethoscope over the trachea instead. Aspirate until you hear a small leak on inspiration, and add just enough air to stop the leak. Record the amount of air needed to inflate the cuff for subsequent monitoring of tracheal dilation or erosion.

● Clearly note the centimeter marking on the tube where it exits the patient's mouth or nose. *By periodically monitoring this mark, you can detect tube displacement.*

● Make sure a chest X-ray is taken *to verify tube position.*

● Place a swivel adapter between the ET tube and the humidified oxygen source *to allow for intermittent suctioning and to reduce tube tension.*

● Place the patient on his side with his head in a comfortable position *to avoid tube kinking and airway obstruction.*

● Auscultate both sides of the chest, and watch chest movement as indicated by the patient's condition *to ensure correct tube placement and full lung ventilation.* Provide frequent oral care to the orally intubated patient, and position the ET tube to prevent the formation of pressure ulcers and to avoid excessive pressure on the sides of the mouth. Provide frequent nasal and oral care to the nasally intubated patient *to prevent formation of pressure ulcers and drying of oral mucous membranes.* **Science**

● Suction secretions through the ET tube as the patient's condition indicates *to clear secretions and to prevent mucus plugs from obstructing the tube.*

Special considerations

● Orotracheal intubation is preferred in emergencies *because insertion is easier and faster than with nasotracheal intubation.* However, maintaining exact tube placement is more difficult, and the tube must be well secured *to avoid kinking and prevent bronchial obstruction or accidental extubation.* Orotracheal intubation is also poorly tolerated by conscious patients *because it stimulates salivation, coughing, and retching.*

● Nasotracheal intubation is preferred for elective insertion when the patient is capable of spontaneous ventilation for a short period. Blind intubation is typically used in conscious patients who risk imminent respiratory arrest or who have cervical spinal injury.

● Although nasotracheal intubation is more comfortable than oral intubation, it's also more difficult to perform. *Because the tube passes blindly through the nasal cavity,* the procedure causes greater tissue trauma, increases the risk of infection by nasal bacteria introduced into the trachea, and risks pressure necrosis of the nasal mucosa. However, exact tube placement is easier, and the risk of dislodgment is lower. The cuff on the ET tube maintains a closed system that permits positive-pressure ventilation and protects the airways from aspiration of secretions and gastric contents.

● Although low-pressure cuffs have significantly reduced the incidence of tracheal erosion and necrosis caused by cuff pressure on the tracheal wall, overinflation of a low-pressure cuff can negate the benefit. Use the minimal-leak technique to avoid these complications. Inflating the cuff a bit more to make a complete seal with the least amount of air is the next most desirable method.

● Always record the volume of air needed to inflate the cuff. A gradual increase in this volume indicates tracheal dilation or erosion. A sudden increase in volume indicates rupture of the cuff and requires immediate reintubation if the patient is being ventilated or if he requires continuous cuff inflation to maintain a high concentration of delivered oxygen. When the cuff has been inflated, measure its pressure at least every 8 hours *to avoid overinflation.* Normal cuff pressure is about 18 mm Hg.

● When neither method of ET intubation is possible, consider retrograde intubation as an alternative. (See *Retrograde intubation,* page 294.)

Nursing diagnoses

● Impaired spontaneous ventilation
● Risk for aspiration

Retrograde intubation

When the patient's airway can't be secured using conventional oral or nasal intubation, retrograde intubation should be considered. In this alternative technique, a wire is inserted through the trachea and out the mouth and is then used to guide the insertion of an endotracheal (ET) tube (as shown below).

Only physicians, nurses, and paramedics who have been specially trained may perform retrograde intubation. However, the procedure has numerous advantages. It requires little or no head movement, it's less invasive than cricothyrotomy or tracheotomy and doesn't leave a permanent scar, and it doesn't require direct visualization of the vocal cords.

Retrograde intubation is contraindicated in patients with complete airway obstruction, coagulopathy, a thyroid tumor, or an enlarged thyroid gland that overlies the cricothyroid ligament. It's also contraindicated in patients whose mouths can't open wide enough to allow the guide wire to be retrieved. Possible complications include minor bleeding and hematoma formation at the puncture site, subcutaneous emphysema, hoarseness, and bleeding into the trachea.

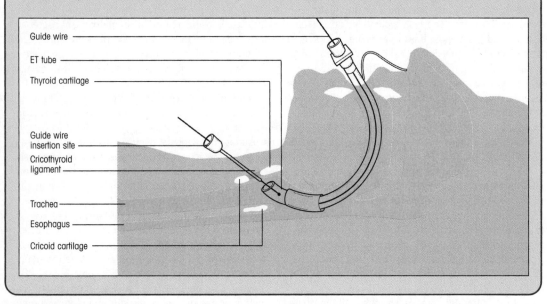

Guide wire
ET tube
Thyroid cartilage
Guide wire insertion site
Cricothyroid ligament
Trachea
Esophagus
Cricoid cartilage

Expected outcomes

The patient will:
• maintain a respiratory rate within 5 breaths/minute of baseline
• maintain normal arterial blood gas levels
• breathe spontaneously after ventilator support is withdrawn
• have no adventitious breath sounds on auscultation.

Complications

• ET intubation can result in apnea caused by reflex breath-holding or interruption of oxygen delivery; bronchospasm; tooth damage or loss; aspiration of blood, secretions, or gastric contents; and injury to the lips, mouth, pharynx, or vocal cords. It also can result in laryngeal edema and erosion and tracheal stenosis, erosion, and necrosis.
• Nasotracheal intubation can result in nasal bleeding, laceration, sinusitis, and otitis media.

Documentation

Record the date and time of the procedure, its indication and success or failure, tube type and size, cuff size, depth of ET tube as marked at the front teeth, amount of inflation and inflation technique, administration of medication, initiation of supplemental oxygen or ventilation therapy, results of chest auscultation and the chest X-ray, any complications and interventions, and the patient's reaction to the procedure.

Supportive references

American Heart Association. "2005 AHA Guidelines for Cardiopulmonary Resuscitation and Emergency Cardiovascular Care: International Consensus on Science," *Circulation* 112(22 Suppl): IV-1-IV-211, November 2005.

Lynn-McHale Wiegand, D.J., and Carlson, K.K. *AACN Procedure Manual for Critical Care,* 5th ed. Philadelphia: W.B. Saunders Co., 2005. **EB**

Wong, E., et al. "Confirmation of Endotracheal Tube Placement: Analysis of 6,294 Emergency Department Intubations," *Annals of Emergency Medicine* 36(4 Part 2):S53, October 2000.

Endotracheal tube care

The intubated patient requires meticulous care to ensure airway patency and prevent complications until he can maintain independent ventilation. This care includes frequent assessment of his airway status, maintenance of proper cuff pressure to prevent tissue ischemia and necrosis, repositioning the tube to avoid traumatic manipulation, and constant monitoring for complications. Endotracheal (ET) tubes are repositioned for patient comfort or if a chest X-ray shows improper placement. Move the tube from one side of the mouth to the other to prevent pressure ulcers.

Equipment
Maintaining the airway
Stethoscope • suction equipment • gloves

Repositioning the ET tube
10-ml syringe • compound benzoin tincture • stethoscope • adhesive or hypoallergenic tape or Velcro tube holder • suction equipment • sedative or 2% lidocaine • gloves • handheld resuscitation bag with mask in case of accidental extubation

Removing the ET tube
10-ml syringe • suction equipment • supplemental oxygen source with mask • cool-mist large-volume nebulizer • handheld resuscitation bag with mask • gloves • equipment for reintubation

Preparation of equipment
Repositioning the ET tube
● Assemble all equipment at the patient's bedside.
● Using sterile technique, set up the suction equipment.

Removing the ET tube
● Assemble all equipment at the patient's bedside.
● Set up the suction and supplemental oxygen equipment.
● Have ready all equipment for emergency reintubation.

Implementation
● Confirm the patient's identity using two patient identifiers according to facility policy. **JCAHO**
● Explain the procedure to the patient even if he doesn't appear to be alert. Provide privacy, wash your hands thoroughly, and put on gloves. **CDC**

Maintaining airway patency
● Auscultate the patient's lungs regularly and at any sign of respiratory distress. If you detect an obstructed airway, determine the cause and treat it accordingly. If secretions are obstructing the ET tube lumen, suction the secretions from the tube. (See "Tracheal suction," page 352.)

▲ **ALERT** *Ongoing monitoring of ET tube placement is recommended, especially when transporting the patient.* **AHA**
● If the ET tube has slipped from the trachea into the right or left mainstem bronchus, breath sounds will be absent over one lung. Obtain a chest X-ray as ordered *to verify tube placement* and, if necessary, reposition the tube.

Repositioning the ET tube
● Get help from a respiratory therapist or another nurse *to prevent accidental extubation during the procedure if the patient coughs.* **Science**
● Hyperoxygenate the patient and then suction the patient's trachea through the ET tube to remove secretions, which can cause the patient to cough during the procedure. Then suction the patient's pharynx to remove secretions that may have accumulated above the ET tube cuff. *This helps to prevent aspiration of secretions during cuff deflation.* **EB1**
● To prevent traumatic manipulation of the tube, instruct the assisting nurse to hold it as you carefully

untape the tube or unfasten the Velcro tube holder. When freeing the tube, locate a landmark, such as a number on the tube, or measure the distance from the patient's mouth to the top of the tube *so that you have a reference point when moving the tube.* **Science**

- Deflate the cuff by attaching a 10-ml syringe to the pilot balloon port and aspirating air until you meet resistance and the pilot balloon deflates. Deflate the cuff before moving the ET tube *because the cuff forms a seal within the trachea and movement of an inflated cuff can damage the tracheal wall and vocal cords.* **AARC**

- Reposition the ET tube as necessary, noting new landmarks or measuring the length. Immediately reinflate the cuff; instruct the patient to inhale, and slowly inflate the cuff using a 10-ml syringe attached to the pilot balloon port. As you do this, use your stethoscope to auscultate the patient's neck *to determine the presence of an air leak.* When air leakage ceases, stop cuff inflation and, while still auscultating the patient's neck, aspirate a small amount of air until you detect a slight leak. *This creates a minimal air leak, which indicates that the cuff is inflated at the lowest pressure possible to create an adequate seal.* If the patient is being mechanically ventilated, aspirate to create a minimal air leak during the inspiratory phase of respiration *because the positive pressure of the ventilator during inspiration will create a larger leak around the cuff.* Note the number of cubic centimeters of air required to achieve a minimal air leak. **AARC**

- Measure cuff pressure, and compare the reading with previous pressure readings *to prevent overinflation.* Then use benzoin and hypoallergenic tape to secure the ET tube in place, or refasten the Velcro tube holder.

  ✓ **CLINICAL IMPACT** *Studies have shown that adhesive or twill tape has been effective in preventing an unplanned extubation and maintaining skin integrity of the oral mucosa and face.* **EB2**

- The ET tube also can be secured with a backboard commercial device. Studies show that using backboard commercial devices better prevent tube displacement when compared to using tape. **AHA**

- Make sure that the patient is comfortable and the airway is patent. Properly clean or dispose of equipment.

- When the cuff is inflated, measure pressure at least every 8 hours *to avoid overinflation.* **AARC**
- Auscultate the lungs *to ensure bilateral breath sounds.* **AARC**

Removing the ET tube

- Explain the procedure to the patient *to reduce his anxiety.*

  ✓ **CLINICAL IMPACT** *When the patient no longer requires mechanical ventilation, his ET tube may be removed. The Agency for Healthcare Research and Quality (AHRQ) selected the McMaster University Evidence-Based Practice Center to investigate issues related to weaning patients from mechanical ventilation. Their recommendations include:*

- *Develop a protocol implemented by nurses and respiratory therapists to begin trials to decrease ventilator support soon after intubation. This ventilator support should be reduced at every opportunity.*
- *When using step-wise reductions in mechanical ventilation, pressure support mode or multiple T-piece trials may be better than using intermittent mandatory ventilation.*
- *When using weaning trials of unassisted breathing, low levels of pressure support may be helpful.*
- *Patients who are alert, cooperative, and ready to breathe without an artificial airway may benefit from early extubation and the use of noninvasive positive-pressure ventilation.* **AHRQ**

- When you're authorized to remove the tube, obtain another nurse's assistance *to prevent traumatic manipulation of the tube when it's untaped or unfastened.*
- Elevate the head of the patient's bed to high Fowler's position, unless contraindicated.
- Suction the patient's oropharynx and nasopharynx to remove accumulated secretions and to help prevent aspiration of secretions when the cuff is deflated. **Science**
- Using a handheld resuscitation bag or the mechanical ventilator, give the patient several deep breaths through the ET tube *to hyperinflate his lungs and to increase his oxygen reserve.*
- Attach a 10-ml syringe to the pilot balloon port, and aspirate air until you meet resistance and the pilot balloon deflates. If you fail to detect an air leak around the deflated cuff, notify the physician imme-

diately and *don't* proceed with extubation. *Absence of an air leak may indicate marked tracheal edema, which can result in total airway obstruction if the ET tube is removed.* **AARC**

● If you detect the proper air leak, untape or unfasten the ET tube while the assisting nurse stabilizes the tube.

● Insert a sterile suction catheter through the ET tube. Then apply suction and ask the patient to take a deep breath and to open his mouth fully and pretend to cry out. *This causes abduction of the vocal cords and reduces the risk of laryngeal trauma during withdrawal of the tube.*

● Simultaneously remove the ET tube and the suction catheter in one smooth, outward and downward motion, following the natural curve of the patient's mouth. *Suctioning during extubation removes secretions retained at the end of the tube and prevents aspiration.* **AARC**

● Give the patient supplemental oxygen. For maximum humidity, use a cool-mist, large-volume nebulizer *to help decrease airway irritation, patient discomfort, and laryngeal edema.*

● Encourage the patient to cough and deep-breathe. Remind him that a sore throat and hoarseness are to be expected and will gradually subside.

● Make sure that the patient is comfortable and the airway is patent. Clean or dispose of equipment.

● After extubation, auscultate the patient's lungs frequently and watch for signs of respiratory distress. Stay especially alert for stridor or other evidence of upper airway obstruction. If ordered, obtain a sample for arterial blood gas (ABG) analysis. **AARC**

Special considerations

● When repositioning an ET tube, be especially careful in patients with highly sensitive airways. Sedation or direct instillation of 2% lidocaine to numb the airway may be indicated in such patients. *Because the lidocaine is absorbed systemically,* you must have a physician's order to use it.

● After extubation of a patient who has been intubated for an extended time, keep reintubation supplies readily available for at least 12 hours or until you're sure he can tolerate extubation. **AARC**

● Never extubate a patient unless someone skilled in intubation is readily available.

● If you inadvertently cut the pilot balloon on the cuff, immediately call the person responsible for intubation in your facility, who will remove the damaged ET tube and replace it with one that's intact. Don't remove the tube *because a tube with an air leak is better than no airway.* **AARC**

Nursing diagnoses

● Impaired gas exchange
● Risk for aspiration
● Risk for trauma

Expected outcomes

The patient will:
● maintain normal ABG levels
● express feelings of comfort in maintaining air exchange
● have no adventitious breath sounds on auscultation
● avoid injury to the larynx or trachea.

Complications

● Traumatic injury to the larynx or trachea may result from tube manipulation, accidental extubation, or tube slippage into the right bronchus.

● Ventilatory failure and airway obstruction due to laryngospasm or marked tracheal edema are the gravest possible complications of extubation.

Documentation

After ET tube repositioning, record the date and time of the procedure, reason for repositioning (such as malposition shown by chest X-ray), new tube position, total amount of air in the cuff after the procedure, any complications and interventions, and the patient's tolerance of the procedure. Document the physical findings and nonphysical examination to confirm tube placement.

After extubation, record the date and time of extubation, presence or absence of stridor or other signs of upper airway edema, type of supplemental oxygen administered, any complications and required subsequent therapy, and the patient's tolerance of the procedure.

Supportive references

Agency for Healthcare Research and Quality. *Criteria for Weaning from Mechanical Ventilation.* Evidence

How ETco_2 monitoring works

The optical portion of an end-tidal carbon dioxide (ETco_2) monitor contains an infrared light source, a sample chamber, a special carbon dioxide (CO_2) filter, and a photodetector. The infrared light passes through the sample chamber and is absorbed in varying amounts, depending on the amount of CO_2 the patient has just exhaled. The photodetector measures CO_2 content and relays this information to the microprocessor in the monitor, which displays the CO_2 value and waveform.

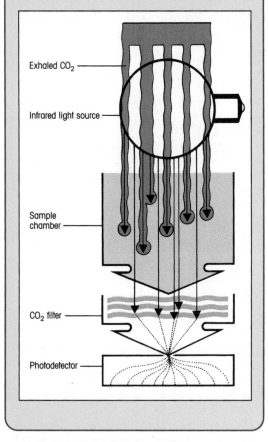

Report/Technology Assessment: Number 23. AHRQ Publication No. 00-E028, June 2000. *www.ahrq.gov/clinic/epcsums/mechsumm.htm*.

American Association for Respiratory Care. "AARC Clinical Practice Guideline: Removal of the Endotracheal Tube," *Respiratory Care* 44(1):85-90, January 1999.

American Heart Association. "2005 AHA Guidelines for Cardiopulmonary Resuscitation and Emergency Cardiovascular Care: International Consensus on Science," *Circulation* 112(22 Suppl):IV-1-IV-211, November 2005.

Lynn-McHale Wiegand, D.J., and Carlson, K.K. *AACN Procedure Manual for Critical Care*, 5th ed. Philadelphia: W.B. Saunders Co., 2005. **EB1**

Moore, A.S. "Clinical Highlights: Does It Matter Whether You Use Twill or Adhesive Tape?" *RN* 62(2):20, February 1999. **EB2**

End-tidal carbon dioxide monitoring

Monitoring end-tidal carbon dioxide (ETco_2) determines the carbon dioxide (CO_2) concentration in exhaled gas. In this technique, a photodetector measures the amount of infrared light absorbed by airway gas during inspiration and expiration. (Light absorption increases along with the CO_2 concentration.) A monitor converts these data to a CO_2 value and a corresponding waveform, or capnogram, if capnography is used. (See *How ETco_2 monitoring works*.)

ETco_2 monitoring provides information about the patient's pulmonary, cardiac, and metabolic status that aids patient management and helps prevent clinical compromise. This technique has become standard during anesthesia administration and mechanical ventilation. Research suggests that ETco_2 monitoring may be used to assess whether a patient will survive after cardiopulmonary arrest. (See *Using ETco_2 to predict survival in cardiopulmonary arrest*. See also "Cardiopulmonary resuscitation," page 217.)

The sensor, which contains an infrared light source and a photodetector, is positioned at one of two sites in the monitoring setup. With a mainstream monitor, it's positioned directly at the patient's airway with an airway adapter, between the endotracheal (ET) tube and the breathing circuit tubing. With a sidestream monitor, the airway adapter is positioned at the airway (regardless of whether the patient is intubated) *to allow aspiration of gas from the patient's airway back to the sensor, which lies either within or close to the monitor.*

Some CO_2 detection devices provide semiquantitative indications of CO_2 concentrations, supplying an approximate range rather than a specific value for $ETco_2$. Other devices simply indicate whether CO_2 is present during exhalation. (See *Analyzing CO_2 levels*, page 300.)

$ETco_2$ monitoring may be used to help wean a patient with a stable acid-base balance from mechanical ventilation. It also reduces the need for frequent arterial blood gas (ABG) measurements, especially when combined with pulse oximetry. Other uses for $ETco_2$ monitoring include assessing resuscitation efforts and identifying the return of spontaneous circulation. This technique also detects apnea because no CO_2 is exhaled when breathing stops.

Advanced cardiac life support guidelines recommend the confirmation of ET tube position using clinical assessment and confirmation devices, such as an $ETco_2$ indicator or esophageal detection device. $ETco_2$ monitoring used during ET intubation can avert neurologic injury and even death by confirming correct tube placement and detecting accidental esophageal intubation because CO_2 isn't normally produced by the stomach. **AHA**

The Society of Critical Care Medicine recommends that every intensive care unit have capnography available. **SCCM**

According to the American Association for Respiratory Care (AARC) guidelines, capnography should be used for all patients on mechanical ventilation. Capnography is also indicated to:
- evaluate exhaled CO_2, especially $ETco_2$, which is the maximum partial pressure of CO_2 exhaled just before the beginning of inspiration (tidal breath)
- monitor the severity of pulmonary disease and to evaluate the response to therapy, especially therapy intended to improve the ratio of dead space to tidal volume, matching of ventilation-perfusion ratio, and therapy intended to increase coronary blood flow
- determine that tracheal rather than esophageal intubation has taken place
- monitor the integrity of the ventilatory circuit, including the artificial airway
- evaluate the efficiency of mechanical ventilatory support by determining the difference between the partial pressure of arterial CO_2 ($Paco_2$) and the partial $PETco_2$
- measure the volume of CO_2 elimination in order to monitor metabolic rate and alveolar ventilation

Using ETco_2 to predict survival in cardiopulmonary arrest **EB1**

Researchers have found that patients with end-tidal carbon dioxide (ETco_2) levels of 10 mm Hg or less after 20 minutes of cardiopulmonary resuscitation aren't likely to survive. The higher the ETco_2 levels, the greater the chances of survival. In fact, the sensitivity, specificity, positive predictive value, and negative predictive value of ETco_2 to predict outcomes following resuscitation procedures was 100%. Some researchers recommend that aggressive resuscitation efforts be continued in patients with ETco_2 values greater than 15 mm Hg.

- monitor adequacy of pulmonary and coronary blood flow
- monitor inspired CO_2 when CO_2 gas is being therapeutically administered as a graphic evaluation of the ventilator-patient interface. **AARC** **EB2**

Ongoing $ETco_2$ monitoring throughout intubation also can prove valuable because an ET tube may become dislodged during manipulation or patient movement or transport.

Equipment
Gloves • mainstream or sidestream CO_2 monitor • CO_2 sensor • airway adapter as recommended by the manufacturer (a neonatal adapter may have a much smaller dead space, making it appropriate for a smaller patient) • $ETco_2$ sensor

Preparation of equipment
- If the monitor you're using isn't self-calibrating, calibrate it as the manufacturer directs. **MFR**
- If you're using a sidestream CO_2 monitor, be sure to replace the water trap between patients, if directed. *The trap allows humidity from exhaled gases to be condensed into an attached container.* Newer sidestream models don't require water traps.

Implementation
- Confirm the patient's identity using two patient identifiers according to facility policy. **JCAHO**

Analyzing CO$_2$ levels

Depending on the end-tidal carbon dioxide (ETco_2) detector you use, the meaning of color changes within the detector dome may differ from the analysis for the Easy Cap detector described below.

- The rim of the Easy Cap is divided into sections A, B, and C. Their control colors range from purple (in section A), signifying the absence of carbon dioxide (CO$_2$), to beige, tan and, finally, yellow (in section C).The numbers in the sections range from 0.03 to 5 and indicate the percentage of exhaled CO$_2$.
- The color in the center rectangle reflects the patient's CO$_2$ level. It should fluctuate during ventilation from purple (matching section A) during inspiration to yellow (matching section C) at the end of expiration. This indicates that the ETco_2 levels are adequate — above 2%.
- An end-expiratory color change from the C range to the B range may be the first sign of hemodynamic instability.
- During cardiopulmonary resuscitation (CPR), an end-expiratory color change from the A or B range to the C range may mean the return of spontaneous ventilation.
- During prolonged cardiac arrest, inadequate pulmonary perfusion leads to inadequate gas exchange. The patient exhales little or no CO$_2$, so the color stays in the purple range even with proper intubation. Ineffective CPR also leads to inadequate pulmonary perfusion.

Color indicators on ETco_2 detector

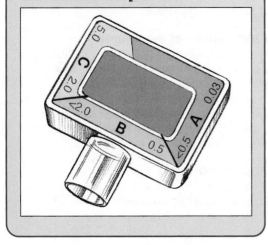

- If the patient requires ET intubation, an ETco_2 detector or monitor is usually applied immediately after the tube is inserted. If he doesn't require intubation or is already intubated and alert, explain the purpose and expected duration of monitoring. Tell an intubated patient that the monitor will painlessly measure the amount of CO$_2$ he exhales. Inform a nonintubated patient that the monitor will track his CO$_2$ concentration to make sure that his breathing is effective.
- Wash your hands. **CDC** After turning on the monitor and calibrating it (if necessary), position the airway adapter and CO$_2$ sensor as the manufacturer directs. **MFR** For an intubated patient, position the adapter directly on the ET tube. For a nonintubated patient, place the adapter at or near the patient's airway. (An oxygen-delivery cannula may have a sample port through which gas can be aspirated for monitoring.) **AARC**
- Turn on all alarms and adjust alarm settings as appropriate for your patient. Make sure that the alarm volume is loud enough to hear. **AARC**

Special considerations

- Wear gloves when handling the airway adapter *to prevent cross-contamination.* **CDC** Make sure that the adapter is changed with every breathing circuit and ET tube change.
- Place the adapter on the ET tube *to avoid contaminating exhaled gases with fresh gas flow from the ventilator.* If you're using a heat and moisture exchanger, you may be able to position the airway adapter between the exchanger and breathing circuit.
- If the patient's ETco_2 values differ from the Paco_2 level, assess him for factors that can influence ETco_2 — especially when the differential between arterial and ETco_2 values (the arterial absolute difference of carbon dioxide [a-ADco_2]) is above normal. Such factors include decreasing CO$_2$ production, increased CO$_2$ removal caused by hyperventilation, and diminished pulmonary perfusion.

✔ **CLINICAL IMPACT** *After the patient is started on ETco_2 monitoring, obtain a sample for ABG analysis to determine baseline values. Note the difference between ETco_2 and Paco_2 values (a-ADco_2). Typically, ETco_2 levels are 1 to 6 mm Hg less than Paco_2 levels. As long as a-ADco_2 is normal, you can estimate the Paco_2 level from the ETco_2 level. Each time ABG values are obtained, note a-ADco_2. If you use ETco_2 values to estimate*

CO₂ waveform

The carbon dioxide (CO_2) waveform, or capnogram, produced in end-tidal carbon dioxide ($ETco_2$) monitoring reflects the course of CO_2 elimination during exhalation. A normal capnogram (shown below) consists of several segments that reflect the various stages of exhalation and inhalation.

Normally, gas eliminated from the airway during early exhalation is dead-space gas that hasn't undergone exchange at the alveolocapillary membrane. Measurements taken during this period contain no CO_2.

As exhalation continues, CO_2 concentration rises sharply and rapidly. The sensor now detects gas that has undergone exchange, producing measurable quantities of CO_2.

The final stages of alveolar emptying occur during late exhalation. During the alveolar plateau phase, CO_2 concentration rises more gradually *because alveolar emptying is more constant.*

The point at which the $ETco_2$ value is derived is the end of exhalation, when CO_2 concentration peaks. Unless an alveolar plateau is present, this value doesn't accurately estimate alveolar CO_2. During inhalation, the CO_2 concentration declines sharply to zero.

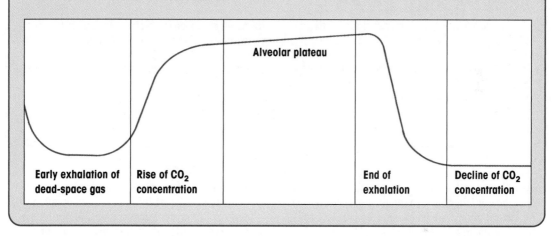

Alveolar plateau

Early exhalation of dead-space gas | **Rise of CO₂ concentration** | **End of exhalation** | **Decline of CO₂ concentration**

---

the $Paco_2$ *level, measure expired ventilation at the same time. If expired ventilation and $ETco_2$ values are constant, the patient's a-$ADco_2$ isn't likely to have changed. Avoid estimating the $Paco_2$ level from the $ETco_2$ level if the expired ventilation has changed. Alert the physician if the patient's a-$ADco_2$ level is above the normal range. He may have a mismatching or shunting problem. Monitor a-$ADco_2$ levels throughout therapy to determine the effectiveness of treatment and detect potential problems. If a-$ADco_2$ increases, the patient may have reduced pulmonary perfusion.*

● The a-$ADco_2$ value, if correctly interpreted, provides useful information about the patient's status. For example, an increased a-$ADco_2$ may mean that the patient has worsening dead space, especially if his tidal volume remains constant.

● Remember that $ETco_2$ monitoring doesn't replace ABG analysis *because it doesn't assess oxygenation or blood pH.* Supplementing $ETco_2$ monitoring with pulse oximetry may provide more complete information. **AARC**

● If the CO_2 waveform is available, assess it for height, frequency, rhythm, baseline, and shape *to help evaluate gas exchange.* Make sure that you know how to recognize a normal waveform and can identify abnormal waveforms in the patient's medical record. (See *CO₂ waveform.*)

● In a nonintubated patient, use $ETco_2$ values to establish trends. Be aware that in this patient, exhaled gas is more likely to mix with ambient air and exhaled CO_2 may be diluted by fresh gas flow from the nasal cannula.

Using a disposable ETco$_2$ detector

Before using a disposable end-tidal carbon dioxide (ETco$_2$) detector, check the instructions and ensure ideal working conditions for the device. Additional guidelines are provided here.

Avoiding high humidity, moisture, and heat
● Watch for changes indicating that the ETco$_2$ detector's efficiency is decreasing—for example, sluggish color changes from breath to breath. A detector may be used for about 2 hours; however, using it with a ventilator that delivers high-humidity ventilation may shorten its usefulness to no more than 15 minutes.
● Don't use the detector with a heated humidifier or nebulizer.
● Keep the detector protected from secretions, which render the device useless. If secretions enter the dome, remove and discard the detector.
● Use a heat and moisture exchanger to protect the detector. In some detectors, this filter fits between the endotracheal (ET) tube and the detector.
● If you're using a heat and moisture exchanger, remember that it will increase the patient's breathing effort.

Stay alert for increased resistance and breathing difficulties, and remove the exchanger, if necessary.

Taking additional precautions
● Instilling epinephrine through the ET tube can damage the detector's indicator (the color may stay yellow). If this happens, discard the device.
● Take care when using an ETco$_2$ detector in a child who weighs less than 30 lb (13.6 kg). A small patient who rebreathes air from the dead air space (about 38 cc) will inhale too much of his own carbon dioxide.
● Frequently spot-check the ETco$_2$ detector you're using for effectiveness. If you must transport the patient to another area for testing or treatment, use another method to verify the tube's placement.
● Never reuse a disposable ETco$_2$ detector. It's intended for one-time, one-patient use only.

● ETco$_2$ monitoring is usually discontinued when the patient has been weaned effectively from mechanical ventilation or when he's no longer at risk for respiratory compromise. Carefully assess the patient's tolerance to weaning.

⚠ **ALERT** *After extubation, continuous ETco$_2$ monitoring may detect the need for reintubation.*

● Disposable ETco$_2$ detectors are available. When using a disposable ETco$_2$ detector, always check its color under fluorescent or natural light *because the dome looks pink under incandescent light* (light provided by ordinary lightbulbs). (See *Using a disposable ETco$_2$ detector.*)

Nursing diagnoses
● Impaired gas exchange

Expected outcomes
The patient will:
● maintain normal ABG values
● have normal breath sounds.

Complications
● Inaccurate measurements—such as from poor sampling technique, calibration drift, contamination of optics with moisture or secretions, or equipment malfunction—can lead to misdiagnosis and improper treatment.
● The effects of manual resuscitation or ingestion of alcohol or carbonated beverages can alter the detector's findings.
● Color changes detected after fewer than six ventilations can be misleading.

Documentation
Document the initial ETco$_2$ value and all ventilator settings. Describe the waveform if one appears on the monitor. If the monitor has a printer, you may want to print out a sample waveform and include it in the patient's medical record.

Document ETco$_2$ values at least as often as vital signs, whenever significant changes in waveform or patient status occur, and before and after weaning, respiratory, and other interventions. Periodically obtain samples for ABG analysis as the patient's condition dictates, and document the corresponding $ETco_2$ values.

Supportive references

Ahrens, T., et al. "End-Tidal Carbon Dioxide Measurements as a Prognostic Indicator of Outcome of Cardiac Arrest," *American Journal of Critical Care* 10(6):391-98, November 2001.

Ahrens, T. "Technology Utilization in the Cardiac Surgical Patient: SvO_2 and Capnography Monitoring," *Critical Care Nursing Quarterly* 21(1):24-40, May 1998.

American Association for Respiratory Care. "AARC Clinical Practice Guideline: Capnography/Capnometry during Mechanical Ventilation," *Respiratory Care* 48(5): 1321-324, May 2003. **EB2**

American Heart Association. "2005 AHA Guidelines for Cardiopulmonary Resuscitation and Emergency Cardiovascular Care: International Consensus on Science," *Circulation* 112(22 Suppl):IV-1-IV-211, November 2005.

Blonshine, S. "Expanding the Knowledge Base: New Applications of Capnography," *AARC Times* 23(2): 51-53, February 1999. **EB1**

Capovilla, J., et al. "Noninvasive Blood Gas Monitoring," *Critical Care Nursing Quarterly* 23(2):79-86, August 2000.

Carroll, P. "Respiratory Monitoring: Evolutions: Capnography," *RN* 62(5):68-71, 78, May 1999.

Esophageal airway insertion and removal

Esophageal airways, such as the esophageal gastric tube airway (EGTA) and the esophageal obturator airway (EOA), are used temporarily (for up to 2 hours) to maintain ventilation in the comatose patient during cardiac or respiratory arrest. These devices avoid tongue obstruction, prevent air from entering the stomach, and keep stomach contents from entering the trachea. They can be inserted only after a patent airway is established.

CONTROVERSIAL ISSUE *According to the American Association for Respiratory Care (AARC) guidelines, controversy exists about the use of the EOA and EGTA in managing airway emergencies. While many believe that these two airways require less time to achieve competency than the endotracheal (ET) tube, this may not be true. Research looking at the effectiveness of the*

EOA is hard to evaluate because of differences in patients and medical supervision. Many studies have reported complications in the use of these airway devices. Some believe the EOA and EGTA should be used as second-line airway adjuncts to prevent stomach distention and aspiration of stomach contents while others believe that more time should be spent training personnel in ET intubation, basic airway maintenance, and ventilation rather than in the use of the EOA.

An esophageal-tracheal tube is an alternative to esophageal airways. This tube has two cuffed lumens—one is sealed at the distal end and has perforations at the level of the pharynx and the other lumen is open at the distal end. If the esophageal-tracheal tube is in the trachea, it functions as an ET tube after the small distal cuff is inflated. If the tube enters the esophagus, the larger cuff on the sealed lumen is inflated and the tube functions as an EOA. This device has the advantage of being able to provide ventilations, unlike the EOA, if the tube is inserted into the trachea. **AARC**

Although health care providers must have special training to insert an EGTA or EOA, insertion of these airways is much simpler than ET intubation. One reason is that these devices don't require visualization of the trachea or hyperextension of the neck. This makes them useful for treating patients with suspected spinal cord injuries.

Esophageal airways shouldn't be used unless the patient is unconscious and not breathing because conscious and semiconscious patients will reject this method. They're also contraindicated if facial trauma prevents a snug mask fit or if the patient has an absent or weak gag reflex, has recently ingested toxic chemicals, has an esophageal disease, or has taken an overdose of opioids that can be reversed by naloxone (Narcan).

ALERT *Because pediatric sizes aren't currently available, these airways shouldn't be used in patients younger than age 16.*

Equipment

Esophageal tube • face mask • #16 or #18 French nasogastric (NG) tube (for EGTA) • 35-ml syringe • intermittent gastric suction equipment • oral suction equipment • gloves and face shield • optional: handheld resuscitation bag, water-soluble lubricant

Types of esophageal airways

Gastric tube airway

A gastric tube airway consists of an inflatable mask and an esophageal tube, as shown. The transparent face mask has two ports: a lower one for insertion of an esophageal tube and an upper one for ventilation, which can be maintained with a handheld resuscitation bag. The inside of the mask is soft and pliable; it molds to the patient's face and makes a tight seal, preventing air loss.

The proximal end of the esophageal tube has a one-way, nonrefluxing valve that blocks the esophagus. This valve prevents air from entering the stomach, thus reducing the risk of abdominal distention and aspiration. The distal end of the tube has an inflatable cuff that rests in the esophagus just below the tracheal bifurcation, preventing pressure on the noncartilaginous tracheal wall. During ventilation, air is directed into the upper port in the mask and, with the esophagus blocked, enters the trachea and lungs.

Esophageal gastric tube airway

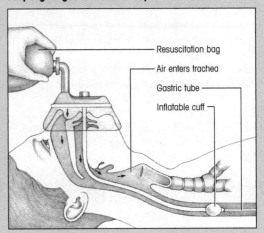

- Resuscitation bag
- Air enters trachea
- Gastric tube
- Inflatable cuff

Obturator airway

An obturator airway consists of an adjustable, inflatable transparent face mask with a single port, attached by a snap lock to a blind esophageal tube, as shown at right. When properly inflated, the transparent mask prevents air from escaping through the nose and mouth.

The esophageal tube has holes at its proximal end, through which air or oxygen introduced into the port of the mask is transferred to the trachea. The tube's distal end is closed and circled by an inflatable cuff. When the cuff is inflated, it occludes the esophagus, preventing air from entering the stomach and acting as a barrier against vomitus and involuntary aspiration.

Esophageal obturator airway

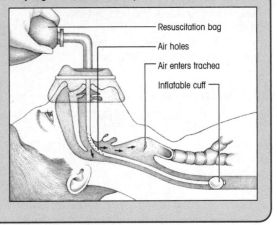

- Resuscitation bag
- Air holes
- Air enters trachea
- Inflatable cuff

Preparation of equipment

- Gather the equipment. (See *Types of esophageal airways*.)
- Fill the face mask with air *to check for leaks.*
- Inflate the esophageal tube's cuff with 35 cc of air *to check for leaks;* then deflate the cuff.
- Connect the esophageal tube to the face mask (the lower opening on an EGTA) and listen for the tube to click *to determine proper placement.*

Implementation

- Lubricate the tube's distal tip with a water-soluble lubricant.
- Assess the patient's condition to determine if he's an appropriate candidate for an esophageal airway. **AARC**
- If the patient's condition permits, place him in the supine position with his neck in a neutral or semi-flexed position. *Hyperextension of the neck may cause*

the tube to enter the trachea instead of the esophagus. Remove his dentures, if applicable. **Science**

● Insert your thumb deeply into the patient's mouth behind the base of his tongue. Place your index finger and middle fingers of the same hand under the patient's chin and lift his jaw straight up.

● With your other hand, grasp the esophageal tube just below the mask in the same way you would grasp a pencil. *This promotes gentle maneuvering of the tube and reduces the risk of pharyngeal trauma.*

● Still elevating the patient's jaw with one hand, insert the tip of the esophageal tube into the patient's mouth. Gently guide the airway over the tongue into the pharynx and then into the esophagus, following the natural pharyngeal curve. No force is required for proper insertion; the tube should easily seat itself. If you encounter resistance, withdraw the tube slightly and readvance it. When the tube is fully advanced, the mask should fit snugly over the patient's mouth and nose. When this is accomplished, the cuff will lie below the level of the carina. If the cuff is above the carina, it may, when inflated, compress the posterior membranous portion of the trachea and cause tracheal obstruction.

● *Because the tube may enter the trachea,* deliver positive-pressure ventilation before inflating the cuff. Watch for the chest to rise *to confirm that the tube is in the esophagus.* **AARC**

● When the tube is properly in place in the esophagus, draw 35 cc of air into the syringe, connect the syringe to the tube's cuff-inflation valve, and inflate the cuff. Avoid overinflation *because this can cause esophageal trauma.* **AARC**

● If you've inserted an EGTA, insert the NG tube through the lower port on the face mask and into the esophageal tube and advance it to the second marking, so it reaches 6″ (15.2 cm) beyond the distal end of the esophageal tube. Suction stomach contents using intermittent gastric suction *to decompress the stomach.* This is particularly necessary after mouth-to-mouth resuscitation, which introduces air into the stomach. Leave the tube in place during resuscitation.

● For both airways, attach a handheld resuscitation bag or a mechanical ventilator to the face mask port (upper port) on the EGTA. Up to 100% of the fraction of inspired oxygen can be delivered this way. **AARC**

● Monitor the patient *to ensure adequate ventilation.* Watch for chest movement, and suction the patient if mucus blocks the EOA tube perforations or in any way interrupts respiration. **AARC**

Removing an esophageal airway

● Assess the patient's condition to determine if airway removal is appropriate. The airway may be removed if respirations are spontaneous and number 16 to 20 breaths/minute. If 2 hours have elapsed since airway insertion and respirations aren't spontaneous and at the normal rate, the patient must be switched to an artificial airway that can be used for long-term ventilation such as an ET tube. **AARC**

● Detach the mask from the esophageal tube.

● Place the patient on his left side, if possible, *to avoid aspiration during the removal of the esophageal airway.* If he's unconscious and requires an ET tube, insert it or assist with its insertion and inflate the cuff of the ET tube before removing the esophageal tube. *With the esophageal tube in place, the ET tube can be guided easily into the trachea, and stomach contents are less likely to be aspirated when the esophageal tube is removed.* **AARC** **Science**

● Deflate the cuff on the esophageal tube by removing air from the inflation valve with the syringe. Don't try to remove the tube with the cuff inflated *because it may perforate the esophagus.*

● Remove the EGTA or EOA with one swift, smooth motion, following the natural pharyngeal curve *to avoid esophageal trauma.*

● Perform oropharyngeal suctioning *to remove residual secretions.*

● Assist the physician as required in monitoring and maintaining adequate ventilation.

Special considerations

● Store EGTAs and EOAs in the manufacturer's package to preserve their natural curve. **MFR**

● To ease insertion, direct the airway along the right side of the patient's mouth *because the esophagus is located to the right and behind the trachea.* Or you may advance the tip upward toward the hard palate, and then invert the tip and glide it along the tongue surface and into the pharynx. *This keeps the tube centered, avoids snagging on the sides of the throat, and eases insertion in the patient with clenched jaws.*

● Watch the unconscious patient as he regains consciousness *because activation of the gag reflex can cause retching.* Evaluate the conscious patient's need for continued ventilatory support and for removal of

the esophageal airway. *To help prevent complications, don't leave the EOA in place for more than 2 hours.*
AARC

● A mechanical ventilator attached to the ET tube or tracheostomy tube maintains more exact tidal volume than a mechanical ventilator attached to an esophageal airway.

Nursing diagnoses

● Impaired spontaneous ventilation
● Risk for trauma

Expected outcomes

The patient will:
● maintain normal arterial blood gas values
● maintain a respiratory rate within 5 breaths/minute of baseline
● remain free from esophageal injuries and other injuries that may result from tongue obstruction.

Complications

● EOAs may be inferior to ET intubation in providing adequate oxygenation and ventilation. They don't prevent aspiration of foreign material from the mouth and pharynx into the trachea and bronchi.
● Esophageal airways may cause esophageal injuries, including rupture, and in semiconscious patients may cause laryngospasm, vomiting, and aspiration.
● Tracheal occlusion can occur if the esophageal airway is inserted in the trachea.

Documentation

Record the date and time of the procedure, type of airway inserted, patient's vital signs and level of consciousness, removal of the airway, any alternative airway inserted after extubation, and any complications and interventions taken.

Supportive references

American Association for Respiratory Care. "AARC Clinical Practice Guideline: Management of Airway Emergencies," *Respiratory Care* 40(7):749-60, July 1995.

Asselin, M.E., and Cullen, H.A. "What You Need to Know about the New ACLS Guidelines," *Nursing2001* 31(4):48-50, April 2001.

Barnes, T.A., et al. "Cardiopulmonary Resuscitation and Emergency Cardiovascular Care: Airway Devices,"

Annals of Emergency Medicine 37(4):S145-51, April 2001.

Blanda, M. "The Difficult Airway: Tools and Techniques for Acute Management," *Journal of Critical Illness* 15(7):358-60, 369-73, July 2000.

Kern, K.B., et al. "New Guidelines for Cardiopulmonary Resuscitation and Emergency Cardiac Care: Changes in the Management of Cardiac Arrest," *JAMA* 285(10): 1267-269, March 2001.

Foreign body airway obstruction

Severe airway obstruction is an uncommon but preventable emergency that can result in death within minutes if not treated. Sudden airway obstruction may occur when a foreign body lodges in the throat or bronchus, when the tongue blocks the pharynx, when the patient experiences traumatic injury, or when the patient aspirates blood, mucus, or vomitus. An obstructed airway can also occur from bronchoconstriction or bronchospasm.

An obstructed airway causes anoxia, which in turn leads to brain damage and death in 4 to 6 minutes. The Heimlich maneuver uses an upper-abdominal thrust to create sufficient diaphragmatic pressure in the static lung below the foreign body to expel the obstruction. The Heimlich maneuver is used in conscious adult patients and in children older than age 1. However, the abdominal thrust is contraindicated in pregnant women, markedly obese patients, and infants younger than age 1. For such patients, a chest thrust, which forces air out of the lungs to create an artificial cough, should be used.

CONTROVERSIAL ISSUE *Studies show that chest thrusts, abdominal thrusts, and back blows are effective for relieving foreign body obstructions in the conscious adult and children age 1 or older. However, to simplify training, the American Heart Association's (AHA) 2005 guidelines for cardiopulmonary resuscitation (CPR) and emergency cardiovascular care recommend abdominal thrusts applied in rapid sequence until the obstruction is cleared. If this maneuver doesn't clear the obstruction, chest thrusts should be considered.*

These maneuvers are contraindicated in a patient with mild airway obstruction, when the patient can maintain adequate ventilation to dislodge the foreign body by effective coughing, and in an infant. However, if the patient has poor air exchange and increased breathing difficulty, a silent cough, cyanosis, or the inability to speak or breathe, immediate action to dislodge the obstruction should be taken. (See also "Cardiopulmonary resuscitation," page 217.)

Implementation

Conscious adult with mild airway obstruction AHA

● Ask the person who's coughing or using the universal distress sign (clutching the neck between the thumb and fingers) if she's choking. If she indicates that she is but can speak and cough forcefully, she has good air exchange and should be encouraged to continue to cough. Remain with the person and monitor her.

Conscious adult with severe airway obstruction AHA

● Ask the person, "Are you choking?" If the patient nods yes and has signs of severe airway obstruction, tell her that you'll help dislodge the foreign body.
● Standing behind the patient, wrap your arms around her waist. Make a fist with one hand, and place the thumb side against her abdomen in the midline, slightly above the umbilicus and well below the xiphoid process. Then grasp your fist with the other hand (as shown below).

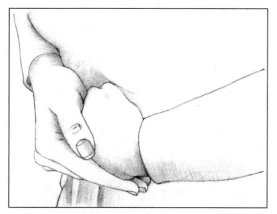

● Squeeze the patient's abdomen with quick inward and upward thrusts. Each thrust should be a separate and distinct movement, forceful enough to create an

artificial cough that will dislodge an obstruction (as shown below).

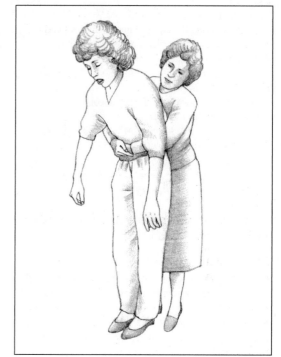

● Make sure that you have a firm grasp on the patient *because she may lose consciousness and need to be lowered to the floor.* Support her head and neck *to prevent injury,* and continue as described below.
● Repeat the thrusts until the foreign body is expelled or if the patient becomes unconscious. At this point, contact the emergency medical service (EMS) and follow the interventions for relieving an obstructed airway in an unconscious person.

⚠ **ALERT** *If the victim of an airway obstruction becomes unconscious, the lay rescuer should lower the patient to the ground and immediately contact EMS and begin CPR. Studies demonstrate that chest thrusts generated higher sustained airway pressure than pressure generated by abdominal thrusts. For this reason, it's believed that chest compressions alone may relieve the obstruction in the unconscious victim.* AHA EB

Unresponsive adult AHA

● Lower the patient to the ground and immediately contact EMS.
● Begin CPR.
● Each time the airway is opened using a head tilt-chin lift, look for an object in the patient's mouth.
● Remove the object if present.
● Attempt to ventilate the patient and follow with 30 chest compressions.

⚠️ **ALERT** *The blind finger sweep is no longer being taught by the AHA. A finger sweep only should be used when a foreign body can be seen in the mouth. Studies have shown that blind finger sweeps may result in injury to the patient's mouth and throat or to the rescuer's fingers, and there's no evidence of its effectiveness. In addition, the tongue-jaw lift is no longer used. The patient's mouth should be opened using a head tilt-chin lift.* AHA

Obese or pregnant adult AHA

● If the patient is conscious, stand behind her and place your arms under her armpits and around her chest.
● Place the thumb side of your clenched fist against the middle of the sternum, avoiding the margins of the ribs and the xiphoid process. Grasp your fist with your other hand and perform a chest thrust with enough force to expel the foreign body. Continue until the patient expels the obstruction or loses consciousness (as shown below).

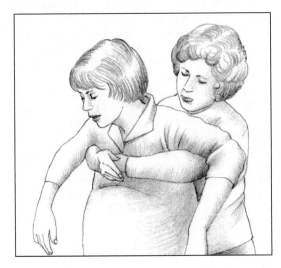

● If the patient loses consciousness, carefully lower her to the floor.
● Then, follow the same steps you would use for the unresponsive adult (as shown below).

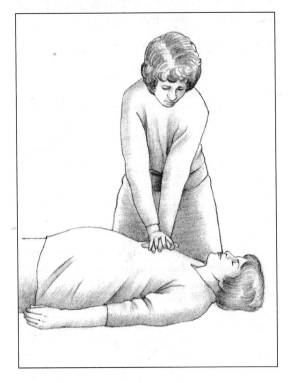

Conscious child with severe airway obstruction AHA

● If the child is conscious and can stand but can't cough or make a sound, perform abdominal thrusts using the same technique as you would with an adult.

Unresponsive child AHA

● Use the same techniques you would for the unresponsive adult.

Conscious infant AHA

● Place the conscious infant face down so that he's straddling your arm with his head lower than his trunk. Rest your forearm on your thigh and deliver five forceful back blows with the heel of your hand between the infant's shoulder blades (as shown at top of next page).

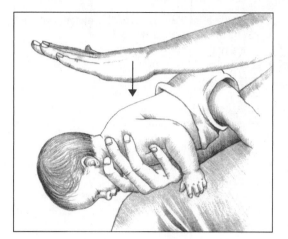

creases, smooth and skeletal muscles relax, making your maneuvers more likely to succeed.

Nursing diagnoses
- Ineffective airway clearance

Expected outcomes
The patient will:
- maintain a patent airway
- cough effectively
- have no adventitious breath sounds
- maintain normal arterial blood gas levels.

Complications
- Nausea, regurgitation, and achiness may develop after the patient regains consciousness and can breathe independently.
- Even when performed correctly, abdominal thrusts can damage internal organs of the abdomen or chest by laceration or rupture.
- Incorrect placement of the rescuer's hands, or osteoporosis or metastatic lesions that increase the risk of fracture, also may cause injury.
- The patient who has received abdominal thrusts should be evaluated by a physician to detect possible complications.

Documentation
Record the date and time of the procedure, the patient's actions before the obstruction, signs and symptoms of airway obstruction, approximate length of time it took to clear the airway, and the type and size of the object removed. Note his vital signs after the procedure, any complications that occurred and interventions taken, and his tolerance of the procedure. Note the time, name of the physician notified, any orders given, and your interventions.

Supportive references
American Heart Association. "2005 Guidelines for Cardiopulmonary Resuscitation and Emergency Cardiovascular Care: International Consensus on Science," *Circulation* (22 Suppl):IV-1-IV-211, November 2005. **EB**

American Heart Association. *Currents in Emergency Cardiovascular Care* 16(4), Winter 2005-2006.

- If you haven't removed the obstruction, place your free hand on the infant's back. Supporting his neck, jaw, and chest with your other hand, turn him over onto your thigh. Keep his head lower than his trunk.
- Position your fingers. To do so, imagine a line between the infant's nipples and place the index finger of your free hand on his sternum, just below this imaginary line. Then place your middle and ring fingers next to your index finger and lift the index finger off his chest. Deliver five quick chest thrusts as you would for chest compression at a rate of approximately one per second.

⚠ ALERT *Never perform a blind finger sweep on a child or an infant because you risk pushing the foreign body farther back into the airway. Also, abdominal thrusts aren't recommended for infants because they may damage the liver.*
- If the airway obstruction persists, repeat the five back blows and five chest thrusts until the obstruction is relieved or the infant becomes unresponsive.

Unresponsive infant **AHA**
- Use the same techniques you would for the unresponsive adult.

Special considerations
- If the patient vomits during abdominal thrusts, quickly wipe out his mouth with your fingers and resume the maneuver as necessary.
- Even if your efforts to clear the airway don't seem to be effective, keep trying. *As oxygen deprivation in-*

Humidifiers

Humidifiers, which deliver a maximum amount of water vapor without producing particulate water, are used to prevent drying and irritation of the upper airway in such conditions as croup, in which the upper airway is inflamed, or when secretions are particularly thick and tenacious. Some humidifiers heat the water vapor, which raises the moisture-carrying capacity of gas and thus increases the amount of humidity delivered to the patient. Room humidifiers add humidity to an entire room, while humidifiers added to ventilation lines humidify only the air being delivered to the patient. (See *Comparing humidifiers.*)

Equipment

Humidifier • sterile distilled water, or tap water if the unit has a demineralizing capability • container for wastewater • bleach • white vinegar • flowmeter • vaporizer • disinfectant

Preparation of equipment

Bedside humidifier

● Open the reservoir and add sterile distilled water to the fill line, and then close the reservoir.
● Keep all room windows and doors closed tightly *to maintain adequate humidification.*
● Plug the unit into the electrical outlet.

Heated vaporizer

● Remove the top and fill the reservoir to the fill line with tap water. Replace the top securely.
● Place the vaporizer about 4′ (1 m) from the patient, directing the steam toward but not directly onto the patient. Place the unit in a spot where it can't be overturned *to avoid hot water burns;* this is especially important if children will be in the room.
● Plug the unit into an electrical outlet. Steam should soon rise from the unit into the air.
● Close all windows and doors to maintain adequate humidification.

Diffusion head humidifier

● Unscrew the humidifier reservoir, and add sterile distilled water to the appropriate level. (If using a disposable unit, screw the cap with the extension onto the top of the unit.)
● Screw the reservoir back onto the humidifier and attach the flowmeter to the oxygen source.

● Screw the humidifier onto the flowmeter until the seal is tight. Then set the flowmeter at a rate of 2 L/minute and check for gentle bubbling.
● Check the positive-pressure release valve by occluding the end valve on the humidifier. The pressure should back up into the humidifier, signaled by a high-pitched whistle. If this doesn't occur, tighten all connections and try again.

Cascade bubble diffusion humidifier

● Unscrew the cascade reservoir and add sterile distilled water to the fill line.
● Screw the top back onto the reservoir. Plug in the heater unit, and set the temperature between 95° and 100.4° F (35° and 38° C).

Implementation

● Confirm the patient's identity using two patient identifiers according to facility policy. **JCAHO**
● Check that the humidifier or vaporizer has been prepared properly.

Bedside humidifier

● Direct the humidifier unit's nozzle away from the patient's face (but toward the patient) *to provide effective treatment.* Check for a fine mist emission from the nozzle, which indicates proper operation.
● Check the unit every 4 hours for proper operation and the water level every 8 hours. When refilling, unplug the unit, discard any old water, wipe with a disinfectant, rinse the reservoir container, and refill with sterile distilled water as necessary. **AARC**
● Keep the unit cleaned and refilled with sterile water to reduce the risk of bacterial growth. Replace the unit every 7 days and send used units for proper decontamination. **AARC**

Heated vaporizer

● Check the unit every 4 hours for proper functioning. **AARC**
● If steam production seems insufficient, unplug the unit, discard the water, and refill with half distilled water and half tap water, or clean the unit well.
● Check the water level in the unit every 8 hours. To refill, unplug the unit, discard any old water, wipe with a disinfectant, rinse the reservoir container, and refill with tap water as necessary.

Comparing humidifiers

The chart below describes the various types of humidifiers and their advantages and disadvantages.

Type	Description and uses	Advantages	Disadvantages
Bedside humidifier	• Spinning disk splashes water against a baffle, creating small drops and increasing evaporation; motor disperses mist to directly humidify room air.	• May be used with all oxygen masks and nasal cannulas • Easy to operate • Inexpensive	• Produces humidity inefficiently • Can't be used for a patient with a bypassed upper airway • May harbor bacteria and molds
Heated vaporizer	• Water that's heated in the reservoir provides direct humidification to room air.	• May be used with all oxygen masks and nasal cannulas • Easy to operate • Inexpensive	• Can't guarantee the amount of humidity delivered • Risk of burn injury occurring if machine knocks over
Diffusion head humidifier	• In-line humidifier is most commonly used with low-flow oxygen delivery systems. Gas flows through the porous diffuser in the reservoir to increase gas-liquid interface, providing humidification to patients using a nasal cannula or oxygen mask (except the Venturi mask).	• Easy to operate • Inexpensive	• Provides only 20% to 30% humidity at body temperature • Can't be used for a patient with bypassed upper airway
Cascade bubble diffusion	• Gas is forced through a plastic grid in a reservoir of warmed water to create fine bubbles. It's commonly used in patients receiving mechanical ventilation or continuous positive airway pressure therapy.	• Delivers 100% humidity at body temperature • Most effective of all evaporative humidifiers	• If correct water level isn't maintained, mucosa possibly becoming irritated

Diffusion head humidifier

• Attach the oxygen delivery device to the humidifier and then to the patient. Then adjust the flowmeter to the appropriate oxygen flow rate.

• Check the reservoir every 4 hours. If the water level drops too low, empty the remaining water, rinse the jar, and refill it with sterile water. (As the reservoir water level decreases, the evaporation of water in the gas decreases, reducing humidification of the delivered gas.) **AARC**

• Change the humidification system regularly *to prevent bacterial growth and invasion.* **AARC** **CDC**

- Periodically assess the patient's sputum; *sputum that's too thick can hinder mobilization and expectoration.* If this occurs, the patient requires a device that can provide higher humidity.

Cascade bubble diffusion humidifier

- Assess the temperature of the inspired gas near the patient's airway every 2 hours when used in critical care and every 4 hours when used in general patient care. If the cascade becomes too hot, drain the water and replace it. *Overheated water vapor can cause respiratory tract burns.* **AARC**
- Check the reservoir's water level every 2 to 4 hours, and fill as necessary. *If the water level falls below the minimum water level mark, humidity will decrease to that of room air.*
- Stay alert for condensation buildup in the tubing, which can result from the very high humidification produced by the cascade.
- Check the tubing frequently, and empty the condensate as necessary *so it can't drain into the patient's respiratory tract, encourage growth of microorganisms, or obstruct dependent sections of tubing.* To do so, disconnect the tubing, drain the condensate into a container, and dispose of it properly. Never drain the condensate into the humidification system. **AARC**
- Change the cascade regularly according to your facility's policy.

Special considerations

- *Because it creates a humidity level comparable to that of ambient air,* the diffusion head humidifier is only used for oxygen flow rates greater than 4 L/minute.
- *Because the bedside humidifier doesn't deliver a precise amount of humidification, assess the patient regularly to determine the effectiveness of therapy.* Ask him if he has noticed an improvement, and evaluate his sputum.
- Like the bedside humidifier, the heated vaporizer doesn't deliver a precise amount of humidification, so assess the patient regularly by asking if he's feeling better and by examining his sputum.
- Keep in mind that a humidifier, if not kept clean, can cause or aggravate respiratory problems, especially for people allergic to mold. Refer to your facility's policy for changing and disposing of humidification equipment.

TEACHING *Make sure that the patient and his family understand the reason for using a humidifier and know how to use the equipment. Give them specific, written guidelines concerning all aspects of home care.*

Instruct a patient using a bedside humidifier at home to fill it with plain tap water and to periodically use sterile distilled water to prevent mineral buildup. Also advise him to run white vinegar through the unit to help clean it, prevent bacterial buildup, and dissolve deposits.

Tell the patient using a heated vaporizer unit to rinse it with bleach and water every 5 days. Also tell him to run white vinegar through it to help clean it, prevent bacterial buildup, and dissolve any deposits.

Nursing diagnoses

- Ineffective breathing pattern

Expected outcomes

The patient will:
- report feeling comfortable when breathing
- achieve maximum lung expansion and adequate ventilation.

Complications

- Cascade humidifiers can cause aspiration of tubal condensation and, if the air is heated, pulmonary burns.
- Humidifiers, if contaminated, can cause infection.

Documentation

Record the date and time when humidification began and was discontinued, the type of humidifier, flow rate (of a gas system), thermometer readings (if heated), any complications and interventions taken, and the patient's reaction to humidification.

Supportive references

American Association for Respiratory Care. "AARC Clinical Practice Guideline: Humidification during Mechanical Ventilation," *Respiratory Care* 37(8):887-90, August 1992.

Bronson, R. "Humidification for Patients with Artificial Airways," *Respiratory Care* 44(6):630-42, June 1999.

Incentive spirometry

Incentive spirometry involves using a breathing device to help the patient achieve maximum ventilation. The device measures respiratory flow or respiratory volume and induces the patient to take a deep breath and hold it for several seconds. This deep breath increases lung volume, boosts alveolar inflation, and promotes venous return. This exercise also establishes alveolar hyperinflation for a longer time than is possible with a normal deep breath, thus preventing and reversing the alveolar collapse that causes atelectasis and pneumonitis.

The American Association for Respiratory Care (AARC) guidelines recommend the use of an incentive spirometer for conditions predisposing to the development of pulmonary atelectasis, such as:
● upper-abdominal surgery
● thoracic surgery
● surgery in patients with chronic obstructive pulmonary disease
● restrictive lung defect associated with quadriplegia or a dysfunctional diaphragm. **AARC**

Five to 10 breaths are suggested per session every hour while awake (approximately 100 breaths per day). **AARC**

Devices used for incentive spirometry provide a visual incentive to breathe deeply. Some are activated when the patient inhales a certain volume of air; the device then estimates the amount of air inhaled. Others contain plastic floats, which rise according to the amount of air the patient pulls through the device when he inhales.

Patients at low risk for developing atelectasis may use a flow incentive spirometer. Patients at high risk may need a volume incentive spirometer, which measures lung inflation more precisely.

Incentive spirometry benefits the patient on prolonged bed rest, especially the postoperative patient who may regain his normal respiratory pattern slowly due to such predisposing factors as abdominal or thoracic surgery, advanced age, inactivity, obesity, smoking, and decreased ability to cough effectively and expel lung secretions.

Equipment

Flow or volume incentive spirometer, as indicated, with sterile disposable flow tube and mouthpiece (the tube and mouthpiece are sterile on first use and clean on subsequent uses) ● stethoscope ● watch ● pencil and paper

Preparation of equipment

● Assemble the ordered equipment at the patient's bedside.
● Read the manufacturer's instructions for spirometer setup and operation. **MFR**
● Remove the sterile flow tube and mouthpiece from the package, and attach them to the device.
● Set the flow rate or volume goal as determined by the physician or respiratory therapist and based on the patient's preoperative performance.
● Turn on the machine, if necessary.

Implementation

● Confirm the patient's identity using two patient identifiers according to facility policy. **JCAHO**
● Assess the patient's condition.
● Explain the procedure to the patient, making sure that he understands the importance of performing this exercise regularly *to maintain alveolar inflation*.
● Wash your hands. **CDC**
● Help the patient into a comfortable sitting or semi-Fowler's position *to promote optimal lung expansion*. If you're using a flow incentive spirometer and the patient can't assume or maintain this position, he can perform the procedure in any position as long as the device remains upright. *Tilting a flow incentive spirometer decreases the required patient effort and reduces the exercise's effectiveness.* **AARC**
● Auscultate the patient's lungs to provide a baseline for comparison with posttreatment auscultation. **AARC**
● Instruct the patient to insert the mouthpiece and close his lips tightly around it *because a weak seal may alter flow or volume readings*.
● Instruct the patient to exhale normally and then inhale as slowly and as deeply as possible. If he has difficulty with this step, tell him to suck as he would through a straw but more slowly. Ask the patient to retain the entire volume of air he inhaled for 3 seconds or, if you're using a device with a light indicator, until the light turns off. This deep breath creates sustained transpulmonary pressure near the end of inspiration and is sometimes called a sustained maximal inspiration. **AARC**
● Tell the patient to remove the mouthpiece and exhale normally. Allow him to relax and take several

normal breaths before attempting another breath with the spirometer. Repeat this sequence 5 to 10 times during every waking hour. Note tidal volumes. **AARC**
- Evaluate the patient's ability to cough effectively, and encourage him to cough after each effort *because deep lung inflation may loosen secretions and facilitate their removal.* Observe any expectorated secretions. **AARC** **Science**
- Auscultate the patient's lungs, and compare findings with the first auscultation.
- Instruct the patient to remove the mouthpiece. Wash the device in warm water and shake it dry. Avoid immersing the spirometer itself *because this enhances bacterial growth and impairs the internal filter's effectiveness in preventing inhalation of extraneous material.*
- Place the mouthpiece in a plastic storage bag between exercises, and label it and the spirometer, if applicable, with the patient's name *to avoid inadvertent use by another patient.*

Special considerations
- If the patient is scheduled for surgery, make a preoperative assessment of his respiratory pattern and capability *to ensure the development of appropriate postoperative goals.* Teach the patient how to use the spirometer before surgery *so that he can concentrate on your instructions and practice the exercise.* A preoperative evaluation will also help in establishing a postoperative therapeutic goal.

- Avoid exercising at mealtime *to prevent nausea.* Provide paper and pencil *so the patient can note exercise times.* Exercise frequency varies with the patient's condition and ability.
- Immediately after surgery, monitor the exercise frequently *to ensure compliance and assess achievement.*

Nursing diagnoses
- Ineffective airway clearance

Expected outcomes
The patient will:
- cough effectively
- have no adventitious breath sounds
- have normal chest X-rays
- maintain a patent airway.

Documentation
Record any preoperative teaching you provided. Document the preoperative flow or volume levels, date and time of the procedure, type of spirometer, flow or volume levels achieved, and number of breaths taken. Also record the patient's condition before and after the procedure, his tolerance of the procedure, and the results of both auscultations. (See *Documenting flow and volume levels.*)

Supportive references
American Association for Respiratory Care. "AARC Clinical Practice Guideline: Directed Cough," *Respiratory Care* 38(5):495-99, May 1993.
American Association for Respiratory Care. "AARC Clinical Practice Guideline: Incentive Spirometry," *Respiratory Care* 36(12):1402-405, December 1991.
Vines, D.L., et al. "Current Respiratory Care, Part 1: Oxygen Therapy, Oximetry, Bronchial Hygiene," *Journal of Critical Illness* 15(9):507-10, 513-15, September 2000.

Latex allergy protocol

Latex — a natural product of the rubber tree — is used in many products in the health care field as well as other areas. With the increased use of latex in barrier protection and medical equipment, many more nurses and patients are becoming hypersensitive to it. Certain groups of people, such as those who have had or will have multiple surgical procedures (especially those with a history of spina bifida), health

Latex allergy screening questionnaire

To determine whether the patient has a latex sensitivity or allergy, ask the following screening questions:

Allergies
- Do you have a history of hay fever, asthma, eczema, allergies, or rashes? If so, what type of reaction do you have?
- Have you experienced an allergic reaction, local sensitivity, or itching following exposure to latex products, such as balloons or condoms?
- Do you have shortness of breath or wheezing after blowing up balloons or after a dental visit? Do you have itching in or around your mouth after eating a banana?
- If you experience shortness of breath or wheezing when blowing up latex balloons, describe your reaction.
- Are you allergic to any foods, especially bananas, avocados, kiwi, or chestnuts? If so, describe your reaction.

Occupation
- What's your occupation?
- Are you exposed to latex in your occupation?
- Do you experience a reaction to latex products at work? If so, describe your reaction.

- If you've had a rash on your hands develop after wearing latex gloves, how long after putting on the gloves did it take for the rash to develop?
- What did the rash look like?

Personal history
- Do you have any congenital abnormalities? If yes, explain.
- Have you ever had itching, swelling, hives, cough, shortness of breath, or other allergic symptoms during or after using condoms or diaphragms or following a vaginal or rectal examination?

Surgical history
- Have you had previous surgical procedures? Did you experience associated complications? If so, describe them.
- Have you had previous dental procedures? Did complications result? If so, describe them.
- Do you have spina bifida or a urinary tract problem that requires surgery or catheterization?

---

care workers (especially those in the emergency department and operating room), and workers who manufacture latex and latex-containing products, are at an increased risk for developing latex allergy. Still others may have a genetic predisposition to latex allergy.

People who are allergic to certain "cross-reactive" foods — including apricots, cherries, grapes, kiwis, passion fruit, bananas, avocados, chestnuts, tomatoes, and peaches — may also be allergic to latex. Exposure to latex elicits an allergic response similar to the one elicited by these foods.

For people with latex allergy, latex becomes a hazard when its protein comes in direct contact with mucous membranes or is inhaled, which happens when powdered latex surgical gloves are used. People with asthma are at a greater risk for developing worsening symptoms from airborne latex.

The diagnosis of latex allergy is based on the patient's history and physical examination. Laboratory testing should be performed to confirm or eliminate the diagnosis. Skin testing can be done, but the AlaSTAT test, Hycor assay, and the Pharmacia CAP test are the only U.S. Food and Drug Administration–approved blood tests available. Some laboratories may also choose to perform an enzyme-linked immunosorbent assay.

Latex allergy can produce myriad symptoms, including a rash, hives, generalized itching (on the hands and arms, for example); sneezing and coughing (hay fever-type signs); bronchial asthma, scratchy throat, or difficulty breathing; itchy, watery, or burning eyes; edema of the face, hands, or neck; and anaphylaxis.

To help identify the patient at risk for latex allergy, ask latex allergy-specific questions during the health history. (See *Latex allergy screening questionnaire.*) If the patient's history reveals a latex sensitivity, he's assigned to one of three categories based on the extent of his sensitization. Group 1 includes patients

Creating a latex-free environment

● Ask all patients about latex sensitivity. Use a screening questionnaire to determine latex sensitivity.
● Teach the patient to treat the latex allergy the same as a food or drug allergy by informing all future health care providers about his allergy.
● Include information about latex allergy on the patient's identification bracelet. Make sure that the information is also noted on the front of the patient's chart and in the facility's database.
● Post a LATEX ALLERGY sign in the patient's room.
● Implement and disseminate latex allergy protocols and lists of nonlatex substitutes that can be used to care for the patient.
● Remove all latex-containing products that may come in contact with the patient.
● Use tubing made of polyvinyl chloride.
● Check adhesives and tapes, including electrocardiogram electrodes and dressing supplies, for latex content.
● Have a special latex-free crash cart outside the room at all times during the patient's hospitalization.
● Notify central supply and pharmacy that the patient has a latex allergy so that latex contact is eliminated from drugs and other materials prepared for the patient.
● Notify dietary staff of relevant food allergies and instruct them to avoid handling the patient's food with powdered latex gloves.

who have a history of anaphylaxis or a systemic reaction when exposed to a natural latex product. Group 2 patients have a clear history of an allergic reaction of a nonsystemic type. Group 3 patients don't have a previous history of latex hypersensitivity but are designated as "high risk" because of an associated medical condition, occupation, or "crossover" allergy.

If you determine that the patient has a latex sensitivity, make sure that he doesn't come in contact with latex *because such contact could result in a life-threatening hypersensitivity reaction.* Also, be sure to record the patient's allergies in his permanent medical record. Creating a latex-free environment is the only way to safeguard him. (See *Creating a latex-free envi-*

ronment.) Hypoallergenic latex gloves contain significant amounts of latex allergens and shouldn't be worn in the vicinity of someone who's allergic to latex. Many health care facilities now designate "latex-free" equipment, which is usually kept on a cart that can be moved into the patient's room.

The National Institute of Occupational Safety and Health (NIOSH) has published an advisory document on natural latex rubber in the workplace. It recommends that nonlatex gloves be used for all activities that aren't likely to involve contact with infectious materials (for example, food preparation, routine housekeeping, and maintenance). **CDC**

Equipment

Latex allergy patient identification bracelet ● latex-free equipment cart with necessary supplies, including room contents ● anaphylaxis kit ● optional: LATEX ALLERGY sign

Preparation of equipment

● After you've determined that the patient has a latex allergy or is sensitive to latex, arrange for him to be placed in a private room. If that isn't possible, make the room latex-free, even if the roommate hasn't been designated as hypersensitive to latex. *This prevents the spread of airborne particles from latex products used on the other patient.*

Implementation

● Assess all patients being admitted to the delivery room or short-procedure unit or having a surgical procedure for possible latex allergy.

Patients in groups 1 and 2

● If the patient has a confirmed latex allergy, bring a cart with latex-free supplies into his room. **CDC**
● Document in the patient's chart (according to your facility's policy) that the patient has a latex allergy. If policy requires that the patient wear a latex allergy patient identification bracelet, place it on the patient. **CDC**

● If the patient will be receiving anesthesia, make sure that "latex allergy" is clearly visible on the front of his chart. Notify the circulating nurse in the surgical unit, the postanesthesia care unit nurses, and other team members that the patient has a latex allergy. (See *Anesthesia induction and latex allergy.*)

Anesthesia induction and latex allergy

Latex allergy can cause signs and symptoms in conscious and anesthetized patients.

Causes of intraoperative reaction	Signs and symptoms in a conscious patient	Signs and symptoms in an anesthetized patient
• Latex contact with mucous membrane • Latex contact with intraperitoneal serosal lining • Inhalation of airborne latex particles during anesthesia • Injection of antibiotics and anesthetic agents through latex ports	• Abdominal cramping • Anxiety • Bronchoconstriction • Diarrhea • Feeling of faintness • Generalized pruritus • Itchy eyes • Nausea • Shortness of breath • Swelling of soft tissue (hands, face, tongue) • Vomiting • Wheezing	• Bronchospasm • Cardiopulmonary arrest • Facial edema • Flushing • Hypotension • Laryngeal edema • Tachycardia • Urticaria • Wheezing

• If the patient must be transported to another area of the facility, make certain the latex-free cart accompanies him and that all health care workers who come in contact with him are wearing nonlatex gloves. The patient should wear a mask with cloth ties when leaving his room *to protect him from inhaling airborne latex particles.*

• If the patient will have an I.V. line, make sure that I.V. access is accomplished using all latex-free products. Post a LATEX ALLERGY sign on the I.V. tubing *to prevent access of the line using latex products.* **CDC**

• Flush I.V. tubing with 50 ml of I.V. solution to rinse the tubing out *because of latex ports in the I.V. tubing.*

• Place a warning label on I.V. bags that says, "Don't use latex injection ports."

• Use a nonlatex tourniquet. If none are available, use a latex tourniquet over clothing.

• Remove the vial stopper to mix and draw up medications.

• Use latex-free oxygen administration equipment. Remove the elastic, and tie equipment on with gauze. **CDC**

• Wrap your stethoscope with a nonlatex product *to protect the patient from latex contact.*

• Wrap Tegaderm over the patient's finger before using pulse oximetry.

• Use latex-free syringes when administering medication through a syringe.

• Make sure that an anaphylaxis kit is readily available. If the patient has an allergic reaction to latex, you must act immediately. **CDC**

Special considerations

• Remember that signs and symptoms of latex allergy usually occur within 30 minutes of anesthesia induction. However, the time of onset can range from 10 minutes to 5 hours.

• Don't forget that, as a health care worker, you're in a position to develop a latex hypersensitivity. If you suspect that you're sensitive to latex, contact the employee health services department concerning facility protocol for latex-sensitive employees. Use latex-free products as often as possible *to help reduce your exposure to latex.*

• Don't assume that if something doesn't look like rubber it isn't latex. Latex can be found in a wide variety of equipment, including electrocardiograph leads, oral and nasal airway tubing, tourniquets, nerve stimulation pads, temperature strips, and blood pressure cuffs.

Nursing diagnoses

• Risk for latex allergy response

Expected outcomes

The patient (and his family) will:
- maintain stable vital signs, especially respiratory status, within his limits
- have skin that's free from erythema, edema, urticaria, and breakdown
- have nasal passages and laryngeal areas that remain clear and free from edema and secretions
- express an understanding of the risk of latex allergy.

Supportive references

Burt, S. "What You Need to Know about Latex Allergy," *Nursing99* 30(8):20-25, November 1999. *www.nursingcenter.com.*

Centers for Disease Control and Prevention. National Institute for Occupational Safety and Health. "Latex Allergy: A Prevention Guide," Department of Health and Human Services (NIOSH) Publication No. 98-113. *www.cdc.gov/niosh/98-113.html.*

Charous, B.L. "Latex Allergy: A New and Common Problem," *American Family Physician* 57(1):42, 47, January 1998.

Reddy, S. "Latex Allergy," *American Family Physician* 57(1):93-102, January 1998. *www.aafp.org.*

Manual ventilation

A handheld resuscitation bag is an inflatable device that can be attached to a face mask or directly to an endotracheal (ET) or tracheostomy tube to allow manual delivery of oxygen or room air to the lungs of a patient who can't breathe by himself or has inadequate ventilation. Typically used in an emergency, manual ventilation also can be performed while the patient is disconnected temporarily from a mechanical ventilator, such as during a tubing change, during transport, or before suctioning. In such instances, the use of a handheld resuscitation bag maintains ventilation. Oxygen administration with a resuscitation bag can help improve a compromised cardiorespiratory system.

The American Heart Association's (AHA) 2005 guidelines on cardiopulmonary resuscitation (CPR) and emergency cardiovascular care developed new evidence-based guidelines for basic life support (BLS) and advanced cardiac life support (ACLS). Follow the 2005 guidelines when performing manual ventilation with a handheld resuscitation bag.

BLS providers should perform manual bag-mask ventilation until ACLS providers arrive to provide alternate airway ventilation measures. If tracheal intubation isn't the best option for the patient, such ventilation methods as the laryngeal mask airway or the esophageal-tracheal Combitube can be used. These alternative measures to ventilation are less likely to result in aspiration of stomach contents. The best method of airway management varies based on the health care provider's experience, emergency medical service or health care system characteristics, and the patient's condition. **AHA**

Equipment

Handheld resuscitation bag (1 to 2 L) • mask • oxygen source (wall unit or tank) • oxygen tubing • nipple adapter attached to oxygen flowmeter • optional: oxygen reservoir, positive end-expiratory pressure (PEEP) valve (see *Using a PEEP valve*)

Preparation of equipment

- The typical bag-mask device used for positive-pressure ventilation has a self-inflating bag with a nonrebreathing valve connected to the face mask. Unless the patient is intubated or has a tracheostomy, select a mask that fits snugly over the mouth and nose. Attach the mask to the resuscitation bag.
- If oxygen is readily available, connect the handheld resuscitation bag to the oxygen.
- Attach one end of the tubing to the bottom of the bag and the other end to the nipple adapter on the flowmeter of the oxygen source.
- Adjust the oxygen to a minimal flow rate of 10 to 12 L/mm, oxygen greater than 40%. Ideally, an oxygen reservoir should be used. This device attaches to an adapter on the bottom of the bag and delivers 100% oxygen.

Implementation

- Before using the handheld resuscitation bag, check the patient's upper airway for foreign matter. If present, remove it *because this alone may restore spontaneous respirations in some instances.* Also, foreign matter or secretions can obstruct the airway and impede resuscitation efforts. Suction the patient to remove secretions that may obstruct the airway. If necessary, insert an oropharyngeal or nasopharyngeal airway *to maintain airway patency.* If the patient has a tracheostomy or ET tube in place, suction the tube.

● If appropriate, remove the bed's headboard and stand at the head of the bed to help keep the patient's neck extended and to free space at the side of the bed for other activities such as CPR.

● Use the head tilt-chin lift to move the tongue away from the base of the pharynx and prevent airway obstruction. If trauma is present, use the jaw thrust method. (See *Using a handheld resuscitation bag and mask,* page 320.)

● Keeping your nondominant hand on the patient's mask, exert downward pressure *to seal the mask against his face.* For the adult patient, use your dominant hand to compress the bag to give 8 to 10 breaths/minute.

● Depress the 1-L bag by about one-half to two-thirds of its volume or a 2-L bag about one-third its volume to deliver a tidal volume sufficient to achieve a visible chest rise.

● Deliver each breath over 1 second. Allow the patient to exhale before giving another ventilation.

ALERT *For infants and children, use a pediatric handheld resuscitation bag with a volume of at least 450 to 500 ml. Deliver 20 breaths/ minute, or one compression of the bag every 3 to 5 seconds. (See* Bag-mask resuscitation in pediatric emergencies, *page 321.)*

● Deliver breaths with the patient's inspiratory effort, if present. Don't attempt to deliver a breath as the patient exhales.

● Observe the patient's chest *to ensure that it rises and falls with each compression.* If ventilation fails to occur, check the fit of the mask and the patency of the patient's airway; if necessary, reposition his head and ensure patency with an oral airway.

ALERT *During CPR health care workers commonly deliver excessive ventilation, especially when an advanced airway is in place. Research shows that delivery of greater than 12 breaths/ minute can lead to increased thoracic pressure, impeding venous return to the heart during chest compressions. This causes diminished cardiac output and decreased coronary and cerebral perfusion. Therefore, be sure to deliver ventilation at a rate of 8 to 10 breaths/minute during CPR.* **AHA**

Special considerations

● Avoid neck hyperextension if the patient has a possible cervical injury; instead, use the jaw-thrust technique to open the airway. **AHA**

Using a PEEP valve

Add positive end-expiratory pressure (PEEP) to manual ventilation by attaching a PEEP valve to the resuscitation bag. *This may improve oxygenation if the patient hasn't responded to increased fraction of inspired oxygen levels.* Always use a PEEP valve to manually ventilate a patient who has been receiving PEEP on the ventilator.

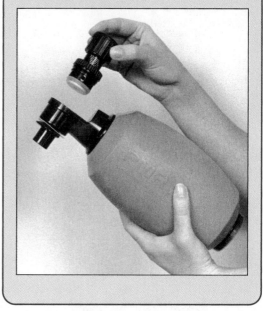

● If you need both hands to keep the patient's mask in place and maintain hyperextension, use the lower part of your arm to compress the bag against your side.

● Observe for vomiting through the clear part of the mask. If vomiting occurs, stop the procedure immediately, lift the mask, turn the patient to his side, wipe and suction vomitus, and resume resuscitation. **AHA**

● Underventilation occurs because the handheld resuscitation bag is difficult to keep positioned tightly on the patient's face while ensuring an open airway. Furthermore, the volume of air delivered to the patient varies with the type of bag used and the hand size of the person compressing the bag. An adult with a small or medium-sized hand may not consistently deliver sufficient air. For these reasons, have someone assist with the procedure, if possible.

Using a handheld resuscitation bag and mask

Bag-mask resuscitation by one rescuer
1. Circle the edges of the mask with the index and first finger of one hand while lifting the jaw with the other fingers. Make sure that there's a tight seal. Use the other hand to compress the bag. Make sure that the chest rises with each breath.

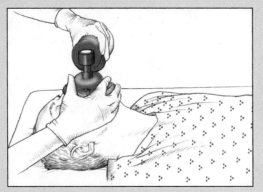

2. Make sure that the patient's mouth remains open underneath the mask. Attach the bag to the mask and to the tubing leading to the oxygen source.

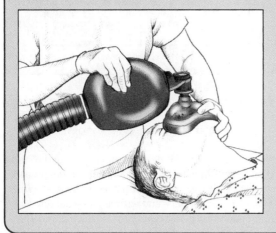

3. Alternatively, if the patient has a tracheostomy or endotracheal tube in place, remove the mask from the bag and attach the handheld resuscitation bag directly to the tube.

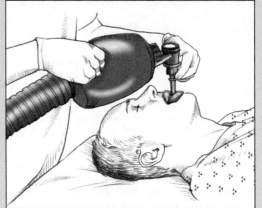

Bag-mask resuscitation by two rescuers
One rescuer stands at the victim's head and uses the thumb and the first finger of both hands to completely seal the edges of the mask. The other fingers lift the jaw and extend the victim's neck. The second rescuer squeezes the bag over 1 second until the chest rises.

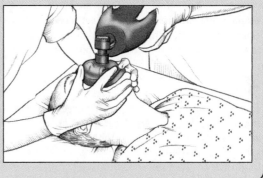

ALERT *The person providing resuscitation with a handheld bag-mask ventilation device may have difficulty providing a tight seal to the face while simultaneously keeping the airway open and squeezing the bag, resulting in a smaller tidal volume. Therefore, bag-mask resuscitation is more efficient when performed by two trained rescuers, with one rescuer providing a seal to the face and the other inflating the bag.* **AHA**

Nursing diagnoses
- Impaired spontaneous ventilation

Expected outcomes

The patient will:
- maintain normal arterial blood gas levels
- breathe spontaneously after ventilator support is withdrawn.

Complications

- Aspiration of vomitus can result in pneumonia, and gastric distention may result from air forced into the patient's stomach.

Documentation

In an emergency, record the date and time you started and stopped the procedure, manual ventilation efforts, oxygen flow rate, any complications and interventions taken, and the patient's response to treatment, according to your facility's policy for respiratory arrest.

In a nonemergency situation, record the date and time of the procedure, reason and length of time the patient was disconnected from mechanical ventilation and received manual ventilation, any complications and interventions taken, and the patient's tolerance of the procedure.

Supportive references

American Heart Association. "2005 AHA Guidelines for Cardiopulmonary Resuscitation and Emergency Cardiovascular Care: International Consensus on Science," *Circulation* 112(22 Suppl):IV-1-IV-211, November 2005.

"Don't Intubate for Peds Emergencies," *AJN* 100(5):19, May 2000.

Little, C. "Manual Ventilation," *Nursing2000* 30(3):50-51, March 2000.

Mechanical ventilation

A mechanical ventilator moves air in and out of a patient's lungs. Although the equipment serves to ventilate a patient, it doesn't ensure adequate gas exchange. Mechanical ventilators may use either positive or negative pressure to ventilate the patient.

Positive-pressure ventilators exert a positive pressure on the airway, which causes inspiration while increasing tidal volume (V_T). The inspiratory cycles of these ventilators may vary in volume, pressure, or time. For example, a volume-cycled ventilator — the type used most commonly — delivers a preset volume

---

Bag-mask resuscitation in pediatric emergencies

Typically, emergency medical workers treat airway emergencies with endotracheal (ET) intubation. However, one study showed that pediatric patients treated with bag-mask resuscitation had the same survival rates and neurologic outcomes as those treated with ET intubation. Moreover, bag-mask resuscitation isn't associated with complications resulting from rushed or difficult intubation. With certain diagnoses, children treated with bag-mask ventilation actually had more favorable survival rates and neurologic outcomes. The researchers recommend that emergency medical workers use bag-mask resuscitation and prompt transportation to a hospital where ET intubation can be performed under more favorable conditions.

---

of air each time, regardless of the amount of lung resistance. A pressure-cycled ventilator generates flow until the machine reaches a preset pressure regardless of the volume delivered or the time required to achieve the pressure. A time-cycled ventilator generates flow for a preset period. A high-frequency ventilator uses high respiratory rates and low V_T to maintain alveolar ventilation.

Negative-pressure ventilators act by creating negative pressure, which pulls the thorax outward and allows air to flow into the lungs. Examples of such ventilators are the iron lung, cuirass (chest shell), and body wrap. Negative-pressure ventilators are used mainly to treat neuromuscular disorders, such as Guillain-Barré syndrome, myasthenia gravis, and poliomyelitis.

Other indications for ventilator use include central nervous system disorders, such as cerebral hemorrhage and spinal cord transsection, acute respiratory distress syndrome, pulmonary edema, chronic obstructive pulmonary disease, flail chest, and acute hypoventilation.

Equipment

Oxygen source • air source that can supply 50 psi • mechanical ventilator • humidifier • ventilator circuit tubing, connectors, and adapters • condensation collection trap • in-line thermometer • gloves • handheld resuscitation bag with reservoir •suction equipment • sterile distilled water •equipment for arterial blood gas (ABG) analysis •optional: oximeter, capnography device

Preparation of equipment

● In most health care facilities, respiratory therapists assume responsibility for setting up the ventilator. If necessary, check the manufacturer's instructions for setting it up. **MFR**

● In most cases, you'll need to add sterile distilled water to the humidifier and connect the ventilator to the appropriate gas source.

Implementation

● Verify the physician's order for ventilator support. If the patient isn't already intubated, prepare him for intubation. (See "Endotracheal intubation," page 289.) **AACN**

● When possible, explain the procedure to the patient and his family *to help reduce anxiety and fear.* Assure them that staff members are nearby to provide care.

● Perform a complete physical assessment and draw blood for ABG analysis *to establish a baseline.* **AARC**

● Suction the patient, if necessary, using a closed suction catheter.

   ALERT *Closed suction catheters should be used to prevent ventilator-associated pneumonia. The catheters don't need to be changed daily for infection control purposes, but the maximum time they can be used is unknown.* **AARC**

● Plug the ventilator into the electrical outlet and turn it on. Adjust the settings on the ventilator as ordered. (See *Mechanical ventilation glossary.*) Make sure that the ventilator's alarms are set, as ordered, and the humidifier is filled with sterile distilled water. Attach a capnographic device to measure carbon dioxide levels *to confirm placement of the endotracheal (ET) tube, detect disconnection from the ventilator, and for early detection of complications.*

● Put on gloves if you haven't already. Connect the ET tube to the ventilator. Observe for chest expansion, and auscultate for bilateral breath sounds *to verify that the patient is being ventilated.* **AACN AARC CDC**

● Monitor the patient's ABG values after the initial ventilator setup (usually 20 to 30 minutes), after changes in ventilator settings, and as the patient's clinical condition indicates *to determine whether the patient is being adequately ventilated and to avoid oxygen toxicity.* Be prepared to adjust ventilator settings depending on ABG values. **AARC**

● Check the ventilator tubing frequently for condensation, *which can cause resistance to airflow and which may also be aspirated by the patient.* As needed, drain the condensate into a collection trap or briefly disconnect the patient from the ventilator (ventilating him with a handheld resuscitation bag, if necessary), and empty the water into an appropriate receptacle. Don't drain the condensate into the humidifier *because the condensation may be contaminated with the patient's secretions and is considered infectious.* Also avoid accidental drainage of condensation into the patient's airway. **AACN AARC**

● Inspect the humidification device regularly and remove condensate as needed. Inspect heat and moisture exchangers, and replace if secretions contaminate the insert or filter. Note humidifier settings. The heated humidifier should be set to deliver an inspired gas temperature of 91.4° F (33° C) plus or minus 3.6° F (2° C) and should provide a minimum of 30 mg/L of water vapor with routine use to an intubated patient.

● If you're using a heated humidifier, monitor the inspired air temperature as close to the patient's airway as possible. The inspiratory gas shouldn't be greater than 98.6° F (37° C) at the opening of the airway. Check that the high temperature alarm is set no higher than 98.6° F and no lower than 86° F (30° C). Observe the amount and consistency of the patient's secretions. If the secretions are copious or increasingly tenacious when a heat and moisture exchanger is used, a heated humidifier should be used instead. **AACN AARC**

● Check the in-line thermometer to make sure that the temperature of the air delivered to the patient is close to body temperature.

● When monitoring the patient's vital signs, count spontaneous breaths as well as ventilator-delivered breaths. **AACN**

● Change, clean, or dispose of the ventilator tubing and equipment according to your facility's policy.

   ALERT *According to the American Association for Respiratory Care's (AARC) standards for ventilator circuit changes, research indicates that ventilator circuits shouldn't be routinely changed for infection control purposes. Studies*

Mechanical ventilation glossary

Although a respiratory therapist usually monitors ventilator settings based on the physician's order, you should understand all of these terms.

Assist-control mode
The ventilator delivers a preset rate; however, the patient can initiate additional breaths, which trigger the ventilator to deliver the preset tidal volume (V_T) at positive pressure.

Continuous positive airway pressure
The continuous positive airway pressure setting prompts the ventilator to deliver positive pressure to the airway throughout the respiratory cycle. It works only on patients who can breathe spontaneously.

Control mode
The ventilator delivers a preset V_T at a fixed rate regardless of whether the patient is breathing spontaneously.

Fraction of inspired oxygen
The fraction of inspired oxygen is the amount of oxygen delivered to the patient by the ventilator. The dial on the ventilator that sets this percentage is labeled as *oxygen concentration* or *oxygen percentage.*

I:E ratio
The I:E ratio compares the duration of inspiration with the duration of expiration. The I:E ratio of normal, spontaneous breathing is 1:2, meaning that expiration is twice as long as inspiration.

Inspiratory flow rate
The inspiratory flow rate denotes the V_T delivered within a certain time. Its value can range from 20 to 120 L/minute.

Minute ventilation or minute volume
The minute ventilation measurement results from multiplying the respiratory rate and V_T.

Peak inspiratory pressure
Measured by the pressure manometer on the ventilator, peak inspiratory pressure reflects the amount of pressure required to deliver a preset V_T.

Positive end-expiratory pressure
In the positive end-expiratory pressure mode, the ventilator is triggered to apply positive pressure at the end of each expiration to increase the area for oxygen exchange by helping to inflate and keep open collapsed alveoli.

Pressure support ventilation
The pressure support ventilation (PSV) mode allows the ventilator to apply a preset amount of positive pressure when the patient inspires spontaneously. PSV increases V_T while decreasing the patient's breathing workload.

Respiratory rate
The respiratory rate is the number of breaths per minute delivered by the ventilator, also called *frequency.*

Sensitivity setting
A sensitivity setting determines the amount of effort the patient must exert to trigger the inspiratory cycle.

Sigh volume
The sigh volume is a ventilator-delivered breath that is 1½ times as large as the patient's V_T.

Synchronized intermittent mandatory ventilation
The ventilator delivers a preset number of breaths at a specific V_T. The patient may supplement these mechanical ventilations with his own breaths, in which case the V_T and rate are determined by his own inspiratory ability.

Tidal volume
V_T refers to the volume of air delivered to the patient with each cycle, usually 8 to 12 ml/kg.

---

show that no patient harm and increased costs savings are associated with extended ventilator circuit change intervals. It isn't known what the maximum time a circuit can safely be used. In addition, there's no evidence related to ventilator-associated pneumonia and the use of heated versus unheated circuits, type of humidifier, method of filling the humidifier, or the technique for emptying condensate from ventilator circuits. The ventilator circuit includes components, such as gas delivery tubing, monitoring tubing, humidifier, heat

Weaning from the ventilator

Successful weaning from the ventilator depends on the patient's ability to breathe on his own. This means that he must have a spontaneous respiratory effort that can keep him ventilated, a stable cardiovascular system, and sufficient respiratory muscle strength and level of consciousness to sustain spontaneous breathing. The patient should meet some or all of the following criteria.

Readiness criteria
- Arterial oxygen saturation (Sao_2) greater than 92% on fraction of inspired oxygen less than or equal to 40%, positive end-expiratory pressure (PEEP) less than or equal to 5 cm H_2O
- Hemodynamically stable, adequately resuscitated and doesn't require vasoactive support
- Serum electrolyte levels and pH within normal range
- Hematocrit greater than 25%
- Core body temperature greater than 96.8° F (36° C) and less than 102.2° F (39° C)
- Pain is adequately managed
- Successful withdrawal of a neuromuscular blocker
- Arterial blood gas values within normal limits or at patient's baseline

Weaning intervention (long term – more than 72 hours)
- Transfer to pressure-support ventilation (PSV) mode and adjust support level to maintian patient's respiratory rate at less than 35 breaths/minute.
- Observe for 30 minutes for signs of early failure, such as:
  - sustained respiratory rate greater than 35 breaths/minute
  - Sao_2 less than 89%
  - tidal volume less than or equal to 5 ml/kg
  - sustained minute ventilation greater than 200 ml/kg/minute

- evidence of respiratory or hemodynamic distress: labored respiratory pattern, increased diaphoresis or anxiety or both, sustained heart rate greater than 20% higher or lower than baseline, systolic blood pressure greater than 180 mm Hg or less than 90 mm Hg higher.
- If tolerated, continue trial for 2 hours, then return patient to "rest" settings by adding ventilator breaths or increasing PSV to achieve a total respiratory rate of less than 20 breaths/minute.
- After 2 hours of rest, repeat trial for 2 to 4 hours at same PSV level as previous trial. If the patient exceeds the tolerance criteria, stop the trial and return to "rest" settings. In this case, the next trial should be performed at a higher support level than the failed trial.
- Record the results after each weaning episode, including specific parameters and the time frame if failure was observed.
- The goal is to increase trial lengths and reduce the PSV level needed in increments.
- With each successful trial, the PSV level may be decreased by 2 to 4 cm H_2O, the time interval may be increased by 1 to 2 hours, or both while keeping the patient within tolerable parameters.
- Ensure nocturnal ventilation at "rest" settings (with a respiratory rate of less than 20 breaths/minute) for at least 6 hours each night until the patient's weaning trials demonstrate readiness to discontinue support. **EB4**

and moisture exchanger, humidifier water reservoir, and water traps. **AARC** **EB1**

The AARC also recommends that passive humidifiers can be used for at least 48 hours and in some patients for up to 1 week. **AARC**

Weaning from the ventilator **AACN** **EB2** **EB3**
- When ordered, begin to wean the patient from the ventilator. (See *Weaning from the ventilator*.) According to the American Association of Critical-Care Nurses' (AACN) Third National Study Group, weaning

from mechanical ventilation is a process consisting of 3 stages: preweaning, weaning, and outcome.
- During the preweaning stage, the events leading up to the need for mechanical ventilation are considered and complications that may interfere with weaning are prevented. The health care team determines the patient's readiness for weaning and chooses a strategy and mode of weaning. As the patient stabilizes, he crosses the readiness threshold into the weaning stage.

● During the weaning stage, the patient may experience progress and setbacks. Factors related to the patient that may affect weaning during this phase include myocardial function and oxygenation, nutrition, electrolyte balance, ventilatory muscle strength, ventilatory drive, and psychological concerns. During weaning, assessment criteria that indicate a weaning trial should be stopped include dyspnea; rapid, shallow breathing; facial expression; accessory muscle use; heart rate; and blood pressure. Facilitative strategies, such as biofeedback, may also be used during this phase.

● The outcome stage includes complete weaning, incomplete weaning where long-term partial or full mechanical ventilatory support may be required, and terminal weaning in which natural death may occur (also called *withdrawal of life support*).

◆ **INNOVATIVE PRACTICE** *Many studies have shown that the ability to successfully wean a patient from mechanical ventilation is determined by a coordinated multidisciplinary team approach rather than the use of a particular weaning protocol. Studies that focused on particular weaning methods failed to show that one weaning approach (such as T-piece, intermittent mandatory ventilation [IMV], and pressure support ventilation [PSV]) was superior to another.*

To facilitate a team approach to weaning, all members of the team should be involved in the development of a weaning protocol even if only the respiratory therapists or nurses will actually be implementing the protocol.

A communication and documentation plan also should be developed. Because documentation in an intensive care unit is usually short term, tracking the progress of weaning over several days or even weeks is typically difficult. Use of communication boards and weaning flow sheets facilitates communication and demonstrates progression to all members of the health care team, the patient, and the patient's family.

The weaning board may be a dry-erase board kept at the patient's bedside. Information on assessment of readiness, the weaning plan, and criteria for stopping a weaning trial should be included. Weaning flow sheets contain variables related to weaning and include space for several days' documentation so that trends can be seen.

Multidisciplinary rounds are also recommended to facilitate weaning. During rounds, patient progress is discussed and plans are communicated to the team. **EB2**

Special considerations

● Make sure the ventilator alarms are on at all times. *These alarms alert the nursing staff to potentially hazardous conditions and changes in the patient's status.* If an alarm sounds and the problem can't be identified easily, disconnect the patient from the ventilator and use a handheld resuscitation bag to ventilate him. (See *Responding to ventilator alarms,* page 326.)

● Provide emotional support to the patient during all phases of mechanical ventilation *to reduce anxiety and promote successful treatment.* Even if the patient is unresponsive, continue to explain all procedures and treatment to him.

● Unless contraindicated, turn the patient from side to side every 1 to 2 hours *to facilitate lung expansion and removal of secretions.* Perform active or passive range-of-motion exercises for all extremities *to reduce the hazards of immobility.* If the patient's condition permits, position him upright at regular intervals *to increase lung expansion.* When moving the patient or the ventilator tubing, be careful to prevent condensation in the tubing from flowing into the lungs *because aspiration of this contaminated moisture can cause infection.* Provide care for the patient's artificial airway as needed. **AACN**

● Assess the patient's peripheral circulation, and monitor his urine output for signs of decreased cardiac output. Watch for signs and symptoms of fluid volume excess or dehydration.

● Place the call button within the patient's reach, and establish a method of communication, such as a communication board, *because intubation and mechanical ventilation impair the patient's ability to speak.* An artificial airway may help the patient to speak by allowing air to pass through his vocal cords.

● Administer a sedative or neuromuscular blocking agent, as ordered, *to relax the patient or eliminate spontaneous breathing efforts that can interfere with the ventilator's action.* Remember that the patient receiving a neuromuscular blocking medication requires close observation *because of his inability to breathe or communicate.* **AACN**

● If the patient is receiving a neuromuscular blocking agent, make sure that he also receives a sedative.

Responding to ventilator alarms

The chart below distinguishes ventilator alarms, their possible causes, and appropriate interventions.

Signal	Possible cause	Interventions
Low-pressure alarm	• Tube disconnected from ventilator	• Reconnect the tube to the ventilator.
	• Endotracheal (ET) tube displaced above vocal cords or tracheostomy tube extubated	• Check tube placement and reposition it, if needed. If extubation or displacement has occurred, ventilate the patient manually and call the physician immediately.
	• Leaking tidal volume from low cuff pressure (from an underinflated or ruptured cuff or a leak in the cuff or one-way valve)	• Listen for a whooshing sound around the tube, indicating an air leak. If you hear one, check cuff pressure. If you can't maintain pressure, call the physician; he may need to insert a new tube.
	• Ventilator malfunction	• Disconnect the patient from the ventilator and ventilate him manually, if necessary. Obtain another ventilator.
	• Leak in ventilator circuitry (from loose connection or hole in tubing, loss of temperature-sensitive device, or cracked humidification jar)	• Make sure that all connections are intact. Check for holes or leaks in the tubing and replace it, if necessary. Check the humidification jar and replace it, if cracked.
High-pressure alarm	• Increased airway pressure or decreased lung compliance caused by worsening disease	• Auscultate the lungs for evidence of increasing lung consolidation, barotrauma, or wheezing. Call the physician, if indicated.
	• Patient biting on oral ET tube	• Insert a bite block, if needed.
	• Secretions in airway	• Listen for secretions in the airway. To remove them, suction the patient or have him cough.
	• Condensate in large-bore tubing	• Check tubing for condensate, and remove any fluid.
	• Intubation of right mainstem bronchus	• Check tube position. If it has slipped, call the physician; he may need to reposition it.
	• Patient coughing, gagging, or attempting to talk	• If the patient fights the ventilator, provide explanations and use a communication board. If these fail, the physician may order a sedative or neuromuscular blocking agent.
	• Chest wall resistance	• Reposition the patient to see if doing so improves chest expansion. If repositioning doesn't help, administer the prescribed analgesic.
	• Failure of high-pressure relief valve	• Have the faulty equipment replaced.
	• Bronchospasm	• Assess the patient for the cause. Report to the physician and treat as ordered.

Neuromuscular blocking agents cause paralysis without altering the patient's level of consciousness (LOC). Reassure the patient and his family that the paralysis is temporary. Also make sure that emergency equipment is readily available in case the ventilator malfunctions or the patient is accidentally extubated. Continue to explain all procedures to the patient, and take extra steps to ensure his safety, such as raising the side rails during turning and covering and lubricating his eyes. **AACN**

● Make sure that the patient gets adequate rest and sleep *because fatigue can delay weaning from the ventilator.* Provide subdued lighting, safely muffle equipment noises, and restrict staff access to the area *to promote quiet during rest periods.*

● When weaning the patient, continue to observe for signs of hypoxia. Schedule weaning to fit comfortably and realistically with the patient's daily regimen. Avoid scheduling sessions after meals, baths, or lengthy therapeutic or diagnostic procedures. Have the patient help you set up the schedule *to give him some sense of control over a frightening procedure.* As the patient's tolerance for weaning increases, help him sit up out of bed *to improve his breathing and sense of well-being.* Suggest diversionary activities *to take his mind off breathing.*

TEACHING *If the patient will be discharged on a ventilator, evaluate the family's or the caregiver's ability and motivation to provide such care. Well before discharge, develop a teaching plan that will address the patient's needs. For example, teaching should include information about ventilator care and settings, artificial airway care, suctioning, respiratory therapy, communication, nutrition, therapeutic exercise, the signs and symptoms of infection, and ways to troubleshoot minor equipment malfunctions.*

● Also evaluate the patient's need for adaptive equipment, such as a hospital bed, wheelchair or walker with a ventilator tray, patient lift, and bedside commode. Determine whether the patient needs to travel; if so, select appropriate portable and backup equipment.

● Before discharge, have the patient's caregiver demonstrate her ability to use the equipment. At discharge, contact a durable medical equipment vendor and a home health nurse to follow up with the patient. Also refer the patient to community resources, if available.

Nursing diagnoses
● Impaired spontaneous ventilation

Expected outcomes
The patient will:
● maintain normal ABG levels
● breathe spontaneously after ventilatory support is withdrawn
● have a partial pressure of arterial oxygen that remains within normal limits as his activity level increases.

Complications
● Mechanical ventilation can cause tension pneumothorax, decreased cardiac output, oxygen toxicity, fluid volume excess caused by humidification, infection, and such GI complications as distention or bleeding from stress ulcers.

Documentation
Document the date and time of initiation of mechanical ventilation. Name the type of ventilator used for the patient, and note its settings. Include ET tube or tracheostomy size, position, and pressure. Describe the patient's subjective and objective response to mechanical ventilation, including his vital signs, breath sounds, accessory muscle use, skin color, chest motion, intake and output, and weight. Note any spontaneous respirations. List any complications and interventions taken. Record all pertinent laboratory data, including ABG analysis results, end-tidal carbon dioxide values, and oxygen saturation levels.

During weaning, record the date and time of each session, the weaning method used, and baseline and subsequent vital signs, oxygen saturation levels, and ABG values. Describe the patient's subjective and objective responses, including LOC, respiratory effort, arrhythmias, skin color, and need for suctioning.

List all complications and interventions taken. If the patient was receiving PSV or using a T-piece or tracheostomy collar, note the duration of spontaneous breathing and the patient's ability to maintain the weaning schedule. If using IMV, with or without PSV, record the control breath rate, the time of each breath reduction, and the rate of spontaneous respirations.

Supportive references
Agency for Healthcare Research and Quality. *Criteria for Weaning from Mechanical Ventilation.* Evidence

Report/Technology Assessment: Number 23. AHRQ Publication No. 00-E028, June 2000. *www.ahrq.gov/clinic/epcsums/mechsumm.htm.*

Ahrens, T., et al. "End-Tidal Carbon Dioxide Measurements as a Prognostic Indicator of Outcome of Cardiac Arrest," *American Journal of Critical Care* 10(6):391-98, November 2001.

American Association for Respiratory Care. "AARC Clinical Practice Guideline: Capnography/Capnometry during Mechanical Ventilation," *Respiratory Care* 48(5):534-39, May 2003.

American Association for Respiratory Care. "AARC Clinical Practice Guideline: Care of the Ventilator Circuit," *Respiratory Care* 48(9):869-79, September 2003. **EB1**

American Association for Respiratory Care. "AARC Clinical Practice Guideline: Evidence-Based Guideline for Weaning and Discontinuing Ventilatory Support," *Respiratory Care* 47(1):69-90, January 2002.

American Association for Respiratory Care. "AARC Clinical Practice Guideline: Patient-Ventilator System Checks," *Respiratory Care* 37(8):882-86, August 1992.

Henneman, E.A. "Liberating Patients from Mechanical Ventilation: A Team Approach," *Critical Care Nurse* 21(3):25, 27-33, June 2001. **EB2**

Knebel, A., et al. "Weaning from Mechanical Ventilatory Support: Refinement of a Model," *American Journal of Critical Care* 7(2):149-52, March 1998. **EB3**

Morton, P.G., et al. *Critical Care Nursing: A Holistic Approach*, 8th ed. Philadelphia: Lippincott Williams & Wilkins, 2005. **EB4**

Tasota, F.J., and Dobbin, K. "Weaning Your Patient from Mechanical Ventilation," *Nursing2000* 30(10):41-46, October 2000.

Nasopharyngeal airway insertion and care

Insertion of a nasopharyngeal airway — a soft rubber or latex uncuffed catheter — establishes or maintains a patent airway. This airway is the typical choice for patients who have had recent oral surgery or facial trauma and for patients with loose, cracked, or avulsed teeth. It's also used to protect the nasal mucosa from injury when the patient needs frequent nasotracheal suctioning. This type of airway may also be tolerated better than an oropharyngeal airway by a patient who isn't deeply unconscious.

According to the 2005 American Heart Association's (AHA) guidelines for cardiopulmonary resuscitation and emergency cardiovascular care, a nasopharyngeal airway is especially useful in patients with such conditions as clenched jaws, which prevent placement of an oral airway. It also may be used in patients with an obstructed airway to deliver ventilations with a bag-mask device. The 2005 guidelines warn that this type of airway should be used cautiously in patients with severe craniofacial injury. They also stress that safe use of nasopharyngeal airways requires adequate training and practice, with regular retraining. **AHA**

The airway follows the curvature of the nasopharynx, passing through the nose and extending from the nostril to the posterior pharynx. The bevel-shaped pharyngeal end of the airway facilitates insertion, and its funnel-shaped nasal end helps prevent slippage.

Insertion of a nasopharyngeal airway is preferred when an oropharyngeal airway is contraindicated or fails to maintain a patent airway. A nasopharyngeal airway is contraindicated if the patient is receiving anticoagulant therapy or has a hemorrhagic disorder, sepsis, or pathologic nasopharyngeal deformity. It's been found that airway bleeding can occur in up to 30% of patients after insertion. **AHA**

Equipment
Insertion
Nasopharyngeal airway of proper size • tongue blade • water-soluble lubricant • gloves • optional: suction equipment

Cleaning
Hydrogen peroxide • water • basin • optional: pipe cleaner

Preparation of equipment
● Measure the diameter of the patient's nostril and the distance from the tip of his nose to his earlobe.
● Select an airway that's a slightly smaller diameter than the nostril and about 1″ (2.5 cm) longer than measured. The sizes for this type of airway are labeled according to their internal diameter. The recommended size for a large adult is 8 to 9 mm; for a medium adult, 7 to 8 mm; for a small adult, 6 to 7 mm.
● Lubricate the distal half of the airway's surface with a water-soluble lubricant *to prevent traumatic injury during insertion.*

Implementation

- Put on gloves. **CDC**
- In a nonemergency situation, explain the procedure to the patient.
- Properly insert the airway. (See *Inserting a nasopharyngeal airway*.)
- After the airway is inserted, check it regularly *to detect dislodgment or obstruction*.
- When the patient's natural airway is patent, remove the airway in one smooth motion. If the airway sticks, apply lubricant around the nasal end of the tube and around the nostril, and then gently rotate the airway until it's free.

Special considerations

- When you insert the airway, remember to use a chin-lift or jaw-thrust technique to anteriorly displace the patient's mandible. Immediately after insertion, assess the patient's respirations. If absent or inadequate, initiate artificial positive-pressure ventilation with a mouth-to-mask technique, a handheld resuscitation bag, or an oxygen-powered breathing device.
- If the patient coughs or gags, the tube may be too long. If so, remove the airway and insert a shorter one.
- At least once every 8 hours, remove the airway to check nasal mucous membranes for irritation or ulceration. **AARC**
- Clean the airway by placing it in a basin and rinsing it with hydrogen peroxide and then with water. If secretions remain, use a pipe cleaner to remove them. Reinsert the clean airway into the other nostril (if it's patent) *to avoid skin breakdown*.

Nursing diagnoses

- Impaired gas exchange
- Risk for injury

Expected outcomes

The patient will:
- maintain respiratory rate within 5 breaths/minute of baseline
- have normal breath sounds
- have mucous membranes remain intact.

Complications

- Sinus infection may result from obstruction of sinus drainage.

Inserting a nasopharyngeal airway

First, hold the airway beside the patient's face *to make sure that it's the proper size* (as shown below). It should be slightly smaller than the patient's nostril diameter and slightly longer than the distance from the tip of his nose to his earlobe.

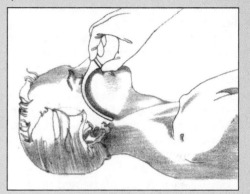

To insert the airway, hyperextend the patient's neck (unless contraindicated). Then push up the tip of his nose and pass the airway into his nostril (as shown below). Avoid pushing against any resistance *to prevent tissue trauma and airway kinking*.

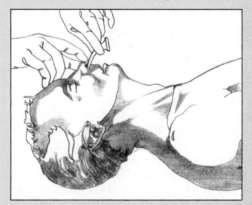

To check for correct airway placement, first close the patient's mouth. Then place your finger over the tube's opening *to detect air exchange*. Depress the patient's tongue with a tongue blade, and look for the airway tip behind the uvula.

● Insertion of the airway may injure the nasal mucosa and cause bleeding and, possibly, aspiration of blood into the trachea. Suction as necessary to remove secretions or blood.

● If the tube is too long, it may enter the esophagus and cause gastric distention and hypoventilation during artificial ventilation. In addition, if the tube is too long, stimulation of the laryngeal or glossopharyngeal reflexes may cause laryngospasm, retching, or vomiting.

● Although semiconscious patients usually tolerate this type of airway better than conscious patients do, they may still experience laryngospasm and vomiting.

Documentation

Record the date and time of the airway's insertion, size of the airway, removal and cleaning of the airway, shifts from one nostril to the other, condition of the mucous membranes, suctioning, any complications and interventions taken, and the patient's tolerance of the procedure.

Supportive references

American Heart Association. "2005 AHA Guidelines for Cardiopulmonary Resuscitation and Emergency Cardiovascular Care: International Consensus on Science," *Circulation* 112(22 Suppl):IV-1-IV-211, November 2005.

Nebulizer therapy

An established component of respiratory care, nebulizer therapy aids bronchial hygiene by restoring and maintaining mucous blanket continuity, hydrating dried, retained secretions, promoting expectoration of secretions, humidifying inspired oxygen, and delivering medications. The therapy may be administered through nebulizers that have a large or small volume, are ultrasonic, or are placed inside ventilator tubing.

Ultrasonic nebulizers are electrically driven and use high-frequency vibrations to break up surface water into particles. The resultant dense mist can penetrate smaller airways and is useful for hydrating secretions and inducing a cough. Large-volume nebulizers are used to provide humidity for an artificial airway, such as a tracheostomy, and small-volume nebulizers are used to deliver medications such as bronchodilators. In-line nebulizers are used to deliver medications to patients who are being mechanically ventilated. In this case, the nebulizer is placed in the inspiratory side of the ventilatory circuit as close to the endotracheal tube as possible.

Standard precautions for body fluid isolation should be used for all patients on nebulizer therapy. **CDC** To control the exposure to tuberculosis (TB) and droplet nuclei from a patient with known or suspected TB, implement the following measures:
● enclose and contain aerosol administration
● filter aerosols that bypass or are exhaled by the patient.

If the release of the aerosol can't be routed through a filter, the Centers for Disease Control and Prevention (CDC) recommends:
● using filtered scavenger systems to remove the aerosols that can't be contained
● using local exhaust ventilation to remove aerosols that are released into room air
● providing frequent air exchange to dilute the concentration of aerosol in the room
● allowing exchange of gas in the room to eliminate 99% of the aerosol before the next patient enters or receives treatment in that area.

If multiple patients are treated in one area, make available booths or stalls that provide airflow to draw aerosol and droplet nuclei into a filtration system. The CDC recommends:
● not reusing nebulizers between disinfection
● considering filters, nebulizers, and other disposable parts hazardous waste after use
● using personal protection devices, such as goggles, masks, gowns, and gloves, when engineering alternatives aren't in place
● minimize exposure to aerosols because data show that adverse effects of certain aerosols on health care workers is incomplete. **AARC** **CDC**

Equipment
Ultrasonic nebulizer
Ultrasonic gas-delivery device ●large-bore oxygen tubing ●nebulizer couplet compartment

Large-volume nebulizer (such as Venturi jet)
Pressurized gas source ●flowmeter ●large-bore oxygen tubing ●nebulizer bottle ●sterile distilled water ● heater (if ordered) ●in-line thermometer (if using heater)

Small-volume nebulizer (such as mini-nebulizer)

Pressurized gas source • flowmeter • oxygen tubing • nebulizer cup • mouthpiece or mask • normal saline solution or water • prescribed medication

In-line nebulizer

Pressurized gas source • flowmeter • nebulizer cup • normal saline solution • prescribed medication

Preparation of equipment

Ultrasonic nebulizer

● Fill the couplet compartment on the nebulizer to the level indicated.

Large-volume nebulizer

● Fill the water chamber to the indicated level with sterile distilled water. Avoid using normal saline solution *to prevent corrosion.*

● Add a heating device if ordered, and place an in-line thermometer between the outlet port and the patient, as close to the patient as possible, *to monitor the actual temperature of the inhaled gas and to avoid burning the patient.*

● If the unit will supply oxygen, analyze the flow at the patient's end of the tubing *to ensure delivery of the prescribed oxygen percentage.*

Small-volume nebulizer

● Draw up the prescribed medication, inject it into the nebulizer cup, and add the prescribed amount of normal saline solution or water.

● Attach the mouthpiece, mask, or other gas-delivery device.

In-line nebulizer

● Draw up the prescribed medication and diluent, remove the nebulizer cup, quickly inject the medication, and then replace the cup.

● If using an intermittent positive-pressure breathing machine, attach the mouthpiece and mask to the machine.

Implementation

● Confirm the patient's identity using two patient identifiers according to facility policy. **JCAHO**

● Explain the procedure to the patient, and wash your hands. **CDC**

● Take the patient's vital signs, and auscultate his lung fields *to establish a baseline.* If possible, place the patient in a sitting or high Fowler's position *to encourage full lung expansion and promote aerosol dispersion.* Encourage the patient to take slow, even breaths during the treatment. **Science**

Ultrasonic nebulizer

● Before beginning, administer an inhaled bronchodilator (metered-dose inhaler or small-volume nebulizer) *to prevent bronchospasm.*

● Turn on the machine, and check the outflow port *to ensure proper misting.*

● Check the patient frequently during the procedure *to observe for adverse reactions.* Watch for labored respirations *because ultrasonic nebulizer therapy may hydrate retained secretions and obstruct airways.* Take the patient's vital signs, and listen to his lung fields.

● Encourage the patient to cough and expectorate, or suction his airway as needed.

Large-volume nebulizer

● Attach the delivery device to the patient.

● Encourage the patient to cough and expectorate, or suction his airway as needed.

● Check the water level in the nebulizer at frequent intervals and refill or replace as indicated. When refilling a reusable container, discard the old water *to prevent infection from bacterial or fungal growth,* and refill the container to the indicator line with sterile distilled water.

● Change the nebulizer unit and the oxygen tubing according to your facility's policy *to prevent bacterial contamination.*

● If the nebulizer is heated, tell the patient to report warmth, discomfort, or hot tubing *because these may indicate a heater malfunction.* Use the in-line thermometer to monitor the temperature of the gas the patient is inhaling. If you turn off the flow for more than 5 minutes, unplug the heater *to avoid overheating the water and burning the patient when the aerosol is resumed.*

Small-volume nebulizer

● After attaching the flowmeter to the gas source, attach the nebulizer to the flowmeter and then adjust the flow to at least 10 L/minute *to ensure adequate functioning* but not more than 14 L/minute *to prevent excess venting.*

- Check the outflow port *to ensure adequate misting.*
- Remain with the patient during the treatment, which lasts 15 to 20 minutes, and take his vital signs *to detect adverse reactions to the medication.*
- Encourage the patient to cough and expectorate, or suction his airway as necessary.
- Change the nebulizer cup and tubing according to your facility's policy *to prevent bacterial contamination.* **CDC**

In-line nebulizer
- Turn on the machine and check the outflow port *to ensure proper misting.*
- Remain with the patient during the treatment, which lasts 15 to 20 minutes, and take his vital signs *to detect adverse reactions to the medication.*
- Encourage the patient to cough, and suction excess secretions as necessary.
- Listen to the patient's lungs *to evaluate the effectiveness of therapy.*

Special considerations
- When using a high-output nebulizer, such as an ultrasonic nebulizer, on pediatric patients or patients with a delicate fluid balance, stay alert for signs of overhydration (exhibited by unexplained weight gain occurring over several days after the beginning of therapy), pulmonary edema, crackles, and electrolyte imbalance.
- If oxygen is being delivered concomitantly, the fraction of inspired oxygen (FIO_2) may be diluted if the flow isn't adequate. Therefore, if the mist disappears when the patient inhales, increase the gas flow.

Nursing diagnoses
- Ineffective breathing pattern

Expected outcomes
The patient will:
- have mobilization of fluids and secretions
- have improved oxygen saturation as indicated by pulse oximetry
- report feeling comfortable when breathing.

Complications
- Nebulized particulates can irritate the mucosa in some patients and cause bronchospasm and dyspnea.
- Other complications include airway burns (when heating elements are used), infection from contaminated equipment (rare), and adverse reactions from medications.

Documentation
Record the date, time, and duration of therapy; type and amount of medication; FIO_2 or oxygen flow, if administered; baseline and subsequent vital signs and breath sounds; and the patient's response to treatment.

Supportive references
American Association for Respiratory Care. "AARC Clinical Practice Guideline: Bland Aerosol Administration," *Respiratory Care* 48(5):529-33, May 2003.
American Association for Respiratory Care. "AARC Clinical Practice Guideline: Selection of Aerosol Delivery Device," *Respiratory Care* 37(8):891-97, August 1992.

Oronasopharyngeal suction

Oronasopharyngeal suction removes secretions from the pharynx by a suction catheter inserted through the mouth or nostril. Performed to maintain a patent airway, this procedure helps the patient who can't clear his airway effectively with coughing and expectoration such as the unconscious or severely debilitated patient. The procedure should be done as often as necessary, depending on the patient's condition.

Oronasopharyngeal suction is an aseptic procedure that requires sterile equipment. However, clean technique may be used for a tonsil tip suction device. In fact, an alert patient can use a tonsil tip suction device himself to remove secretions.

Nasopharyngeal suctioning should be used with caution in patients who have nasopharyngeal bleeding or spinal fluid leakage into the nasopharyngeal area, in trauma patients, in patients receiving anticoagulant therapy, and in those who have blood diseases because these conditions increase the risk of bleeding.

Equipment
Wall suction or portable suction apparatus • collection bottle • connecting tubing • water-soluble lubricant • sterile normal saline solution • disposable sterile container • sterile suction catheter (#12 or #14 French

catheter for an adult, #8 or #10 French catheter for a child, or pediatric feeding tube for an infant) • sterile gloves • clean gloves • nasopharyngeal or oropharyngeal airway (optional for frequent suctioning) • overbed table or bedside stand • waterproof trash bag • mask and goggles or face shield • optional: tongue blade, tonsil tip suction device

A commercially prepared kit contains a sterile catheter, disposable container, and sterile gloves.

Preparation of equipment

• Before beginning, check your facility's policy to determine whether a physician's order is required for oronasopharyngeal suctioning.
• Review the patient's arterial blood gas (ABG) or oxygen saturation values, and check his vital signs.
• Evaluate the patient's ability to cough and deep breathe *to determine his ability to move secretions up the tracheobronchial tree.*
• Check the patient's history for a deviated septum, nasal polyps, nasal obstruction, traumatic injury, epistaxis, or mucosal swelling.
• If no contraindications exist, gather and place the suction equipment on the patient's overbed table or bedside stand.
• Position the table or stand on your preferred side of the bed *to facilitate suctioning.*
• Attach the collection bottle to the suctioning unit, and attach the connecting tubing to it.
• Date and then open the bottle of sterile normal saline solution.
• Open the waterproof trash bag.

Implementation AARC

• Confirm the patient's identity using two patient identifiers according to facility policy. JCAHO
• Explain the procedure to the patient, even if he's unresponsive. Inform him that suctioning may stimulate transient coughing or gagging, but tell him that coughing helps to mobilize secretions. Reassure him throughout the procedure *to minimize anxiety and fear, which can increase oxygen consumption.* Assess nasal patency.
• Wash your hands. CDC
• Assess the patient for other signs of respiratory compromise, such as labored breathing, tachypnea, or cyanosis.

• Place the patient in semi-Fowler's or high Fowler's position, if tolerated, *to promote lung expansion and effective coughing.*
• Put on goggles and a mask or a face shield. CDC
• Turn on the suction from the wall or portable suction apparatus, and set the pressure according to your facility's policy. The American Association for Respiratory Care (AARC) recommends that pressure be set at 100 to 150 mm Hg for adults and 100 to 120 mm Hg for children *because higher pressures cause excessive trauma, hypoxemia, and atelectasis without enhancing secretion removal.* Occlude the end of the connecting tubing *to check suction pressure.*
• Using strict aseptic technique, open the suction catheter kit or the packages containing the sterile catheter, container, and gloves. Put on the gloves; consider your dominant hand sterile and your nondominant hand nonsterile. Using your nondominant hand, pour the saline solution into the sterile container.
• With your nondominant hand, place a small amount of water-soluble lubricant on the sterile area. *The lubricant is used to facilitate passage of the catheter during nasopharyngeal suctioning.*
• Pick up the catheter with your dominant (sterile) hand and attach it to the connecting tubing. Use your nondominant hand to control the suction valve while your dominant hand manipulates the catheter.
• Instruct the patient to cough and breathe slowly and deeply several times before beginning suction. Coughing helps loosen secretions and may decrease the amount of suction necessary, while deep breathing helps minimize or prevent hypoxia. (See *Airway clearance tips,* page 334.) Science

Nasal insertion AARC

• Raise the tip of the patient's nose with your nondominant hand *to straighten the passageway and facilitate catheter insertion.* Without applying suction, gently insert the sterile suction catheter into the patient's nostril. Roll the catheter between your fingers *to help it advance through the turbinates.* Continue to advance the catheter approximately 5″ to 6″ (12.5 to 15 cm) until you reach the pool of secretions or the patient begins to cough.

Oral insertion

• Without applying suction, gently insert the catheter into the patient's mouth. Advance it 3″ to 4″ (7.5 to

TEACHING

Airway clearance tips

Deep breathing and coughing are vital for removing secretions from the airways. Other techniques used to help clear the airways include diaphragmatic breathing and forced expiration. Here's how to teach these techniques to your patients.

Diaphragmatic breathing

First, tell the patient to lie supine, with his head elevated 15 to 20 degrees on a pillow. Tell him to place one hand on his abdomen and then inhale so that he can feel his abdomen rise. Explain that this is known as *breathing with the diaphragm.*

Next, instruct the patient to exhale slowly through his nose — or, even better, through pursed lips — while letting his abdomen collapse. Explain that this action decreases his respiratory rate and increases his tidal volume.

Suggest that the patient perform this exercise for 30 minutes several times per day. After he becomes accustomed to the position and has learned to breathe using his diaphragm, he may apply abdominal weights of 8.8 to 11 lb (4 to 5 kg). *The weights enhance the movement of the diaphragm toward the head during expiration.*

To enhance the effectiveness of exercise, the patient may also manually compress the lower costal margins, perform straight-leg lifts, and coordinate the breathing technique with a physical activity such as walking.

Forced expiration

Explain to the patient that forced expiration (also known as *huff coughing*) helps clear secretions while causing less traumatic injury than does a cough. To perform the technique, tell the patient to forcefully expire without closing his glottis, starting with a middle to low lung volume. Tell him to follow this expiration with a period of diaphragmatic breathing and relaxation.

10 cm) along the side of the patient's mouth until you reach the pool of secretions or the patient begins to cough. Suction both sides of the patient's mouth and pharyngeal area.

● Using intermittent suction, withdraw the catheter from either the mouth or the nose with a continuous rotating motion *to minimize invagination of the mucosa into the catheter's tip and side ports.* Apply suction for no longer than 10 to 15 seconds at a time *to minimize tissue trauma and hypoxia.* **Science**

● Between passes, wrap the catheter around your dominant hand *to prevent contamination.*

● If secretions are thick, clear the catheter lumen by dipping it in sterile normal saline solution and applying suction.

● Repeat the procedure a second time, if necessary.

● After completing suctioning, pull your sterile glove off over the coiled catheter and discard it and the nonsterile glove along with the container of water. **CDC**

● Flush the connecting tubing with sterile normal saline solution.

● Replace the reusable items *so they're ready for the next suctioning,* and wash your hands.

● Assist the patient with mouth care.

Special considerations

● If the patient has no history of nasal problems, alternate suctioning between nostrils *to minimize traumatic injury.* If repeated oronasopharyngeal suctioning is required, the use of a nasopharyngeal or oropharyngeal airway will help with catheter insertion, reduce traumatic injury, and promote a patent airway. *To facilitate catheter insertion for oropharyngeal suctioning,* depress the patient's tongue with a tongue blade, or ask another nurse to do so. *This helps you to visualize the back of the throat and also prevents the patient from biting the catheter.*

● If the patient has excessive oral secretions, consider using a tonsil tip catheter *because this allows the patient to remove oral secretions independently.*

● Let the patient rest after suctioning while you continue to observe him. The frequency and duration of suctioning depend on the patient's tolerance of the procedure and on any complications.

● Remember that oronasopharyngeal suctioning is just one component of bronchial hygiene. The patient's lungs should be auscultated before suctioning to determine the presence of secretions in the airways.

● Perform suctioning only when necessary and when other methods of removing secretions haven't been effective.

TEACHING *Oronasopharyngeal suctioning may be performed in the home using a portable suction machine. Under these circumstances, suctioning is a clean rather than a sterile procedure. Properly cleaned catheters can be reused, putting less financial strain on patients.*

Catheters should be cleaned by first washing them in water with a detergent, followed by one of the following: a 60-minute soak in solution of vinegar and water with an acetic acid content of 1.25% and greater, quaternary ammonium compound, glutaraldehyde, or boiling when equipment can withstand it. The catheters should then be rinsed with normal saline solution or tap water. **AARC**

Whether the patient requires disposable or reusable suction equipment, you should make sure that the patient and his caregivers have received proper teaching and support.

Teach the patient proper coughing techniques and tell him to drink lots of fluids to help facilitate the removal of secretions. **AARC** **Science**

Nursing diagnoses

● Ineffective airway clearance

Expected outcomes

The patient will:
● remove secretions
● maintain normal ABG levels and pulse oximetry
● have improved breath sounds.

Complications

● Increased dyspnea caused by hypoxia and anxiety may result from oronasopharyngeal suctioning. Hypoxia can result *because oxygen from the oronasopharynx is removed with the secretions.* The amount of oxygen removed varies, depending upon the duration of the suctioning, suction flow and pressure, the size of the catheter in relation to the size of the patient's airway, and his physical condition.

● Bloody aspirate can result from prolonged or traumatic suctioning. Water-soluble lubricant can help to minimize traumatic injury.

Documentation

Record the date, time, reason for suctioning, and technique used; amount, color, consistency, and odor (if any) of the secretions; the patient's respiratory status before and after the procedure; any complications and interventions taken; and the patient's tolerance of the procedure.

Supportive references

American Association for Respiratory Care. "AARC Clinical Practice Guideline: Directed Cough," *Respiratory Care* 38(5):495-99, May 1993.

American Association for Respiratory Care. "AARC Clinical Practice Guideline: Nasotracheal Suctioning," *Respiratory Care* 49(9):1080-1084, September 2004.

American Association for Respiratory Care. "AARC Clinical Practice Guideline: Suctioning of the Patient in the Home," *Respiratory Care* 44(1):99-104, January 1999.

Joanna Briggs Institute. "Tracheal Suctioning of Adults with an Artificial Airway," *Best Practice* 4(4):1-6, 2000.

Oropharyngeal airway insertion and care

An oropharyngeal airway, a curved rubber or plastic device, is inserted into the mouth to the posterior pharynx to establish or maintain a patent airway. In an unconscious patient, the tongue usually obstructs the posterior pharynx. The oropharyngeal airway conforms to the curvature of the palate, removing the obstruction and allowing air to pass around and through the tube. It also facilitates oropharyngeal suctioning. The oropharyngeal airway is intended for short-term use, as in the postanesthesia or postictal stage. It may be left in place longer as an airway adjunct to prevent the orally intubated patient from biting the endotracheal tube.

The oropharyngeal airway isn't the airway of choice for the patient with loose or avulsed teeth or recent oral surgery. Inserting this airway in the conscious or semiconscious patient may stimulate vomiting, laryngospasm, and retching as a result of gag reflex stimulation; therefore, you'll usually insert the airway only in an unconscious patient.

According to the 2005 American Heart Association's (AHA) guidelines for cardiopulmonary resuscitation

Inserting an oral airway

Unless this position is contraindicated, hyperextend the patient's head (as shown below) before using either the cross-finger or tongue blade insertion method.

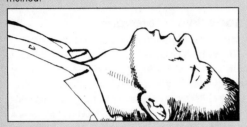

To insert an oral airway using the cross-finger method, place your thumb on the patient's lower teeth and your index finger on his upper teeth. Gently open his mouth by pushing his teeth apart (as shown below).

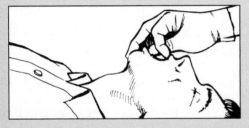

Insert the airway upside down *to avoid pushing the tongue toward the pharynx,* and slide it over the tongue toward the back of the mouth. Rotate the airway as it approaches the posterior wall of the pharynx so that it points downward (as shown below).

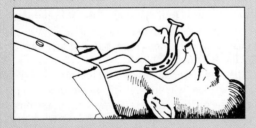

To use the tongue blade technique, open the patient's mouth and depress the tongue with the blade. Guide the airway over the back of the tongue as described in the cross-finger technique.

and emergency cardiovascular care, an oropharyngeal airway should be reserved for the unconscious patient with no cough or gag reflex. The 2005 guidelines state that the oropharyngeal airway should be inserted only by someone trained in its use. **AHA**

Equipment
Insertion
Oral airway of appropriate size • tongue blade • padded tongue blade • gloves • optional: suction equipment, handheld resuscitation bag or oxygen-powered breathing device

Cleaning
Hydrogen peroxide • water • basin • optional: pipe cleaner

Reflex testing
Cotton-tipped applicator

Preparation of equipment
● Select an oral airway of appropriate size for your patient; an oversized airway can obstruct breathing by depressing the epiglottis into the laryngeal opening.
● Usually, you'll select a small size (size 1 or 2) for an infant or child, a medium size (size 4 or 5) for an average adult, and a large size (size 6) for a large adult.
● Be sure to confirm the correct size of the airway by placing the airway flange beside the patient's cheek, parallel to his front teeth. If the airway is the right size, the airway curve should reach to the angle of the jaw.

Implementation
● Explain the procedure to the patient even though he may not appear to be alert. Provide privacy and put on gloves *to prevent contact with body fluids.* If the patient is wearing dentures, remove them *so they don't cause further airway obstruction.*
● Suction the patient, if necessary.
● Place the patient in the supine position with his neck hyperextended if this isn't contraindicated.
● Insert the airway using the cross-finger or tongue blade technique. (See *Inserting an oral airway.*)
● Auscultate the lungs *to ensure adequate ventilation.*
● After the airway is inserted, position the patient on his side *to decrease the risk of aspiration of vomitus.*

● Perform mouth care every 2 to 4 hours, as needed. Begin by holding the patient's jaws open with a padded tongue blade and gently removing the airway. Place the airway in a basin, and rinse it with hydrogen peroxide and then water. If secretions remain, use a pipe cleaner to remove them. Complete standard mouth care, and reinsert the airway.

● While the airway is removed for mouth care, observe the mouth's mucous membranes *because tissue irritation or ulceration can result from prolonged airway use.* **Science**

● Frequently check the position of the airway *to ensure correct placement.*

● When the patient regains consciousness and can swallow, remove the airway by pulling it outward and downward, following the mouth's natural curvature. After the airway is removed, test the patient's cough and gag reflexes *to ensure that removal of the airway wasn't premature and that the patient can maintain his own airway.*

● To test for the gag reflex, use a cotton-tipped applicator to touch both sides of the posterior pharynx. To test for the cough reflex, gently touch the posterior oropharynx with the cotton-tipped applicator.

Special considerations

● Bilateral breath sounds on auscultation indicate that the airway is the proper size and in the correct position.

● Avoid taping the airway in place *because untaping it could delay airway removal, thus increasing the patient's risk of aspiration.*

● Evaluate the patient's behavior *to provide the cue for airway removal.* The patient is likely to gag or cough as he becomes more alert, indicating that he no longer needs the airway.

Nursing diagnoses

● Impaired spontaneous ventilation

Expected outcomes

The patient will:
● achieve ventilation through a patent airway
● maintain normal arterial blood gas levels and an improved partial pressure of arterial oxygen.

Complications

● Tooth damage or loss, tissue damage, and bleeding may result from airway insertion.

● If the airway is too long, it may press the epiglottis against the entrance of the larynx, producing complete airway obstruction.

● If the airway isn't inserted properly, it may push the tongue posteriorly, aggravating the problem of upper airway obstruction. *To prevent traumatic injury,* make sure that the patient's lips and tongue aren't between his teeth and the airway.

● Immediately after inserting the airway, check for respirations. If respirations are absent or inadequate, initiate artificial positive-pressure ventilation by using a mouth-to-mask technique, a handheld resuscitation bag, or an oxygen-powered breathing device. (See "Manual ventilation," page 318.)

Documentation

Record the date and time of the airway's insertion, size of the airway, removal and cleaning of the airway, condition of mucous membranes, any suctioning, any adverse reactions and interventions taken, and the patient's tolerance of the procedure. Also document breath sounds and respiratory assessment findings.

Supportive references

American Association for Respiratory Care. "Clinical Practice Guideline: Management of Airway Emergencies," *Respiratory Care* 40(7):749-60, July 1995.

American Association for Respiratory Care. "Clinical Practice Guideline: Resuscitation and Defibrillation in the Health Care Setting," *Respiratory Care* 49(9): 1085-1099, September 2004.

American Heart Association. "2005 AHA Guidelines for Cardiopulmonary Resuscitation and Emergency Cardiovascular Care: International Consensus on Science," *Circulation* 112(22 Suppl):IV-1-IV-211, November 2005.

Oxygen administration

A patient will need oxygen therapy when hypoxemia results from a respiratory or cardiac emergency or an increase in metabolic function.

In a respiratory emergency, oxygen administration enables the patient to reduce his ventilatory effort. When such conditions as atelectasis or acute respiratory distress syndrome impair diffusion or when lung volumes are decreased from alveolar hypoventilation, this procedure boosts alveolar oxygen levels.

In a cardiac emergency, oxygen therapy helps meet the increased myocardial workload as the heart tries to compensate for hypoxemia. Oxygen administration is particularly important for a patient whose myocardium is already compromised — perhaps from a myocardial infarction (MI) or cardiac arrhythmia.

When metabolic demand is high (for example, in cases of massive trauma, burns, or high fever), oxygen administration supplies the body with enough oxygen to meet its cellular needs. This procedure also increases oxygenation in the patient with a reduced blood oxygen–carrying capacity, perhaps from carbon monoxide poisoning or sickle cell crisis.

The American Association for Respiratory Care (AARC) recommends careful monitoring of the patient receiving oxygen therapy. Clinical assessment should include examination of the pulmonary, cardiac, and neurologic systems. At the beginning of oxygen therapy, oxygen saturation and tension should be measured. These parameters should also be measured again within 8 to 12 hours of initiating therapy with a fraction of inspired oxygen greater than or equal to 0.4. The parameters also should be measured within 2 hours of starting therapy for a patient with a primary diagnosis of chronic obstructive pulmonary disease and within 72 hours in a patient with an MI. Oxygen saturation and tension should be measured in neonates within 1 hour of birth. **AARC**

The adequacy of oxygen therapy is determined by arterial blood gas (ABG) analysis, oximetry monitoring, and clinical examination. The patient's disease, physical condition, and age will help determine the most appropriate method of administration.

Equipment

The equipment needed depends on the type of delivery system ordered. (See *Guide to oxygen delivery systems.*)

Equipment includes selections from the following list: oxygen source (wall unit, cylinder, liquid tank, or concentrator)• flowmeter adapter, if using a wall unit, or a pressure-reduction gauge, if using a cylinder• sterile humidity bottle and adapters• sterile distilled water• OXYGEN PRECAUTION sign• appropriate oxygen delivery system (nasal cannula, simple mask, partial rebreather mask, or nonrebreather mask for low-flow and variable oxygen concentrations; a Venturi mask, aerosol mask, T tube, tracheostomy collar,

tent, or oxygen hood (for high-flow and specific oxygen concentrations)• small- and large-diameter connection tubing• flashlight (for nasal cannula)• water-soluble lubricant• gauze pads and tape (for oxygen masks)• jet adapter for Venturi mask (if adding humidity)• optional: oxygen analyzer

Preparation of equipment

● Although a respiratory therapist is typically responsible for setting up, maintaining, and managing the equipment, you'll need a working knowledge of the oxygen system being used.

● Check the oxygen outlet port *to verify flow.*

● Pinch the tubing near the prongs *to ensure that an audible alarm will sound if the oxygen flow stops.*

Implementation

● Confirm the patient's identity using two patient identifiers according to facility policy. **JCAHO**

● Assess the patient's condition. In an emergency, verify that he has an open airway before administering oxygen. **AARC** **Science**

● Explain the procedure to the patient, and let him know why he needs oxygen *to ensure his cooperation.*

● Check the patient's room *to make sure it's safe for oxygen administration.* Whenever possible, replace electrical devices with nonelectric ones.

⚠ **ALERT** *If the patient is a child and is in an oxygen tent, remove all toys that may produce a spark. Oxygen supports combustion, and the smallest spark can cause a fire.*

● Place an OXYGEN PRECAUTION sign over the patient's bed and on the door to his room.

● Help place the oxygen delivery device on the patient. Make sure that it fits properly and that it's stable.

● Monitor the patient's response to oxygen therapy. Check his ABG values during initial adjustments of oxygen flow. When the patient is stabilized, you may use pulse oximetry instead. Check the patient frequently for signs of hypoxia, such as decreased level of consciousness, increased heart rate, arrhythmias, restlessness, perspiration, dyspnea, accessory muscle use, yawning or flared nostrils, cyanosis, and cool, clammy skin. **AARC**

● Check the patient's skin *to prevent skin breakdown on pressure points from the oxygen delivery device.*

(Text continues on page 342.)

Guide to oxygen delivery systems

Patients may receive oxygen through one of several administration systems. Each has its own benefits, drawbacks, and indications for use. The advantages and disadvantages of each system are compared here.

Nasal cannula

Oxygen is delivered through plastic cannulas placed in the patient's nostrils.

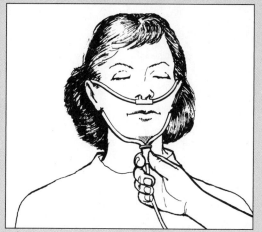

Advantages: Safe and simple, comfortable and easily tolerated, nasal prongs can be shaped to fit any face, effective for low oxygen concentrations, inexpensive and disposable, allows for movement, eating, and talking

Disadvantages: Can't deliver concentrations higher than 40%, can't be used in patients with complete nasal obstruction, may cause headaches or dry mucous membranes if flow rate exceeds 6 L/minute, can dislodge easily

Administration guidelines: Ensure patency of the patient's nostrils with a flashlight. If patent, hook the cannula tubing behind the patient's ears and under the chin. Slide the adjuster upward under the chin to secure the tubing. If using an elastic strap to secure the cannula, position it over the ears and around the back of the head. Avoid applying it too tightly, which can result in excess pressure on facial structures and cannula occlusion as well. With a nasal cannula, oral breathers achieve the same oxygen delivery as nasal breathers. Oxygen can be administered without humidification at flow at less than or equal to 4 L/minute.

Simple mask

Oxygen flows through an entry port at the bottom of the mask and exits through large holes on the sides of the mask.

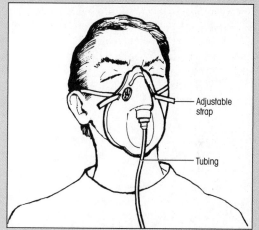

Adjustable strap

Tubing

Advantages: Can deliver concentrations of 35% to 50%

Disadvantages: Hot and confining, may irritate the patient's skin, interferes with talking and eating, impractical for long-term therapy because of imprecision, tight seal required for higher oxygen concentration may cause discomfort

Administration guidelines: Select the mask size that offers the best fit. Place the mask over the patient's nose, mouth, and chin, and mold the flexible metal edge to the bridge of the nose. Adjust the elastic band around the head to hold the mask firmly but comfortably over the cheeks, chin, and bridge of the nose. For an elderly or a cachectic patient with sunken cheeks, tape gauze pads to the mask over the cheek area to try to create an airtight seal. Without this seal, room air dilutes the oxygen, preventing delivery of the prescribed concentration. A minimum of 5 L/minute is required in all masks to flush expired carbon dioxide from the mask so that the patient doesn't rebreathe it.

(continued)

Guide to oxygen delivery systems *(continued)*

Partial rebreather mask

The patient inspires oxygen from a reservoir bag along with atmospheric air and oxygen from the mask. The first third of exhaled tidal volume enters the bag; the rest exits the mask. Because air entering the reservoir bag comes from the trachea and bronchi, where no gas exchange occurs, the patient rebreathes the oxygenated air he just exhaled.

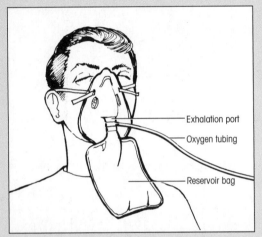

Exhalation port
Oxygen tubing
Reservoir bag

Advantages: Effectively delivers concentrations of 40% to 70%, openings in the mask allow the patient to inhale room air if oxygen source fails

Disadvantages: Tight seal required for accurate oxygen concentration may cause discomfort, interferes with eating and talking, hot and confining, may irritate skin, bag may twist or kink, impractical for long-term therapy

Administration guidelines: Follow the procedures listed for the simple mask. If the reservoir bag collapses more than slightly during inspiration, raise the flow rate until you see only a slight deflation. Marked or complete deflation indicates insufficient oxygen flow; carbon dioxide may accumulate in the mask and bag. Keep the reservoir bag from twisting or kinking. Ensure free expansion by making sure that the bag lies outside the patient's gown and bedcovers.

Nonrebreather mask

On inhalation, the one-way valve opens, directing oxygen from a reservoir bag into the mask. On exhalation, gas exits the mask through the one-way expiratory valve and enters the atmosphere. The patient only breathes air from the bag.

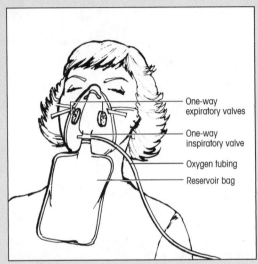

One-way expiratory valves
One-way inspiratory valve
Oxygen tubing
Reservoir bag

Advantages: Delivers the highest possible oxygen concentration (60% to 80%) short of intubation and mechanical ventilation, effective for short-term therapy, doesn't dry mucous membranes, can be converted to a partial rebreather mask, if necessary, by removing the one-way valve

Disadvantages: Requires a tight seal that may cause discomfort and be difficult to maintain, may irritate the patient's skin, interferes with talking and eating, impractical for long-term therapy

Administration guidelines: Follow procedures listed for the simple mask. Make sure that the mask fits very snugly and the one-way valves are secure and functioning. *Because the mask excludes room air, valve malfunction can cause carbon dioxide buildup and suffocate an unconscious patient.* If the reservoir bag collapses more than slightly during inspiration, raise the flow rate until you see only a slight deflation. *Marked or complete deflation indicates an insufficient flow rate.* Keep the reservoir bag from twisting or kinking. Ensure free expansion by making sure that the bag lies outside the patient's gown and bedcovers.

Guide to oxygen delivery systems *(continued)*

CPAP mask

This system allows the spontaneously breathing patient to receive continuous positive airway pressure (CPAP) with or without an artificial airway.

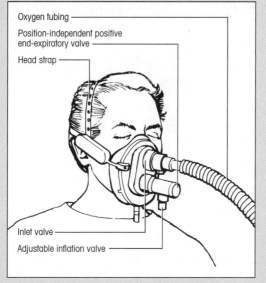

Oxygen tubing
Position-independent positive end-expiratory valve
Head strap
Inlet valve
Adjustable inflation valve

Advantages: Noninvasively improves arterial oxygenation by increasing functional residual capacity, alleviates the need for intubation, allows the patient to talk and cough without interrupting positive pressure

Disadvantages: Requires a tight fit that may cause discomfort; interferes with eating and talking; heightened risk of aspiration if the patient vomits; increased risk of pneumothorax, diminished cardiac output, and gastric distention; contraindicated in patients with chronic obstructive pulmonary disease, bullous lung disease, low cardiac output, or tension pneumothorax

Administration guidelines: Place one strap behind the patient's head and the other strap over his head *to ensure a snug fit.* Attach one latex strap to the connector prong on one side of the mask. Then, use one hand to position the mask on the patient's face while using the other hand to connect the strap to the other side of the mask. After the mask is applied, assess the patient's respiratory, circulatory, and GI function every hour. Watch for signs of pneumothorax, decreased cardiac output, a drop in blood pressure, and gastric distention.

Transtracheal oxygen

The patient receives oxygen through a catheter inserted into the base of his neck in a simple outpatient procedure.

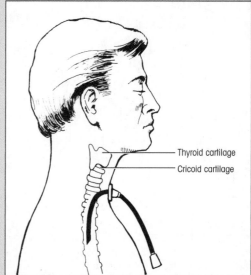

Thyroid cartilage
Cricoid cartilage

Advantages: Supplies oxygen to the lungs throughout the respiratory cycle, provides continuous oxygen without hindering mobility, doesn't interfere with eating or talking, doesn't dry mucous membranes, catheter can easily be concealed by a shirt or scarf

Disadvantages: Not suitable for use in patients at risk for bleeding or those with severe bronchospasm, uncompensated respiratory acidosis, pleural herniation into the base of the neck, or high corticosteroid dosages

Administration guidelines: After insertion, obtain a chest X-ray *to confirm placement.* Monitor the patient for bleeding, respiratory distress, pneumothorax, pain, coughing, or hoarseness. Don't use the catheter for about 1 week after insertion *to decrease the risk of subcutaneous emphysema.*

(continued)

Guide to oxygen delivery systems *(continued)*

Venturi mask

The mask is connected to a Venturi device, which mixes a specific volume of air and oxygen.

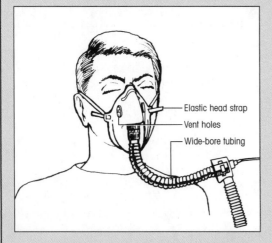

Elastic head strap
Vent holes
Wide-bore tubing

Advantages: Delivers highly accurate oxygen concentration despite the patient's respiratory pattern because the same amount of air is always entrained, has dilute jets that can be changed or a dial that changes oxygen concentration, doesn't dry mucous membranes, allows addition of humidity or aerosol

Disadvantages: Confining and may irritate skin, interferes with eating and talking, condensate possibly collecting and dripping on the patient if humidification is used, possible oxygen concentration alteration if mask fits loosely, tubing kinks, oxygen intake ports become blocked, flow is insufficient, or patient is hyperpneic

Administration guidelines: Make sure that the oxygen flow rate is set at the amount specified on each mask and the Venturi valve is set for the desired fraction of inspired oxygen.

Aerosols

A face mask, hood, tent, or tracheostomy tube or collar is connected to wide-bore tubing that receives aerosolized oxygen from a jet nebulizer. The jet nebulizer, which is attached near the oxygen source, adjusts air entrainment in a manner similar to the Venturi device.

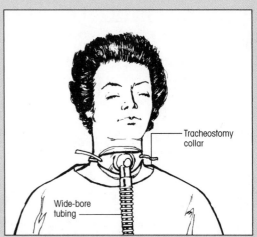

Tracheostomy collar
Wide-bore tubing

Advantages: Administers high humidity, allows gas to be heated (when delivered through artificial airway) or cooled (when delivered through a tent)

Disadvantages: Condensate collected in the tracheostomy collar or T tube possibly draining into the tracheostomy, weight of the T tube possibly putting stress on the tracheostomy tube

Administration guidelines: Guidelines vary with the type of nebulizer used: the ultrasonic, large-volume, small-volume, or in-line. When using a high-output nebulizer, watch for signs of overhydration, pulmonary edema, crackles, and electrolyte imbalance.

Wipe moisture or perspiration from the patient's face and from the mask as needed. **Science**

● If the patient is receiving oxygen at a concentration above 60% for more than 24 hours, watch carefully for signs and symptoms of oxygen toxicity (fatigue, lethargy, weakness, restlessness, nausea, vomiting, anorexia, coughing, and dyspnea progressing to severe dyspnea, tachypnea, tachycardia, decreased breath sounds, crackles, and cyanosis). Remind the patient to cough and deep-breathe frequently *to prevent atelectasis.* Also, *to prevent the development of serious lung damage,* measure ABG values repeatedly *to determine whether high oxygen concentrations are still necessary.*

Special considerations

ALERT *Never administer oxygen by nasal cannula at more than 2 L/minute to a patient with chronic lung disease unless you have a specific order to do so because he may have become dependent on a state of hypercapnia and hypoxia to stimulate his breathing, and supplemental oxygen could cause him to stop breathing. However, long-term oxygen therapy of 12 to 17 hours daily may help the patient with chronic lung disease sleep better, survive longer, and experience a reduced incidence of pulmonary hypertension.*

● When monitoring a patient's response to a change in oxygen flow, check the pulse oximetry monitor or measure ABG values 20 to 30 minutes after adjusting the flow. In the interim, monitor the patient closely for an adverse response to the change in oxygen flow.

Nursing diagnoses

● Impaired gas exchange

Expected outcomes

The patient will:
● express comfort in maintaining air exchange
● have normal breath sounds
● maintain normal ABG values
● cough effectively.

TEACHING *Before discharging a patient who will receive oxygen therapy at home, make sure that you know the types of oxygen therapy, the kinds of services that are available, and the service schedules offered by local home suppliers. Together with the physician and the patient, choose the device best-suited to the patient. (See* Types of home oxygen therapy.*)*

If the patient is receiving transtracheal oxygen therapy, teach him how to properly clean and care for the catheter. Advise him to keep the skin surrounding the insertion site clean and dry to prevent infection.

No matter which device the patient uses, you'll need to evaluate his and his family members' ability and motivation to administer oxygen therapy at home. Make sure that they understand the reason the patient is receiving oxygen and the safety issues involved in oxygen administration. Teach them how to properly use and clean the equipment and supplies.

If the patient will be discharged with oxygen for the first time, make sure that his health insurance covers home oxygen. If it doesn't, find out what criteria he must meet to obtain coverage. Without a third-party payer, the patient may not be able to afford home oxygen therapy.

Types of home oxygen therapy

Oxygen therapy can be administered at home using an oxygen tank, an oxygen concentrator, or liquid oxygen.

Oxygen tank
Commonly used for patients who need oxygen on a standby basis or who need a ventilator at home, the oxygen tank has several disadvantages, including its cumbersome design and the need for frequent refills. Because oxygen is stored under high pressure, the oxygen tank also poses a potential hazard.

Oxygen concentrator
The oxygen concentrator extracts oxygen molecules from room air. It can be used for low oxygen flow (less than 4 L/minute) and doesn't need to be refilled with oxygen. However, because the oxygen concentrator runs on electricity, it won't function during a power failure.

Liquid oxygen
Liquid oxygen is commonly used by patients who are oxygen-dependent but still mobile. The system includes a large liquid reservoir for home use. When the patient wants to leave the house, he fills a portable unit worn over the shoulder; this supplies oxygen for up to several hours, depending on the liter flow.

Documentation

Record the date and time of oxygen administration, the delivery device used, oxygen flow rate, patient's vital signs, skin color, respiratory effort, lung sounds, subjective patient response before and after initiation of therapy, and any patient or family teaching.

Supportive references

American Association for Respiratory Care. "AARC Clinical Practice Guidelines: Oxygen Therapy for Adults in the Acute Care Hospital," *Respiratory Care* 47(6):717-20, June 2002.

Wright, J., and White, J. "Continuous Positive Airway Pressure for Obstructive Sleep Apnea," *Cochrane Database of Systematic Reviews* 2(2):CD001106, 2000.

Peak flow meter

A peak flow meter is a portable, inexpensive, hand-held device used to measure how air flows from the patient's lungs. The meter measures the ability to push air out of the lungs. Peak flow meters are available in two ranges: a low range peak flow meter is for small children, and a standard range meter is used for older children, teenagers, and adults.

The patient with asthma benefits most from the use of a peak flow meter. The meter can be used to determine the necessity for adjustments in his daily asthma medication, and can be an important part of his asthma management plan. For example, peak flow readings can help a patient to decide to start taking his medication early, before he develops symptoms.

The peak flow meter can also determine whether the patient's asthma is getting worse and can reveal the gradual changes that sometimes occur in asthma before the patient actually feels them. These measurements can help a patient realize that he may need to take his asthma medication for a longer period, until the medicine has worked and his asthma is better. It can allow the physician to adjust a patient's treatment and alleviate the need for emergency room visits and hospitalizations.

Three zones of measurement are commonly used to interpret peak flow rates. (See *Measuring peak flow rates*.) The colors red, green, and yellow are used to depict the zones. (See *Understanding zone symptoms*.) In general, a normal peak flow rate can vary as much as 20%.

Children as young as age 3 can use a peak flow meter and in some instances patients with chronic bronchitis and emphysema may also benefit from the use of a peak flow meter.

A peak flow meter can help the patient and physician identify causes of asthma attacks at home, work, or play. It can assist parents in determining what might trigger their child's asthma and when to administer medications. Using peak flow rates may help make treatment decisions easier.

Equipment

Adult standard peak flow meter, operating range 60 to 880 L/minute • pediatric peak flow meter, operating range 50 to 385 L/minute

Implementation ALA

● Confirm the patient's identity using two patient identifiers according to facility policy. JCAHO

● Explain the procedure to the patient and the indications for use.

● Before each use, make sure that the sliding marker or arrow on the peak flow meter is at the bottom of the numbered scale (zero or the lowest number on the scale).

● Make sure that the patient is standing up straight and has removed any food or gum from his mouth. Tell the patient to take a deep breath and place the peak flow meter in his mouth and to tightly close his

---

Measuring peak flow rates EB

A peak flow meter uses green, yellow, and red zones to measure the patient's flow rates, as described below.

All clear
Green zone: 80% to 100% of the patient's usual or "normal" peak flow rate signals all clear. A reading in this zone means that the patient's asthma is under reasonably good control. The patient should continue his current prescribed management program.

Caution
Yellow zone: 50% to 80% of the patient's "normal" peak flow rate signals caution. The patient's airways are narrowing and extra treatment may be required. The patient's symptoms may improve or worsen depending on what he does, or how and when he uses his medication. His physician should be notified.

Medical alert
Red zone: Less than 50% of the patient's "normal" peak flow rate signals a medical alert. Immediate intervention is necessary *because severe airway narrowing may be occurring.* The patient's physician should be notified immediately.

lips around the mouthpiece. Make sure that the patient's tongue is away from the mouthpiece.
● Tell the patient to blow as hard and as quickly as possible until he has blown nearly all of the air from his lungs. *Remember:* It's important that the patient blow a "fast hard blast" rather than "slowly blowing" *to get an accurate reading.*
● The force of air coming out of the patient's lungs causes the marker to move along the numbered scale. Note the number on a piece of paper.
● Repeat the entire process three times. If the numbers from each time are close together, the patient has done the routine properly.
● Because a patient can't breathe out too much air but may not breathe in enough, be sure to record the highest rating to ensure an accurate reading. Don't calculate the average of all three readings.
● Make sure that the peak flow rate is done close to the same time each day *to ensure consistency.* One suggestion is to have the patient perform the rate around the time of his medication (either before or after taking his medication). It's important that the peak flow reading is performed under similar conditions each time.
● Tell the patient to keep a chart of his peak flow rates and be sure to discuss his readings with the physician at the time of his next visit.

Special considerations

● Use of a peak flow meter depends on several factors. Its use should be discussed with the physician.
● It's important for the patient to know his peak flow reading, and even more important for him to know what to do based on those readings.
● Tell the patient to record the peak flow readings that his physician recommends for his green, yellow, and red zones. Work with the patient to develop a management plan that follows the green-yellow-red guidelines.
● If a patient's asthma is well controlled and he knows his "normal" rate, tell him that he only needs to measure his peak flow rate when he senses his asthma is getting worse. More severe asthma may require several measurements per day.
● Remind the patient that the peak flow meter needs care and regular cleaning. Dirt collected in the meter may make his peak flow measurements inaccurate. If the patient has a cold or other respiratory infection, germs or mucus may also collect in the meter.

Understanding zone symptoms

The green, yellow, and red zones indicate how well the patient's asthma is managed.

Green zone
The patient reports no symptoms or occasional signs or symptoms that include:
● coughing
● wheezing
● shortness of breath
● chest tightness
● interrupted sleep.

Yellow zone
The patient reports some signs or symptoms, including:
● coughing
● wheezing
● chest tightness
● increased use of inhaler
● being awakened at night by symptoms
● taking occasional time off from work or school
● not participating in certain activities because of asthma symptoms.

Red zone
The patient reports more noticeable, frequent, or serious signs or symptoms, including:
● increased breathlessness
● difficulty walking or talking
● using inhaler frequently without relief.

● Instruct the patient to properly clean the peak flow meter in hot water, with a mild detergent, to keep it working accurately and keep him healthier.

Nursing diagnoses
● Deficient knowledge (use of peak flow meter)

Expected outcomes
The patient will:
● state an understanding of the use of the peak flow meter
● demonstrate the proper use of the peak flow meter

● keep a chart of rates and discuss them with his physician.

Complications

● Because a peak flow meter isn't medicine, it has no major adverse effects. Inform the patient that sometimes pushing the air out of his lungs in a "fast blast" may cause him to cough or wheeze and that this is normal.

Documentation

Record the date and time of the measurement and the highest of the three readings in the patient's chart. Be sure to indicate the patient's current medications, the time he last took his medication, and when the reading occurred in relation to this. Document the patient's vital signs, note any changes in the patient's color and rate and depth of respirations, and record breath sounds before and after the measurement. If the measurement falls in the "yellow" or "red" zones, be sure to document interventions done and changes in the patient's medications.

Supportive references

American Lung Association. "Peak Flow Meters," March 2002. *www.lungusa.org/asthma/astpeakflow.htm.* **EB**
Professional Guide to Diseases, 8th ed. Philadelphia: Lippincott Williams & Wilkins, 2005.

Pulse and ear oximetry

Performed intermittently or continuously, oximetry is a relatively simple procedure used to monitor arterial oxygen saturation noninvasively. Arterial oxygen saturation values obtained by pulse oximeters are denoted with the symbol SpO_2, whereas invasively measured arterial oxygen saturation values are denoted by the symbol SaO_2.

The American Association for Respiratory Care (AARC) has developed clinical guidelines for performing pulse oximetry. Indications for pulse oximetry include:
● monitoring the adequacy of arterial oxyhemoglobin saturation
● measuring and recording the response of arterial oxyhemoglobin saturation to therapeutic intervention or to a diagnostic procedure such as bronchoscopy

● complying with facility policy or unit protocol. Staff caring for a patient on pulse oximetry should be trained in pulse oximetry and equipment use. **AARC**

CONTROVERSIAL ISSUE *Continuous pulse oximetry monitoring has become the standard of care during surgery, in the immediate postoperative recovery period, and in intensive care units. However, the Child Health Corporation of America's Cooperative Pulse Oximetry FORUM believes that continuous pulse oximetry has limited benefits when used on general nursing units and by untrained staff.*

Pulse oximetry readings obtained by untrained personnel can be inaccurate. Untrained personnel may not be aware of how technical factors, such as probe size and placement, movement, and bright lights, affect readings. Moreover, untrained staff may turn off alarm monitors of the patient receiving continuous oximetry monitoring without the patient being properly assessed.

The FORUM recommends that the physician document the rationale for continuous pulse oximetry monitoring for a patient breathing room air. They also suggest that periodic pulse oximetry readings are more appropriate than continuous monitoring for a patient on an apnea monitor and a cardiac monitor. The FORUM further recommends that the nurse understand the oximetry equipment, technical and physiologic limitations, alarm settings, and clinical appropriateness of each type of monitor. The nurse must also interpret pulse oximetry results in relation to the patient's clinical condition and other physiologic data. The patient receiving continuous pulse oximetry monitoring should be in a location where the alarms can be heard and immediately assessed. Moreover, the nurse should question the physician about inappropriate use of pulse oximetry. **EB1** **FORUM**

In this procedure, two diodes send red and infrared light through a pulsating arterial vascular bed such as the one in the fingertip. A photodetector slipped over the finger measures the transmitted light as it passes through the vascular bed, detects the relative amount of color absorbed by arterial blood, and calculates the exact mixed venous oxygen saturation without interference from surrounding venous blood, skin, connective tissue, or bone. Ear oximetry works by monitoring the transmission of light waves through the vascular bed of a patient's earlobe. Results will be inaccurate if the patient's earlobe is poorly perfused, as in the case of a patient with a low cardiac output. (See *How oximetry works*.)

Equipment

Oximeter • finger or ear transducer probe • alcohol pads • nail polish remover, if necessary

Preparation of equipment

● Review the manufacturer's instructions for assembling the oximeter. **MFR**
● Choose the appropriate probe for the site you're using.

Implementation

● Confirm the patient's identity using two patient identifiers according to facility policy. **JCAHO**
● Explain the procedure to the patient. **PCP**
● Validate pulse oximetry readings by comparing Spo_2 readings with Sao_2 values obtained by arterial blood gas (ABG) analysis. Obtain these two measurements simultaneously at the beginning of pulse oximetry monitoring, and then reevaluate periodically according to the patient's condition. **AARC**
● If pulse oximetry readings are being monitored continuously, set the high and low alarms according to the patient's clinical condition.

Pulse oximetry

● Select a finger for the test. Although the index finger is commonly used, a smaller finger may be selected if the patient's fingers are too large for the equipment. Make sure that the patient isn't wearing false fingernails, and remove any nail polish from the test finger. Place the transducer (photodetector) probe over the patient's finger so that light beams and sensors oppose each other. If the patient has long fingernails, position the probe perpendicular to the finger, if possible, or clip the fingernail. Always position the patient's hand at heart level *to eliminate venous pulsations and to promote accurate readings.* **AARC**

⚠ **ALERT** *If you're testing a neonate or small infant, use probes specifically designed for them. For a large infant, use a probe that fits on the great toe and secure it to the foot.*

● Turn on the power switch. If the device is working properly, a beep will sound, a display will light momentarily, and the pulse searchlight will flash. Initially, the Spo_2 and pulse rate displays will show stationary zeros. After four to six heartbeats, the displays

How oximetry works

The pulse oximeter allows noninvasive monitoring of the percentage of hemoglobin saturated by oxygen, or Spo_2, levels by measuring the absorption (amplitude) of light waves as they pass through areas of the body that are highly perfused by arterial blood. Oximetry also monitors pulse rate and amplitude.

Light-emitting diodes in a transducer (photodetector) attached to the patient's body (shown here on the index finger) send red and infrared light beams through tissue. The photodetector records the relative amount of each color absorbed by arterial blood and transmits the data to a monitor, which displays the information with each heartbeat. If the Spo_2 level or pulse rate varies from preset limits, the monitor triggers visual and audible alarms.

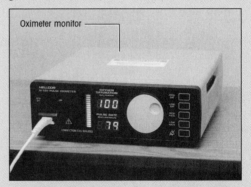

Oximeter monitor

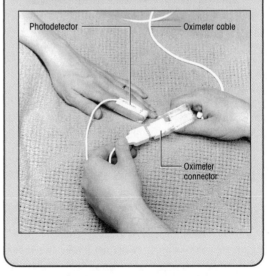

Photodetector

Oximeter cable

Oximeter connector

will supply information with each beat and the pulse amplitude indicator will begin tracking the pulse.

Ear oximetry

● Using an alcohol pad, massage the patient's earlobe for 10 to 20 seconds. Mild erythema indicates adequate vascularization. Following the manufacturer's instructions, attach the ear probe to the patient's earlobe or pinna. **MFR** Use the ear probe stabilizer for prolonged or exercise testing. Be sure to establish good contact on the ear *because an unstable probe may set off the low-perfusion alarm.* After the probe has been attached for a few seconds, a saturation reading and pulse waveform will appear on the oximeter's screen.

● Leave the ear probe in place for 3 or more minutes, until readings stabilize at the highest point, or take three separate readings and average them. Make sure that you revascularize the patient's earlobe each time. **AARC**

● After the procedure, remove the probe, turn off and unplug the unit, and clean the probe by gently rubbing it with an alcohol pad.

Special considerations

● Use clinical judgment in evaluating pulse oximetry readings. Validate the readings with a clinical assessment of the patient.

● If oximetry has been performed properly, readings are typically accurate. However, certain factors may interfere with accuracy. For example, an elevated bilirubin level may falsely lower Spo_2 readings, while elevated carboxyhemoglobin or methemoglobin levels (such as occur in heavy smokers and urban dwellers) can cause a falsely elevated Spo_2 reading.

● Certain intravascular substances, such as lipid emulsions and dyes, can also prevent accurate readings. Other factors that may interfere with accurate results include excessive light (for example, from phototherapy, surgical lamps, direct sunlight, and excessive ambient lighting), excessive patient movement, excessive ear pigment, hypothermia, hypotension, and vasoconstriction.

● Pulse oximetry may be used to monitor Spo_2 during respiratory arrest. *Because pulse oximetry relies on perfusion,* it shouldn't be used during cardiac arrest.

● Know whether your facility's policy allows nurses to initiate pulse oximetry without a physician's order.

The Joint Commission on Accreditation of Healthcare Organizations (JCAHO) requires a physician's order for pulse oximetry in the home care setting. According to a JCAHO Standards Clarification, oximetry isn't without risk to the patient, and indications and contraindications for oximetry must be distinctly related to the patient's assessment and monitoring needs. JCAHO recommends that home care nurses must receive training in performing and interpreting pulse oximetry results and must be aware of pulse oximetry limitations so that false results don't lead to inappropriate intervention. Other professional organizations, such as the AARC, also recommend that home care nurses should perform pulse oximetry only with a physician's order. **EB2** **JCAHO**

● If the patient has compromised circulation in his extremities, you can place a photodetector across the bridge of his nose.

● If Spo_2 is used to guide weaning the patient from forced inspiratory oxygen, obtain an ABG analysis occasionally to correlate Spo_2 readings with Sao_2 levels.

● If an automatic blood pressure cuff is used on the same extremity that's used for measuring Spo_2, the cuff will interfere with Spo_2 readings during inflation.

● If light is a problem, cover the probes; if patient movement is a problem, move the probe or select a different probe; and if ear pigment is a problem, reposition the probe, revascularize the site, or use a finger probe. (See *Diagnosing pulse oximeter problems.*)

● Normal Spo_2 readings for ear and pulse oximetry are 95% to 100% for adults and 93.8% to 100% by 1 hour after birth for healthy, full-term neonates. Lower levels may indicate hypoxemia, which warrants intervention. For such patients, follow your facility's policy or the physician's order, which may include increasing oxygen therapy. If Spo_2 readings decrease suddenly, perform a clinical assessment of the patient. Notify the physician of any significant change in the patient's condition.

● When the Sao_2 level is greater than 80%, pulse oximetry is highly accurate in healthy people. In patients on mechanical ventilation, however, accuracy is reduced when the Sao_2 level is 90% or lower.

Nursing diagnoses

● Impaired gas exchange

Expected outcomes

The patient will:

Diagnosing pulse oximeter problems

To maintain a continuous display of arterial oxygen saturation (Spo_2) levels, you'll need to keep the monitoring site clean and dry. Make sure that the skin doesn't become irritated from adhesives used to keep disposable probes in place. You may need to change the site if this happens. Disposable probes that irritate the skin also can be replaced by nondisposable models that don't need tape.

Another common problem with pulse oximeters is the failure of the devices to obtain a signal. Your first reaction if this happens should be to check the patient's vital signs. If they're sufficient to produce a signal, check for the following problems.

Venous pulsations

Erroneous readings may be obtained if the pulse oximeter detects venous pulsations. This may occur in patients with tricuspid regurgitation or pulmonary hypertension or if a finger probe is taped too tightly to the finger.

Poor concentration

See if the sensors are properly aligned. Make sure that the wires are intact and securely fastened and that the pulse oximeter is plugged into a power source.

Inadequate or intermittent blood flow to the site

Check the patient's pulse rate and capillary refill time and take corrective action if blood flow to the site is decreased. This may mean loosening restraints, removing tight-fitting clothes, taking off a blood pressure cuff, or checking arterial and I.V. lines. If none of these interventions work, you may need to find an alternate site. Finding a site with proper circulation may also prove challenging when a patient is receiving vasoconstrictive drugs.

Equipment malfunction

If you think the equipment might be malfunctioning, remove the pulse oximeter from the patient, set the alarm limits at 85% and 100%, and try the instrument on yourself or another healthy person. This will tell you if it's working correctly.

Penumbra effect

The penumbra effect may occur when an adult oximetry probe is placed on an infant's or a small child's finger. Because of a different path length of tissue for each of the wavelengths, the oximeter can underread or overread the Spo_2 level. To avoid the penumbra effect, use probes specifically designed for infants and children.

- have pulse oximetry results that reflect his clinical condition
- state an understanding of the procedure.

Documentation

Document the procedure, including the date, time, procedure type, oximetry measurement, and any action taken. Chart other relevant patient assessments performed to validate the oximetry reading. Record the inspired oxygen concentrated and the type of oxygen delivery device used. Record ABG values obtained. Record readings in appropriate flowcharts, if indicated.

CLINICAL IMPACT *If you detect a discrepancy between Spo_2 and Sao_2 levels and the patient's clinical appearance, look for possible causes before you report the results. If troubleshooting measures, such as choosing an alternate monitoring site or changing the probe, don't reduce the discrepancy; the AARC pulse oximetry guidelines recommend that you don't document the Spo_2 reading. Rather, document the corrective actions you performed and the Sao_2 level obtained by ABG analysis. The acceptable amount of discrepancy varies with the patient's condition and the oximetry device being used. Always exercise sound clinical judgment.* **AARC** **EB3**

Supportive references

American Association for Respiratory Care. "AARC Clinical Practice Guideline: Pulse Oximetry," *Respiratory Care* 36(12):1406-409, December 1991. **EB3**

Child Health Corporation of America's Cooperative Pulse Oximetry FORUM. "The FORUM Offers Recommendations on Best Practices in Pediatric Pulse Oximetry," *AARC Times* 24(4):36-38, 40-44, April 2000. **EB1**

Duarte, A.G., and Bidani, A. "Monitoring Patients with ARDS, Part 2: Pulmonary Oxygen Uptake," *Journal of Critical Illness* 16(1):38-46, January 2001.

Joint Commission for Accreditation of Healthcare Organizations. "Standards Clarification: Physician's Order to Perform Pulse Oximetry," March 2002. *www.jcaho.org/standards_frm.html.* **EB2**

Stoddart, S., et al. "Pulse Oximetry: What It Is and How to Use It," *Journal of Neonatal Nursing* 3(4):10, 12-14, July 1997.

Tate, J., and Tasota, F.J. "Using Pulse Oximetry," *Nursing2000* 30(9):30, September 2000.

Vines, D.L., et al. "Current Respiratory Care, Part 1: Oxygen Therapy, Oximetry, Bronchial Hygiene," *Journal of Critical Illness* 15(9):507-10, 513-15, September 2000.

Tracheal cuff pressure measurement

An endotracheal (ET) or tracheostomy cuff provides a closed system for mechanical ventilation, allowing a desired tidal volume to be delivered to the patient's lungs. To function properly, the cuff must exert enough pressure on the tracheal wall to seal the airway without compromising the blood supply to the tracheal mucosa.

The ideal pressure (known as *minimal occlusive volume*) is the lowest amount needed to seal the airway. Many authorities recommend maintaining a cuff pressure lower than venous perfusion pressure — usually about 16 to 24 cm H_2O. (More than 24 cm H_2O may exceed venous perfusion pressure.) Actual cuff pressure will vary with each patient, however. To keep pressure within safe limits, measure minimal occlusive volume at least once per shift or as directed by your facility's policy. Cuff pressure can be measured by a respiratory therapist or by the nurse.

Equipment

Cuff pressure manometer • 10-ml syringe • three-way stopcock • stethoscope • suction equipment • gloves

Preparation of equipment

● Assemble all equipment at the patient's bedside.
● If measuring with a blood pressure manometer, attach the syringe to one stopcock port, and then attach the tubing from the manometer to another port of the stopcock.
● Turn off the stopcock port where you'll be connecting the pilot balloon cuff *so that air can't escape from the cuff.*
● Use the syringe to instill air into the manometer tubing until the pressure reading reaches 10 mm Hg. *This will prevent sudden cuff deflation when you open the stopcock to the cuff and the manometer.*

Implementation

● Confirm the patient's identity using two patient identifiers according to facility policy. **JCAHO**
● Explain the procedure to the patient. Put on gloves and suction the ET or tracheostomy tube and the patient's oropharynx to remove accumulated secretions above the cuff. Then attach the cuff pressure manometer to the pilot balloon port. **CDC** **PCP**
● Place the diaphragm of the stethoscope over the trachea and listen for an air leak (as shown below). Keep in mind that a smooth, hollow sound indicates a sealed airway; a loud, gurgling sound indicates an air leak. **AARC**

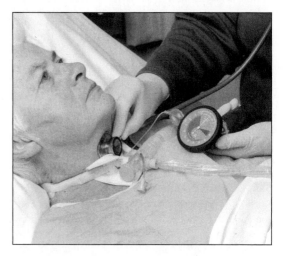

● If you don't hear an air leak, press the red button under the dial of the cuff pressure manometer to slowly release air from the balloon on the tracheal tube (as shown at top of next page). Auscultate for an air leak.

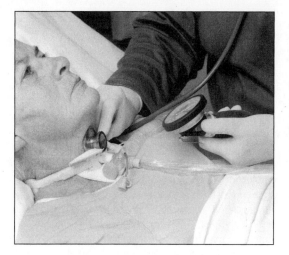

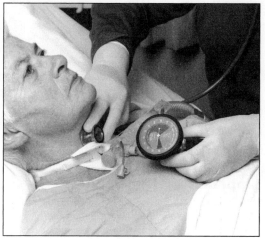

● As soon as you hear an air leak, release the red button and gently squeeze the handle of the cuff pressure manometer to inflate the cuff (as shown below). Continue to add air to the cuff until you no longer hear an air leak.

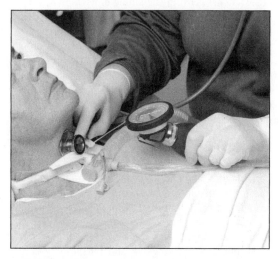

● When the air leak ceases, read the dial on the cuff pressure manometer (as shown at top of next column). This is the minimal pressure required to effectively occlude the trachea around the tracheal tube. In many cases, this pressure will fall within the green area (16 to 24 cm H_2O) on the manometer dial.

● Disconnect the cuff pressure manometer from the pilot balloon port. Document the pressure value.

Special considerations

● Measure cuff pressure at least every 8 hours *to avoid overinflation*.

● Keep in mind that some patients require less pressure, whereas others — for example, those with tracheal malacia (an abnormal softening of the tracheal tissue) — require more pressure. Maintaining the cuff pressure at the lowest possible level will minimize cuff-related problems.

● When measuring cuff pressure, keep the connection between the measuring device and the pilot balloon port tight *to avoid an air leak that could compromise cuff pressure*. If you're using a stopcock, don't leave the manometer in the off position *because air will leak from the cuff if the syringe accidentally comes off*. Also, note the volume of air needed to inflate the cuff. A gradual increase in this volume indicates tracheal dilation or erosion. A sudden increase in volume indicates cuff rupture and requires immediate reintubation if the patient is being ventilated.

Nursing diagnoses

● Risk for injury

Expected outcomes

The patient will:
● not develop trauma to the trachea.

Complications

• Aspiration of upper airway secretions, underventilation, or coughing spasms may occur if a leak is created during cuff pressure measurement.

Documentation

After cuff pressure measurement, record the date and time of the procedure, cuff pressure, total amount of air in the cuff after the procedure, any complications and interventions taken, and the patient's tolerance of the procedure.

Supportive references

Schreiber, D. "Trach Care at Home," *RN* 64(7):43-46, July 2001.

Serra, A. "Tracheostomy Care," *Nursing Standard* 14(42):45-52, 54-55, July 2000.

Tamburri, L.M. "Care of the Patient with a Tracheostomy," *Orthopaedic Nursing* 19(2):49-60, March-April 2000.

Tracheal suction

Tracheal suction involves the removal of secretions from the trachea or bronchi by means of a catheter inserted through the mouth or nose, tracheal stoma, a tracheostomy tube, or an endotracheal (ET) tube. In addition to removing secretions, tracheal suctioning also stimulates the cough reflex. This procedure helps maintain a patent airway to promote optimal exchange of oxygen and carbon dioxide and to prevent pneumonia that results from pooling of secretions. Performed as frequently as the patient's condition warrants, tracheal suction calls for strict aseptic technique.

According to American Association for Respiratory Care (AARC) guidelines, the need to remove accumulated pulmonary secretions is evidenced by one of the following:

• breath sounds that are coarse or "noisy" on auscultation, such as gurgling, rhonchi, or diminished breath sounds

• increased peak inspiratory pressures during volume-controlled ventilation or decreased tidal volume during pressure-controlled ventilation

• the patient's inability to generate an effective spontaneous cough

• visible secretions in the airway

• suspected aspiration of gastric or upper airway secretions

• clinically apparent increased work of breathing

• deterioration of arterial blood gas (ABG) values

• restlessness

• feelings of secretions in the chest (tactile fremitus)

• chest X-ray that shows atelectasis or consolidation. **AARC**

According to AARC guidelines, before suctioning the patient, hyperoxygenate him with 100% oxygen for at least 30 seconds. Sterile technique should be employed. The duration of each suctioning should be approximately 10 to 15 seconds. Suction pressure should be set as low as possible and yet effectively clear secretions. Following suctioning, the patient should be hyperoxygenated again for 1 minute or longer by the same technique used to preoxygenate the patient. **AARC**

Tracheal suction is only one component of bronchial hygiene. Encourage the patient to clear his airways by coughing and teach him proper cough techniques. Push adequate hydration to facilitate removal of secretions. Perform suctioning only when necessary and when other methods of removing secretions haven't been effective. Suctioning shouldn't be performed as a routine procedure. Assess the patient for clinical signs that suctioning is necessary, such as coarse breath sounds on auscultation, noisy respirations, prolonged expiratory breath sounds, and increased or decreased heart rate, respiratory rate, or blood pressure.

Equipment

Oxygen source (mechanical ventilator, wall or portable unit, and handheld resuscitation bag with a mask, 15-mm adapter, or a positive end-expiratory pressure valve, if indicated) • wall or portable suction apparatus • collection container • connecting tube • suction catheter kit, or a sterile suction catheter, one sterile glove, one clean glove, and a disposable sterile solution container • 1-L bottle of sterile water or normal saline solution • sterile water-soluble lubricant (for nasal insertion) • syringe for deflating cuff of ET or tracheostomy tube • waterproof trash bag • goggles and face mask or face shield • optional: sterile towel

Preparation of equipment

- Choose a sterile suction catheter of appropriate size. The diameter should be no larger than half the inside diameter of the tracheostomy or ET tube *to minimize hypoxia during suctioning.* (A #12 or #14 French catheter may be used for an 8-mm or larger tube.)
- Place the suction apparatus on the patient's overbed table or bedside stand.
- Position the table or stand on your preferred side of the bed *to facilitate suctioning.*
- Attach the collection container to the suction unit and the connecting tube to the collection container.
- Label and date the normal saline solution or sterile water.
- Open the waterproof trash bag.

Implementation

- Confirm the patient's identity using two patient identifiers according to facility policy. **JCAHO**
- Before suctioning, determine whether your facility requires a physician's order and obtain one, if necessary.
- Assess the patient's vital signs, breath sounds, and general appearance *to establish a baseline for comparison after suctioning.* Review the patient's ABG values and oxygen saturation levels if they're available. Evaluate the patient's ability to cough and deep-breathe *because this will help move secretions up the tracheobronchial tree.* If you'll be performing nasotracheal suctioning, check the patient's history for a deviated septum, nasal polyps, nasal obstruction, nasal trauma, epistaxis, or mucosal swelling. **AARC**
- Wash your hands. Explain the procedure to the patient. Tell him that suctioning usually causes transient coughing or gagging but that coughing is helpful for removing secretions. Continue to reassure the patient throughout the procedure *to minimize anxiety, promote relaxation, and decrease oxygen demand.* **AARC CDC**
- Unless contraindicated, place the patient in semi-Fowler's or high Fowler's position *to promote lung expansion and productive coughing.*
- Remove the top from the normal saline solution or water bottle.
- Put on the face mask and goggles. **CDC**
- Open the package containing the sterile solution container.

- Using strict aseptic technique, open the suction catheter kit, and put on the gloves. If using individual supplies, open the suction catheter and the gloves, placing the nonsterile glove on your nondominant hand and the sterile glove on your dominant hand. **AARC CDC**
- Using your nondominant (nonsterile) hand, pour the normal saline solution or sterile water into the solution container.
- Place a small amount of sterile water-soluble lubricant on the sterile area. *Lubricant may be used to facilitate passage of the catheter during nasotracheal suctioning.*
- Place a sterile towel over the patient's chest, if desired, *to provide an additional sterile area.*
- Using your dominant (sterile) hand, remove the catheter from its wrapper. Keep it coiled so it can't touch a nonsterile object. Using your other hand to manipulate the connecting tubing, attach the catheter to the tubing (as shown below). **AARC**

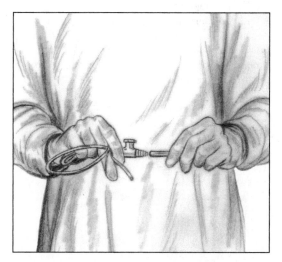

- Using your nondominant hand, set the suction pressure according to your facility's policy. Typically, pressure may be set between 100 and 150 mm Hg. *Higher pressures don't enhance secretion removal and may cause traumatic injury.* Occlude the suction port *to assess suction pressure* (as shown at top of next page).

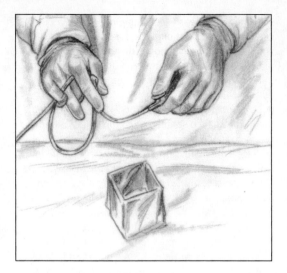

● Dip the catheter tip in the saline solution *to lubricate the outside of the catheter and reduce tissue trauma during insertion.*

● With the catheter tip in the sterile solution, occlude the control valve with the thumb of your nondominant hand. Suction a small amount of solution through the catheter (as shown below) *to lubricate the inside of the catheter,* thus facilitating passage of secretions through it.

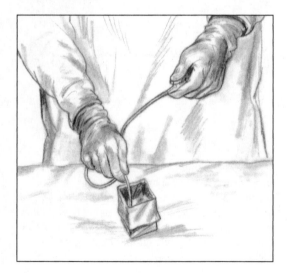

● For nasal insertion of the catheter, lubricate the tip of the catheter with the sterile, water-soluble lubricant to reduce tissue trauma during insertion. **AARC**

● If the patient isn't intubated or is intubated but not receiving supplemental oxygen or aerosol, instruct him to take three to six deep breaths to help minimize or prevent hypoxia during suctioning.

● If the patient isn't intubated but is receiving oxygen, evaluate his need for preoxygenation. If indicated, instruct the patient to take three to six deep breaths while using his supplemental oxygen. (If needed, the patient may continue to receive supplemental oxygen during suctioning by leaving his nasal cannula in one nostril or by keeping the oxygen mask over his mouth.)

● If the patient is being mechanically ventilated, preoxygenate him *to minimize hypoxia after suctioning.* Use the ventilator rather than a handheld resuscitation bag to hyperoxygenate and hyperinflate the lungs before suctioning. Be aware that providing hyperoxygenation on some ventilators requires a washout time of up to 2 minutes to ensure a higher oxygen concentration to travel through the tubing and reach the patient. Newer models may be able to provide increased oxygen concentrations to the patient in less time. **AARC**

● To preoxygenate using the ventilator, first adjust the fraction of inspired oxygen (FIO_2) and tidal volume according to your facility's policy and the patient's needs. **EB1** Then, use the sigh mode to deliver three to six breaths. If you have an assistant for the procedure, the assistant can manage the patient's oxygen needs while you perform suctioning. **AARC**

⚑ **CLINICAL IMPACT** *The instillation of a normal saline bolus into the ET tube before suctioning has been a traditional nursing practice. This practice may have originated when mechanical ventilators couldn't adequately humidify the airway. However, research indicates that this practice isn't beneficial and that saline and secretions are immiscible even after vigorous shaking, so that tenacious secretions aren't thinned. While saline may cause the person to cough, mobilizing secretions, the cough produced may be uncontrollable and may damage the respiratory mucosa. Research also suggests that bacteria from an ET tube may be forced into the airway with the instillation of saline. Current evidence suggests that saline* *shouldn't be routinely used before suctioning. Nursing interventions that improve patient hydration can facilitate mobilization of respiratory secretions.* **EB2**

Nasotracheal insertion in the nonintubated patient

● Disconnect the oxygen from the patient, if applicable.
● Using your nondominant hand, raise the tip of the patient's nose *to straighten the passageway and facilitate catheter insertion.*
● Insert the catheter into the patient's nostril while gently rolling it between your fingers *to help it advance through the turbinates.*
● As the patient inhales, quickly advance the catheter as far as possible. *To avoid oxygen loss and tissue trauma,* don't apply suction during insertion. **AARC**
● If the patient coughs as the catheter passes through the larynx, briefly hold the catheter still and then resume advancement when the patient inhales.

Insertion in the intubated patient

● If you're using a closed system, see *Closed tracheal suctioning,* pages 356 and 357.
● Using your nonsterile hand, disconnect the patient from the ventilator.
● Using your sterile hand, gently insert the suction catheter into the artificial airway (as shown below). Advance the catheter, without applying suction, until you meet resistance. If the patient coughs, pause briefly and then resume advancement.

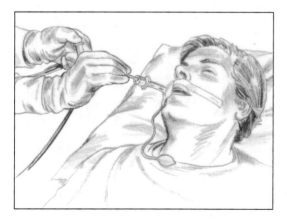

Suctioning the patient

● After inserting the catheter, apply suction intermittently by removing and replacing the thumb of your nondominant hand over the control valve. Simultaneously use your dominant hand to withdraw the catheter as you roll it between your thumb and forefinger. **AARC** *This rotating motion prevents the catheter from pulling tissue into the tube as it exits, thus avoiding tissue trauma.*
● Never suction more than 10 to 15 seconds at a time *to prevent hypoxia.* Don't pass the catheter more than twice *to reduce trauma to the tracheal mucosa.* **AARC**
● If the patient is intubated, use your nondominant hand to stabilize the tip of the ET tube as you withdraw the catheter *to prevent mucous membrane irritation or accidental extubation.*
● If applicable, resume oxygen delivery by reconnecting the source of oxygen or ventilation, and hyperoxygenating the patient's lungs before continuing *to prevent or relieve hypoxia.* **AARC**
● Observe the patient, and allow him to rest for a few minutes before the next suctioning. The timing of each suctioning and the length of each rest period depend on his tolerance of the procedure and the absence of complications. *To enhance secretion removal,* encourage the patient to cough between suctioning attempts. **AARC** **Science**
● Observe the secretions. If they're thick, clear the catheter periodically by dipping the tip in the saline solution and applying suction. Normally, sputum is watery and tends to be sticky. Tenacious or thick sputum usually indicates dehydration. Watch for color variations. White or translucent color is normal; yellow indicates pus; green indicates retained secretions or *Pseudomonas* infection; brown usually indicates old blood; red indicates fresh blood; and a "red currant jelly" appearance indicates *Klebsiella* infection. When sputum contains blood, note whether it's streaked or well mixed. Also indicate how often blood appears. **Science**
● Monitor the patient's heart rate and rhythm. If the patient is being monitored, observe for arrhythmias. Should they occur, stop suctioning and ventilate the patient.
● Patients who can't mobilize secretions effectively may need to perform tracheal suctioning after discharge. (See *Tracheal suctioning at home,* page 358.)

Closed tracheal suctioning

The closed tracheal suction system can ease removal of secretions and reduce patient complications. Consisting of a sterile suction catheter in a clear plastic sleeve, the system permits the patient to remain connected to the ventilator during suctioning. With this system, the patient can maintain the tidal volume, oxygen concentration, and positive end-expiratory pressure (PEEP) delivered by the ventilator while being suctioned. In turn, this reduces the occurrence of suction-induced hypoxemia.

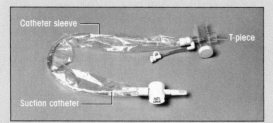

Because the catheter remains in a protective sleeve, another advantage of this system is a reduced risk of infection, even when the same catheter is used many times. The caregiver doesn't need to touch the catheter and the ventilator circuit remains closed.

A closed tracheal suction device allows the patient to remain connected to the ventilator during suctioning. As a result, the patient may continue to be oxygenated and receive PEEP while being suctioned. In patients receiving intermittent mandatory mechanical ventilation, closed tracheal suctioning may reduce arterial desaturation and eliminate the need for preoxygenation.

Because suction catheters are considered contaminated after a single use, researchers studied whether closed tracheal suctioning increased the rate of health care-associated pneumonia in mechanically ventilated patients. They found that patients receiving closed tracheal suctioning had lower rates of health care-associated pneumonia than those receiving open suctioning. Moreover, researchers

found that changing closed tracheal suction catheters as needed was just as effective in preventing ventilator-associated pneumonia as daily catheter changes.

On the negative side, closed tracheal suctioning has been found to produce increased negative airway pressure when certain ventilatory modes are used, increasing the risk of atelectasis and hypoxemia.

Implementation

To perform the procedure, gather the closed suction system that consists of a control valve, a T-piece to connect the artificial airway to the ventilator breathing circuit, and a catheter sleeve that encloses the catheter and has connections at each end for the control valve and the T-piece. Then follow these steps:

● Wash your hands. **CDC**
● Remove the closed suction system from its wrapping. Attach the control valve to the connecting tubing.
● Depress the thumb suction control valve, and keep it depressed while setting the suction pressure to the desired level.
● Connect the T-piece to the ventilator breathing circuit; make sure that the irrigation port is closed. Then connect the T-piece to the patient's endotracheal or tracheostomy tube (as shown below).
● Hyperoxygenate and hyperinflate the patient using the ventilator. **EB1**

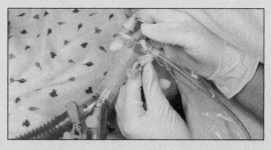

After suctioning

● After suctioning, hyperoxygenate the patient being maintained on a ventilator by using the ventilator's sigh mode, as described above. **Science**
● Readjust the FIO_2 and, for ventilated patients, the tidal volume to the ordered settings.

● After suctioning the lower airway, assess the patient's need for upper airway suctioning. If the cuff of the ET or tracheostomy tube is inflated, suction the upper airway before deflating the cuff with a syringe. (See "Oronasopharyngeal suction," page 332, and "Endotracheal tube care," page 295.) Always change the catheter and sterile glove before resuctioning the

● Put on clean gloves. **CDC** Steadying the T-piece, use the thumb and index finger of the other hand to advance the catheter through the tube and into the patient's tracheobronchial tree (as shown below). It may be necessary to gently retract the catheter sleeve as you advance the catheter.

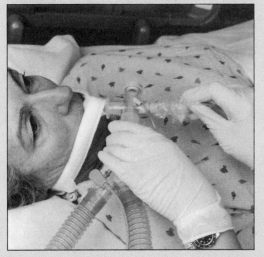

● While continuing to hold the T-piece and control valve, apply intermittent suction and withdraw the catheter until it reaches its fully extended length in the sleeve. Repeat the procedure only if necessary.
● After you've finished suctioning, flush the catheter by maintaining suction while slowly introducing normal saline solution or sterile water into the irrigation port.
● Place the thumb control valve in the OFF position.
● Dispose of and replace the suction equipment and supplies according to your facility's policy.
● Remove your gloves and wash your hands. **CDC**
● Change the closed suction system every 24 hours to minimize the risk of infection.

lower airway *to avoid introducing microorganisms into the lower airway.*
● Discard the gloves and catheter in the waterproof trash bag. Clear the connecting tubing by aspirating the remaining saline solution or water. Discard and replace suction equipment and supplies according to your facility's policy. Wash your hands. **CDC**

● Auscultate the lungs bilaterally and take the patient's vital signs, if indicated, *to assess the procedure's effectiveness.* Note his skin color, breathing pattern, and respiratory rate. **AARC**

Special considerations
● Raising the patient's nose into the sniffing position helps align the larynx and pharynx and may facilitate passing the catheter during nasotracheal suctioning. If the patient's condition permits, have an assistant extend the patient's head and neck above his shoulders. The patient's lower jaw may need to be moved up and forward. If the patient is responsive, ask him to stick out his tongue *so he can't swallow the catheter during insertion.*
● During suctioning, the catheter typically is advanced as far as the mainstem bronchi. However, because of tracheobronchial anatomy, the catheter tends to enter the right mainstem bronchi instead of the left. Using an angled catheter, such as a catheter coudé, may help you guide the catheter into the left mainstem bronchus. Rotating the patient's head to the right seems to have a limited effect.
● In addition to the closed tracheal method, oxygen insufflation offers a new approach to suctioning. This method uses a double-lumen catheter that allows oxygen insufflation during the suctioning procedure.
● Don't allow the collection container on the suction machine to become more than three-quarters full *to keep from damaging the machine.*

Nursing diagnoses
● Anxiety
● Ineffective airway clearance

Expected outcomes
The patient will:
● state less anxiety and have decreased work of breathing
● have improved breath sounds
● have a normal chest X-ray
● have normal oxygen levels.

Complications
● *Because oxygen is removed along with secretions, the patient may experience hypoxemia and dyspnea.*
● Anxiety and pain may alter respiratory patterns.

Tracheal suctioning at home

If a patient can't mobilize secretions effectively by coughing, he may have to perform tracheal suctioning at home using either clean or aseptic technique. Most patients use clean technique, which consists of thorough hand washing and possibly wearing a clean glove. However, a patient with poor hand-washing technique, recurrent respiratory infections or a compromised immune system or one who has had recent surgery, may need to use aseptic technique.

Clean technique

Because the cost of disposable catheters can be prohibitive, many patients reuse disposable catheters, but the practice remains controversial. If the catheter has thick secretions adhering to it, the patient may clean it with Control III, a quaternary compound.

An alternative to disposable catheters is to use nondisposable, red rubber catheters. These catheters contain latex, so use with caution. Consult your facility's policy regarding the care and cleaning of suction catheters in the home setting.

Supplies needed

The supplies needed vary with the technique used. If the patient will be using clean technique, he'll need suction catheter kits (or clean gloves, suction catheters, and a basin) and distilled water. If he'll be using sterile technique, everything must be sterile: suction catheters, gloves, basin, and water (or normal saline solution).

The type of suction machine necessary will depend on the patient's needs. You'll need to evaluate the amount of suction the machine provides, how easy it is to clean, the volume of the collection bottles, how much it costs, and whether the machine has an overflow safety device to prevent secretions from entering the compressor. You'll also need to determine whether the patient needs a machine that operates on batteries and, if so, how long the batteries will last and whether and how they can be recharged.

Nursing goals

Before discharge, the patient and his family should demonstrate the suctioning procedure. They also need to recognize the indications for suctioning, the signs and symptoms of infection, the importance of adequate hydration, and when to use adjunct therapy, such as aerosol therapy, chest physiotherapy, oxygen therapy, or a handheld resuscitation bag. At discharge, arrange for a home health care provider and a durable medical equipment vendor to follow up with the patient.

● Cardiac arrhythmias can result from hypoxia and stimulation of the vagus nerve in the tracheobronchial tree.
● Tracheal or bronchial trauma can result from traumatic or prolonged suctioning.
● Patients with compromised cardiovascular or pulmonary status are at risk for hypoxemia, arrhythmias, hypertension, or hypotension.
● Patients with a history of nasopharyngeal bleeding, those who are taking anticoagulants, those who have recently had a tracheostomy, and those who have a blood disease are at increased risk for bleeding as a result of suctioning.
● Use caution when suctioning patients who have increased intracranial pressure because it may increase pressure further.
● If the patient experiences laryngospasm or bronchospasm (rare complications) during suctioning, discuss with the patient's physician the use of bronchodilators or lidocaine (Xylocaine) to reduce the risk of this complication.

Documentation

Record the date and time of the procedure; technique used; reason for suctioning; amount, color, consistency, and odor (if any) of secretions; any complications and interventions taken; and the patient's subjective response to the procedure. Chart preprocedure and postprocedure breath sounds and vital signs.

Supportive references

American Association for Respiratory Care. "AARC Clinical Practice Guideline: Directed Cough," *Respiratory Care* 38(5):495-99, May 1993.
American Association for Respiratory Care. "AARC Clinical Practice Guideline: Endotracheal Suctioning of

Mechanically Ventilated Adults and Children with Artificial Airways," *Respiratory Care* 38(5):500-504, May 1993.

American Association for Respiratory Care. "AARC Clinical Practice Guideline: Nasotracheal Suctioning," *Respiratory Care* 49(9):1080-1084, September 2004.

American Association for Respiratory Care. "AARC Clinical Practice Guideline: Suctioning of the Patient in the Home," *Respiratory Care* 44(1):99-104, January 1999.

"As-needed In-line Suction Catheter Changes Were as Safe as and Less Expensive than Daily Scheduled Catheter Changes during Mechanical Ventilation," *Evidence-Based Nursing* 1(3):82, July 1998.

Joanna Briggs Institute for Evidence-Based Nursing and Midwifery. "Best Practice: Tracheal Suctioning of Adults with an Artificial Airway," 4(4):1-6, 2000. *www.joannabriggs.edu.au/bpmenu.html.* **EB2**

Lynn-McHale Wiegand, D.J., and Carlson, K.K. *AACN Procedure Manual for Critical Care,* 5th ed. Philadelphia: W.B. Saunders Co., 2005. **EB1**

Paul-Allen, J., and Ostrow, C.L. "Survey of Nursing Practices with Closed-System Suctioning," *American Journal of Critical Care* 9(1):9-17, January 2000.

Tracheostomy care

Whether a tracheotomy is performed in an emergency or after careful preparation, as a permanent measure or as temporary therapy, the goal is the same: to ensure airway patency by keeping the tube free from mucus buildup, to maintain mucous membrane and skin integrity, and to prevent infection.

The patient may have one of three types of tracheostomy tube — uncuffed, cuffed, or fenestrated. Tube selection depends on the patient's condition and the physician's preference. An uncuffed tube, which may be plastic or metal, allows air to flow freely around the tracheostomy tube and through the larynx, reducing the risk of tracheal damage. Uncuffed tubes may be used for a permanent tracheostomy. A cuffed tube, made of plastic, is disposable. It's used for patients on mechanical ventilation and patients at risk for aspiration. A plastic fenestrated tube permits speech through the upper airway when the external opening is capped and the cuff is deflated. It also allows for easy removal of the inner cannula for cleaning. However, a fenestrated tube may become occluded.

If the patient is on a ventilator, a tube with an inflated cuff must be used to seal the space between the trachea and the tube so that air moves through the tube to the lungs. The patient who's breathing normally on his own may need the cuff inflated when he takes nutrition orally.

Tracheostomy care should be performed using aseptic technique until the stoma has healed *to prevent infection.* For recently performed tracheotomies — less than 7 days postoperatively — or unhealed tracheostomies, the site should be assessed at least every 4 hours and the stoma should be cleaned and redressed every 8 hours. Tracheostomy care should be performed at least every shift on a healed tracheostomy. **Science** Sterile gloves should be worn for all manipulations at the tracheostomy site. After the stoma has healed, clean gloves may be substituted for sterile ones.

◀ **INNOVATIVE PRACTICE** *To prepare nurses on general units to care for the increasing number of patients with tracheostomies transferred from the intensive care unit (ICU) and specialty units, nurses from the University of Pittsburgh Medical Center Presbyterian Hospital implemented a program to improve tracheostomy care and increase nurses' competencies. Using the Society of Otorhinolaryngology and Head-Neck Nurses guidelines, they developed standards to ensure consistent care between the ICU and general units.*

A self-learning module was created to teach tracheostomy care. After completing the module, the nurse's skills were peer reviewed. Problem-solving skills were evaluated through the use of a case study. As a result of this innovative educational program, patients with tracheostomies are cared for on a general nursing unit rather than being admitted or transferred to a specialty unit. Competence in tracheostomy care is evaluated annually.

Provide safety measures for the patient, such as admitting him to a room close to the nurses' station, keeping an emergency tracheostomy tray on the unit, and a label at the nurses' station near the call unit if the patient can't speak.

Keep with the patient at all times (especially when traveling for tests) an emergency replacement tracheostomy tube of the present size and one size smaller, a curved hemostat or tracheal dilator/obturator for the current tube, and a large-bore suction catheter and suction machine. Make sure that the areas the patient may travel to (such as X-ray) have working suction equipment.

Equipment
Aseptic stoma and outer-cannula care
Waterproof trash bag • two sterile solution containers • normal saline solution • hydrogen peroxide • sterile cotton-tipped applicators • sterile 4″ × 4″ gauze pads • sterile gloves • prepackaged sterile tracheostomy dressing (or 4″ × 4″ gauze pad) • equipment and supplies for suctioning and mouth care • water-soluble lubricant or topical antibiotic cream • materials as needed for cuff procedures and changing tracheostomy ties (see below)

Aseptic inner-cannula care
All of the preceding equipment plus a prepackaged commercial tracheostomy care set, or sterile forceps • sterile nylon brush • sterile 6″ (15-cm) pipe cleaners • clean gloves • a third sterile solution container • disposable temporary inner cannula (for a patient on a ventilator)

Changing tracheostomy ties
30″ (76-cm) length of tracheostomy twill tape • bandage scissors • sterile gloves • hemostat

Emergency tracheostomy tube replacement
Sterile tracheal dilator or sterile hemostat • sterile obturator that fits the tracheostomy tube in use • two extra sterile tracheostomy tubes and obturators in the appropriate size • suction equipment and supplies

Keep these supplies in full view in the patient's room at all times for easy access in case of an emergency. Consider taping an emergency sterile tracheostomy tube in a sterile wrapper to the head of the bed for easy access in an emergency.

Cuff procedures
5- or 10-ml syringe • padded hemostat • stethoscope

Preparation of equipment
● Wash your hands, and assemble all equipment and supplies in the patient's room. **CDC** Check the expiration date on each sterile package and inspect the package for tears.

● Open the waterproof trash bag, and place it next to you *so that you can avoid reaching across the sterile field or the patient's stoma when discarding soiled items.*

● Establish a sterile field near the patient's bed (usually on the overbed table), and place equipment and supplies on it.

● Pour sterile normal saline solution, hydrogen peroxide, or a mixture of equal parts of both solutions into one of the sterile solution containers, and then pour normal saline solution into the second sterile container for rinsing.

● For inner-cannula care, you may use a third sterile solution container to hold the gauze pads and cotton-tipped applicators saturated with cleaning solution.

● If you're replacing the disposable inner cannula, open the package containing the new inner cannula while maintaining sterile technique.

● Obtain or prepare new tracheostomy ties, if indicated.

Implementation
● Confirm the patient's identity using two patient identifiers according to facility policy. **JCAHO**

● Assess the patient's condition *to determine his need for care.*

● Explain the procedure to the patient even if he's unresponsive. Provide privacy. **PCP**

● Place the patient in semi-Fowler's position (unless it's contraindicated) *to decrease abdominal pressure on the diaphragm and promote lung expansion.*

● Remove any humidification or ventilation device.

● If the patient is being mechanically ventilated, administer hyperoxygenation and hyperinflation using the ventilator settings. If he's breathing on his own, evaluate the need for preoxygenation and instruct him to take deep breaths.

● Using sterile technique, suction the entire length of the tracheostomy tube *to clear the airway of any secretions that may hinder oxygenation.* (See "Tracheal suction," page 352.)

● Reconnect the patient to the humidifier or ventilator, if necessary.

Cleaning a stoma and outer cannula
● Put on sterile gloves. **CDC**

● With your dominant hand, saturate a sterile gauze pad or cotton-tipped applicator with the cleaning solution. Squeeze out the excess liquid *to prevent accidental aspiration.* Wipe the patient's neck under the tracheostomy tube flanges and twill tapes.

● Saturate a second pad or applicator, and wipe until the skin surrounding the tracheostomy is cleaned. Use additional pads or cotton-tipped applicators to clean the stoma site and the tube's flanges. Wipe only once with each pad or applicator, and then discard it *to prevent contamination of a clean area with a soiled pad or applicator.* **Science**

● Rinse debris and peroxide (if used) with one or more sterile 4″ × 4″ gauze pads dampened in normal saline solution. Dry the area thoroughly with additional sterile gauze pads, and then apply a new sterile tracheostomy dressing.

● Remove and discard your gloves. **CDC**

Cleaning a nondisposable inner cannula

● Put on sterile gloves. **CDC**

● Using your nondominant hand, remove and discard the patient's tracheostomy dressing. With the same hand, disconnect the ventilator or humidification device, and unlock the tracheostomy tube's inner cannula by rotating it counterclockwise. Place the inner cannula in the container with hydrogen peroxide.

● Working quickly, use your dominant hand to scrub the cannula with the sterile nylon brush. If the brush doesn't slide easily into the cannula, use a sterile pipe cleaner.

● Immerse the cannula in the container of normal saline solution, and agitate it for about 10 seconds *to rinse it thoroughly because hydrogen peroxide can irritate the tracheal mucosa.*

● Inspect the cannula for cleanliness. Repeat the cleaning process, if necessary. If it's clean, tap it gently against the inside edge of the sterile container *to remove excess liquid and prevent aspiration.* Don't dry the outer surface *because a thin film of moisture acts as a lubricant during insertion.*

● Reinsert the inner cannula into the patient's tracheostomy tube. Lock it in place and then gently pull on it *to make sure that it's positioned securely.* Reconnect the mechanical ventilator. Apply a new sterile tracheostomy dressing.

● If the patient can't tolerate being disconnected from the ventilator for the time it takes to clean the inner cannula, replace the existing inner cannula with a clean one and reattach the mechanical ventilator. Then clean the cannula just removed from the patient, and store it in a sterile container for use the next time.

Caring for a disposable inner cannula

● Put on clean gloves. **CDC**

● Using your dominant hand, remove the patient's inner cannula. After evaluating the secretions in the cannula, discard it properly.

● Pick up the new inner cannula, touching only the outer locking portion. Insert the cannula into the tracheostomy and, following the manufacturer's instructions, lock it securely. **MFR**

Changing tracheostomy ties

● Change the ties as necessary and when soiled after the first change by the surgeon. **AACN**

● Obtain assistance from another nurse or a respiratory therapist *because of the risk of accidental tube expulsion during this procedure.* Patient movement or coughing can dislodge the tube.

● Wash your hands thoroughly, and put on sterile gloves. **CDC**

● If you aren't using commercially packaged tracheostomy ties, prepare new ties from a 30″ (76-cm) length of twill tape by folding one end back 1″ (2.5 cm) on itself. With the bandage scissors, cut a ¹/₂″ (1.3-cm) slit down the center of the tape from the folded edge.

● Prepare the other end of the tape the same way.

● Hold both ends together and, using scissors, cut the resulting circle of tape so that one piece is approximately 10″ (25 cm) long and the other is about 20″ (51 cm) long.

● Assist the patient into semi-Fowler's position, if possible.

● After your assistant puts on gloves, instruct her to hold the tracheostomy tube in place *to prevent its expulsion during replacement of the ties.* If you must perform the procedure without assistance, fasten the clean ties in place before removing the old ties *to prevent tube expulsion.*

● With the assistant's gloved fingers holding the tracheostomy tube in place, cut the soiled tracheostomy ties and discard them. If using scissors, be careful not to cut the tube of the pilot balloon.

● Thread the slit end of one new tie a short distance through the eye of one tracheostomy tube flange from the underside; use the hemostat, if needed, to pull the tie through. Thread the other end of the tie completely through the slit end, and pull it taut so it loops firmly through the flange. *This avoids knots that can cause throat discomfort, tissue irritation, pressure, and necrosis at the patient's throat.*

● Fasten the second tie to the opposite flange in the same manner.

● Instruct the patient to flex his neck while you bring the ties around to the side, and tie them together with a square knot. *Flexion produces the same neck circumference as coughing and helps prevent an overly tight tie.* Instruct your assistant to place one finger under the tapes as you tie them *to ensure that they're tight enough to avoid slippage but loose enough to prevent choking or jugular vein constriction. Placing the closure on the side allows easy access and prevents pressure necrosis at the back of the neck when the patient is recumbent.*

● After securing the ties, cut off the excess tape with the scissors and instruct your assistant to release the tracheostomy tube.

● Make sure that the patient is comfortable and can reach the call button easily.

● Check tracheostomy-tie tension frequently on patients with traumatic injury, radical neck dissection, or cardiac failure *because neck diameter can increase from swelling and cause constriction;* also check neonatal or restless patients frequently *because ties can loosen and cause tube dislodgment.*

Concluding tracheostomy care

● Replace any humidification device.

● Provide oral care as needed because the oral cavity can become dry and malodorous or develop sores from encrusted secretions.

● Observe soiled dressings and any suctioned secretions for amount, color, consistency, and odor.

● Properly clean or dispose of all equipment, supplies, solutions, and trash, according to your facility's policy.

● Remove and discard your gloves. **CDC**

● Make sure that the patient is comfortable and can easily reach the call button.

● Make sure that all necessary supplies are readily available at the bedside.

● Repeat the procedure at least once every 8 hours or as needed. Change the dressing as often as necessary regardless of whether you also perform the entire cleaning procedure *because a wet dressing with exudate or secretions predisposes the patient to skin excoriation, breakdown, and infection.*

Deflating and inflating a tracheostomy cuff

● Read the cuff manufacturer's instructions because cuff types and procedures vary widely. **MFR** (See *Comparing tracheostomy tubes.*)

● Assess the patient's condition, explain the procedure to him, and reassure him. Wash your hands thoroughly. **CDC**

● Help the patient into semi-Fowler's position, if he's able.

● Suction the oropharyngeal cavity to prevent pooled secretions from descending into the trachea after cuff deflation.

● Release the padded hemostat clamping the cuff inflation tubing, if a hemostat is present.

● Insert a 5- or 10-ml syringe into the cuff pilot balloon, and very slowly withdraw all air from the cuff. Leave the syringe attached to the tubing for later reinflation of the cuff. Slow deflation allows positive lung pressure to push secretions upward from the bronchi. Cuff deflation may also stimulate the patient's cough reflex, producing additional secretions.

● Remove any ventilation device. Suction the lower airway through any existing tube to remove all secretions. Reconnect the patient to the ventilation device.

● While the cuff is deflated, observe the patient for adequate ventilation, and suction as necessary. If the patient has difficulty breathing, reinflate the cuff immediately by depressing the syringe plunger very slowly. Use a stethoscope to listen over the trachea for the air leak, and then inject the least amount of air necessary to achieve an adequate tracheal seal.

● When inflating the cuff, you may use the minimal-leak technique or the minimal occlusive volume technique to help gauge the proper inflation point. (For more information, see "Endotracheal intubation," page 289, and "Endotracheal tube care," page 295.)

● Be careful not to exceed 20 mm Hg. If pressure exceeds 20 mm Hg, notify the physician because you may need to change to a larger-size tube, use higher inflation pressures, or permit a larger air leak. The

Comparing tracheostomy tubes

Made of plastic or metal, tracheostomy tubes come in uncuffed, cuffed, and fenestrated varieties. Tube selection depends on the patient's condition and the physician's preference. This chart lists the advantages and disadvantages of some commonly used tubes.

Type	Advantages	Disadvantages
Uncuffed (plastic or metal) 	• Permits air to flow freely around the tracheostomy tube and through the larynx • Reduces the risk of tracheal damage • Is a safer choice for children	• Increases the risk of aspiration in adults • May require adapter for mechanical ventilation
Cuffed (plastic) 	• Is disposable • Stops the cuff and the tube from separating accidentally inside the trachea because the cuff is bonded to the tube • Doesn't require periodic deflating to lower pressure because the cuff pressure is low and evenly distributed against the tracheal wall • Reduces the risk of tracheal damage	• May cost more than other tubes
Fenestrated (plastic) 	• Permits speech through the upper airway when the external opening is capped and the cuff is deflated • Allows breathing by mechanical ventilation with the inner cannula in place and the cuff inflated • Allows easy removal of the inner cannula for cleaning	• May have possible occlusion of the fenestrations • May allow the inner cannula to dislodge

patient may also have a fistula if more air is needed to inflate the cuff. The recommended cuff pressure is about 18 mm Hg.

• After you've inflated the cuff, if the tubing doesn't have a one-way valve at the end, clamp the inflation line with a padded hemostat (to protect the tubing) and remove the syringe.

• Check for a minimal-leak cuff seal. Place your stethoscope over the trachea and listen while injecting air with a syringe into the pilot balloon until you no longer hear an air leak. Then slowly remove air until you hear a slight hiss at the end of inspiration. You shouldn't feel air coming from the patient's mouth, nose, or tracheostomy site, and a conscious patient shouldn't be able to speak.

• Stay alert for air leaks from the cuff itself. Suspect a leak if injection of air fails to inflate the cuff or increase cuff pressure, if you're unable to inject the amount of air you withdrew, if the patient can speak, if ventilation fails to maintain adequate respiratory movement with pressures or volumes previously considered adequate, or if air escapes during the ventilator's inspiratory cycle.

• Note the exact amount of air used to inflate the cuff *to detect tracheal malacia if more air is consistently needed.*

● Make sure that the patient is comfortable and can easily reach the call button and communication aids.
● Properly clean or dispose of all equipment, supplies, and trash according to your facility's policy.
● Replenish any used supplies, and make sure that all necessary emergency supplies are at the bedside.

Special considerations

● Keep appropriate equipment at the patient's bedside for immediate use in an emergency.
● Consult the physician about first-aid measures you can use for your tracheostomy patient should an emergency occur. Follow your facility's policy regarding procedure if a tracheostomy tube is expelled or if the outer cannula becomes blocked. If the patient's breathing is obstructed — for example, when the tube is blocked with mucus that can't be removed by suctioning or by withdrawing the inner cannula — call the appropriate code, and provide manual resuscitation with a handheld resuscitation bag or reconnect the patient to the ventilator. Don't remove the tracheostomy tube entirely *because this may allow the airway to close completely.* Use extreme caution when attempting to reinsert an expelled tracheostomy tube *because of the risk of tracheal trauma, perforation, compression, and asphyxiation.* Reassure the patient until the physician arrives (usually 1 minute or less in this type of code or emergency).
● Refrain from changing tracheostomy ties unnecessarily during the immediate postoperative period before the stoma track is well formed (usually 4 days) *to avoid accidental dislodgment and expulsion of the tube.* Unless secretions or drainage is a problem, ties can be changed once per day.
● Refrain from changing a single-cannula tracheostomy tube or the outer cannula of a double-cannula tube. *Because of the risk of tracheal complications,* the physician usually changes the cannula, with the frequency of change depending on the patient's condition.
● If the patient's neck or stoma is excoriated or infected, apply a water-soluble lubricant or topical antibiotic cream as ordered. Remember not to use a powder or an oil-based substance on or around a stoma *because aspiration can cause infection and abscess.*

● Replace all equipment, including solutions, regularly according to your facility's policy *to reduce the risk of nosocomial infections.*

TEACHING *If the patient is being discharged with a tracheostomy, start self-care teaching as soon as he's receptive. Teach the patient how to change and clean the tube. If he's being discharged with suction equipment (a few patients are), make sure that he and his family feel knowledgeable and comfortable about using the equipment. Make appropriate referrals for home care.*

Nursing diagnoses

● Risk for infection

Expected outcomes

The patient will:
● have respiratory secretions that remain clear and odorless
● show no evidence of skin breakdown.

Complications

● Complications that may occur within the first 48 hours after tracheostomy tube insertion include hemorrhage at the operative site, causing drowning; bleeding or edema in tracheal tissue, causing airway obstruction; aspiration of secretions; introduction of air into the pleural cavity, causing pneumothorax; hypoxia or acidosis, triggering cardiac arrest; and introduction of air into surrounding tissues, causing subcutaneous emphysema.
● Late complications include tracheal stenosis, tracheomalacia, and fistula formation.
● Secretions collecting under dressings and twill tape can encourage skin excoriation and infection.
● Hardened mucus or a slipped cuff can occlude the cannula opening and obstruct the airway.
● Tube displacement can stimulate the cough reflex if the tip rests on the carina, or it can cause blood vessel erosion and hemorrhage.
● The presence of the tube or cuff pressure can produce tracheal erosion and necrosis.

Documentation

Record the date, time, and type of the procedure; the amount, consistency, color, and odor of secretions; stoma and skin condition; the patient's respiratory status before, during, and after the procedure; change of the tracheostomy tube by the physician; duration of any cuff deflation; amount of any cuff inflation; and cuff pressure readings and specific body position. Note any complications and interventions taken, any patient or family teaching and their comprehension and progress, and the patient's tolerance of the treatment.

Supportive references

McConnell, E. "Providing Tracheostomy Care," *Nursing2002* 32(1):17, January 2002.

Schreiber, D. "Trach Care at Home," *RN* 64(7):43-46, July 2001.

Serra, A. "Tracheostomy Care," *Nursing Standard* 14(42):45-52, 54-55, July 2000.

Tamburri, L.M. "Care of the Patient with a Tracheostomy," *Orthopaedic Nursing* 19(2):49-60, March-April 2000.

7

Neurologic and sensory care

A neurologic examination provides a record of vital information regarding the patient's neurologic function. Its purpose is to determine the presence of nervous system dysfunction. A skilled examiner knows the proper technique for testing function and is familiar with the expected normal responses to testing. Effective neurologic care aims to preserve and restore optimal nervous system function. Precise nursing skills and meticulous attention to detail are indispensable to achieving effective care. It's also important that you're aware of the standards of care endorsed by the American Academy of Neurology **AAN**, the American Association of Neuroscience Nurses **AANN**, the American Association of Neurological Surgeons **AANS**, the American Heart Association **AHA**, the American Pain Society **APS**, the Infusion Nurses Society **INS**, and the National Institute of Neurological Disorders and Stroke **NINDS**. In addition to being supported by evidence-based **EB** data and fundamental principles of science **Science**, the best practices presented in this chapter are supported by guidelines of the Centers for Disease Control and Prevention **CDC**, the National Institutes of Health **NIH**, the Joint Commission on Accreditation of Healthcare Organizations **JCAHO**, and the tenets of the American Hospital Association's Patient Care Partnership **PCP**. For points on equipment, manufacturers **MFR** may recommend specific guidelines. Together, they'll provide you with the information necessary to care for patients with neurologic deficits or injury.

Neurologic assessment and examination

A neurologic physical examination may be conducted by the physician or by an advanced practice nurse. For nursing purposes, this examination is used to de-termine whether nervous system dysfunction is present and to determine the patient's responses to actual or potential health problems precipitated by the dysfunction. The neurologic examination is typically preceded by a physical examination and history. It should be conducted in a systematic, hierarchical approach from the highest level of function (cerebral cortex) to the lowest (reflexes) and should include a review of mental state, cranial nerve, motor and sensory systems, and cerebellar function and reflexes.

The first step in a neurologic examination is to assess neurologic vital signs, starting with the patient's level of consciousness and orientation level. Many patients with neurologic disorders experience changes in perception — from confusion to psychosis — from neurologic dysfunction. Unaddressed, such disorientation further impairs the patient's ability to participate in recovery. Recognizing this will help you intervene properly.

To record or track assessment findings, use special flowcharts or neurologic assessment forms. In common use at most health care facilities, these charts and forms separate and grade components of a neurologic assessment, assisting the nurse and other caregivers to quickly recognize changes in neurologic status and to plan subsequent patient care.

Respiratory assessment constitutes an important part of an overall neurologic assessment because patients with neurologic damage — especially those with traumatic brain or spinal cord injuries — are at considerable risk for respiratory complications. Such injuries may depress the respiratory control center and paralyze the muscles used for breathing. As a result, brain tissue, which is especially sensitive to blood oxygen levels, can quickly be damaged by inadequate oxygenation.

Thorough respiratory care goes hand in hand with neurologic care. Frequent position changes, chest physiotherapy, and tracheal suctioning are typical interventions. Additional techniques for preventing complications and promoting comfort include pain management and maintaining a quiet, stress-free environment.

Rehabilitation

Neurologic rehabilitation begins on admission and touches all aspects of daily care. Because neurologic impairment can alter every area of function, the patient's identity may change. Consequently, rehabilitation procedures must address the psychosocial and physiologic changes associated with the patient's condition — a task that requires enormous time and patience.

The success of rehabilitation efforts may hinge largely on a patient's ability to adapt to significant — even profound — changes. A few of the factors that influence this ability to adapt include the patient's age, the deficit itself, and available support systems. Another ingredient needed for effective rehabilitation is sensitive and skilled nursing care. Such care can dramatically improve the patient's prospects for positive adaptation and recovery.

Cerebrospinal fluid drains

Cerebrospinal fluid (CSF) drainage aims to reduce CSF pressure to the desired level and then to maintain it at that level. Fluid is withdrawn from the lateral ventricle (ventriculostomy). Ventricular drainage is used to reduce increased intracranial pressure (ICP). External CSF drainage is used most commonly to manage increased ICP and to facilitate spinal or cerebral dural healing after traumatic injury or surgery. In either case, CSF is drained by a catheter or a ventriculostomy tube in a sterile, closed drainage collection system.

Other therapeutic uses include ICP monitoring via the ventriculostomy, direct instillation of medications, contrast media, or air for diagnostic radiology, and aspiration of CSF for laboratory analysis.

To place the ventricular drain, the physician inserts a ventricular catheter through a burr hole in the patient's skull. Usually, this is done in the operating room, with the patient receiving a general anesthetic. (See *CSF drainage,* page 368.)

Equipment

Overbed table • sterile gloves • sterile cotton-tipped applicators • chlorhexidine solution • alcohol pads • sterile fenestrated drape • 3-ml syringe for local anesthetic • 25G ³/₄″ needle for injecting anesthetic • local anesthetic (usually 1% lidocaine [Xylocaine]) • 18G or 20G sterile spinal needle or Tuohy needle • #5 French whistle-tip catheter or ventriculostomy tube • external drainage set (includes drainage tubing and sterile collection bag) • suture material • 4″ × 4″ dressings • paper tape • lamp or another light source • I.V. pole • ventriculostomy tray and twist drill • sterile marker • sterile labels • optional: pain medication (such as an analgesic) and antiinfective agent (such as an antibiotic)

Preparation of equipment

● Open all equipment using sterile technique.
● Check all packaging for breaks in seals and for expiration dates.
● After the physician places the catheter, connect it to the external drainage system tubing.
● Secure connection points with tape or a connector.
● Place the collection system, including drip chamber and collection bag, on an I.V. pole.

Implementation

● Explain the procedure to the patient and his family. Consent should be obtained by the physician from the patient or a responsible family member and should be documented according to your facility's policy. **PCP**
● Perform a baseline neurologic assessment, including vital signs, *to help detect alterations or signs of deterioration.* **AANN**
● Wash your hands thoroughly. **CDC**

Inserting a ventricular drain

● Place the patient in a supine position.
● Place the equipment tray on the overbed table, and unwrap the tray. Label all medications, medication containers, and other solutions on and off the sterile field. **JCAHO**
● Adjust the height of the bed *so that the physician can perform the procedure comfortably.*
● Illuminate the area of the catheter insertion site.
● The physician will clean the insertion site and administer a local anesthetic. He'll put on sterile gloves and drape the insertion site.

CSF drainage

Cerebrospinal fluid (CSF) drainage aims to control intracranial pressure (ICP) during treatment for traumatic injury or other conditions that cause a rise in ICP. A ventricular drain using a closed drainage system is detailed below.

Ventricular drain

For a ventricular drain, the physician makes a burr hole in the patient's skull and inserts the catheter into the ventricle. The distal end of the catheter is connected to a closed drainage system.

Closed drainage system

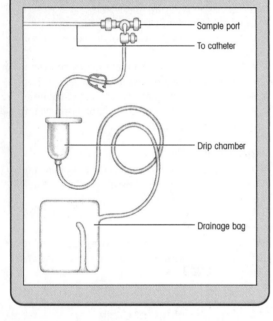

Sample port

To catheter

Drip chamber

Drainage bag

● To insert the drain, the physician will request a ventriculostomy tray with a twist drill. After completing the ventriculostomy, he'll connect the drainage system and suture the ventriculostomy in place. He'll then cover the insertion site with a sterile dressing.

Monitoring CSF drainage

● Maintain a continuous hourly output of CSF. Ensure that the flow chamber of the ICP monitoring set-up remains positioned as ordered. **AANN** **NIH**
● To drain CSF as ordered, put on sterile gloves, and then turn the main stopcock on to drainage. *This al-*

lows CSF to collect in the graduated flow chamber. Document the time and the amount of CSF obtained. Turn the stopcock off to drainage. To drain the CSF from this chamber into the drainage bag, release the clamp below the flow chamber. *Never empty the drainage bag. Instead, replace it when full using sterile technique.* **AANN** **CDC** **NIH**
● Check the dressing frequently for drainage, *which could indicate CSF leakage.* **AANN** **NIH**
● Check the tubing for patency by watching the CSF drops in the drip chamber.
● Observe CSF for color, clarity, amount, blood, and sediment. CSF specimens for laboratory analysis should be obtained from the collection port attached to the tubing, not from the collection bag.
● Change the collection bag when it's full or every 24 hours, according to your facility's policy. **AANN**

Special considerations

● Maintenance of a continual hourly output of CSF is essential *to prevent overdrainage or underdrainage.* Underdrainage or lack of CSF may reflect kinked tubing, catheter displacement, or a drip chamber placed higher than the catheter insertion site. Overdrainage can occur if the drip chamber is placed too far below the catheter insertion site.
● Raising or lowering the head of the bed can affect the CSF flow rate. When changing the patient's position, reset the system to zero. **AANN**
● If the patient is ambulatory or is allowed out of bed, advise him that he must call for assistance before getting out of bed. *The drain must be closed before getting the patient out of bed.*
● The patient may experience chronic headache during continuous CSF drainage. Reassure him that this isn't unusual; administer analgesics as appropriate. **AANN**
● For ventricular drains, make sure ICP waveforms are being monitored at all times. **AANN**

Nursing diagnoses

● Decreased intracranial adaptive capacity
● Risk for infection

Expected outcomes

The patient will:
● maintain ICP within normal limits
● show no evidence of neurologic compromise
● remain free from infection.

Treatment and adverse effects of ICP control

Listed below are the common medications and nursing interventions used to decrease elevated (greater than 20 mm Hg) intracranial pressure (ICP) and the adverse effects of each treatment.

Treatment	Application	Adverse effects
Barbiturates	To induce barbiturate coma as a last resort	Hypotension, loss of neurologic examination, cardiac abnormalities
Hyperventilation	To reduce carbon dioxide and dilate cerebral vasculature to lower ICP	Reduced cerebral blood flow and oxygenation
Hypothermia	To possibly benefit moderately severe head injuries	Cardiac suppression, renal dysfunction
Mannitol (Osmitrol)	To reduce acute ICP elevation; given as an I.V. bolus	Dehydration, renal failure
Neuromuscular paralysis	To reduce activity that could elevate ICP; given in conjunction with sedatives	Respiratory compromise
Sedation	To reduce elevated breakthrough ICP in conjunction with paralysis	Hypotension

Complications

● Signs of excessive CSF drainage include headache, tachycardia, diaphoresis, and nausea.
● Acute overdrainage may result in collapsed ventricles, tonsillar herniation, and medullary compression.

ALERT *If drainage accumulates too rapidly, clamp the system and immediately notify the physician because this constitutes a potential neurosurgical emergency.*

● Cessation of drainage may indicate clot formation. If you can't quickly identify the cause of the obstruction, notify the physician. If drainage is blocked, the patient may develop signs of increased ICP.
● Infection may cause meningitis. To prevent this, administer antibiotics as ordered.

Documentation

Record the time and date of the insertion procedure and the patient's response. Record routine vital signs and neurologic assessment findings at least every 4 hours.

Document the color, clarity, and amount of CSF at least every 8 hours. Record hourly and 24-hour CSF output, and describe the condition of the dressing.

Supportive references

American Association of Neuroscience Nurses. *Core Curriculum for Neuroscience Nursing,* 4th ed. Philadelphia: W.B. Saunders Co., 2004.

Barker, E. *Neuroscience Nursing,* 2nd ed. St. Louis: Mosby–Year Book, Inc., 2002.

Hickey, J.V. *The Clinical Practice of Neurological and Neurosurgical Nursing,* 5th ed. Philadelphia: Lippincott Williams & Wilkins, 2003.

Lynn-McHale Wiegand, D.J., and Carlson, K.K. (eds.) *AACN Procedure Manual for Critical Care,* 5th ed. Philadelphia: W.B. Saunders Co., 2005.

Intracranial pressure monitoring

Intracranial pressure (ICP) monitoring measures pressure exerted by the brain, blood, and cerebrospinal fluid (CSF) against the inside of the skull. Normal ICP is 0 to 15 mm Hg, with the ICP threshold of 20 to 25 mm Hg as the highest acceptable limit before instituting treatment. **AANS** Indications for monitoring ICP include head trauma with bleeding or edema, overproduction or insufficient absorption of CSF, cerebral hemorrhage, and space-occupying brain lesions. ICP monitoring can detect elevated ICP early,

Understanding ICP monitoring

Intracranial pressure (ICP) can be monitored using one of four systems.

Intraventricular catheter monitoring

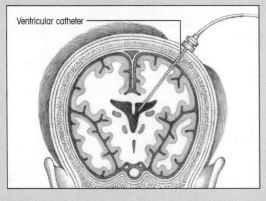

Ventricular catheter

Subarachnoid bolt monitoring

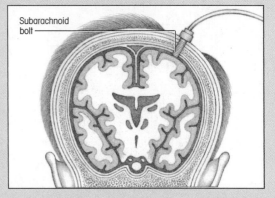

Subarachnoid bolt

In intraventricular catheter monitoring, which monitors ICP directly, the physician inserts a small polyethylene or silicone rubber catheter into the lateral ventricle through a burr hole.

Although this method measures ICP most accurately, it carries the greatest risk of infection. This is the only type of ICP monitoring that allows evaluation of brain compliance and drainage of significant amounts of cerebrospinal fluid (CSF).

Contraindications usually include stenotic cerebral ventricles, cerebral aneurysms in the path of catheter placement, and suspected vascular lesions.

Subarachnoid bolt monitoring involves insertion of a special bolt into the subarachnoid space through a twist-drill burr hole that's positioned in the front of the skull behind the hairline.

Placing the bolt is easier than placing an intraventricular catheter, especially if a computed tomography scan reveals that the cerebrum has shifted or the ventricles have collapsed. This type of ICP monitoring also carries less risk of infection and parenchymal damage because the bolt doesn't penetrate the cerebrum.

---

before clinical danger signs develop. Prompt intervention can then help avert or diminish neurologic damage caused by cerebral hypoxia and shifts of brain mass. (See *Treatment and adverse effects of ICP control,* page 369.)

The four basic ICP monitoring systems are intraventricular catheter, subarachnoid bolt, epidural sensor, and intraparenchymal pressure monitoring. (See *Understanding ICP monitoring.*)

Regardless of which system is used, the procedure is typically performed by a neurosurgeon in the operating room, emergency department, or intensive care unit. Insertion of an ICP monitoring device requires sterile technique to reduce the risk of central nervous system (CNS) infection. Setting up equipment for the monitoring systems also requires strict asepsis. **AANN AANS**

Equipment

Monitoring unit and transducers as ordered • 16 to 20 sterile 4″ × 4″ gauze pads • linen-saver pads • shave preparation tray or hair scissors • sterile drapes • chlorhexidine solution • sterile gown • surgical mask • sterile gloves • head dressing supplies (two rolls of 4″ elastic gauze dressing, one roll of 4″ roller gauze, adhesive tape) • sterile marker • sterile labels • optional: suction apparatus, I.V. pole, and yardstick

Preparation of equipment

● Monitoring units and setup protocols are varied and complex and differ among health care facilities. Check your facility's guidelines for your particular unit.

● Various types of preassembled ICP monitoring units are available, each with its own setup protocols.

Epidural or subdural sensor monitoring

Intraparenchymal monitoring

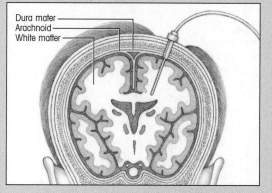

Epidural sensor

Dura mater
Arachnoid
White matter

ICP can also be monitored from the epidural or subdural space. For epidural monitoring, a fiber-optic sensor is inserted into the epidural space through a burr hole. This system's main drawback is its questionable accuracy because ICP isn't being measured directly from a CSF-filled space.

For subdural monitoring, a fiber-optic transducer-tipped catheter is tunneled through a burr hole, and its tip is placed on brain tissue under the dura mater. The main drawback to this method is its inability to drain CSF.

In intraparenchymal monitoring, the physician inserts a catheter through a small subarachnoid bolt and, after puncturing the dura, advances the catheter a few centimeters into the brain's white matter. There's no need to balance or calibrate the equipment after insertion.

Although this method doesn't provide direct access to CSF, measurements are accurate because brain tissue pressure correlates well with ventricular pressures. Intraparenchymal monitoring may be used to obtain ICP measurements in patients with compressed or dislocated ventricles.

These units are designed to reduce the risk of infection by eliminating the need for multiple stopcocks, manometers, and transducer dome assemblies. Some facilities use units that have miniaturized transducers rather than transducer domes.

Implementation

● Explain the procedure to the patient or his family. Make sure the patient or a responsible family member has signed a consent form. **PCP**
● Determine whether the patient is allergic to iodine preparations.
● Provide privacy if the procedure is being done in an open emergency department or intensive care unit. **PCP**
● Wash your hands. **CDC**

● Obtain baseline routine and neurologic vital signs *to aid in prompt detection of decompensation during the procedure.* **AANN**
● Place the patient in the supine position, and elevate the head of the bed 30 degrees (or as ordered). **AANN**
● Place linen-saver pads under the patient's head. Clip his hair at the insertion site, as indicated by the physician, *to decrease the risk of infection.* Carefully fold and remove the linen-saver pads *to avoid spilling loose hair onto the bed.* Drape the patient with sterile drapes. Scrub the insertion site for 2 minutes with chlorhexidine solution. **CDC**
● The physician puts on the sterile gown, mask, and sterile gloves. He then opens the interior wrap of the sterile supply tray and proceeds with insertion of the catheter or bolt. Label all medications, medication

Setting up an ICP monitoring system

To set up an intracranial pressure (ICP) monitoring system, follow these steps, using strict sterile technique. **CDC**

- Begin by opening a sterile towel. On the sterile field, place a 20-ml luer-lock syringe, an 18G needle, a 250-ml bag filled with normal saline solution (with outer wrapper removed), and a disposable transducer.
- Put on sterile gloves and gown, and fill the 20-ml syringe with normal saline solution from the I.V. bag. **CDC**
- Remove the injection cap from the patient line and attach the syringe. Turn the system stopcock off to the short end of the patient line, and flush through to the drip chamber (as shown). Allow a few drops to flow through the flow chamber (the manometer), the tubing, and the one-way valve into the drainage bag. (Fill the tubing and the manometer slowly to minimize air bubbles. If any air bubbles surface, be sure to force them from the system.)

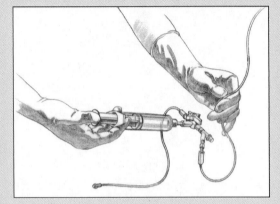

- Attach the manometer to the I.V. pole at the head of the bed.
- Slide the drip chamber onto the manometer, and align the chamber to the zero point (as shown).
- Next, connect the transducer to the monitor.
- Put on a clean pair of sterile gloves. **CDC**
- Keeping one hand sterile, turn the patient stopcock off to the patient.

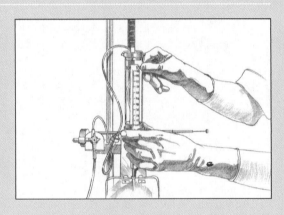

containers, and other solutions on and off the sterile field. **JCAHO**

- *To facilitate placement of the device,* hold the patient's head in your hands or attach a long strip of 4" roller gauze to one side rail, and bring it across the patient's forehead to the opposite rail. Reassure the conscious patient *to help ease his anxiety.* Talk to him frequently *to assess his level of consciousness (LOC) and detect signs of deterioration.* Watch for cardiac arrhythmias and abnormal respiratory patterns.
- After insertion, put on sterile gloves and apply chlorhexidine solution and a sterile dressing to the site. If not done by the physician, connect the catheter to the appropriate monitoring device, depending on the system used. **CDC** (See *Setting up an ICP monitoring system.*)

- If the physician has set up a ventriculostomy drainage system, attach the drip chamber to the headboard or bedside I.V. pole as ordered.
- Inspect the insertion site at least every 24 hours (or according to your facility's policy) for redness, swelling, and drainage. Clean the site, reapply chlorhexidine solution, and apply a fresh sterile dressing.
- Assess the patient's clinical status, and take routine and neurologic vital signs every hour, or as ordered.

● Align the zero point with the center line of the patient's head, level with the middle of the ear (as shown).
● Lower the flow chamber to zero, and turn the stopcock off to the dead-end cap. With a clean hand, balance the system according to monitor guidelines.

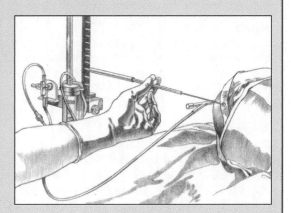

● Turn the system stopcock off to drainage, and raise the flow chamber to the ordered height (as shown).
● Return the stopcock to the ordered position, and observe the monitor for the return of ICP patterns.

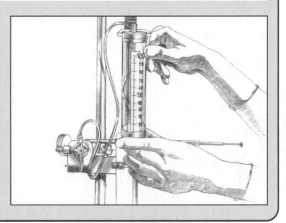

Make sure you've obtained orders for waveforms and pressure parameters from the physician.
● Calculate cerebral perfusion pressure (CPP) hourly; use the equation: CPP = MAP − ICP (MAP refers to *mean arterial pressure*).
● Observe digital ICP readings and waves. Remember, *the pattern of readings is more significant than any single reading.* (See *Interpreting ICP waveforms,* page 374.) If you observe continually elevated ICP readings, note how long they're sustained. If they last several minutes, notify the physician immediately. Finally, record and describe any CSF drainage.

Special considerations

ALERT *In infants, ICP monitoring can be performed without penetrating the scalp. In this external method, a photoelectric transducer with a pressure-sensitive membrane is taped to the anterior fontanel. The transducer responds to pressure at the site and transmits readings to a bedside monitor and recording system. The external method is restricted to infants because pressure readings can be obtained only at fontanels, the incompletely ossified areas of the skull.*
● Osmotic diuretic agents such as mannitol (Osmitrol) reduce cerebral edema by shrinking intracra-

Interpreting ICP waveforms

Three waveforms — A, B, and C — are used to monitor intracranial pressure (ICP). A (plateau) waves are an ominous sign of intracranial decompensation and poor compliance. B waves correlate with changes in respiration, and C waves correlate with changes in arterial pressure.

Normal waveform

A normal ICP waveform typically shows a steep upward systolic slope followed by a downward diastolic slope with a dicrotic notch. In most cases, this waveform occurs continuously and indicates an ICP between 0 and 15 mm Hg — normal pressure.

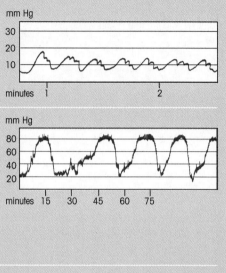

A waves

The most clinically significant ICP waveforms are A waves (shown at right), which may reach elevations of 50 to 100 mm Hg, persist for 5 to 20 minutes, then drop sharply — signaling exhaustion of the brain's compliance mechanisms. A waves may come and go, spiking from temporary rises in thoracic pressure or from any condition that increases ICP beyond the brain's compliance limits. Activities, such as sustained coughing or straining during defecation, can cause temporary elevations in thoracic pressure.

B waves

B waves, which appear sharp and rhythmic with a sawtooth pattern, occur every 1½ to 2 minutes and may reach elevations of 50 mm Hg. The clinical significance of B waves isn't clear, but the waves correlate with respiratory changes and may occur more frequently with decreasing compensation. Because B waves sometimes precede A waves, notify the physician if B waves occur frequently.

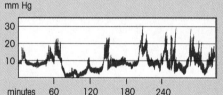

C waves

Like B waves, C waves are rapid and rhythmic, but they aren't as sharp. Clinically insignificant, they may fluctuate with respirations or systemic blood pressure changes.

Waveform showing equipment problem

A waveform that looks like the one shown at right signals a problem with the transducer or monitor. Check for line obstruction, and determine if the transducer needs rebalancing.

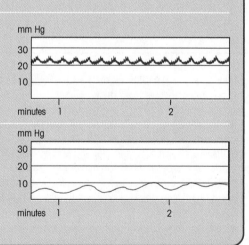

Managing increased ICP

By performing nursing care gently, slowly, and cautiously, you can best help manage — or even significantly reduce — increased intracranial pressure (ICP). If possible, urge your patient to participate in his own care. Here are some steps you can take to manage increased ICP.

- Plan your care to include rest periods between activities. This allows the patient's ICP to return to baseline, thus avoiding lengthy and cumulative pressure elevations.
- Speak to the patient before attempting any procedures, even if he appears comatose. Touch him on an arm or leg first before touching him in a more personal area, such as the face or chest. This is especially important if the patient doesn't know you or if he's confused or sedated.
- Suction the patient 10 seconds or less and only when needed to remove secretions and maintain airway patency. Avoid depriving him of oxygen for long periods while suctioning; always hyperventilate the patient with oxygen before and after the procedure. Monitor his heart rate while suctioning. If multiple catheter passes are needed to clear secretions, hyperventilate the patient between them to bring ICP as close to baseline as possible.
- To promote venous drainage, keep the patient's head in the midline position, even when he's positioned on his side. Avoid flexing the neck or hip more than 90 degrees, and keep the head of the bed elevated 30 to 45 degrees.

- To avoid increasing intrathoracic pressure, which raises ICP, discourage Valsalva's maneuver and isometric muscle contractions. To avoid isometric contractions, distract the patient when giving him painful injections (by asking him to wiggle his toes and by massaging the area before injection to relax the muscle) and have him concentrate on breathing through difficult procedures such as bed-to-stretcher transfers. To keep the patient from holding his breath when moving around in bed, tell him to relax as much as possible during position changes. If necessary, administer a stool softener to help prevent constipation and unnecessary straining during defecation.
- If the patient is heavily sedated, monitor his respiratory rate and blood gas levels. Depressed respirations will compromise ventilations and oxygen exchange. Maintaining adequate respiratory rate and volume helps reduce ICP.
- If you're in a specialty unit, you may be able to routinely hyperventilate the patient to counter sustained ICP elevations. This procedure is one of the best ways to reduce high ICP at bedside for short periods. Consult your facility's protocol.

---

nial contents. Given by I.V. drip or bolus, mannitol draws water from tissues into plasma; it doesn't cross the blood-brain barrier. Monitor serum electrolyte levels and osmolality readings closely *because the patient may become dehydrated very quickly.* Be aware that a rebound increase in ICP may occur. (See *Managing increased ICP.*) **Science**

- To avoid rebound increased ICP, 50 ml of albumin may be given with the mannitol bolus. Note, however, that you'll see a residual rise in ICP before it decreases. If your patient has heart failure or severe renal dysfunction, monitor for problems in adapting to the increased intravascular volumes.
- Fluid restriction, usually 1,200 to 1,500 ml/day, prevents cerebral edema from developing or worsening.
- Barbiturate-induced coma depresses the reticular activating system and reduces the brain's metabolic demand. Reduced demand for oxygen and energy reduces cerebral blood flow, thereby lowering ICP. **EB** **Science**

- Hyperventilation with oxygen from a handheld resuscitation bag or ventilator helps rid the patient of excess carbon dioxide, thereby constricting cerebral vessels and reducing cerebral blood volume and ICP. However, only normal brain tissues respond because blood vessels in damaged areas have reduced vasoconstrictive ability. **Science**

ALERT *Hyperventilation with a handheld resuscitation bag or a ventilator should be performed with care because hyperventilation can cause ischemia.*

- Before tracheal suctioning, hyperventilate the patient with 100% oxygen as ordered. Apply suction for a maximum of 10 seconds. Avoid inducing hypoxia *because this condition greatly increases cerebral blood flow.* **AANN**

● Because fever raises brain metabolism, which increases cerebral blood flow, fever reduction (achieved by administering acetaminophen [Tylenol], sponge baths, or a hypothermia blanket) also helps to reduce ICP. However, *rebound increases in ICP and brain edema may occur if rapid rewarming takes place after hypothermia or if cooling measures induce shivering.*

● Withdrawal of CSF through the drainage system reduces CSF volume and thus reduces ICP. Although less commonly used, surgical removal of a skull-bone flap provides room for the swollen brain to expand. If this procedure is performed, keep the site clean and dry *to prevent infection* and maintain sterile technique when changing the dressing. **AANN**

Nursing diagnoses

● Decreased intracranial adaptive capacity
● Risk for infection

Expected outcomes

The patient will:
● maintain ICP within normal limits
● show no evidence of neurologic compromise
● remain free from infection.

Complications

● CNS infection, the most common hazard of ICP monitoring, can result from contamination of the equipment setup or of the insertion site.

ALERT *Be especially cautious when positioning the ventriculostomy; if the drip chamber is too high, it may raise ICP; if it's too low, it may cause excessive CSF drainage. Such loss can rapidly decompress the cranial contents and damage bridging cortical veins, leading to hematoma formation. Decompression can also lead to rupture of existing hematomas or aneurysms, causing hemorrhage.*

● Watch for signs of impending or overt decompensation: pupillary dilation (unilateral or bilateral), decreased pupillary response to light, decreasing LOC, rising systolic blood pressure and widening pulse pressure, bradycardia, slowed, irregular respirations and, in late decompensation, decerebrate posturing.

Documentation

Record the time and date of the insertion procedure and the patient's response. Note the insertion site and the type of monitoring system used. Record ICP digital readings and waveforms and CPP hourly in your notes, on a flowchart, or directly on readout strips, depending on your facility's policy. Document any factors that may affect ICP (for example, drug therapy, stressful procedures, or sleep).

Record routine and neurologic vital signs hourly, and describe the patient's clinical status. Note the amount, character, and frequency of any CSF drainage (for example, "between 6 p.m. and 7 p.m., 15 ml of blood-tinged CSF"). Record the ICP reading in response to drainage.

Supportive references

American Association of Neuroscience Nurses. *Core Curriculum for Neuroscience Nursing,* 4th ed. Philadelphia: W.B. Saunders Co., 2004.

Barker, E. *Neuroscience Nursing,* 2nd ed. St. Louis: Mosby–Year Book, Inc., 2002.

Hickey, J.V. *The Clinical Practice of Neurological and Neurosurgical Nursing,* 5th ed. Philadelphia: Lippincott Williams & Wilkins, 2003.

Kirkness, C.J., et al. "Intracranial Pressure Waveform Analysis: Clinical and Research Implications," *Journal of Neuroscience Nursing* 32(5):271-77, October 2000.

Lynn-McHale Wiegand, D.J., and Carlson, K.K. (eds.) *AACN Procedure Manual for Critical Care,* 5th ed. Philadelphia: W.B. Saunders Co., 2005.

March, K. "Intracranial Pressure Monitoring and Assessing Intracranial Compliance in Brain Injury," *Critical Care Nursing Clinics of North America* 12(4):429-35, December 2000.

Morton, P.G., et al. *Critical Care Nursing: A Holistic Aproach,* 8th ed. Philadelphia: Lippincott Williams & Wilkins, 2005. **EB**

Jugular venous oxygen saturation monitoring

Jugular venous oxygen saturation ($SjvO_2$) monitoring measures the venous oxygenation saturation of blood as it leaves the brain. It reflects the oxygen saturation of blood after cerebral perfusion has taken place. After comparing $SjvO_2$ with the arterial venous oxygenation, you can determine if blood flow to the brain matches the brain's metabolic demand.

$SjvO_2$ monitoring is often used with other types of cerebral hemodynamic monitoring, such as intracranial pressure (ICP) monitoring, to provide better information about pressure and perfusion during treatment. Treatment regimens can be titrated to enhance pressure and perfusion.

The normal range for $SjvO_2$ is 55% to 70%. Values higher than 70% indicate hyperperfusion. Values between 40% and 54% indicate relative hypoperfusion. Values lower than 40% indicate ischemia.

Data from monitoring can also be used to calculate cerebral extraction of oxygen (CeO_2 = oxygen saturation in arterial blood [SaO_2] − $SjvO_2$), cerebral arterial oxygen content (CaO_2 = 1.34 × hemoglobin [Hb] × SaO_2 − 0.0031 × partial pressure of arterial oxygen [PaO_2]), the global cerebral content saturation ($CjvO_2$ = 1.34 × Hb × $SjvO_2$ + 0.0031 × $PjvO_2$), arteriovenous jugular oxygen content ($AVjDO_2$ = CaO_2 − $CjvO_2$), which help determine cerebral oxygen use, metabolic demand, and adequacy of oxygen delivery.

Monitoring of $SjvO_2$ allows the nurse to maximize the balance between cerebral perfusion, oxygenation, and metabolism. Criteria for $SjvO_2$ monitoring include any neurologic injury where ischemia is a threat and may include intra-operative monitoring, subarachnoid hemorrhage, and post-acute head injury with increased ICP.

Equipment
Insertion of $SjvO_2$ monitor
Sterile towels • sterile drapes • surgical caps • gowns • sterile gloves • masks • chlorhexidine scrub • chlorhexidine solution • central venous catheter (CVC) insertion kit • 1% or 2% lidocaine without epinephrine (Xylocaine) • 5- or 10-cc syringe, with an 18G and 23G needle • 5 French percutaneous introducer • 4 French fiber-optic $SjvO_2$ catheter • oximetric monitor with cable • 500 cc normal saline solution (heparinized or nonheparinized based on facility policy) • pressure tubing with continuous flush device • pressure bag or device • sterile occlusive dressing • sterile marker • sterile labels

Removal of $SjvO_2$ monitor
Sterile gloves • suture removal set • sterile hemostat • sterile scissors • chlorhexidine solution • sterile occlusive dressing

Implementation
● Explain the procedure to the patient and provide privacy. **PCP**

● Wash your hands and put on sterile gloves. **CDC**
● Using aseptic technique, prime the pressure tubing system, removing all air bubbles and maintaining sterility of the system for insertion. **MFR**
● Position the patient with the head elevated at 30 to 45 degrees and the neck in a neutral position. Document baseline intracranial pressure (ICP).
● Turn the head laterally, away from the site chosen for catheter insertion. Note and document any change in ICP.
● Follow facility guidelines for the dressing procedure for insertion of central lines.
● Put on new sterile gloves. Using sterile technique, open and prepare the CVC insertion kit, and add a 5 French sterile introducer and a 4 French fiber-optic $SjvO_2$ catheter. Label all medications, medication containers, and other solutions on and off the sterile field. **JCAHO**
● Scrub the insertion site with chlorhexidine scrub solution. **CDC**
● Position the sterile drapes over the upper thorax and neck, exposing only the insertion site.
● Assist the physician during insertion, as needed.
● Monitor neurologic status, vital signs, ICP, and pain during insertion.
● After the line is in place, attach the pressure tubing and confirm patency of both jugular catheter lumens by aspirating and flushing.
● Obtain a lateral cervical spine or lateral skull X-tray *to confirm catheter placement at the level of the jugular bulb.*

 ALERT *Optimum placement of the $SvjO_2$ catheter tip is at the level of the jugular bulb of the internal jugular vein. The tip of the catheter should be viewed at the upper border of the second cervical vertebra.*

Draw a jugular venous blood gas sample and perform in vivo calibration according to the manufacturer's guidelines. **MFR**

ALERT *In vivo calibration is necessary to ensure reliability of the data.*

Monitoring and care
● Assess neurologic status, vital signs, and ICP immediately after insertion.

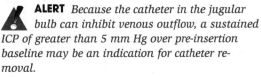 **ALERT** *Because the catheter in the jugular bulb can inhibit venous outflow, a sustained ICP of greater than 5 mm Hg over pre-insertion baseline may be an indication for catheter removal.*

- Record baseline parameters for continuously monitored $SjvO_2$. Calculate $AvjDO_2$, CeO_2, and global cerebral oxygen extraction ratio (O_2ER) as a baseline.

ALERT *Repeated patterns of desaturation are reliable indicators of poor outcomes in patients with severe head injury.*

- Continuously monitor $SjvO_2$.
- Verify the accuracy of the reading by drawing $SjvO_2$ every 8 to 12 hours. The blood sample reading should be within 4% of the reading shown on the monitor.
- Record $SjvO_2$ and ICP values hourly and note trends. Assess ICP in relation to $SjvO_2$. Notify the physician of any deviation from the trend.
- Calculate CeO_2 and O_2ER as indicated.
- Maintain a safe environment during monitoring *to prevent accidental dislodgment of the catheter.*
- Use sedation of analgesia as indicated to maintain the monitor and enhance cerebral perfusion pressure (CPP).
- Perform in vivo calibration with jugular blood gas sample as recommended by the monitor manufacturer (usually performed each shift).
- Change the dressing using aseptic technique if it becomes soiled or loosened, or as indicated by facility policy for central line redressing.
- Change the I.V. solution and tubing for the catheter according to facility policy. **INS**
- Replace an $SjvO_2$ catheter with low light intensity. Check the fiber-optic catheter for obstruction and occlusion. Aspirate the catheter until blood can be freely sampled and normal light intensity is displayed. If you can't aspirate a blood sample, the catheter needs to be replaced.

ALERT *Low light intensity may indicate catheter occlusion or drainage to the fiber-optics.* **EB**

For an $SjvO_2$ catheter with low light intensity, adjust the patient's head to ensure neutral neck position.

ALERT *High light intensity indicates vessel wall artifact, which is usually encountered during repositioning of the patient.* **EB**

To prevent catheter coiling, identify rhythmic fluctuations in $SjvO_2$ trends. Obtain a lateral cervical spine or lateral skull X-ray to assess the position of the catheter in the external jugular vein (compare to the X-ray done on insertion). If coiling is confirmed, consider replacing the catheter. **EB**

ALERT *Rhythmic fluctuation of trends that are unrelated to changes in ICP, CPP, or systemic blood pressure signify coiling of the catheter.* **EB**

- Identify $SjvO_2$ desaturations and notify the physician. (See *Common causes of desaturation.*)
- Assess for a change in ICP. In patients with brain injury, increased ICP is a frequent cause of desaturation.

ALERT *Desaturations are emergencies that require immediate interventions to restore cerebral blood flow and oxygen delivery.*

- Confirm the $SjvO_2$ data by obtaining a jugular venous blood gas sample.
- Perform in vivo calibration.

ALERT *Significant change in readings following sampling can signify errors related to aspiration of blood. Avoid errors by aspirating blood slowly during the sampling procedure (1 ml per minute).*

Removing $SjvO_2$ monitor

- Explain the procedure to the patient and provide privacy. **PCP**
- Wash your hands and prepare the equipment. **CDC**
- Inactivate alarms.
- Turn stopcocks off, position the patient properly, monitor vital signs, put on sterile gloves, and assist the physician with catheter removal as needed.
- Apply direct pressure to the site until there are no signs of active bleeding.
- Put on new sterile gloves. Apply chlorhexidine solution and the sterile occlusive dressing to the catheter site. **CDC**
- Assess the site for signs of bleeding every 15 minutes for 1 hour, then every 30 minutes for 1 hour, and then 1 hour later.

Nursing diagnoses

- Risk for infection
- Risk for injury

Expected outcomes

The patient will:
- remain free from infection
- remain free from injury.

Common causes of desaturation

Causes	Interventions
Anemia (hemoglobin less than 90 g/L)	• Report abnormal results to the physician, and administer a blood transfusion, if ordered.
Increased intracranial pressure (over 20 mm Hg)	• Elevate the head of the bed 30 degrees, decrease external stimuli, administer prescribed osmotic diuretics such as mannitol, and adjust ventilator settings to produce mild hyperventilation (partial pressure of arterial carbon dioxide 30 to 35 mm Hg), as ordered. Other measures may include drainage of cerebrospinal fluid and methods to reduce cerebral oxygen demand, such as sedation, neuromuscular blockade, or barbiturate coma.
Systemic hypotension (mean blood pressure less than 70 mm Hg)	• Report abnormal results to the physician, and administer a fluid challenge or vasopressors, if ordered.
Systemic hypoxemia (one of the most common causes of cerebral hypoxia)	• If the oxygen saturation is less than 90%, increase the oxygen percentage or fraction of inspired oxygen and adjust the ventilator settings, as ordered.

Complications

• Complications associated with $SjvO_2$ monitoring are similar to complications that can occur with any central line. The most common is sepsis.
• Pneumothorax, carotid artery puncture, internal jugular thrombosis, and excessive bleeding are all risk with catheter placement.
• In rare instances, the catheter also can cause impaired cerebral venous drainage and increased ICP.

Documentation

Document difficulties encountered during insertion, depth (in centimeters) of the catheter, patient tolerance of the procedure, and the ICP reading during insertion. Record the baseline $SjvO_2$ reading and the initial CeO_2 and $AvjDO_2$ calculations.

Record $SjvO_2$ and ICP hourly. Record CeO_2, $AvjDO_2$, and O_2ER when indicated. Document your assessment of the insertion site, expected and unexpected outcomes, interventions taken, and patient and family education provided.

Supportive references

American Association of Neuroscience Nurses. *Core Curriculum for Neuroscience Nursing,* 4th ed. Philadelphia: W.B. Saunders Co., 2004.

Barker, E. Neuroscience Nursing, 2nd ed. St. Louis: Mosby–Year Book, Inc., 2002.

Hickey, J.V. *The Clinical Practice of Neurological and Neurosurgical Nursing,* 5th ed. Philadelphia: Lippincott Williams & Wilkins, 2003.

Lynn-McHale Wiegand, D.J., and Carlson, K.K. (eds.) *AACN Procedure Manual for Critical Care,* 5th ed. Philadelphia: W.B. Saunders Co., 2005. **EB**

Ricci, M., et al. "Near-infrared Spectroscopy to Monitor Cerebral Oxygen Saturation in Single-ventricle Physiology," *Journal of Thoracic and Cardiovascular Surgery* 131(2):395-402, February 2006.

Neurologic assessment

Neurologic assessment supplements the routine measurement of temperature, pulse rate, and respirations by evaluating the patient's level of consciousness (LOC), pupillary activity, and orientation to time, place, and person. These findings provide a simple,

Using the Glasgow Coma Scale

The Glasgow Coma Scale provides a standard reference for assessing or monitoring level of consciousness in a patient with a suspected or confirmed brain injury. This scale measures three responses to stimuli — eye opening, motor response, and verbal response — and assigns a number to each of the possible responses within these categories.

A score of 3 is the lowest possible score, reflecting that the patient is in a deep coma; 15 is the highest score, indicating that the patient is fully intact. A score of 7 or less indicates coma. This scale is commonly used in the emergency department, at the scene of an accident, and for evaluation of the hospitalized patient.

Characteristic	Response and score
Eye opening	• Spontaneous — 4 • To verbal command — 3 • To pain — 2 • Doesn't open eyes to painful stimuli — 1

Best motor response	• Obeys commands — 6
	• To painful stimuli
	  – Localizes pain; pushes stimulus away — 5
	  – Flexes and withdraws — 4
	  – Abnormal flexion — 3
	  – Abnormal extension response — 2
	  – No motor response — 1

Best verbal response (Arouse patient with painful stimuli if necessary.)	• Oriented and converses — 5 • Disoriented and converses — 4 • Uses inappropriate words — 3 • Makes incomprehensible sounds — 2 • No verbal response — 1
	Total: 3 to 15

indispensable tool for quickly checking the patient's neurologic status.

If the patient's condition and circumstances of admission allow, the first neurologic assessment should occur at the time of admission *to establish a baseline.* The frequency and extent of the neurologic assessment will depend on the stability of the patient and the underlying condition. For a stable patient who's doing well, an assessment may be ordered every 4 to 8 hours. For an unstable patient, it may be ordered as frequently as every 5 minutes *to monitor changes and the need for intervention.*

LOC, a measure of environmental awareness and self-awareness, reflects cortical function and usually provides the first sign of central nervous system deterioration. Changes in pupillary activity (pupil size, shape, equality, and response to light) may signal increased intracranial pressure (ICP) associated with a space-occupying lesion. Evaluating muscle strength and tone, reflexes, and posture may also help identify nervous system damage.

Finally, changes in vital signs alone don't indicate possible neurologic compromise. Alterations in LOC or papillary changes are the early signs that indicate neurologic problems. Therefore, any changes in vital signs should be evaluated in light of a complete neurologic assessment. Because vital signs are controlled at the medullary level, changes noted after the deterioration of neurologic status are too late and irreversible neurologic damage should be suspected.

Equipment

Penlight • thermometer • sterile cotton ball or cotton-tipped applicator • stethoscope • sphygmomanometer • pupil size chart • pencil or pen

Implementation

• Confirm the patient's identity using two patient identifiers according to facility policy. **JCAHO**
• Explain the procedure to the patient, even if he's unresponsive. **PCP**
• Wash your hands and provide privacy. **CDC**

Assessing LOC and orientation **AAN** **AANN**

• Assess the patient's LOC by evaluating his responses. Use standard methods such as the Glasgow Coma Scale and the Rancho Los Amigos Cognitive Scale. (See *Using the Glasgow Coma Scale,* and *Using the Rancho Los Amigos Cognitive Scale.*)
• Begin by measuring the patient's response to verbal, light tactile (touch), or painful (nail bed pressure) stimuli, or if there's no response to stimuli. First, ask the patient his full name. If he responds appropriately, assess his orientation to time, place, and person. Ask him where he is, and then what day, season, and year it is. (Expect disorientation to affect the

Using the Rancho Los Amigos Cognitive Scale

Widely used to classify brain-injured patients according to their behavior, the Rancho Los Amigos Cognitive Scale describes the phases of recovery — from coma to dependent functioning — on a scale of I (unresponsive) to VIII (purposeful, appropriate, alert, and oriented). This chart is useful when assessing patients with posttraumatic amnesia.

Level	Response	Characteristics
I	None	The patient is unresponsive to any stimulus.
II	Generalized	The patient makes limited, inconsistent, nonpurposeful responses, typically to pain only.
III	Localized	The patient can localize and withdraw from painful stimuli, can make purposeful responses and focus on presented objects, and may follow simple commands, but inconsistently and in a delayed manner.
IV	Confused and agitated	The patient is alert but agitated, confused, disoriented, and aggressive. He can't perform self-care and has no awareness of present events. Bizarre behavior is likely; agitation appears related to internal confusion.
V	Confused and inappropriate	The patient is alert and responds to commands but is easily distracted and can't concentrate on tasks or learn new information. He becomes agitated in response to external stimuli, and his behavior and speech are inappropriate. His memory is severely impaired and he can't carry over learning from one situation to another.
VI	Confused and appropriate	The patient has some awareness of himself and others but is inconsistently oriented. He can follow simple directions consistently with cueing and can relearn some old skills, such as activities of daily living, but continues to have serious memory problems (especially with short-term memory).
VII	Automatic and appropriate	The patient is consistently oriented with little or no confusion but frequently appears robotlike when performing daily routines. His awareness of himself and his interaction with his environment increase, but he lacks insight, judgment, problem-solving skills, and the ability to plan realistically.
VIII	Purposeful and appropriate	The patient is alert and oriented, recalls and integrates past events, learns new activities, and performs activities of daily living independently; however, deficits in stress tolerance, judgment, and abstract reasoning persist. He may function in society at a reduced level.

sense of date first, then time, place, caregivers and, finally, self.) When he responds verbally, assess the quality of replies. For example, garbled words indicate difficulty with the motor nerves that govern speech muscles. Rambling responses indicate difficulty with thought processing and organization.

● Assess the patient's ability to understand and follow one-step commands that require a motor response. For example, ask him to open and close his eyes or stick out his tongue. Note whether the patient remains awake. If you must gently shake him to keep him focused on your verbal commands, he may be neurologically compromised.

● If the patient doesn't respond to commands or touch, apply a painful stimulus. With moderate pressure, squeeze the nail beds on fingers and toes, and note his response. Check motor responses bilaterally *to rule out monoplegia (paralysis of a single area) and hemiplegia (paralysis of one side of the body).*

Pupil gauge

The pupils are typically equal in size, with an average diameter of 3.5 mm. To ensure accurate evaluation of pupil size, compare your patient's pupils to the scale below. Keep in mind that maximum constriction may be less than 1 mm and maximum dilation greater than 9 mm.

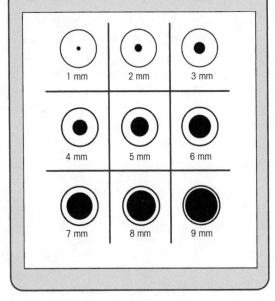

6 mm). Remember, pupil size varies considerably, and unequal pupils (anisocoria) are normal in some patients. See if the pupils are positioned in, or deviated from, the midline. (See *Pupil gauge.*)

● Test the patient's direct light response. First, darken the room. Hold each eyelid open in turn, keeping the other eye covered. Swing the penlight from the patient's ear toward the midline of the face. Shine the light directly into the eye. Normally, the pupil constricts immediately. When you remove the penlight, the pupil should dilate immediately. Wait about 20 seconds before testing the other pupil *to allow it to recover from reflex stimulation.* **Science**

● Next, test consensual light response. Hold both eyelids open, but shine the light into one eye only. Watch for constriction in the other pupil, *which indicates proper nerve function of the optic chiasm.* **Science**

● Brighten the room and have the conscious patient open his eyes. Observe the eyelids for ptosis or drooping. Check extraocular movements. Hold up one finger, and ask the patient to follow it with his eyes alone. As you move the finger up, down, laterally, and obliquely, see if the patient's eyes track together to follow your finger (conjugate gaze). Watch for involuntary jerking or oscillating eye movements (nystagmus).

● Check the patient's accommodation-convergence reflex. Hold up one finger midline to the patient's face and several feet away. Have the patient focus on your finger. Gradually move your finger toward his nose while he focuses on your finger or a pencil or pen. This should cause his eyes to converge and both pupils to constrict equally.

● If the patient is comatose, test the corneal reflex by touching a wisp of cotton ball to the cornea. This normally causes an immediate blink reflex. Repeat for the other eye.

● If the patient is unconscious, test the oculocephalic (doll's eye) reflex. Hold the patient's eyelids open. Quickly but gently turn the patient's head to one side and then the other. If the patient's eyes move in the opposite direction from the side to which you turn the head, the reflex is intact.

⚠ **ALERT** *Never use the doll's eye reflex test if you know or suspect that the patient has a cervical spine injury because permanent spinal cord damage may result.*

● A patient's response to painful stimuli should be described as one of the following: *localization*—the patient withdraws from the pain, attempts to push away the painful stimulus, and can localize where the pain originates; *withdrawal*—the patient moves slightly, but makes no attempt to push the painful stimulus away; or *unresponsive*—the patient doesn't react to the application of painful stimulus (commonly seen in patients in a deep coma). **AANN**

Examining pupils and eye movement **AANN** **AANS**

● Ask the patient to open his eyes. If he doesn't respond, gently lift his upper eyelids. Inspect each pupil for size and shape, and compare the two for equality. *To evaluate pupil size more precisely,* use a chart showing the various pupil sizes (in increments of 1 mm, with the normal diameter ranging from 2 to

Evaluating motor function AANN AANS

● Identify the patient's strength on a scale of 0 to 5 with 0 being no muscle strength and 5 being full muscle strength.

● If the patient is conscious, test his grip strength in both hands at the same time. Extend your hands, ask him to squeeze your fingers as hard as he can, and compare the strength of each hand. Grip strength is usually slightly stronger in the dominant hand.

● Test arm strength by having the patient close his eyes and hold his arms straight out in front of him with the palms up for 20 to 30 seconds. See if either arm drifts downward or pronates, *indicating muscle weakness.*

● Test leg strength by having the patient raise his legs, one at a time, against gentle downward pressure from your hand. Gently push down on each leg at the midpoint of the thigh *to evaluate muscle strength.*

⚠ **ALERT** *If decorticate or decerebrate posturing develops in response to noxious stimuli, notify the physician immediately. (See* Identifying warning postures.*)*

● Flex and extend the extremities on both sides *to evaluate muscle tone.*

● Test the plantar reflex. To do so, stroke the lateral aspect of the sole of the patient's foot with your thumbnail or another moderately sharp object. Normally, this elicits flexion of all toes. Watch for a positive Babinski's sign — dorsiflexion of the great toe with fanning of the other toes — *which indicates an upper motor neuron lesion.* AANS

Completing the neurologic examination

● Taking the patient's temperature, pulse rate, respiratory rate, and blood pressure are important facets of a full assessment. However, when changes in the pulse pressure (the difference between systolic pressure and diastolic pressure) are noted, a widening pulse pressure is a late sign of increased ICP.

Special considerations

⚠ **ALERT** *If a previously stable patient suddenly develops a change in neurologic or routine vital signs, further assess his condition and immediately notify the physician.*

Nursing diagnoses

● Impaired environmental interpretation syndrome

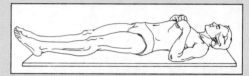
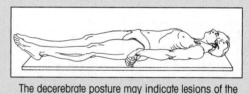
Expected outcomes

The patient will:

● remain oriented to his environment to the fullest extent

● remain free from injury.

Documentation

Baseline data require detailed documentation; subsequent notes can be brief unless the patient's condition changes. Record the patient's LOC and orientation, pupillary activity, motor function, and routine vital signs, as your facility's policy directs. To save time while keeping complete records, you may be allowed to use abbreviations. Use only commonly understood abbreviations and terms to avoid misinterpretation. Examples include:

● A + O × 3 = alert and oriented to time, place, and person
● PERRLA = pupils equal, round, reactive to light and accommodation
● PERL = pupils equal, reactive to light
● EOM = extraocular movements.

Also describe the patient's behavior — for example, "difficult to arouse by gentle shaking," "sleepy," or "unresponsive to painful stimuli."

Supportive references

American Association of Neuroscience Nurses. *Core Curriculum for Neuroscience Nursing,* 4th ed. Philadelphia: W.B. Saunders Co., 2004.

Barker, E. *Neuroscience Nursing,* 2nd ed. St. Louis: Mosby–Year Book, Inc., 2002.

Hickey, J.V. *The Clinical Practice of Neurological and Neurosurgical Nursing,* 5th ed. Philadelphia: Lippincott Williams & Wilkins, 2003.

Lynn-McHale Wiegand, D.J., and Carlson, K.K. (eds.) *AACN Procedure Manual for Critical Care,* 5th ed. Philadelphia: W.B. Saunders Co., 2005.

Pain management

Pain is defined as the sensory and emotional experience associated with actual or potential tissue damage. Thus, pain includes not only the perception of an uncomfortable stimulus, but also the response to that perception.

In health care, the physician's role is to identify and treat the cause of pain, and prescribe medications and other interventions to relieve pain, whereas nurses have traditionally been responsible for assessing and managing a patient's pain.

✔ **CLINICAL IMPACT** **JCAHO** *According to JCAHO standards, health care facilities are required to develop policies and procedures for pain control, which include developing policies and procedures supporting the appropriate use of analgesics and other pain control therapies. Health care providers are expected to be knowledgeable about pain assessment and management. The new standards also state that:*

● *Pain should be assessed on admission and regularly reassessed.*
● *Patients should be informed of relevant providers in pain assessment and management.*
● *Patients and their families should be educated regarding their roles in pain management as well as the potential limitations and adverse effects of pain treatments.*
● *Pain assessment should include personal, cultural, spiritual, and ethnic beliefs.*
● *Patients will be involved in making care decisions.*
● *Routine and as needed analgesics are to be administered.*

Several interventions can be used to manage pain. These include analgesics, emotional support, comfort measures, and cognitive techniques to distract the patient. Severe pain usually requires an opioid analgesic. Invasive measures, such as epidural analgesia or patient-controlled analgesia (PCA), may also be required.

Equipment

Pain assessment tool or scale • oral hygiene supplies • water • nonopioid analgesic (such as aspirin or acetaminophen [Tylenol]) • optional: PCA device; mild opioid (such as oxycodone or codeine); strong opioid (such as methadone [Dolophine], levorphanol [Levo-Dromoron], morphine [Duramorph], or hydromorphone [Dilaudid])

Implementation

● Explain to the patient how pain medications work together with other pain management therapies to provide relief. Explain that management aims to keep pain at a low level to permit optimal bodily function. **PCP**

● Assess the patient's pain by using a pain assessment tool or scale or by asking him key questions and noting his response to the pain. For instance, ask him to describe its duration, severity, and source. Look for physiologic or behavioral clues to the pain's severity. (See *Assessing pain.*) **JCAHO**

● Develop nursing diagnoses. Appropriate nursing diagnostic categories include acute or chronic pain, anxiety, activity intolerance, fear, risk for injury, deficient knowledge, and powerlessness.

• Work with the patient to develop a nursing care plan using interventions appropriate to his lifestyle. These may include prescribed medications, emotional support, comfort measures, cognitive techniques, and education about pain and its management. Emphasize the importance of maintaining good bowel habits, respiratory functions, and mobility *because pain may exacerbate any problems in these areas.* **Science**

• Implement your care plan. Because individuals respond to pain differently, you'll find that what works for one person may not work for another.

Giving medications
• If the patient is allowed oral intake, begin with a nonopioid analgesic, such as acetaminophen or aspirin, every 4 to 6 hours as ordered. **JCAHO**
• If the patient needs more relief than a nonopioid analgesic provides, you may give a mild opioid (such as oxycodone or codeine) as ordered. **JCAHO**
• If the patient needs still more pain relief, you may administer a strong opioid (such as methadone, levorphanol, morphine, or hydromorphone) as prescribed. Administer oral medications if possible. Check the appropriate drug information for each medication given.
• If ordered, teach the patient how to use a PCA device. *Such a device can help the patient manage his pain and decrease his anxiety.* **JCAHO**

Providing emotional support
• Show your concern by spending time talking with the patient. Because of his pain and his inability to manage it, he may be anxious and frustrated. *Such feelings can worsen his pain.* **EB**

Performing comfort measures
• Periodically reposition the patient *to reduce muscle spasms and tension and to relieve pressure on bony prominences.* Increasing the angle of the bed can reduce pull on an abdominal incision, diminishing pain. If appropriate, elevate a limb *to reduce swelling, inflammation, and pain.* **Science**
• Give the patient a back massage *to help reduce tense muscles.*
• Perform passive range-of-motion exercises *to prevent stiffness and further loss of mobility, relax tense muscles, and provide comfort.* **Science**

Assessing pain

To assess pain properly, you'll need to consider the patient's description and your own observations of his physical and behavioral responses. Start by asking this series of key questions (bearing in mind that the patient's responses will be shaped by his prior experiences, self-image, and beliefs about his condition):
• Where is the pain located? How long does it last? How often does it occur?
• Can you describe the pain?
• What relieves the pain or makes it worse?
  Ask the patient to rank his pain on a scale of 0 to 10, with 0 denoting lack of pain and 10 denoting the worst pain level. This helps the patient verbally evaluate pain therapies. Observe the patient's behavioral and physiologic responses to pain. Physiologic responses may be sympathetic or parasympathetic.

Behavioral responses
Behavioral responses include altered body position, moaning, sighing, grimacing, withdrawal, crying, restlessness, muscle twitching, and immobility.

Sympathetic responses
Sympathetic responses are commonly associated with mild to moderate pain and include pallor, elevated blood pressure, dilated pupils, skeletal muscle tension, dyspnea, tachycardia, and diaphoresis.

Parasympathetic responses
Parasympathetic responses are commonly associated with severe, deep pain and include pallor, decreased blood pressure, bradycardia, nausea and vomiting, weakness, dizziness, and loss of consciousness.
  Assess pain at least every 2 hours and during rest, during activity, and through the night when pain is usually heightened. Keep in mind that the ability to sleep doesn't indicate absence of pain.

• Provide oral hygiene. Keep a fresh water glass or cup at the bedside *because many pain medications tend to dry the mouth.*
• Wash the patient's face and hands *to soothe the patient, which may reduce his perception of pain.*

Visual pain rating scale

You can evaluate pain in a nonverbal manner for pediatric patients age 3 and older and for adults with language difficulties. One instrument is the Wong-Baker FACES pain rating scale; another, two simple faces such as the ones shown below. Ask the patient to choose the face that describes how he's feeling — either happy because he has no pain, or sad because he has some or a lot of pain. Alternatively, to pinpoint varying levels of pain, you can ask the patient to draw a face.

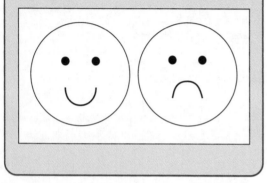

Using cognitive therapy

● Help the patient enhance the effect of analgesics by using such techniques as distraction, guided imagery, deep breathing, and relaxation. You can easily use these "mind-over-pain" techniques at the bedside. Choose the method the patient prefers. If possible, start these techniques when the patient feels little or no pain. If he feels persistent pain, begin with short, simple exercises. Before beginning, dim the lights, remove the patient's restrictive clothing, and eliminate noise from the environment.

● For *distraction,* have the patient recall a pleasant experience or focus his attention on an enjoyable activity. For instance, have him use music as a distraction by turning on the radio when the pain begins. Tell him to close his eyes and concentrate on listening, raising or lowering the volume as his pain increases or subsides. Note, however, that distraction is usually effective only against brief episodes of pain lasting less than 5 minutes.

● For *guided imagery,* help the patient concentrate on a peaceful, pleasant image such as walking on the beach. Encourage him to concentrate on the details of

the image he has selected by asking about its sight, sound, smell, taste, and touch. The positive emotions evoked by this exercise minimize pain.

● For *deep breathing,* have the patient stare at an object, then slowly inhale and exhale as he counts aloud to maintain a comfortable rate and rhythm. Tell him to concentrate on the rise and fall of his abdomen. Encourage him to feel more and more weightless with each breath while he concentrates on the rhythm of his breathing or on any restful image.

● For *muscle relaxation,* have the patient focus on a particular muscle group. Ask him to tense the muscles and note the sensation. After 5 to 7 seconds, tell him to relax the muscles and concentrate on the relaxed state. Tell him to note the difference between the tense and relaxed states. After he tenses and relaxes one muscle group, have him proceed to another and another until he has covered his entire body.

Special considerations

● Evaluate your patient's response to pain management. If he's still in pain, reassess him and alter your care plan as appropriate.

● Remind the patient that results of cognitive therapy techniques improve with practice. Help him through the initial sessions.

● Remember that patients receiving opioid analgesics are at risk for developing tolerance, dependence, or addiction. Patients with acute pain may have a smaller risk of dependence or addiction than patients with chronic pain.

● If a patient receiving an opioid analgesic experiences abstinence syndrome when the drug is withdrawn abruptly, suspect physical dependence. The signs and symptoms include anxiety, irritability, chills and hot flashes, excessive salivation and tearing, rhinorrhea, sweating, nausea, vomiting, and seizures. These signs and symptoms are likely to begin in 6 to 12 hours and to peak in 24 to 72 hours. *To reduce the risk of dependence,* discontinue an opioid by decreasing the dose gradually each day. You may switch to an oral opioid and decrease its dose gradually.

● If a patient becomes addicted, his behavior will be characterized by compulsive drug use and a craving for the drug to experience effects other than pain relief. A patient demonstrating such behavior usually has a preexisting problem that's exacerbated by the opioid use. Discuss the addicted patient's problem with supportive personnel, and make appropriate referrals to experts.

● During periods of intense pain, the patient's ability to concentrate diminishes. If your patient is in severe pain, help him to select a cognitive technique that's simple to use. After he selects a technique, encourage him to use it consistently.

● If your patient has dementia or some other cognitive impairment, don't assume that he can't understand a pain scale or communicate about his pain. Experiment with several pain scales, a scale featuring faces such as the Wong-Baker FACES scale is a good choice for many cognitively impaired patients and those with limited language skills. (See *Visual pain rating scale.*)

Nursing diagnoses

● Acute pain
● Chronic pain

Expected outcomes

The patient will:
● identify characteristics of pain
● state and carry out interventions for pain relief
● express comfort and relief from pain.

Complications

The most common adverse effects of analgesics include respiratory depression (the most serious), sedation, constipation, nausea, and vomiting.

Documentation

Document each step of the nursing process. Describe the subjective information you elicited from the patient, using his own words. Note the location, quality, and duration of the pain as well any precipitating factors.

Record your nursing diagnoses, and include the pain-relief method selected. Use a flow sheet to document pain assessment findings. Summarize your actions and the patient's response, including vital signs. If the patient's pain wasn't relieved, note alternative treatments to consider the next time pain occurs. Record any complications of drug therapy.

Supportive references

Acello, B. "Meeting JCAHO Standards for Pain Control," *Nursing2000* 30(3):52–54, March 2000.

Joint Commission on the Accreditation of Healthcare Organizations. *Comprehensive Accreditation Manual for Hospitals: Pain Management Standards.* Chicago: JCAHO, 2002.

McCaffery, M., and Pasero, C. *Pain: Clinical Manual,* 2nd ed. St. Louis: Mosby–Year Book, Inc., 1999. **EB**

McCaffery, M., and Pasero, C. *Pain Management. Part 1: Assessment and Overview of Analgesics.* Version 1.0. Philadelphia: Lippincott Williams & Wilkins, 2001.

McCaffery, M., and Pasero, C. *Pain Management. Part 2: The Nurse's Active Role in Opioid Administration.* Version 1.0. Philadelphia: Lippincott Williams & Wilkins, 2001.

Wong, D.L., et al. *Whaley and Wong's Essentials of Pediatric Nursing,* 6th ed. St. Louis: Mosby–Year Book, Inc., 2001.

Seizure management

Seizures are paroxysmal events associated with abnormal electrical discharges of neurons in the brain. Partial seizures are usually confined to one cerebral hemisphere, involving a localized or focal area of the brain. Generalized seizures involve the entire brain. (See *Differentiating among seizure types,* page 388.) When a patient has a generalized seizure, nursing care aims to protect him from injury and prevent serious complications. Appropriate care also includes observation of seizure characteristics to help determine the area of the brain involved. **AAN**

Patients considered at risk for seizures are those with a history of seizures and those with conditions that predispose them to seizures. Such conditions include metabolic abnormalities, such as hypocalcemia, hypoglycemia, and pyridoxine deficiency; brain tumors or other space-occupying lesions; infections, such as meningitis, encephalitis, and brain abscess; traumatic injury, especially if the dura mater was penetrated; ingestion of toxins, such as mercury, lead, or carbon monoxide; genetic abnormalities, such as tuberous sclerosis and phenylketonuria; perinatal injuries; and stroke. Patients at risk for seizures need precautionary measures to help prevent injury if a seizure occurs. (See *Precautions for generalized seizures,* page 389.) **AAN**

Most major seizures (generalized or tonic-clonic) last only 1 to 2 minutes and demand little of the person observing the seizure. All that's needed is to let the seizure run its course, to ensure that the patient is

Differentiating among seizure types

The hallmark of epilepsy is recurring seizures, which can be classified as partial or generalized. Some patients may be affected by more than one type of seizure.

Partial seizures (focal, local seizures)

Arising from a localized area in the brain, partial seizures cause specific symptoms. Categories of partial seizures include simple partial seizures (consciousness is intact), complex partial seizures (some loss of consciousness occurs), and partial seizures in which seizure activity may be spread to the entire brain, thereby causing a generalized seizure.

Simple partial seizures

A simple partial seizure can be present in several ways depending upon the focal point of the seizure in the brain.
- Motor symptoms (jerking of the thumb or the cheek)
- Somatosensory symptoms (visual, vestibular, gustatory, olfactory or auditory hallucinations or sensations)
- Autonomic symptoms (such as tachycardia, sweating, pupillary dilation)
- Psychic symptoms (which rarely occur without some changes in consciousness such as feelings of déjà-vu or dreamy states).

Complex partial seizures

Consciousness becomes impaired with a complex partial seizure. This type of seizure begins as a simple partial seizure in which the consciousness isn't impaired and evolves to an impairment of consciousness. The same symptoms that present during a simple partial seizure are still seen as the seizure develops into a complex partial seizure.

Partial seizures evolving to generalized tonic-clonic seizures

A partial seizure can be either a simple partial or a complex partial seizure that progresses to a generalized seizure. An aura may precede the progression. Loss of consciousness occurs immediately or within 1 to 2 minutes of the start of the progression.

Generalized seizures (convulsive or nonconvulsive)

As the term suggests, generalized seizures cause a general electrical abnormality within the brain. They include several distinct types.

Absence (petit mal) seizures

An absence seizure occurs commonly in children, but it may also affect adults. It usually begins with a brief change in the level of consciousness, indicated by blinking or rolling of the eyes, or a blank stare, and slight mouth movements. Typically, the seizure lasts 1 to 10 seconds. The impairment is so brief that the patient (or parent) is sometimes unaware of it. If not properly treated, these seizures can recur as often as 100 times per day and may result in learning difficulties.

Myoclonic seizures

A myoclonic seizure is marked by brief bilateral muscular jerks of the body extremities. They may occur in a rhythmic manner and may be accompanied by brief loss of consciousness.

Generalized tonic-clonic (grand mal) seizures

Typically, a generalized tonic-clonic seizure begins with a loud cry, precipitated by air rushing from the lungs through the vocal cords. The patient falls to the ground, losing consciousness. The body stiffens (tonic phase) and then alternates between episodes of muscle spasm and relaxation (clonic phase). Tongue biting, incontinence, labored breathing, apnea, and subsequent cyanosis may also occur. The seizure stops in 2 to 5 minutes, when abnormal electrical conduction of the neurons is completed. The patient then regains consciousness but is somewhat confused and may have difficulty talking. If he can talk, he may complain of drowsiness, fatigue, headache, muscle soreness, and arm or leg weakness. He may fall into a deep sleep after the seizure.

Atonic seizures (drop attacks)

Characterized by a general loss of postural tone and a temporary loss of consciousness, an atonic seizure occurs in young children. It's sometimes called a "drop attack" because it causes the child to fall.

in no physical danger, and to maintain a patent airway. However, a patient with status epilepticus, in which he experiences repeated seizures without regaining consciousness, requires immediate medical intervention. **AAN**

Equipment

Oral airway • suction equipment • side rail pads • seizure activity record • additional equipment: I.V. line, normal saline solution, oxygen, endotracheal (ET) intubation equipment

Implementation **AAN** **AANN**

● If you're with a patient when he experiences an aura, help him into bed, raise the side rails, and adjust the bed flat. If he's away from his room, lower him to the floor and place a pillow, blanket, or other soft material under his head *to keep it from hitting the floor.* **PCP**

● Provide privacy if possible.

● When you have a patient in the hospital who has a known seizure history, maintain I.V. access or a heparin lock so that if he does have a seizure, there's I.V. access *to administer medications* (for example, diazepam [Valium]).

● Stay with the patient during the seizure, and be ready to intervene if complications such as airway obstruction develop. If necessary, have another staff member obtain the appropriate equipment and notify the physician of the obstruction.

● Depending on your facility's policy, if the patient is in the beginning of the tonic phase of the seizure, you may insert an oral airway into his mouth *so his tongue doesn't block his airway.* If an oral airway isn't available, don't try to hold his mouth open or place your hands inside *because you may be bitten.* After the patient's jaw becomes rigid, don't force the airway into place *because you may break his teeth or cause another injury.* Turn the patient to his side *to allow secretions to drain and the tongue to fall forward.* *Never* force any objects into the patient's mouth unless his airway is compromised.

● Move hard or sharp objects out of the patient's way and loosen his clothing.

● Don't forcibly restrain the patient or restrict his movements during the seizure *because the force of the patient's movements against restraints could cause muscle strain or even joint dislocation.*

● Continually assess the patient during the seizure. Observe the earliest symptom, such as head or eye

Precautions for generalized seizures

Taking appropriate precautions will help you protect a patient from injury, aspiration, and airway obstruction should he have a seizure. Plan your precautions using information obtained from the patient's history. What kind of seizure has the patient had before? Is he aware of exacerbating factors? Sleep deprivation, missed doses of anticonvulsants, and even upper respiratory tract infections can increase seizure frequency in some people who have had seizures. Was his previous seizure an acute episode or did it result from a chronic condition?

Equipment preparation

Based on answers provided in the patient's history, you can tailor your precautions to his needs. Start by gathering the appropriate equipment, including a hospital bed with full-length side rails, commercial side rail pads or six bath blankets (four for a crib), adhesive tape, an oral airway, and oral or nasal suction equipment.

Bedside preparation

Carry out the precautions you think appropriate for the patient. Remember that a patient with preexisting seizures who's being admitted for a change in medication, treatment of an infection, or detoxification may have an increased risk of seizures.

● Explain the reasons for the precautions to the patient.

● *To protect the patient's limbs, head, and feet from injury if he has a seizure while in bed,* cover the side rails, headboard, and footboard with side rail pads or bath blankets. If you use blankets, keep them in place with adhesive tape. Be sure to keep the side rails raised while the patient is in bed *to prevent falls.* Keep the bed in a low position *to minimize any injuries that may occur if the patient climbs over the rails.*

● Place an airway at the patient's bedside or tape it to the wall above the bed, according to your facility's protocol. Keep suction equipment nearby *in case you need to establish a patent airway.* Explain to the patient how the airway will be used.

● If the patient has frequent or prolonged seizures, prepare an I.V. heparin lock *to facilitate administration of emergency medications.*

Understanding status epilepticus

A seizure state that continues unless interrupted by emergency interventions, status epilepticus can occur in all seizure types. The most life-threatening example is generalized tonic-clonic status epilepticus, a continuous generalized tonic-clonic seizure without intervening return of consciousness.

Status epilepticus, always an emergency, is accompanied by respiratory distress. It can result from abrupt withdrawal of anticonvulsant medications, hypoxic or metabolic encephalopathy, acute head trauma, or septicemia secondary to encephalitis or meningitis.

Emergency treatment of status epilepticus usually consists of diazepam (Valium), phenytoin (Dilantin), or phenobarbital (Solfoton), dextrose 50% in water I.V. (when seizures are secondary to hypoglycemia), and thiamine I.V. (in the presence of chronic alcoholism or withdrawal).

---

deviation, as well as how the seizure progresses, what form it takes, and how long it lasts. *Your description may help determine the seizure's type and cause.*
- If this is the patient's first seizure, notify the physician immediately. If the patient has had seizures before, notify the physician only if the seizure activity is prolonged or if the patient fails to regain consciousness. (See *Understanding status epilepticus.*)
- If ordered, establish an I.V. line and infuse normal saline solution at a keep-vein-open rate.
- If the seizure is prolonged and the patient becomes hypoxemic, administer oxygen as ordered. Some patients may require ET intubation.
- For a patient with diabetes, administer 50 ml of dextrose 50% in water by I.V. push as ordered. For a patient who's an alcoholic, a 100-mg bolus of thiamine may be ordered to stop the seizure.
- After the seizure, turn the patient on his side and apply suction if necessary *to facilitate drainage of secretions and maintain a patent airway.* Insert an oral airway if needed.
- Check for injuries.
- Reorient and reassure the patient as necessary.

- When the patient is comfortable and safe, document what happened during the seizure.
- Place side rail pads on the bed in case the patient experiences another seizure.
- After the seizure, monitor vital signs and mental status every 15 to 20 minutes for 2 hours.
- Ask the patient about his aura and activities preceding the seizure. The type of aura (auditory, visual, olfactory, gustatory, or somatic) helps pinpoint the site in the brain where the seizure originated.

Special considerations
Because a seizure commonly indicates an underlying disorder such as meningitis or a metabolic or electrolyte imbalance, a complete diagnostic workup will be ordered if the cause of the seizure isn't evident.

Nursing diagnoses
- Ineffective airway clearance
- Risk for injury

Expected outcomes
The patient will:
- maintain a patent airway
- maintain an oxygen level within normal limits
- remain free from injury.

Complications
- The patient who experiences a seizure may experience an injury, respiratory difficulty, and decreased mental capability.
- Common injuries include scrapes and bruises suffered when the patient hits objects during the seizure and traumatic injury to the tongue caused by biting.
- If you suspect a serious injury, such as a fracture or deep laceration, notify the physician and arrange for appropriate evaluation and treatment.
- Changes in respiratory function may include aspiration, airway obstruction, and hypoxemia.
- After the seizure, complete a respiratory assessment and notify the physician if you suspect a problem.
- Expect most patients to experience a postictal period of decreased mental status lasting 30 minutes to 24 hours. Reassure the patient that this doesn't indicate incipient brain damage.

Documentation

Document that the patient requires seizure precautions, and record all precautions taken. Record the date and the time the seizure began as well as its duration and any precipitating factors. Identify any sensation that may be considered an aura. If the seizure was preceded by an aura, have the patient describe what he experienced.

Record any involuntary behavior that occurred at the onset, such as lip smacking, chewing movements, or hand and eye movements. Describe where the movement began and the parts of the body involved. Note any progression or pattern to the activity. Document whether the patient's eyes deviated to one side and if the pupils changed in size, shape, equality, or reaction to light. Note if the patient's teeth were clenched or open. Record any incontinence, vomiting, or salivation that occurred during the seizure.

Note the patient's response to the seizure. Was the patient aware of what happened? Did he fall into a deep sleep following the seizure? Was he upset or ashamed? Note any medications given, any complications experienced during the seizure, and any interventions performed. Finally, note the patient's post-seizure mental status.

Supportive references

American Association of Neuroscience Nurses. *Core Curriculum for Neuroscience Nursing,* 4th ed. Philadelphia: W.B. Saunders Co., 2004.

Barker, E. *Neuroscience Nursing,* 2nd ed. St. Louis: Mosby–Year Book, Inc., 2002.

Brodie, M.J., et al. *Epilepsy, Fast Facts,* 2nd ed. Oxford, England: Health Press Limited, 2001.

Hickey, J.V. *The Clinical Practice of Neurological and Neurosurgical Nursing,* 5th ed. Philadelphia: Lippincott Williams & Wilkins, 2003.

Lynn-McHale Wiegand, D.J., and Carlson, K.K. (eds.) *AACN Procedure Manual for Critical Care,* 5th ed. Philadelphia: W.B. Saunders Co., 2005.

Stroke management

A stroke is a sudden impairment of cerebral circulation in one or more of the blood vessels supplying the brain. A stroke interrupts or diminishes oxygen supply and commonly causes serious damage or necrosis in brain tissues. The sooner circulation returns to normal after stroke, the better chances are for complete recovery. However, about one-half of those who survive a stroke remain permanently disabled and experience a recurrence within weeks, month, or years. **AHA**

The major causes of stroke are thrombosis, embolism, and hemorrhage. *Thrombosis* is the most common cause in middle-age and elderly people, who have a higher incidence of atherosclerosis, diabetes, and hypertension. Thrombosis causes ischemia in brain tissue supplied by the affected vessel as well as congestion and edema; the latter may produce more clinical adverse effects than the thrombosis itself, but these symptoms subside with the edema.

Embolism, the second most common cause of stroke, is an occlusion of a blood vessel caused by a fragmented clot, a tumor, fat, bacteria, or air. It can occur at any age, especially among patients with a history of rheumatic heart disease, endocarditis, post-traumatic valvular disease, or myocardial fibrillation and other cardiac arrhythmias. It can also occur after open-heart surgery.

Hemorrhagic stroke results from chronic hypertension or aneurysms, which cause sudden rupture of a cerebral artery, thereby diminishing blood supply to the area served by the artery. In addition, blood accumulates deep within the brain, further compressing neural tissue and causing even greater damage.

Early treatment of a stroke relies heavily on early recognition and detection of signs and symptoms of a stroke and prompt activation of the emergency medical service (EMS) system. Stroke and transient ischemic shock can be correctly identified in three of four people using the Cincinnati Prehospital Stroke Scale. Nurses and physicians can evaluate the patient using this scale in less than 1 minute. (See *Cincinnati Prehospital Stroke Scale,* page 392.)

EMS providers should establish the precise time and onset of stroke signs and symptoms. The time of onset must be obtained to evaluate the patient for fibrinolytic therapy. Early notification of emergency department personnel enables them to prepare for the arrival of a stroke patient and shortens the time required to determine whether the patient has indications for acute stroke therapy. **AHA** **NINDS**

Nursing management **AHA**

● During the acute phase, focus efforts on survival needs and prevention of further complications. Emergency department personnel should access a patient

Cincinnati Prehospital Stroke Scale AHA

This scale identifies a high percentage of acute strokes in patients by focusing on three physical findings.

Facial droop
Ask the patient to smile or show his teeth.
- Normal — both sides of the patient's face move equally
- Abnormal — one side of the face doesn't move or move as well as the other side

Arm drift
Ask the patient to close his eyes and extend his arms out in front of him for 10 seconds.
- Normal — both arms move the same or not at all
- Abnormal — one arm doesn't move, or one arm drifts compared with the other

Abnormal speech
Ask the patient to repeat the sentence "You can't teach an old dog new tricks."
- Normal — the patient can say the sentence with no slurring and uses the correct words
- Abnormal — words are slurred, the patient can't speak, or he uses the wrong words

If the patient experiences any one of the three abnormal physical findings, the probability that he's had a stroke is 72%.

Source: American Heart Association in collaboration with the International Liaison Committee on Resuscitation. 2005 AHA Guidelines for Cardiopulmonary Resuscitation and Emergency Cardiovascular Care. *Circulation* 112(Suppl. 22):IV-1-IV-211, November 2005.

and nutritional status. Patient care must also include measures to prevent complications such as infection.

- Maintain a patent airway and oxygenation. Loosen constricting clothing. Watch for ballooning of the cheek with respiration. The side that balloons is usually the side affected by the stroke. If the patient is unconscious, keep him in a lateral position *to allow secretions to drain naturally,* or suction secretions, as needed. Insert an artificial airway and start mechanical ventilation, if necessary.
- Check vital signs and neurologic status, record observations and be sure to report any significant changes to the physician. Monitor blood pressure, level of consciousness, pupillary changes, motor function (voluntary and involuntary), sensory function, speech, skin color, temperature, and signs of increased intracranial pressure (ICP), nuchal rigidity, or flaccidity.
- Remember that if a stroke is impending, blood pressure rises suddenly, pulse is rapid and bounding, and the patient may complain of a headache.
- Maintain fluid and electrolyte balance. If the patient can take liquids orally, offer them as often as fluid limitations permit. Administer I.V. fluids as ordered. Be sure never to give too much I.V. fluid too fast *because doing so can increase ICP.*
- Offer the urinal or bedpan every 2 hours. If the patient is incontinent, he may need an indwelling catheter, but this should be avoided, if possible, *because indwelling catheters increase risk of infection.*
- Check for gag reflex before offering small oral feedings of semisolid foods. Place the food tray within the patient's visual field because loss of peripheral vision is common. If oral feedings aren't possible, insert a nasogastric tube. (See chapter 8, Gastrointestinal care.)
- Be alert for signs that the patient is straining during elimination because this also raises ICP. Modify diet and administer stool softeners and laxatives, as ordered.
- Provide meticulous mouth care. Clean and irrigate the patient's mouth to remove food particles. Care for his dentures as needed.
- Provide meticulous eye care. Remove secretions with a cotton ball and sterile normal saline solution. Instill eye drops as ordered. Patch the patient's affected eye if he can't close his lid.
- Maintain correct body alignment and positioning. Use high-topped sneakers *to prevent footdrop and*

suspected of having a stroke within 10 minutes. (See *Suspected stroke algorithm.*) Be prepared for the possible administration of tissue plasminogen activator (tPA). (See *Fibrinolytic therapy for ischemic stroke,* page 394.) Effective care emphasizes continuing neurologic assessment, support of respiration, continuous monitoring of vital signs, careful positioning to prevent aspiration and contractures, management of GI problems, and careful monitoring of fluid, electrolyte,

Suspected stroke algorithm AHA

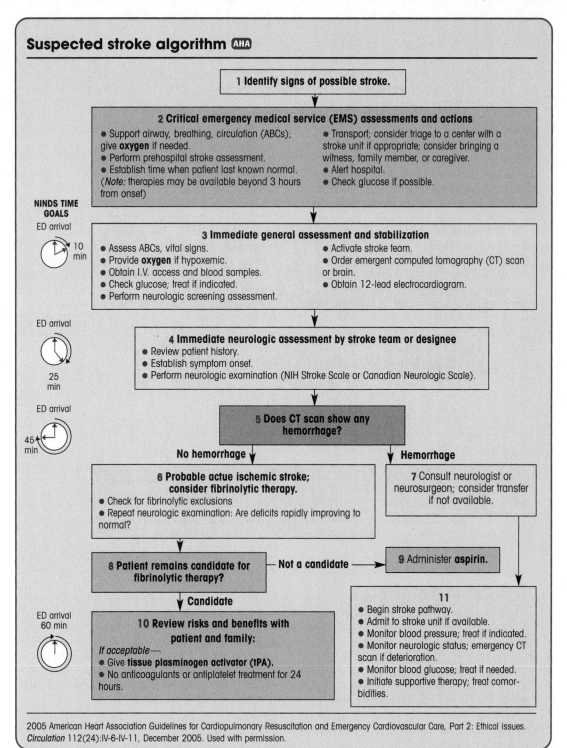

1 Identify signs of possible stroke.

2 Critical emergency medical service (EMS) assessments and actions
- Support airway, breathing, circulation (ABCs); give **oxygen** if needed.
- Perform prehospital stroke assessment.
- Establish time when patient last known normal. (*Note:* therapies may be available beyond 3 hours from onset)
- Transport; consider triage to a center with a stroke unit if appropriate; consider bringing a witness, family member, or caregiver.
- Alert hospital.
- Check glucose if possible.

NINDS TIME GOALS

ED arrival
10 min

3 Immediate general assessment and stabilization
- Assess ABCs, vital signs.
- Provide **oxygen** if hypoxemic.
- Obtain I.V. access and blood samples.
- Check glucose; treat if indicated.
- Perform neurologic screening assessment.
- Activate stroke team.
- Order emergent computed tomography (CT) scan or brain.
- Obtain 12-lead electrocardiogram.

ED arrival
25 min

4 Immediate neurologic assessment by stroke team or designee
- Review patient history.
- Establish symptom onset.
- Perform neurologic examination (NIH Stroke Scale or Canadian Neurologic Scale).

ED arrival
45 min

5 Does CT scan show any hemorrhage?

No hemorrhage

Hemorrhage

6 Probable actue ischemic stroke; consider fibrinolytic therapy.
- Check for fibrinolytic exclusions
- Repeat neurologic examination: Are deficits rapidly improving to normal?

7 Consult neurologist or neurosurgeon; consider transfer if not available.

8 Patient remains candidate for fibrinolytic therapy?

— Not a candidate —→

9 Administer **aspirin.**

Candidate

ED arrival
60 min

10 Review risks and benefits with patient and family:
If acceptable—
- Give **tissue plasminogen activator (tPA).**
- No anticoagulants or antiplatelet treatment for 24 hours.

11
- Begin stroke pathway.
- Admit to stroke unit if available.
- Monitor blood pressure; treat if indicated.
- Monitor neurologic status; emergency CT scan if deterioration.
- Monitor blood glucose; treat if needed.
- Initiate supportive therapy; treat comorbidities.

2005 American Heart Association Guidelines for Cardiopulmonary Resuscitation and Emergency Cardiovascular Care, Part 2: Ethical issues. *Circulation* 112(24):IV-6-IV-11, December 2005. Used with permission.

Fibrinolytic therapy for ischemic stroke

Current recommendations of the American Heart Association (AHA) state that the tissue plasminogen activator (tPA) (Activase) should be administered to carefully selected patients, with strict adherence to treatment protocols, after contraindications to fibrinolytic therapy have been ruled out.

Contraindications

AHA guidelines contraindicate fibrinolytic therapy in a patient with any of the following factors:

❑ evidence of intracranial bleeding on pretreatment noncontrast computed tomography (CT) scan

❑ suspicion of a subarachnoid hemorrhage despite normal findings on CT scan

❑ CT scan shows multilobal infarction (denser than one-third of cerebral hemisphere)

❑ history of intracranial hemorrhage

❑ uncontrolled hypertension (at time of treatment, systolic pressure remains greater than 185 mm Hg or diastolic pressure remains greater than 110 mm Hg despite repeated measurements)

❑ active internal bleeding or acute trauma (fracture)

❑ platelet count less than 100,000 mm^3

❑ heparin received within 48 hours resulting in partial thromboplastin time (PTT) greater than upper limit of normal

❑ recent use of an anticoagulant and elevated International Normalized Ration (INR) greater than 1.7 or prothrombin time (PT) greater than 15 seconds

❑ previous stroke, head trauma, or intracranial or intraspinal surgery that occurred within 3 months of the current condition

❑ arterial puncture at a noncompressible site within past 7 days

❑ history of arteriovenous malformation, neoplasm, or aneurysm

❑ witnessed seizure at onset of stroke.

Relative contraindications and precautions

Recent experience suggests that under some circumstances — with careful consideration and weighing of risk-to-benefit ratio — patients may receive fibrinolytic therapy despite one or more relative contraindications. Consider the pros and cons of tPA administration carefully if any of these relative contraindications is present:

❑ Only minor or rapidly improving stroke symptoms (clearing spontaneously)

❑ Within 14 days of major surgery or serious trauma

❑ Recent GI or urinary tract hemorrhage (within previous 21 days)

❑ Recent acute myocardial infarction (MI) (within previous 3 months)

❑ Post-MI pericarditis

❑ Abnormal blood glucose level (less than 50 or greater than 400 mg/dl [less than 2.8 or greater than 22.2 mmol/L])

*In patients without recent use of oral anticoagulants or heparin, treatment with tPA can be initiated before availability of coagulation study results but should be discontinued if the INR is greater than 1.7 or the PTT is elevated by local laboratory standards.

Adapted from the American Heart Association. Available at: http://circ.ahajournals.org/cgi/content/full/112/24_suppl/IV-111/TBL3 and http://circ.ahajournals.org/cgi/content/full/112/24_suppl/IV-111/TBL4. Accessed January 4, 2006. Used with permission of the publisher.

---

contracture, and convoluted foam, floatation, sheepskin, or pulsating mattresses *to prevent pressure ulcers.* Elevate affected limbs *to control dependent edema.* **Science**

● *To prevent pneumonia,* turn the patient at least every 2 hours. **Science**

● Assist the patient with exercise. Perform range-of-motion exercises for the affected and unaffected sides. Teach and encourage the patient to use his unaffected side and to exercise his affected side. **Science**

● Give medications as ordered, and watch for and report adverse effects.

● Establish and maintain communication with the patient. If he's aphasic, set up a simple method of communicating basic needs. Phrase your questions so he can answer using this system. Repeat yourself quietly and calmly and use gestures if necessary *to help him understand.*

- Provide psychological support. Set realistic short-term goals. Involve the patient's family in his care when possible, and explain his deficits and strengths.

TEACHING *Teach the patient and his family about the disorder. Explain the diagnostic tests, treatments, and rehabilitation he'll have to undergo.*

If surgery is scheduled, provide preoperative teaching. Make sure the patient and his family understand the surgery and its possible adverse effects.

Review ways to decrease the risk of future stroke, such as smoking cessation, maintenance of ideal weight with prescribed diet, control of diabetes and hypertension and minimization of stress, and avoidance of prolonged bed rest.

Teach the patient and his family about the schedule, dosage actions, and adverse effects of prescribed drugs. Make sure the patient taking aspirin realizes that he can't substitute acetaminophen (Tylenol) for aspirin.

Review signs and symptoms of impending stroke, and advise the patient to seek prompt treatment if signs occur.

Nursing diagnoses
- Deficient knowledge (disorder and procedure)
- Ineffective tissue perfusion: Cardiovascular

Expected outcomes
The patient will:
- state an understanding of care that's given
- have an improved level of consciousness
- maintain blood pressure within normal limits.

Documentation
Document the patient's vital signs and neurologic assessment findings on a special flowchart. If the patient was started on tPA, be sure to record date, time, and patient reaction to the medication as well as any patient teaching you performed.

Supportive references
American Heart Association. "2005 AHA Guidelines for Cardiopulmonary Resuscitation and Emergency Cardiovascular Care. Part 9: Adult Stroke," *Circulation* 112(Suppl 22):IV-111-IV-120, November 2005.

Hickey, J.V. *The Clinical Practice of Neurological and Neurosurgical Nursing,* 5th ed. Philadelphia: Lippincott Williams & Wilkins, 2003.

Lynn-McHale Wiegand, D.J., and Carlson, K.K. (eds.) *AACN Procedure Manual for Critical Care,* 5th ed. Philadelphia: W.B. Saunders Co., 2005.

Transcranial Doppler monitoring

Transcranial Doppler ultrasonography is a noninvasive method of monitoring blood flow in the intracranial vessels, specifically the circle of Willis. This procedure is used in the intensive care unit to monitor patients who have experienced cerebrovascular disorders, such as stroke, head trauma, or subarachnoid hemorrhage. It can help detect intracranial stenosis, vasospasm, and arteriovenous malformations as well as assess collateral pathways. Because it has the advantage of monitoring a continuous waveform, it can be used in intraoperative monitoring of cerebral circulation. **AAN** The transcranial Doppler unit transmits pulses of low-frequency ultrasound, which are then reflected back to the transducer by the red blood cells moving in the vessel being monitored. This information is then processed by the instrument into an audible signal and a velocity waveform, which is displayed on the monitor. The displayed waveform is actually a moving graph of blood flow velocities with TIME displayed along the horizontal axis, VELOCITY displayed along the vertical axis, and AMPLITUDE represented by various colors or intensities within the waveform. The heart's contractions speed up the movement of blood cells during systole and slow it down during diastole, resulting in a waveform that varies in velocity over the cardiac cycle.

Transcranial Doppler monitoring provides instantaneous, real-time information about cerebral blood flow and is noninvasive and painless for the patient. The unit itself is portable and easy to use. The method's disadvantage is the reliance on the ability of the ultrasound waves to penetrate thin areas of the cranium; this is difficult if the patient has thickening of the temporal bone, which increases with age.

The transcranial Doppler unit should always be used with its power set at the lowest level needed to provide an adequate waveform. This procedure requires specialized training *to ensure accurate vessel identification and correct interpretation of the signals.*

Equipment

Transcranial Doppler unit • transducer with an attachment system • terry cloth headband • ultrasonic coupling gel • marker

Implementation

● Confirm the patient's identity using two patient identifiers according to facility policy. **JCAHO**

● Explain the procedure to the patient, and answer any questions he has as thoroughly as possible. Place him in the proper position — usually the supine position. **AANN** **PCP**

● Turn the Doppler unit on and observe as it performs a self-test. The screen should show six parameters: PEAK (CM/S), MEAN (CM/S), DEPTH (M/M), DELTA (%), EMBOLI (AGR), and PI + .

● Enter the patient's name and identification number in the appropriate place on the Doppler unit. Depending on the unit you're using, you may need to enter additional information, such as the patient's diagnosis or the physician's name. **MFR**

● Indicate the vessel that you wish to monitor (usually the right or left middle cerebral artery [MCA]). You'll also need to set the approximate depth of the vessel within the skull (50 mm for the MCA). **AAN**

● Use the keypad to increase the power level to 100% to initially locate the signal. You can later decrease the level as needed, depending on the thickness of the patient's skull.

● Examine the temporal region of the patient's head, and mentally identify the three windows of the transtemporal access route: posterior, middle, and anterior (as shown below). **AAN**

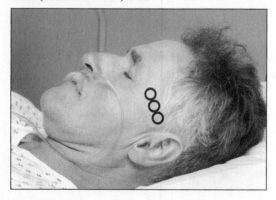

● Apply a generous amount of ultrasonic gel at the level of the temporal bone between the tragus of the ear and the end of the eyebrow, over the area of the three windows.

● Place the transducer on the posterior window. Angle the transducer slightly in an anterior direction, and slowly move it in a narrow circle. This movement is commonly called the *flashlighting technique.* As you hold the transducer at an angle and perform flashlighting, also begin to very slowly move the transducer forward across the temporal area. As you do this, listen for the audible signal with the highest pitch. This sound corresponds to the highest velocity signal, which corresponds to the signal of the vessel you're assessing. You can also use headphones *to help you better evaluate the audible signal and provide patient privacy.*

● After you've located the highest-pitched signal, use a marker to draw a circle around the transducer head on the patient's temple (as shown below). Note the angle of the transducer *so that you can duplicate it after the transducer attachment system is in place.* **AAN**

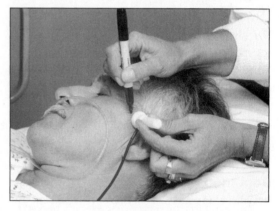

● Place the transducer system on the patient. To do this, first place the plate of the transducer attachment system over the patient's temporal area; match the circular opening in the plate exactly with the circle drawn on the patient's head. Holding the plate in place, encircle the patient's head with the straps attached to the system. Finally, tighten the straps *so that the transducer attachment system will stay in place on the patient's head.*

● Fill the circular opening in the plate with the ultrasonic gel.

● Place the transducer in the gel-filled opening in the attachment system plate. Using the plastic screws provided, loosely secure the two plates together. *This will hold the transducer in place but allow it to rotate for the best angle.*

● Adjust the position and angle of the transducer until you again hear the highest-pitched audible signal. When you hear this signal, look at the waveform on the monitor screen. You should see a clear waveform with a bright white line (called an *envelope*) at the upper edge of the waveform. The envelope exactly follows the contours of the waveform itself. **AAN**

● If the envelope doesn't follow the waveform's contours, adjust the GAIN setting. If the signal is wrapping around the screen, use the SCALE key to increase the scale and the BASELINE key to drop the baseline.

● When you've determined that you have the strongest, highest-pitched signal and the best waveform, lock the transducer in place by tightening the plastic screws (as shown below). The tightened plates will hold the transducer at the angle you've chosen. Disconnect the transducer handle.

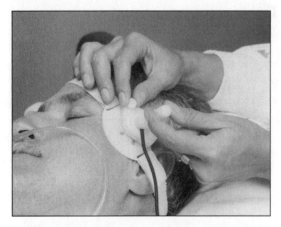

● Place a wide terry cloth headband over the transducer attachment system, and secure it around the patient's head *to provide additional stability for the transducer.*

● Look at the monitor screen. You should be able to see a waveform and read the numeric values of the peak, mean velocities, and pulsatility index (PI +) above the displayed waveform. The shape of the waveform reveals more information. (See *Comparing velocity waveforms,* page 398.) **AAN**

Special considerations

● Velocity changes in the transcranial Doppler signal correlate with changes in cerebral blood flow. The parameter that most clearly reflects this change is the mean velocity. First, establish a baseline for the mean velocity. As the patient's velocity increases or decreases, the value (%) will change negatively or positively from the baseline.

● Emboli appear as high-intensity transients occurring randomly during the cardiac cycle. Emboli make a distinctive "clicking," "chirping," or "plunking" sound. You can set up an emboli counter to count either the total number of emboli aggregates or the rate of embolic events per minute.

● Various screens can be stored on the system's hard drive and can be recalled or printed.

● Before using the transcranial Doppler system, be sure to remove turban head dressings or thick dressings over the test site.

Nursing diagnoses

● Decreased intracranial adaptive capacity

Expected outcomes

The patient will:

● maintain intracranial pressure within normal limits in response to stimulation

● show no evidence of neurologic compromise.

Documentation

Record the date and the time that the monitoring began and which artery is being monitored. Document any patient teaching as well as the patient's tolerance of the procedure.

Supportive references

Lupetin, A.R., et al. "Transcranial Doppler Sonography. Part 1: Principles, Technique and Normal Appearances," *Radiographics* 15(1):179-91, January 1995.

Lupetin, A.R., et al. "Transcranial Doppler Sonography. Part 2: Evaluation of Intracranial and Extracranial Abnormalities and Procedural Monitoring," *Radiographics* 15(1):193-209, January 1995.

Lynn-McHale Wiegand, D.J., and Carlson, K.K. (eds.) *AACN Procedure Manual for Critical Care,* 5th ed. Philadelphia: W.B. Saunders Co., 2005.

Sloan, M.A., et al. "Assessment: Transcranial Doppler Ultrasonography," *Neurology* 62(1):1468-481, January 2004.

Comparing velocity waveforms

A normal transcranial Doppler signal is usually characterized by mean velocities that fall within the normal reported values. Additional information can be gathered by evaluating the shape of the velocity waveform.

Effect of significant proximal vessel obstruction
A delayed systolic upstroke can be seen in a waveform when significant proximal vessel obstruction is present.

Normal

Proximal vessel obstruction

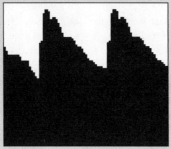
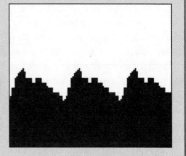

Effect of increased cerebrovascular resistance
Changes in cerebrovascular resistance, as occur with increased intracranial pressure, cause a decrease in diastolic flow.

Normal   **Increased resistance**

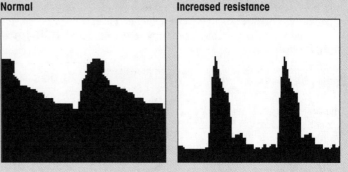

Taormina, M.A., and Nicholes, F.T., "Use of Transcranial Doppler Sonography to Evaluate Patients with Cerebrovascular Disease," *Neurosurgery Clinics of North America* 7(4):589-603, October 1996.

TENS application, use, and removal

Transcutaneous electrical nerve stimulation (TENS) is defined as the application of electrical stimulation to the skin for pain relief. It's based on the gate control theory of pain, which proposes that painful impulses pass through a "gate" in the brain. TENS is performed with a portable, battery-powered device that transmits painless electric current to peripheral nerves or directly to a painful area over relatively large nerve fibers. This treatment effectively alters the patient's perception of pain by blocking painful stimuli traveling over smaller fibers.

Used for postoperative patients and those with chronic pain, TENS reduces the need for analgesic drugs and may allow the patient to resume normal activities. Typically, a course of TENS treatments lasts 3 to 5 days. Some conditions, such as phantom limb pain, may require continuous stimulation; other conditions, such as a painful arthritic joint, require shorter periods (3 to 4 hours). (See *Current uses of TENS.*) **APS**

TENS is contraindicated for patients with cardiac pacemakers because it can interfere with pacemaker function. The procedure is also contraindicated for pregnant patients because its effect on the fetus is unknown. It's also contraindicated in patients with dementia. TENS should be used cautiously in all patients with cardiac disorders. TENS electrodes shouldn't be placed on the head or neck of patients with vascular disorders or seizure disorders.

Equipment

TENS device • alcohol pads • electrodes • electrode gel • warm water and soap • leadwires • charged battery pack • battery recharger • adhesive patch or hypoallergenic tape

Commercial TENS kits are available. They include the stimulator, leadwires, electrodes, spare battery pack, battery recharger, and sometimes the adhesive patch.

Preparation of equipment

Before beginning the procedure, always test the battery pack to make sure it's fully charged.

Implementation

● Confirm the patient's identity using two patient identifiers according to facility policy. **JCAHO**
● Wash your hands and follow standard precautions, as appropriate. Provide privacy. If the patient has never seen a TENS unit, show him the device and explain the procedure. **CDC** **PCP**

Before TENS treatment

● With an alcohol pad, thoroughly clean and dry the skin where the electrode will be applied.
● Apply electrode gel to the bottom of each electrode.
● Place the ordered number of electrodes on the proper skin area, leaving at least 2″ (5 cm) between them. (See *Positioning TENS electrodes,* page 400.) Secure them with the adhesive patch or hypoallergenic tape. Tape all sides evenly *so that the electrodes are firmly attached to the skin.*
● Plug the pin connectors into the electrode sockets. *To protect the cords,* hold the connectors — not the cords themselves — during insertion.
● Turn the channel controls to the OFF position or as recommended in the operator's manual. **MFR**
● Plug the leadwires into the jacks in the control box.
● Turn the amplitude and rate dials slowly as the manual directs. (The patient should feel a tingling sensation.) Adjust the controls on this device to the

Current uses of TENS

Transcutaneous electrical nerve stimulation (TENS) must be prescribed by a physician and is most successful if it's administered and taught to the patient by a therapist skilled in its use. TENS has been used for temporary relief of acute pain, such as postoperative incision pain, and for ongoing relief of chronic pain such as sciatica. Other types of pain that respond to TENS include:

● arthritis
● bone fracture pain
● bursitis
● cancer-related pain
● lower back pain
● musculoskeletal pain
● myofascial pain
● neuralgia and neuropathy
● phantom limb pain
● whiplash.

prescribed settings or to settings that are most comfortable. Most patients select stimulation frequencies of 60 to 100 Hz.
● Attach the TENS control box to part of the patient's clothing, such as a belt, pocket, or bra.
● *To make sure the device is working effectively,* monitor the patient for signs of excessive stimulation, such as muscle twitches, and for signs of inadequate stimulation, signaled by the patient's inability to feel any mild tingling sensation.

After TENS treatment

● Turn off the controls, and unplug the electrode leadwires from the control box.
● If another treatment will be given soon, leave the electrodes in place; if not, remove them.
● Clean the electrodes with soap and water, and clean the patient's skin with alcohol pads. (Don't soak the electrodes in alcohol *because it will damage the rubber.*)
● Remove the battery pack from the unit, and replace it with a charged battery pack.
● Recharge the used battery pack *so it's always ready for use.*

Positioning TENS electrodes

In transcutaneous electrical nerve stimulation (TENS), electrodes placed around peripheral nerves (or an incisional site) transmit mild electrical pulses to the brain. The current is thought to block pain impulses. The patient can influence the level and frequency of his pain relief by adjusting the controls on the device.

Typically, electrode placement varies even though patients may have similar complaints. Electrodes can be placed in several ways:

● to cover the painful area or surround it, as with muscle tenderness or spasm or painful joints

● to "capture" the painful area between electrodes, as with incisional pain.

In peripheral nerve injury, electrodes should be placed proximal to the injury (between the brain and the injury site) to avoid increasing pain. Placing electrodes in a hypersensitive area also increases pain. In an area lacking sensation, electrodes should be placed on adjacent dermatomes.

The illustrations below show combinations of electrode placement (solid squares) and areas of nerve stimulation (shaded area) for lower back and leg pain.

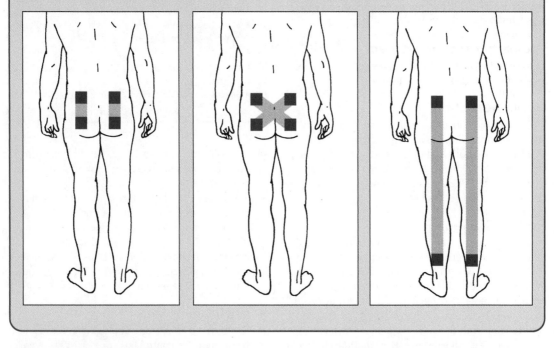

Special considerations

● If you must move electrodes during the procedure, turn off controls first. Follow the physician's orders regarding electrode placement and control settings. *Incorrect placement of the electrodes will result in inappropriate pain control. Setting the controls too high can cause pain; setting them too low will fail to relieve pain.*

⚠ ALERT *Never place electrodes near the patient's eyes or over nerves that innervate the carotid sinus or laryngeal or pharyngeal muscles to avoid interference with critical nerve function.*

● If TENS is used continuously for postoperative pain, remove the electrodes at least daily *to check for skin irritation, and provide skin care.* **Science**

● If appropriate, let the patient study the operator's manual. Teach him how to place the electrodes properly and how to take care of the TENS unit.

Nursing diagnoses

● Acute pain
● Chronic pain

Expected outcomes

The patient will:
- identify characteristics of pain and pain behaviors
- experience relief from pain.

Documentation

On the patient's medical record and the nursing care plan, record the electrode sites and the control settings. Document the patient's tolerance of treatment. Also evaluate pain control.

Supportive references

Barker, E. *Neuroscience Nursing,* 2nd ed. St. Louis: Mosby–Year Book, Inc., 2002.

Hickey, J.V. *The Clinical Practice of Neurological and Neurosurgical Nursing,* 5th ed. Philadelphia: Lippincott Williams & Wilkins, 2003.

"How the TENS Pain Control Units Work." Available at: *www.vitalityweb.com/backstore/tenswork.htm.*

Sluka, K.A. "The Basic Science Mechanisms of TENS and Clinical Implications," *APS Bulletin* 11(2), March-April 2001.

8

Gastrointestinal care

GI conditions affect just about everyone at one time or another. These conditions, so intimately tied to psychological health and stability, range from simple changes in bowel habits to life-threatening disorders requiring major surgery and radical lifestyle changes. GI conditions may be acute or chronic. Patient care for GI conditions also varies widely. For example, the patient with simple constipation may need only brief teaching about diet and exercise. However, the patient with colorectal cancer may need ongoing nursing care — from encouragement and support during the diagnostic workup to meticulous colostomy care during recovery.

Therapeutic GI procedures reflect the wide spectrum of systemic abnormalities. They may involve feeding a patient through a tube, teaching him how to use a gastrostomy feeding button, or minimizing his anxiety before abdominal surgery or his discomfort after it.

To carry out responsibilities like these successfully, you need to address the patient's emotional and physical needs. Where to place the incision or what colostomy to use has important emotional implications for him. Your knowledge of anatomy and physiology as well as your familiarity with surgical procedures will influence your care plan and, ultimately, how your patient responds. The best practices recommended by organizations, such as the Wound Ostomy and Continence Nurses Society **WOCN**, the American Society for Gastrointestinal Endoscopy **ASGE**, the American Academy of Clinical Toxicology **AACT**, American College of Gastroenterology **ACG**, and the American Gastroenterological Association **AGA**, will significantly enhance your ability to care for your patient. In addition to evidence-based **EB** practices and those stemming from standard principles of science **Science**, many of the best practices in this chapter also reflect mandates of the Centers for Disease Control and Prevention **CDC**, the U.S. Food and Drug Ad-

ministration **FDA**, the American Cancer Society **ACS**, the American Dental Association **ADA**, the American Hospital Association's Patient Care Partnership **PCP**, the American Society for Parenteral and Enteral Nutrition **ASPEN**, and the Joint Commission on Accreditation of Healthcare Organizations **JCAHO**. For points related to equipment, manufacturers **MFR** may recommend specific guidelines.

Patients undergoing certain GI procedures, especially those that are uncomfortable or embarrassing, require considerable emotional support. Helping such patients maintain their sense of dignity, while at the same time eliciting their cooperation, requires a skillful blend of compassion and judgment.

For many GI procedures, you'll need to work cooperatively with other staff members, including the pharmacist, physicians, laboratory personnel, diagnostic technicians, dietitians, and the case manager.

Colorectal cancer screening

In the United States and Europe, colorectal cancer is the second most common visceral neoplasm. Many studies show that screening reduces mortality from colorectal cancer.

Colorectal malignant tumors are almost always adenocarcinomas. About one-half of these are sessile lesions of the rectosigmoid area; the rest are polypoid lesions. Colorectal cancer tends to progress slowly and remains localized for a long time; consequently, it's potentially curable in 75% of patients if early diagnosis allows resection before nodal involvement. With early diagnosis, the overall 5-year survival rate is nearing 50%.

The exact cause of colorectal cancer is unknown, but studies showing concentrated occurrences in areas of higher economic development suggest a relationship to diets containing excess animal fat. For example, a diet including high beef consumption and little fiber has been implicated in increasing the risk of colorectal cancer. Other factors that increase the risk of developing colorectal cancer include:

- other disease of the digestive tract
- age (over 40)
- history of ulcerative colitis
- familial polyposis.

Signs and symptoms ACS

The early stages of colon cancer typically produce no symptoms — an individual can have colon cancer and not know it. That's why it's important to be tested regularly. Of course, colon cancer can sometimes produce symptoms:

- blood in or on stools
- a change in bowel habits — diarrhea or constipation
- stools that are thinner than usual
- unexplained pain, aches, or cramps in the abdomen
- frequent gas pains
- unexplained weight loss.

Screening tests CDC

Screening for colorectal cancer is the best intervention to prevent this disease. The Centers for Disease Control and Prevention's campaign to increase public awareness of colorectal cancer screening includes recommendations for the following tests (see *Recommendations for colorectal screening,* page 404)

- *Fecal occult blood test (FOBT)* — The FOBT is used to look for hidden blood in stools. The patient is instructed to place a small stool specimen on a card after three consecutive bowel movements. The card is returned to the physician, who tests to see whether blood is present in the stools. Although blood in the stools can be a sign of colon cancer, other causes exist, too, including eating meats before the test, bleeding from the stomach or other organs, and the presence of *Helicobacter pylori.*
- *Sigmoidoscopy* — A sigmoidoscopy is used to determine the presence of polyps in the lower part of the colon. A short, flexible tube is inserted into the anus and lower colon, allowing the physician to see any polyps. Typically, this test should be performed every 5 years for patients with no known risk factors. Pa-

tients at risk typically undergo colonoscopy, during which any polyps are removed.

- *Colonoscopy* — A colonoscopy is used to determine the presence of polyps in the entire colon. A long, flexible tube is inserted into the anus and upward into the colon, allowing the physician to see any polyps. Most polyps can be removed during the test. This test is usually done every 10 years for patients whose test results are negative, more frequently for patients whose results are positive.
- *Double contrast barium enema* — The double contrast barium enema is an X-ray of the lower GI tract. The patient is given an enema containing barium, a contrast material, after which the physician takes an X-ray. The presence of barium enables the physician to see the outline of the colon on the X-ray. This test is usually done every 5 to 10 years for patients whose test results are negative.
- *Virtual colonoscopy* — Research has shown that virtual colonoscopy is accurate compared to conventional colonoscopy for detection of polyps less than 6 mm in size with few false-positive results. EB1 It's a computed tomography procedure that can produce 3-dimensional images of the colon. Virtual colonoscopy is performed after a standard bowel preparation and air insufflation. The patient is exposed to some radiation but the procedure is noninvasive and has no known complications.

Equipment
Fecal occult blood test
Test kit • gloves • glass or porcelain plate • tongue blade or other wooden applicator

Sigmoidoscopy
Sigmoidoscope

Colonoscopy
Enemas (such as Fleet) • oral laxative (such as bisacodyl or magnesium citrate) • gloves

Double-contrast barium enema
Barium enema • linen-saver pad • bath blanket • bedpan or commode • disposable gloves • lubricant

Implementation

- Bowel preparation is essential for adequate visualization during sigmoidoscopy or colonoscopy. Different regimens may be used, but thorough emptying of

Recommendations for colorectal screening `ACS` `AGA` `ASGE` `EB2`

The guidelines below for colorectal screening are based on the recommendations of the U.S. Multisociety Task Force on Colorectal Cancer that includes the American College of Gastroenterology, the American Society for Gastrointestinal Endoscopy, the American Gastroenterological Association, the American College of Physicians/Society of Internal Medicine, and the American Cancer Society.

Risk category	Risk factors	Recommendations
Average risk	• Age 50 or older but asymptomatic and without any of the characteristics or situations indicating increased risk	• Fecal occult blood screening yearly • Flexible sigmoidoscopy every 5 years or colonoscopy every 10 years or double contrast barium enema every 5 years • Know that patients should be given a choice of the above tests to increase the likelihood that screening will occur
Increased risk	• Close relatives have had colorectal cancer or an adenomatous polyp • Two or more close relatives with colorectal cancer or adenomatous polyps diagnosed at younger than age 60 • Family history of familial adenomatous polyposis	• Same recommendations as above, but screening initiated when the patient is age 40 • Colonoscopy every 5 years, beginning at age 40, or 10 years younger than earliest diagnosis in the family, whichever occurs first • Genetic counseling or testing • In a gene carrier or in someone who hasn't had genetic testing, flexible sigmoidoscopy every 12 months, beginning at puberty
	• Family history of hereditary nonpolyposis colorectal cancer	• Genetic counseling or testing • Examination of the entire colon every 1 to 2 years, starting when the patient is age 20 to 30, or 10 years earlier than the youngest age of colon cancer diagnosis in the family
	• Personal history of adenomatous polyps	• Colonoscopy 3 years after initial examination, with subsequent examinations, depending on the types of polyps detected • In patients with 1 to 2 small adenomas (less than 1 cm), colonoscopy follow-up after 5 years of initial examination
	• Personal history of colorectal cancer	• Complete examination at initial diagnosis or 6 months after surgery; if normal, reexamination of colon in 3 years; if still normal, reexamination in 5 years
	• Inflammatory bowel disease	• Surveillance colonoscopy every 1 to 2 years, beginning after 8 years of disease in the patient with pancolitis and after 15 years in the patient with left colon involvement only

the left side of the colon (for sigmoidoscopy) or entire colon (for colonoscopy) should be achieved. In most patients, this involves administering two Fleet enemas on the morning of the examination. Better results are achieved by adding an oral cathartic. An oral regimen alone, such as two 10-mg bisacodyl tablets or one bottle of magnesium citrate, also provides good bowel preparation.

• For all of the tests, be sure to provide a detailed explanation to the patient about the test ordered and provide educational materials, if possible. For colonoscopy, obtain the necessary consent forms. `PCP`

• *Because these tests are intrusive and usually embarrassing for the patient,* the nurse should strive to maintain patient privacy and dignity.

- Provide privacy for the patient.
- Wash your hands and put on gloves. **CDC**

Fecal occult blood test

- If the patient is going to use a hemoccult slide test, instruct him to open the flap on the slide packet, use the wooden applicator to apply a thin stool specimen to the guaiac-impregnated filter paper to Box A, and apply a second specimen to the filter paper in Box B.
- If you're going to perform the test using the Hematest reagent tablet test, use a wooden applicator to smear a thin stool specimen on the filter paper supplied with the test kit. Or, after performing a digital rectal examination, wipe the finger used for the examination on a square of the filter paper, and place the filter paper on a glass plate.
- Remove a reagent tablet from the bottle and immediately replace the cap tightly. Place the tablet in the center of the stool smear.
- Add one drop of water to the tablet and allow it to soak in for 5 to 10 seconds. Add a second drop, letting it run from the tablet onto the specimen and filter paper. If necessary, tap the plate gently to dislodge any water from the top of the tablet.
- After 2 minutes, the filter paper will turn blue if the test is positive. Don't read the color that appears on the tablet itself or that develops on the filter paper after the 2-minute period.
- Note the results and discard the filter paper.
- Remove and discard your gloves and wash your hands thoroughly.
- Allow the specimens to dry for 3 to 5 minutes, then open the flap on the reverse side of the slide packet and place 2 drops of Hemoccult developing solution over each specimen smear on the paper. If the test is positive for occult blood, a blue reaction will appear in 30 to 60 seconds.
- Record the results and discard the slide package.

Sigmoidoscopy

TEACHING *Tell the patient that he'll experience moderate discomfort, gas, or cramping during the procedure as his lower colon is inflated with air.*

Explain that he also may have sigmoid discomfort after the procedure.

Colonoscopy

TEACHING *Inform the patient to expect moderate discomfort, gas, or cramping, during preparation and after the procedure is completed. Explain that the procedure is performed under sedation and will last 30 to 45 minutes. Tell the patient that he'll need to arrange for a ride home and shouldn't operate any heavy machinery for the next 24 hours.*

Barium enema

TEACHING *Before administering the enema, be sure to ask the patient about any allergy to barium. Explain the procedure.* **PCP**

Tell the patient that he may experience a sensation of fullness and gas or cramping while the solution is being administered.

- Help the patient into the left lateral position, with his right leg flexed.
- Place the linen-saver pad under the patient's buttocks and drape him with the bath blanket.
- Lubricate about 2″ (5 cm) of the enema's rectal tube if necessary. Run some solution through the connecting tube *to expel any air in the tubing,* then close the clamp.
- Put on gloves. **CDC**
- Lift the patient's upper buttock and insert the rectal tube smoothly and slowly about 3″ to 4″ (7.5 to 10 cm) into the rectum, directing it toward the umbilicus. If you feel resistance, ask the patient to take a deep breath; then, run a small amount of the solution through the tube *to relax the anal sphincter.* If you still feel resistance, notify the physician immediately; never force the tube to enter.
- With the tube in place, slowly administer the enema solution either by raising the solution container and opening the clamp, or by compressing the pliable container by hand.
- After instilling all of the solution or when the patient has the urge to defecate, close the clamp and remove the rectal tube.
- *To help the patient retain the enema as ordered,* keep him in the side-lying position as long as possible before assisting him onto the bedpan or commode.

Special considerations

- The most effective treatment for colorectal cancer is surgery to remove the tumor and the adjacent tissues as well as any lymph nodes that may contain cancer cells.

● The type of surgery depends on the location of the tumor.

● Chemotherapy and radiation therapy may be used for patients with metastasis, residual disease, or a recurrent inoperable tumor.

Nursing diagnoses

● Anxiety

Expected outcomes

The patient will:

● cope with GI procedure without severe signs of anxiety

● recognize need for preparation of GI procedure and complete it successfully.

Complications

Complications of sigmoidoscopy and colonoscopy include bleeding and adverse reactions to anesthesia.

Documentation

Be sure to document the date and time of the test and record the results, the patient's vital signs and, in colonoscopy, his response to anesthesia.

Supportive references

Johnson, B.A. "Flexible Sigmoidoscopy: Screening for Colorectal Cancer," *American Family Physician* 59(2):313-27, January 1999.

O'Hare, A. and Fenlon, H. "Virtual Colonoscopy in the Detection of Colonic Polyps and Neoplasms," *Best Practice Research. Clinical Gastroenterology.* 20(1):79-92, February 2006. **EB1**

Winawer, S., et al. "Colorectal Cancer Screening and Surveillance: Clinical Guidelines and Rationale — Update Based on New Evidence," *Gastroenterology* 124(2):544-60, February 2003. **EB2**

Colostomy and ileostomy care

A patient with an ascending or transverse colostomy or an ileostomy must wear an external pouch to collect emerging fecal matter, which will be watery or pasty. Besides collecting waste matter, the pouch helps to control odor and to protect the stoma and peristomal skin. Most disposable pouching systems can be used for 2 to 7 days; some models last even longer.

All pouching systems need to be changed immediately if a leak develops, and every pouch needs emptying when it's one-third to one-half full. The patient with an ileostomy may need to empty his pouch 4 or 5 times daily.

Naturally, the best time to change the pouching system is when the bowel is least active, usually between 2 and 4 hours after meals. After a few months, most patients can predict the best changing time.

The selection of a pouching system should take into consideration which system provides the best adhesive seal and skin protection for the individual patient. The type of pouch selected also depends on the stoma's location and structure, availability of supplies, wear time, consistency of effluent, personal preference, and finances.

Equipment

Pouching system ● stoma measuring guide ● stoma paste (if drainage is watery to pasty or stoma secretes excess mucus) ● scissors ● washcloth and towel ● closure clamp ● toilet or bedpan ● water or pouch cleaning solution ● gloves ● facial tissues ● optional: ostomy belt, paper tape, mild nonmoisturizing soap, skin shaving equipment, liquid skin sealant, and pouch deodorant

Pouching systems may be drainable or closed-bottomed, disposable or reusable, adhesive-backed, and one-piece or two-piece. (See *Comparing ostomy pouching systems.*)

Implementation

● Provide privacy and emotional support. **CDC**

Fitting the pouch and skin barrier

● For a pouch with an attached skin barrier, measure the stoma with the stoma measuring guide. Select the opening size that matches the stoma.

● For an adhesive-backed pouch with a separate skin barrier, measure the stoma with the measuring guide and select the opening that matches the stoma. Trace the selected size opening onto the paper back of the skin barrier's adhesive side. Cut out the opening. (If the pouch has precut openings, which can be handy for a round stoma, select an opening that's 1/8" larger than the stoma. If the pouch comes without an open-

Comparing ostomy pouching systems

Manufactured in many shapes and sizes, ostomy pouches are fashioned for comfort, safety, and easy application. For example, a disposable closed-end pouch may meet the needs of a patient who irrigates his ostomy, who wants added security, or who wants to discard the pouch after each bowel movement. Another patient may prefer a reusable, drainable pouch. Some commonly available pouches are described below.

Disposable pouches

The patient who must empty his pouch often (because of diarrhea or a new colostomy or ileostomy) may prefer a one-piece, drainable, disposable pouch with a closure clamp attached to a skin barrier (as shown below). These transparent or opaque, odor-proof, plastic pouches come with attached adhesive or karaya seals. Some pouches have microporous adhesive or belt tabs. The bottom opening allows for easy draining. This pouch may be used permanently or temporarily, until stoma size stabilizes.

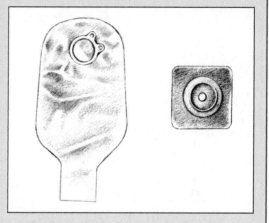

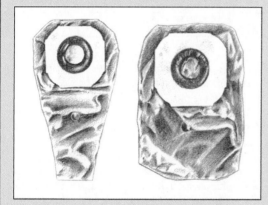

Also disposable and also made of transparent or opaque odor-proof plastic, a one-piece disposable closed-end pouch (as shown) may come in a kit with adhesive seal, belt tabs, skin barrier, or carbon filter for gas release. A patient with a regular bowel elimination pattern may choose this style for additional security and confidence.

A two-piece, drainable, disposable pouch with separate skin barrier (as shown) permits frequent changes and also minimizes skin breakdown. Also made of transparent or opaque odor-proof plastic, this style comes with belt tabs and usually snaps to the skin barrier with a flange mechanism.

Reusable pouches

Typically manufactured from sturdy, opaque, hypoallergenic plastic, the reusable pouch comes with a separate custom-made faceplate and O-ring, (as shown below). Some pouches have a pressure valve for releasing gas. The device has a 1- to 2-month life span, depending on how frequently the patient empties the pouch.

Reusable equipment may benefit a patient who needs a firm faceplate or who wishes to minimize cost. However, many reusable ostomy pouches aren't odor-proof.

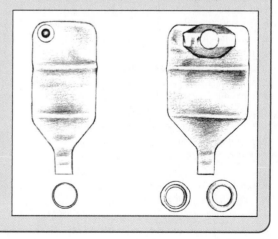

Applying a skin barrier and pouch

Fitting a skin barrier and ostomy pouch properly can be done in a few steps. Shown below is a two-piece pouching system with flanges, which is in common use.

1. Measure the stoma using a measuring guide.

2. Trace the appropriate circle carefully on the back of the skin barrier.

3. Cut the circular opening in the skin barrier. Bevel the edges to keep them from irritating the patient.

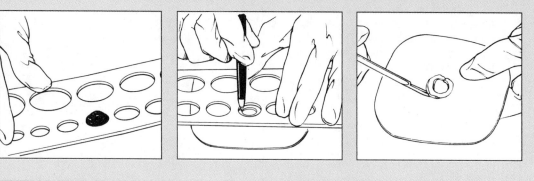

ing, cut the hole ⅛″ wider than the measured tracing.) The cut-to-fit system works best for an irregularly shaped stoma. **WOCN**

● For a two-piece pouching system with flanges, see *Applying a skin barrier and pouch.*

● Avoid fitting the pouch too tightly *because the stoma has no pain receptors. A constrictive opening could injure the stoma or skin tissue without the patient feeling warning discomfort.* Avoid cutting the opening too big *because this may expose the skin to fecal matter and moisture.* **WOCN**

● The patient with a descending or sigmoid colostomy who has formed stools and whose ostomy doesn't secrete much mucus may choose to wear only a pouch. In this case, make sure the pouch opening closely matches the stoma size.

● Between 6 weeks and 1 year after surgery, the stoma will shrink to its permanent size. At that point, pattern-making preparations will be unnecessary unless the patient gains weight, has additional surgery, or injures the stoma.

Applying or changing the pouch
● Collect all equipment.
● Provide privacy, wash your hands, and put on gloves. **CDC**

● Confirm the patient's identity using two patient identifiers according to facility policy. **JCAHO**
● Explain the procedure to the patient. As you perform each step, explain what you're doing and why *because the patient will eventually perform the procedure himself.* **PCP**
● Remove and discard the old pouch. Wipe the stoma and peristomal skin gently with a facial tissue.
● Carefully wash with mild soap and water and dry the peristomal skin by patting gently. Allow the skin to dry thoroughly. Inspect the peristomal skin and stoma. If necessary, shave surrounding hair (in a direction away from the stoma) *to promote a better seal and avoid skin irritation from hair pulling against the adhesive.* **WOCN**
● If applying a separate skin barrier, peel off the paper backing of the prepared skin barrier, center the barrier over the stoma, and press gently to ensure adhesion.
● You may want to outline the stoma on the back of the skin barrier (depending on the product) with a thin ring of stoma paste *to provide extra skin protection.* (Skip this step if the patient has a sigmoid or descending colostomy, formed stools, and little mucus.)

4. Remove the backing from the skin barrier and moisten it or apply barrier paste, as needed, along the edge of the circular opening.

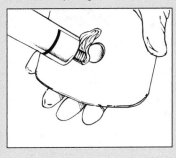

5. Center the skin barrier over the stoma, adhesive side down, and gently press it to the skin.

6. Gently press the pouch opening onto the ring until it snaps into place.

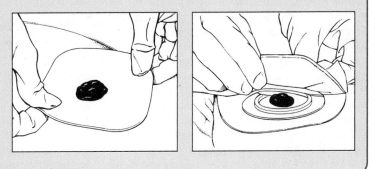

● Remove the paper backing from the adhesive side of the pouching system and center the pouch opening over the stoma. Press gently to secure.

● For a pouching system with flanges, align the lip of the pouch flange with the bottom edge of the skin barrier flange. Gently press around the circumference of the pouch flange, beginning at the bottom, until the pouch securely adheres to the barrier flange. (The pouch will click into its secured position.) Holding the barrier against the skin, gently pull on the pouch *to confirm the seal between flanges.*

● Encourage the patient to stay quietly in position for about 5 minutes *to improve adherence. The patient's body warmth also helps to improve adherence and soften a rigid skin barrier.* **Science** **WOCN**

● Attach an ostomy belt to further secure the pouch, if desired. (Some pouches have belt loops, and others have plastic adapters for belts.)

● Leave a bit of air in the pouch *to allow drainage to fall to the bottom.*

● Apply the closure clamp, if necessary.

● If desired, apply paper tape in a picture-frame fashion to the pouch edges *for additional security.*

Emptying the pouch **WOCN**
● Put on gloves. **CDC**

● Tilt the bottom of the pouch upward and remove the closure clamp.

● Turn up a cuff on the lower end of the pouch and allow it to drain into the toilet or bedpan.

● Wipe the bottom of the pouch and reapply the closure clamp.

● If desired, the bottom portion of the pouch can be rinsed with cool tap water. Don't aim water up near the top of the pouch *because this may loosen the seal on the skin.*

● A two-piece flanged system can also be emptied by unsnapping the pouch. Let the drainage flow into the toilet.

● Release flatus through the gas release valve if the pouch has one. Otherwise, release flatus by tilting the pouch bottom upward, releasing the clamp, and expelling the flatus. To release flatus from a flanged system, loosen the seal between the flanges. (Some pouches have gas release valves.)

● Never make a pinhole in a pouch to release gas. *This destroys the odor-proof seal.*

● Remove and discard gloves. **CDC**

Special considerations

● After performing and explaining the procedure to the patient, encourage the patient's increasing involvement in self-care.
● Use adhesive solvents and removers only after patch-testing the patient's skin *because some products may irritate the skin or produce hypersensitivity reactions.* Consider using a liquid skin sealant, if available, *to give skin tissue additional protection from drainage and adhesive irritants.*
● Remove the pouching system if the patient reports burning or itching beneath it or purulent drainage around the stoma. Notify the physician or therapist of any skin irritation, breakdown, rash, or unusual appearance of the stoma or peristomal area.
● Use commercial pouch deodorants if desired. However, most pouches are odor-free, and odor should be evident only when you empty the pouch or if it leaks. Before discharge, suggest that the patient avoid odor-causing foods, such as fish, eggs, onions, and garlic.
● If the patient wears a reusable pouching system, suggest that he obtain two or more systems *so he can wear one while the other dries after cleaning with soap and water or a commercially prepared cleaning solution.*

Nursing diagnoses

● Disturbed body image
● Effective therapeutic regimen management
● Impaired skin integrity

Expected outcomes

The patient will:
● acknowledge change in body image and communicate feelings about change
● recognize potential problems in the management of his stoma and identify needs
● explain skin care regimen.

Complications

● Failure to fit the pouch properly over the stoma or improper use of a belt can injure the stoma.
● Be alert for a possible allergic reaction to adhesives and other ostomy products.

Documentation

Record the date and time of the pouching system change and note the character of drainage, including color, amount, type, and consistency. Describe the appearance of the stoma and the peristomal skin. Document patient teaching. Describe the teaching content. Record the patient's response to self-care, and evaluate his learning progress.

Supportive references

Craven, R., and Hirnle, C. *Fundamentals of Nursing: Human Health and Function,* 4th ed. Philadelphia: Lippincott Williams & Wilkins, 2002.

Feeding tube insertion and removal

Inserting a feeding tube nasally or orally into the stomach or duodenum allows a patient who can't or won't eat to receive nourishment. The feeding tube also permits supplemental feedings in a patient who has very high nutritional requirements, such as an unconscious patient or one with extensive burns. Typically, the procedure is done by a nurse, as ordered. The preferred feeding tube route is nasal, but the oral route may be used for patients with such conditions as a head injury, deviated septum, or other nose injury.

The physician may order duodenal feeding when the patient can't tolerate gastric feeding or when he expects gastric feeding to produce aspiration. Absence of bowel sounds or possible intestinal obstruction contraindicates using a feeding tube. **AGA**

Feeding tubes differ somewhat from standard nasogastric tubes. Made of silicone, rubber, or polyurethane, feeding tubes have small diameters and great flexibility. This reduces oropharyngeal irritation, necrosis from pressure on the tracheoesophageal wall, distal esophageal irritation, and discomfort from swallowing. To facilitate passage, some feeding tubes are weighted with tungsten, and some need a guide wire to keep them from curling in the back of the throat.

These small-bore tubes usually have radiopaque markings and a water-activated coating, which provides a lubricated surface.

Equipment
For insertion

Feeding tube (#6 to #18 French, with or without guide) ● linen-saver pad ● gloves ● hypoallergenic tape ● water-soluble lubricant ● cotton-tipped applicators • skin preparation (such as compound benzoin tincture) • facial tissues • penlight • small cup of water with straw, or ice chips • emesis basin • 60-ml syringe • pH test strip • water

During use

Mouthwash or normal saline solution • toothbrush

For removal

Linen-saver pad • tube clamp

Preparation of equipment

● Have the proper size tube available. Usually, the physician orders the smallest-bore tube that will allow free passage of the liquid feeding formula.
● Read the instructions on the tubing package carefully *because tube characteristics vary according to the manufacturer.* (For example, some tubes have marks at the appropriate lengths for gastric, duodenal, and jejunal insertion.) **MFR**
● Examine the tube to make sure it's free from defects, such as cracks or rough or sharp edges.
● Next, run water through the tube. This checks for patency, activates the coating, and facilitates removal of the guide.

Implementation

● Confirm the patient's identity using two patient identifiers according to facility policy. **JCAHO**
● Explain the procedure to the patient and show him the tube *so he knows what to expect and can cooperate more fully.* **PCP**
● Provide privacy. Wash your hands and put on gloves. **CDC**
● Assist the patient into semi-Fowler's or high Fowler's position. **AGA**
● Place a linen-saver pad across the patient's chest *to protect him from spills.*
● *To determine the tube length needed to reach the stomach,* first extend the distal end of the tube from the tip of the patient's nose to his earlobe. Coil this portion of the tube around your fingers *so the end stays curved until you insert it.* Then extend the uncoiled portion from the earlobe to the xiphoid process. Use a small piece of hypoallergenic tape to mark the total length of the two portions.

Inserting the tube nasally

● Using the penlight, assess nasal patency. Inspect nasal passages for a deviated septum, polyps, or other obstructions. Occlude one nostril, then the other, *to determine which has the better airflow.* Assess the patient's history of nasal injury or surgery. **Science**
● Lubricate the curved tip of the tube (and the feeding tube guide, if appropriate) with a small amount of water-soluble lubricant *to ease insertion and prevent tissue injury.*
● Ask the patient to hold the emesis basin and facial tissues in case he needs them.
● *To advance the tube,* insert the curved, lubricated tip into the more patent nostril and direct it along the nasal passage toward the ear on the same side. When it passes the nasopharyngeal junction, turn the tube 180 degrees *to aim it downward into the esophagus.* Instruct the patient to lower his chin to his chest *to close the trachea.* Then give him a small cup of water with a straw or ice chips. Direct him to sip the water or suck on the ice and swallow frequently. *This will ease the tube's passage.* Advance the tube as he swallows. **Science**

Inserting the tube orally

● Have the patient lower his chin *to close his trachea,* and ask him to open his mouth.
● Place the tip of the tube at the back of the patient's tongue, give water, and instruct the patient to swallow, as above. Remind him to avoid clamping his teeth down on the tube. Advance the tube as he swallows.

Positioning the tube

● Keep passing the tube until the tape marking the appropriate length reaches the patient's nostril or lips. Tube placement should be confirmed by X-ray. **ASPEN**
● After confirming proper tube placement, remove the tape marking the tube length.
● Tape the tube to the patient's nose and remove the guide wire.
● *To advance the tube to the duodenum,* especially a tungsten-weighted tube, position the patient on his right side. *This lets gravity assist tube passage through the pylorus.* Move the tube forward 2″ to 3″ (5 to 7.5 cm) hourly until X-ray studies confirm duodenal placement. (An X-ray must confirm placement before feeding begins *because duodenal feeding can cause*

nausea and vomiting if accidentally delivered to the stomach.) **AGA** **EB**

● Apply a skin preparation to the patient's cheek before securing the tube with tape. *This helps the tube adhere to the skin and prevents irritation.*

● Tape the tube securely to the patient's cheek *to avoid excessive pressure on his nostrils.*

Removing the tube

● Protect the patient's chest with a linen-saver pad.

● Flush the tube with air, clamp or pinch it *to prevent fluid aspiration during withdrawal,* and withdraw it gently but quickly.

● Promptly cover and discard the used tube.

Special considerations

● Check gastric residual contents before each feeding. Feeding should be held if residual volumes are greater than 200 ml on two successive assessments. **ASPEN** Successful aspiration also confirms correct tube placement before feeding by testing the pH of the gastric aspirate. Attach the syringe to the tube and gently aspirate stomach contents. Examine the aspirate and place a small amount on the pH test strip. Probability of gastric placement is increased if the aspirate has a typical gastric fluid appearance (grassy-green, clear and colorless with mucus shreds, or brown) and the pH is less than or equal to 5.

● Ideally, tube tip placement should be confirmed by X-ray. **ASPEN**

● If no gastric secretions return, the tube may be in the esophagus. You'll need to advance the tube or reinsert it and check placement again before proceeding.

● Flush the feeding tube every 4 hours with up to 20 to 30 ml of normal saline solution or warm water *to maintain patency.* Retape the tube at least daily and as needed. Alternate taping the tube toward the inner and outer side of the nose *to avoid constant pressure on the same nasal area.* Inspect the skin for redness and breakdown. **AGA**

● Provide nasal hygiene daily using the cotton-tipped applicators and water-soluble lubricant *to remove crusted secretions.* Help the patient brush his teeth, gums, and tongue with mouthwash or saline solution at least twice daily.

● If the patient can't swallow the feeding tube, use a guide *to aid insertion.*

● Precise feeding-tube placement is especially important *because small-bore feeding tubes may slide into the trachea without causing immediate signs or symptoms of respiratory distress, such as coughing, choking, gasping, or cyanosis.* However, the patient will usually cough if the tube enters the larynx. To make sure the tube clears the larynx, ask the patient to speak. If he can't, the tube is in the larynx. Withdraw the tube immediately and reinsert.

● When aspirating gastric contents to check tube placement, pull gently on the syringe plunger *to prevent trauma to the stomach lining or bowel.* If you meet resistance during aspiration, stop the procedure *because resistance may result simply from the tube lying against the stomach wall.* If the tube coils above the stomach, you'll be unable to aspirate stomach contents. To rectify this, change the patient's position or withdraw the tube a few inches, readvance it, and try to aspirate again. If the tube was inserted with a guide wire, don't use the guide wire to reposition the tube. The physician may do so, using fluoroscopic guidance.

TEACHING *If your patient will use a feeding tube at home, make appropriate home care nursing referrals and teach the patient and caregivers how to use and care for a feeding tube. Teach them how to obtain equipment, insert and remove the tube, prepare and store feeding formula, and solve problems with tube position and patency.*

Nursing diagnoses

● Imbalanced nutrition: Less than body requirements

Expected outcomes

The patient will:

● remain at or above specified weight

● not develop adverse reactions from feedings such as aspiration, diarrhea, or hyperglycemia.

Complications

Prolonged intubation may lead to skin erosion at the nostril, sinusitis, esophagitis, esophagotracheal fistula, gastric ulceration, and pulmonary and oral infection. (See *Managing tube feeding problems.*)

Documentation

For tube insertion, record the date, time, tube type and size, insertion site, area of placement, confirma-

Managing tube feeding problems

Complication	Interventions
Aspiration of gastric secretions	• Discontinue feeding immediately. • Perform tracheal suction of aspirated contents if possible. • Notify the physician. Prophylactic antibiotics and chest physiotherapy may be ordered. • Check tube placement before feeding *to prevent complication.*
Tube obstruction	• Flush the tube with warm water. If necessary, replace the tube. • Flush the tube with 50 ml of water after each feeding *to remove excess sticky formula, which could occlude the tube.* • When possible, use liquid forms of medications. Otherwise, crush medications well, if not contraindicated.
Oral, nasal, or pharyngeal irritation or necrosis	• Provide frequent oral hygiene using mouthwash or sponge-tipped swabs. Use petroleum jelly on cracked lips. • Change the tube's position. If necessary, replace the tube.
Vomiting, bloating, diarrhea, or cramps	• Reduce the flow rate. • Verify tube placement. • Administer metoclopramide (Reglan) *to increase GI motility.* • Warm the formula *to prevent GI distress.* • For 30 minutes after feeding, position the patient on his right side with his head elevated *to facilitate gastric emptying.* • Notify the physician. He may want to reduce the amount of formula being given during each feeding.
Constipation	• Provide additional fluids if the patient can tolerate them. • Have the patient participate in an exercise program if possible. • Administer a bulk-forming laxative. • Review medications. Discontinue medications that have a tendency to cause constipation. • Increase fruit, vegetable, or sugar content of the feeding.
Electrolyte imbalance	• Monitor serum electrolyte levels. • Notify the physician. He may want to adjust the formula content to correct the deficiency.
Hyperglycemia	• Monitor blood glucose levels. • Notify the physician of elevated levels. • Administer insulin if ordered. • The physician may adjust the sugar content of the formula.

tion of proper placement. Record the name of the person performing the procedure. For tube removal, record the date and time and the patient's tolerance of the procedure.

Supportive references

American Society for Parenteral and Enteral Nutrition. "Access for Administration of Nutrition Support," *Journal of Parenteral Enteral Nutrition* 26(Suppl 1):33SA-41SA, January-February 2002. Available at: *www.guideline.gov.*

Bowers, S. "All About Tubes: Your Guide to Enteral Feeding Devices," *Nursing2000* 30(12):41-47, December 2000. **EB**

Craven, R., and Hirnle, C. *Fundamentals of Nursing: Human Health and Function,* 4th ed. Philadelphia: Lippincott Williams & Wilkins, 2002.

Using wide-bore gastric tubes

If you need to deliver a large volume of fluid rapidly through a gastric tube (when irrigating the stomach of a patient with profuse gastric bleeding or poisoning, for example), a wide-bore gastric tube usually serves best. Typically inserted orally, these tubes remain in place only long enough to complete the lavage and evacuate stomach contents.

Ewald tube
In an emergency, using the Ewald tube, a single-lumen tube with several openings at the distal end, allows you to aspirate large amounts of gastric contents quickly.

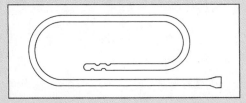

Lavacuator tube
The lavacuator tube has two lumens. Use the larger lumen for evacuating gastric contents; the smaller, for instilling an irrigant.

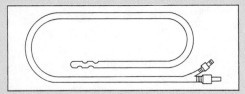

Edlich tube
The Edlich tube is a single-lumen tube that has four openings near the closed distal tip. A funnel or syringe may be connected at the proximal end. Like the Ewald tube, the Edlich tube lets you withdraw large quantities of gastric contents quickly.

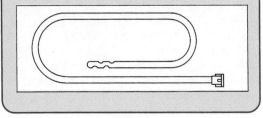

Guenter, P., and Silkroski, M. *Tube Feeding: Practical Guidelines and Nursing Protocols.* Gaithersburg, Md.: Aspen Pubs., Inc., 2001.

Stone, S.J., et al. "Bedside Placement of Postpyloric Feeding Tubes," *AACN Clinical Issues* 11(4):517-30, November 2000.

Gastric lavage

After poisoning or a drug overdose, especially in patients who have central nervous system depression or an inadequate gag reflex, gastric lavage flushes the stomach and removes ingested substances through a gastric lavage tube. The procedure is also used to empty the stomach in preparation for endoscopic examination. For patients with gastric or esophageal bleeding, lavage with tepid or iced water or normal saline solution may be used to stop bleeding. However, some controversy exists over the effectiveness of iced lavage for this purpose.

According to the American Academy of Clinical Toxicology, gastric lavage shouldn't be used routinely in the management of poisoned patients. In experimental studies, the amount of marker removed by gastric lavage was highly variable and diminished with time, indicating that the method doesn't improve clinical outcome. In fact, it's believed that in many cases gastric lavage may cause or increase morbidity. Gastric lavage shouldn't be used unless the patient has ingested a life-threatening amount of the poison and lavage can occur within 60 minutes of ingestion. Even in this situation, clinical improvement hasn't been proved in controlled studies. **AACT**

CONTROVERSIAL ISSUE *Most experts question the effectiveness of using an iced irrigant for gastric lavage to treat GI bleeding because iced irrigating solutions stimulate the vagus nerve, which triggers increased hydrochloric acid secretion. In turn, this stimulates gastric motility, which can irritate the bleeding site.*

Most physicians prefer to use unchilled normal saline solution (which may prevent rapid electrolyte loss) or even water if the patient must avoid sodium. They point out that no research exists to support the use of iced irrigant to stop acute GI bleeding.

Gastric lavage can be continuous or intermittent. Typically, this procedure is done in the emergency department or intensive care unit by a physician, gastroenterologist, or nurse; a wide-bore lavage tube is almost always inserted by a gastroenterologist.

Gastric lavage is contraindicated after ingestion of a corrosive substance (such as lye, petroleum distillates, ammonia, alkalis, or mineral acids) *because the lavage tube may perforate the already compromised esophagus.*

Equipment

Lavage setup (two graduated containers for drainage, three pieces of large-lumen rubber tubing, Y-connector, and a clamp or hemostat) • 2 to 3 L of normal saline solution, tap water, or appropriate antidote as ordered • I.V. pole • basin of ice, if ordered • Ewald tube or any large-lumen gastric tube, typically #36 to #40 French (see *Using wide-bore gastric tubes*) • water-soluble lubricant or anesthetic ointment • stethoscope • $\frac{1}{2}$" hypoallergenic tape • 50-ml bulb or catheter-tip syringe • gloves • face shield • linen-saver pad or towel • Yankauer or tonsil-tip suction device • suction apparatus • labeled specimen container • laboratory request form • norepinephrine (Levophed) • optional: patient restraints, charcoal tablets

A prepackaged, syringe-type irrigation kit may be used for intermittent lavage. For poisoning or a drug overdose, however, the continuous lavage setup may be more appropriate to use because it's a faster and more effective means of diluting and removing the harmful substance.

Preparation of equipment

• Set up the lavage equipment. (See *Preparing for gastric lavage.*)
• If iced lavage is ordered, chill the desired irrigant (water or normal saline solution) in a basin of ice.
• Lubricate the end of the lavage tube with the water-soluble lubricant or anesthetic ointment.

Implementation

ALERT *Correct lavage tube placement is essential for patient safety because accidental misplacement (in the lungs, for example) followed by lavage can be fatal.*
• Explain the procedure to the patient, provide privacy, and wash your hands. **CDC** **PCP**
• Put on gloves and a face shield. **CDC**
• Drape the towel or linen-saver pad over the patient's chest *to protect him from spills.*

Preparing for gastric lavage

Prepare the lavage setup as follows:
• Connect one of the three pieces of the large-lumen tubing to the irrigant container.
• Insert the Y-connector stem in the other end of the tubing.
• Connect the remaining two pieces of tubing to the free ends of the Y-connector.
• Place the unattached end of one of the tubes into one of the drainage containers. (Later, you'll connect the other piece of tubing to the patient's gastric tube.)
• Clamp the tube leading to the irrigant.
• Suspend the entire setup from the I.V. pole, hanging the irrigant container at the highest level.

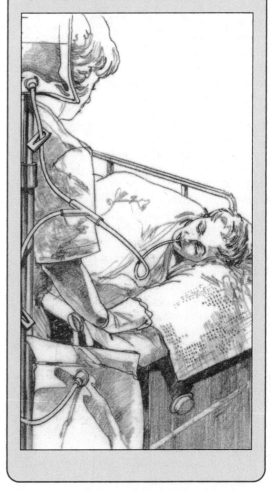

- The physician inserts the lavage tube nasally or orally and advances it slowly and gently *because forceful insertion may injure tissues and cause epistaxis.* He checks the tube's placement by injecting about 30 cc of air into the tube with the bulb syringe and then auscultating the patient's abdomen with a stethoscope. If the tube is in place, he'll hear the sound of air entering the stomach. **Science**
- *Because the patient may vomit when the lavage tube reaches the posterior pharynx during insertion,* be prepared to suction the airway immediately with either a Yankauer or a tonsil-tip suction device.
- After the lavage tube passes the posterior pharynx, assist the patient into Trendelenburg's position and turn him toward his left side in a three-quarter prone posture. *This position minimizes passage of gastric contents into the duodenum and may prevent the patient from aspirating vomitus.* **Science**
- After securing the lavage tube nasally or orally with tape and making sure the irrigant inflow tube on the lavage setup is clamped, connect the unattached end of this tube to the lavage tube. Check tube placement by injecting air into the tube while listening over the stomach or by testing pH of the aspirate. **AACT** Allow the stomach contents to empty into the drainage container before instilling any irrigant. *This confirms proper tube placement and decreases the risk of overfilling the stomach with irrigant and inducing vomiting.* If you're using a syringe irrigation set, aspirate stomach contents with a 50-ml bulb or catheter-tip syringe before instilling the irrigant. **Science**
- After you confirm proper tube placement, begin gastric lavage by instilling about 200 to 300 ml of fluid for an adult. Water or normal saline solution should be used, preferably warmed to 68.4° F (20.2° C) to avoid the risk of hypothermia. **AACT**
- Clamp the inflow tube and unclamp the outflow tube *to allow the irrigant to flow out.* If you're using the syringe irrigation kit, aspirate the irrigant with the syringe and empty it into a calibrated container. Measure the outflow amount to make sure it equals at least the amount of irrigant you instilled. *This prevents accidental stomach distention and vomiting.* If the drainage amount falls significantly short of the instilled amount, reposition the tube until sufficient solution flows out. Gently massage the abdomen over the stomach *to promote outflow.*
- Repeat the inflow-outflow cycle until returned fluids appear clear. *This signals that the stomach no longer holds harmful substances or that bleeding has stopped.*
- Assess the patient's vital signs, urine output, and level of consciousness (LOC) every 15 minutes. Notify the physician of any changes.
- If ordered, remove the lavage tube.

Special considerations

- *To control GI bleeding,* the physician may order continuous irrigation of the stomach with an irrigant and a vasoconstrictor such as norepinephrine. After the stomach absorbs norepinephrine, the portal system delivers the drug directly to the liver, where it's metabolized. *This prevents the drug from circulating systemically and initiating a hypertensive response.* Or the physician may direct you to clamp the outflow tube for a prescribed period after instilling the irrigant and the vasoconstrictive medication and before withdrawing it. *This allows the mucosa time to absorb the drug.*
- Never leave a patient alone during gastric lavage. Observe continuously for any changes in LOC, and monitor vital signs frequently *because the natural vagal response to intubation can depress the patient's heart rate.*
- If you need to restrain the patient, secure restraints on the same side of the bed or stretcher *so you can free him quickly without moving to the other side of the bed.*
- Remember also to keep tracheal suctioning equipment nearby and watch closely for airway obstruction caused by vomiting or excess oral secretions. Throughout gastric lavage, you may need to suction the oral cavity frequently *to ensure an open airway and prevent aspiration.* For the same reasons, and if he doesn't exhibit an adequate gag reflex, the patient may require an endotracheal tube before the procedure.
- When aspirating the stomach for ingested poisons or drugs, save the contents in a labeled container to send to the laboratory for analysis along with a laboratory request form. If ordered, after lavage to remove poisons or drugs, mix charcoal tablets with the irrigant (water or normal saline solution) and administer the mixture through the nasogastric (NG) tube. The charcoal will absorb remaining toxic substances. The tube may be clamped temporarily, allowed to drain via gravity, attached to intermittent suction, or removed.

● When performing gastric lavage to stop bleeding, keep precise intake and output records *to determine the amount of bleeding.* When large volumes of fluid are instilled and withdrawn, serum electrolyte and arterial blood gas levels may be measured during or at the end of lavage.

Nursing diagnoses
● Ineffective tissue perfusion: GI
● Risk for aspiration

Expected outcomes
The patient will:
● maintain normal intake and output
● maintain laboratory values and vital signs within normal limits
● not aspirate stomach contents
● have respiratory secretions that remain clear and odorless.

Complications
● Vomiting and subsequent aspiration, the most common complication of gastric lavage, typically occurs in a groggy patient.
● Bradyarrhythmias may also occur.
● After iced lavage especially, the patient's body temperature may drop, thereby triggering cardiac arrhythmias.

Documentation
Record the date and time of lavage, the size and type of NG tube used, the volume and type of irrigant, and the amount of drained gastric contents. Record this information on the intake and output record sheet, and include your observations, including the color and consistency of drainage. Keep precise records of the patient's vital signs and LOC, any drugs instilled through the tube, the time the tube was removed, and how well the patient tolerated the procedure.

Supportive references
American Academy of Clinical Toxicology, European Association of Poison Centres and Clinical Toxicologists. "Position paper: Gastric Lavage," *Journal of Toxicology, Clinical Toxicology* 42(7):933-43, July 2004.

Blazys, D. "Tips on Gastric Lavage," *Journal of Emergency Nursing* 25(3):200, June 1999.

Blazys, D. "Use of Lavage in Treating Overdose," *Journal of Emergency Nursing* 26(4):394-98, August 2000.

Clegg, T., and Hope, K. "The First Line Response for People Who Self-Poison: Exploring the Options for Gut Decontamination," *Journal of Advanced Nursing* 30(6):1360-367, December 1999.

Craven, R., and Hirnle, C. *Fundamentals of Nursing: Human Health and Function,* 4th ed. Philadelphia: Lippincott Williams & Wilkins, 2002.

Gastrostomy feeding button care

A gastrostomy feeding button serves as an alternative feeding device for an ambulatory patient who's receiving long-term enteral feedings.

Approved by the U.S. Food and Drug Administration for 6-month implantation, feeding buttons can be used to replace gastrostomy tubes if necessary. **FDA**

The button has a mushroom dome at one end and two wing tabs and a flexible safety plug at the other. When inserted into an established stoma, the button lies almost flush with the skin, with only the top of the safety plug visible.

The button can usually be inserted into a stoma in less than 15 minutes. Besides its cosmetic appeal, the device is easily maintained, reduces skin irritation and breakdown, and is less likely to become dislodged or migrate than an ordinary feeding tube. A one-way, antireflux valve mounted just inside the mushroom dome prevents accidental leakage of gastric contents. The device usually requires replacement after 3 to 4 months, typically because the antireflux valve wears out.

Equipment
Gastrostomy feeding button of the correct size (all three sizes, if the correct one isn't known) ● obturator ● water-soluble lubricant ● gloves ● feeding accessories, including adapter, feeding catheter, food syringe or bag, and formula ● catheter clamp ● cleaning equipment, including water, a syringe, cotton-tipped applicator, pipe cleaner, and mild soap or povidone-iodine solution ● optional: I.V. pole, pump to provide continuous infusion over several hours

Implementation
● Explain the insertion, reinsertion, and feeding procedure to the patient. Tell him the physician will perform the initial insertion. **PCP**

Reinserting a gastrostomy feeding button

If your patient's gastrostomy feeding button pops out (with coughing, for instance), either you or he will need to reinsert the device. Here are some steps to follow.

Prepare the equipment
Collect the feeding button, an obturator, and water-soluble lubricant. If the button will be reinserted, wash it with soap and water and rinse it thoroughly.

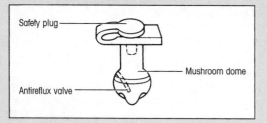

Safety plug

Mushroom dome

Antireflux valve

Insert the button
● Check the depth of the patient's stoma to make sure you have a feeding button of the correct size. Then clean around the stoma.
● Lubricate the obturator with a water-soluble lubricant, and distend the button several times *to ensure patency of the antireflux valve within the button.*
● Lubricate the mushroom dome and the stoma. Gently push the button through the stoma into the stomach.

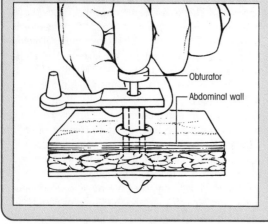

Obturator

Abdominal wall

● Remove the obturator by gently rotating it as you withdraw it *to keep the antireflux valve from adhering to it.* If the valve sticks nonetheless, gently push the obturator back into the button until the valve closes.
● After removing the obturator, make sure the valve is closed. Then close the flexible safety plug, which should be relatively flush with the skin surface.

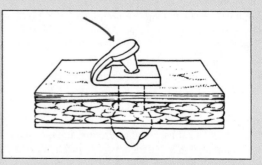

● If you need to administer a feeding right away, open the safety plug and attach the feeding adapter and feeding tube. Deliver the feeding as ordered.

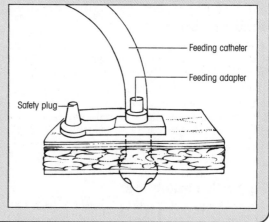

Feeding catheter

Feeding adapter

Safety plug

● Wash your hands, and put on gloves. (See *Reinserting a gastrostomy feeding button.*) **CDC**
● Confirm the patient's identity using two patient identifiers according to facility policy. **JCAHO**
● Elevate the head of the bed 30 to 45 degrees.

● Check for residual with the syringe. If greater than 50 to 100 cc, report to the health care provider and hold feeding until reassessment.
● Attach the adapter and feeding catheter to the syringe or feeding bag. Clamp the catheter and fill the

syringe or bag and catheter with formula. Refill the syringe before it's empty. *These steps prevent air from entering the stomach and distending the abdomen.* `Science`

● Open the safety plug and attach the adapter and feeding catheter to the button. Elevate the syringe or feeding bag above stomach level, and gravity-feed the formula for 15 to 30 minutes, varying the height as needed *to alter the flow rate.* Use a pump for continuous infusion or for feedings lasting several hours. `AGA`

● After the feeding, flush the button with 10 ml of water and clean the inside of the feeding catheter with a cotton-tipped applicator and water *to preserve patency and to dislodge formula or food particles,* and lower the syringe or bag below stomach level *to allow burping.* Remove the adapter and feeding catheter. The antireflux valve should prevent gastric reflux. Then snap the safety plug in place *to keep the lumen clean and prevent leakage if the antireflux valve fails.* If the patient feels nauseated or vomits after the feeding, vent the button with the adapter and feeding catheter *to control emesis.* `Science`

● Maintain head of bed elevation of 30 to 45 degrees for at least 1 hour after feeding.

● Wash the catheter and syringe or feeding bag in warm soapy water and rinse thoroughly. Clean the catheter and adapter with a pipe cleaner. Rinse well before using for the next feeding. Soak the equipment once per week according to manufacturer's recommendations. `MFR`

Special considerations

● If the button pops out while feeding, reinsert it, estimate the formula already delivered, and resume feeding.

● Once daily, clean the peristomal skin with mild soap and water or povidone-iodine, and let the skin air-dry for 20 minutes *to avoid skin irritation.* Clean the site whenever spillage from the feeding bag occurs.

● As the patient's weight or body mass index increases, monitor the site for embedded bumper (external). Report skin irritation and increased tension between exit site and bumper to the physician.

🔳 **TEACHING** *Before discharge, make sure the patient can insert and care for the gastrostomy feeding button. If necessary, teach him or a family member how to reinsert the button by first practicing on a model. Offer written instructions and answer his questions on obtaining replacement supplies.*

Nursing diagnoses

● Imbalanced nutrition: Less than body requirements
● Impaired skin integrity

Expected outcomes

The patient will:
● maintain adequate nutrition and fluid needs as measured by weight and laboratory tests
● maintain skin integrity and remain free from infection at the site.

Documentation

Record feeding time and duration, amount and type of feeding formula used, and patient tolerance. Maintain intake and output records as necessary. Note the appearance of the stoma and surrounding skin.

Supportive references

American Society for Gastrointestinal Endoscopy. "Percutaneous Endoscopic Gastrostomy (PEG)." Available at: *www.askasge.org/pages/ brochures/peg.cfm.*

Craven, R., and Hirnle, C. *Fundamentals of Nursing: Human Health and Function,* 4th ed. Philadelphia: Lippincott Williams & Wilkins, 2002.

Guenter, P., and Silkroski, M. *Tube Feeding: Practical Guidelines and Nursing Protocols.* Gaithersburg, Md.: Aspen Pubs., Inc., 2001.

Shattner, M., et al. "Long-term Enteral Nutrition Facilitates Optimization of Body Weight," *Journal of Parenteral and Enteral Nutrition* 29(3):198-203, March 2005.

Mouth care

Given in the morning, at bedtime, or after meals, mouth care entails brushing and flossing the teeth and inspecting the mouth. It removes soft plaque deposits and calculus from the teeth, cleans and massages the gums, reduces mouth odor, and helps prevent infection. By freshening the patient's mouth, mouth care also enhances appreciation of food, thereby aiding appetite and nutrition.

Although the ambulatory patient can usually perform mouth care alone, the bedridden patient may re-

Using a pediatric toothbrush for oral care

The foam stick applicator commonly used to provide oral care has been proven to be ineffective in removing particles from teeth. Research has shown that only 20% of patients prefer the foam sticks.

A soft-bristle or pediatric-sized toothbrush should be used to provide oral care, and tap water should be used to rinse the mouth. Research has shown that the traditional lemon-glycerin swab used for oral care dries the mouth and also contributes to tooth erosion.

quire partial or full assistance. The comatose or intubated patient requires use of suction equipment *to prevent aspiration during oral care.*

✓ **CLINICAL IMPACT** *Frequent mouth care is key to the prevention of tooth and gum disease in seriously ill patients. Mouth care should be performed every 2 to 6 hours. If the patient is on nasal oxygen, fluid restriction, nothing by mouth status, or mouth breathing, mouth care should be given more frequently.*

Equipment

Towel or facial tissues • emesis basin • trash bag • mouthwash • soft toothbrush and toothpaste containing fluoride • pitcher and glass • drinking straw • dental floss • gloves • dental floss holder if available • small mirror if necessary • optional: oral irrigating device

Comatose or debilitated patient (as needed)

Linen-saver pad • bite-block • gloves • petroleum jelly • mineral oil • sponge-tipped mouth swab • oral suction equipment or gauze pads • soft toothbrush • tongue blade, 4″ × 4″ gauze pads, adhesive tape (see *Using a pediatric toothbrush for oral care*)

Preparation of equipment

● Fill a pitcher with water and bring it and other equipment to the patient's bedside.
● If you'll be using oral suction equipment, connect the tubing to the suction bottle and suction catheter, insert the plug into an outlet, and check for correct operation.
● If necessary, devise a bite-block to protect yourself from being bitten during the procedure.
● Wrap a gauze pad over the end of a tongue blade, fold the edge in, and secure it with adhesive tape.

Implementation

● Confirm the patient's identity using two patient identifiers according to facility policy. **JCAHO**
● Wash your hands thoroughly, put on gloves, explain the procedure to the patient, and provide privacy. **CDC** **PCP**

Supervising mouth care

● For the bedridden patient capable of self-care, encourage him to perform his own mouth care.
● If allowed, place the patient in Fowler's position. Place the overbed table in front of the patient, and arrange the equipment on it. Open the table and set up the built-in mirror, if available, or position a small mirror on the table.
● Drape a towel over the patient's chest *to protect his gown.* Instruct him to floss his teeth while looking into the mirror.
● Observe the patient *to make sure he's flossing correctly,* and correct him if necessary. Tell him to wrap the floss around the second or third fingers of both hands. Starting with his back teeth and without injuring the gums, he should insert the floss as far as possible into the space between each pair of teeth. Then he should clean the surfaces of adjacent teeth by pulling the floss up and down against the side of each tooth. After the patient flosses a pair of teeth, remind him to use a clean 1″ (2.5-cm) section of floss for the next pair. **ADA**
● After the patient flosses, mix mouthwash and water in a glass, place a straw in the glass, and position the emesis basin nearby. Then instruct the patient to brush his teeth and gums while looking into the mirror. Encourage him to rinse frequently during brushing, and provide facial tissues for him to wipe his mouth.

Performing mouth care

● For the comatose patient or the conscious patient incapable of self-care, you'll perform mouth care. If the patient wears dentures, clean them thoroughly. (See *Dealing with dentures.*) Some patients may ben-

Dealing with dentures

Dentures are prostheses, made of acrylic resins, vinyl composites, or both, that replace some or all of the patient's natural teeth. Dentures require proper care to remove soft plaque deposits and calculus and to reduce mouth odor. Such care involves removing and rinsing dentures after meals, daily brushing and removal of tenacious deposits, and soaking in a commercial denture cleaner. Dentures must be removed from the comatose or presurgical patient to prevent possible airway obstruction.

Equipment and preparation

Start by assembling the following equipment at the patient's bedside: emesis basin • labeled denture cup • toothbrush or denture brush • gloves • toothpaste • commercial denture cleaner • paper towel • cotton-tipped mouth swab • mouthwash • gauze • optional: adhesive denture liner.

Wash your hands, and put on gloves. **CDC**

Removing dentures

● To remove a full upper denture, grasp the front and palatal surfaces of the denture with your thumb and forefinger. Position the index finger of your opposite hand over the upper border of the denture, and press *to break the seal between denture and palate.* Grasp the denture with gauze *because saliva can make it slippery.*
● To remove a full lower denture, grasp the front and lingual surfaces of the denture with your thumb and index finger, and gently lift up.
● To remove partial dentures, first ask the patient or a caregiver how the prosthesis is retained and how to remove it. If the partial denture is held in place with clips or snaps, then exert equal pressure on the border of each side of the denture. Avoid lifting the clasps, *which easily bend or break.*

Oral and denture care

● After removing dentures, place them in a properly labeled denture cup. Add warm water and a commercial denture cleaner *to remove stains and hardened deposits.* Follow package directions. Avoid soaking dentures in mouthwash containing alcohol *because it may damage a soft liner.*
● Instruct the patient to rinse with mouthwash *to remove food particles and reduce mouth odor.* Then stroke the palate, buccal surfaces, gums, and tongue with a soft toothbrush or sponge-tipped mouth swab or soft washcloth *to clean the mucosa and stimulate circulation.* Inspect for irritated areas or sores *because they may indicate a poorly fitting denture.*
● Carry the denture cup, emesis basin, toothbrush, and toothpaste to the sink. After lining the basin with a paper towel, fill it with water *to cushion the dentures in case you drop them.* Hold the dentures over the basin, wet them with warm water, and apply toothpaste to a denture brush or long-bristled toothbrush. Clean the dentures using only moderate pressure *to prevent scratches* and warm water *to prevent distortion.*
● Clean the denture cup, and place the dentures in it. Rinse the brush, and clean and dry the emesis basin. Return all equipment to the patient's bedside stand.

Wearing dentures

● If the patient desires, apply adhesive liner to the dentures. Moisten them with water, if necessary, *to reduce friction and ease insertion.*
● Encourage the patient to wear his dentures *to enhance his appearance (thereby contributing to his well-being), facilitate eating and speaking, and prevent changes in the gum line that may affect denture fit.*

---

efit from using an oral irrigating device such as a Water Pik. (See *Using an oral irrigation device,* page 422.)
● Raise the bed to a comfortable working height *to prevent back strain.* Then lower the head of the bed, and position the patient on his side, with his face extended over the edge of the pillow *to facilitate drainage and prevent fluid aspiration.* **Science**

● Arrange the equipment on the overbed table or bedside stand, including the oral suction equipment, if necessary. Turn on the machine. If a suction machine isn't available, wipe the inside of the patient's mouth frequently with a moist, sponge-tipped swab.
● Place a linen-saver pad under the patient's chin and an emesis basin near his cheek *to absorb or catch drainage.*

Using an oral irrigation device

An oral irrigating device, such as the Water Pik, directs a pulsating jet of water around the teeth to massage gums and remove food particles and debris. It's especially useful for cleaning areas missed by brushing, such as around bridgework, crowns, and dental wires. Because this device enhances oral hygiene, it benefits patients undergoing head and neck irradiation, which can damage teeth and cause severe caries. The device also maintains oral hygiene in a patient with a fractured jaw or with mouth injuries that limit standard mouth care.

Equipment and preparation

To use the device, first assemble the following equipment: oral irrigating device • towel • emesis basin • gloves • pharyngeal suction apparatus • salt solution or mouthwash, if ordered • soap.

Wash your hands, and put on gloves. **CDC**

Implementation

● Turn the patient to his side *to prevent aspiration of water.* Then place a towel under his chin and an emesis basin next to his cheek *to absorb or catch drainage.*
● Insert the oral irrigating device's plug into a nearby electrical outlet.
● Remove the device's cover, turn it upside down, and fill it with lukewarm water or with a mouthwash or salt solution, as ordered. When using a salt solution, dissolve the salt beforehand in a separate container, and then pour the solution into the cover.
● Secure the cover to the base of the device. Remove the water hose handle from the base, and snap the jet tip into place. If necessary, wet the grooved end of the tip *to ease insertion.* Adjust the pressure dial to the setting

most comfortable for the patient. If his gums are tender and prone to bleed, choose a low setting.
● Adjust the knurled knob on the handle *to direct the water jet,* place the jet tip in the patient's mouth, and turn on the device. Instruct the alert patient to keep his lips partially closed *to avoid spraying water.*
● Direct the water at a right angle to the gum line of each tooth and between teeth (as shown below). Avoid directing water under the patient's tongue *because this may injure sensitive tissue*
● After irrigating each tooth, pause briefly and instruct the patient to expectorate the water or solution into the

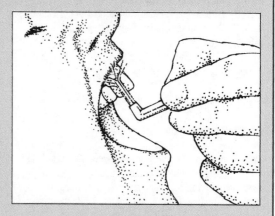

emesis basin. If he can't do so, suction it from the sides of the mouth with the pharyngeal suction apparatus. After irrigating all teeth, turn off the device and remove the jet tip from the patient's mouth.
● Empty the remaining water or solution from the cover, remove the jet tip from the handle, and return the handle to the base. Clean the jet tip with soap and water, rinse the cover, and dry them both and return them to storage.

● Lubricate the patient's lips with petroleum jelly *to prevent dryness and cracking.* Reapply lubricant, as needed, during oral care. **Science**
● If necessary, insert the bite-block *to hold the patient's mouth open during oral care.*
● Using a dental floss holder, hold the floss against each tooth and direct it as close to the gum as possible without injuring the sensitive tissues around the tooth.

● After flossing the patient's teeth, mix mouthwash and water in a glass and place the straw in it.
● Wet the toothbrush with water. If necessary, use hot water *to soften the bristles.* Apply toothpaste.
● Brush the patient's lower teeth from the gum line up; the upper teeth, from the gum line down. Place the brush at a 45-degree angle to the gum line, and press the bristles gently into the gingival sulcus. Using short, gentle strokes *to prevent gum damage,*

brush the facial surfaces (toward the cheek) and the lingual surfaces (toward the tongue) of the bottom teeth. Use just the tip of the brush for the lingual surfaces of the front teeth. Then, using the same technique, brush the facial and lingual surfaces of the top teeth. Next, brush the biting surfaces of the bottom and top teeth, using a back-and-forth motion. If possible, ask the patient to rinse frequently during brushing by taking the mouthwash solution through the straw. Hold the emesis basin steady under the patient's cheek, and wipe his mouth and cheeks with facial tissues, as needed. **ADA**

● After brushing the patient's teeth, dip a sponge-tipped mouth swab into the mouthwash solution. Press the swab against the side of the glass to remove excess moisture. Gently stroke the gums, buccal surfaces, palate, and tongue *to clean the mucosa and stimulate circulation.* Replace the swab as necessary for thorough cleaning. Avoid inserting the swab too deeply *to prevent gagging and vomiting.*

After mouth care

● Assess the patient's mouth for cleanliness and tooth and tissue condition.
● Rinse the toothbrush, and clean the emesis basin and glass. Empty and clean the suction bottle, if used. Remove and discard gloves. **CDC**
● Place a clean suction catheter on the tubing. Return reusable equipment to the appropriate storage location, and properly discard disposable equipment in the trash bag.

Special considerations

● Use sponge-tipped mouth swabs to clean the teeth of a patient with sensitive gums. *These swabs produce less friction than a toothbrush but don't clean as well.*
● Clean the mouth of a toothless comatose patient by wrapping a gauze pad around your index finger, moistening it with mouthwash, and gently swabbing the oral tissues. If necessary, moisten gauze pads in an equal mixture of hydrogen peroxide and water *to remove tenacious mucus.*
● Remember that mucous membranes dry quickly in the patient breathing through his mouth or receiving oxygen therapy. Moisten his mouth and lips regularly with mineral oil, moistened sponge-tipped swabs, or water. If you use water as the lubricant, place a short straw in a glass of water and stop the open end with your finger. Remove the straw from the water and,

with your finger in place, position it in the patient's mouth. Release your finger slightly to let the water flow out gradually. If the patient is comatose, suction excess water *to prevent aspiration.*

Nursing diagnoses

● Impaired oral mucous membrane
● Ineffective therapeutic regimen management

Expected outcomes

The patient will:
● effectively manage daily oral hygiene
● have pink, moist oral mucous membranes.

Complications

Signs of poor dentition and oral hygiene include blood, food matter, odor, dry mucous membranes, loss of teeth, infection, and loss of mucosa integrity.

Documentation

Record the date and time of mouth care in your notes. Document any unusual conditions, such as bleeding, edema, mouth odor, excessive secretions, or plaque on the tongue.

Supportive references

American Dental Association. "Oral Health Topic: Cleaning Your Teeth and Gums (Oral Hygiene)." Available at: *www.ada.org/public/topics/cleaning.html.* Updated January 2002.
Craven, R., and Hirnle, C. *Fundamentals of Nursing: Human Health and Function,* 4th ed. Philadelphia: Lippincott Williams & Wilkins, 2002.
Smeltzer, S.C., and Bare, B.G. *Brunner & Suddarth's Textbook of Medical-Surgical Nursing,* 10th ed. Philadelphia: Lippincott Williams & Wilkins, 2004.

Nasogastric tube care

Providing effective nasogastric (NG) tube care requires meticulous monitoring of the patient and the equipment. Monitoring the patient involves checking drainage from the NG tube and assessing GI function. Monitoring the equipment involves verifying correct tube placement and irrigating the tube to ensure patency and to prevent mucosal damage.

Specific care varies only slightly for the most commonly used NG tubes: the single-lumen Levin tube and the double-lumen Salem sump tube.

Common gastric suction devices

Various suction devices are available for applying negative pressure to nasogastric (NG) and other drainage tubes. Two common types are shown here.

Portable suction machine

In the portable suction machine, a vacuum created intermittently by an electric pump draws gastric contents up the NG tube and into the collecting bottle.

Stationary suction machine

A stationary wall-unit apparatus can provide intermittent or continuous suction. On-off switches and variable power settings let you set and adjust the suction force on either machine.

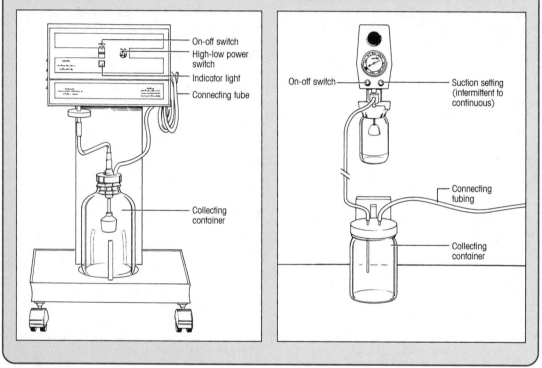

Equipment

Irrigant (usually normal saline solution) • irrigant container • 60-ml catheter-tip syringe • bulb syringe • suction equipment • lemon-glycerin swabs, sponge-tipped swabs, or toothbrush and toothpaste • petroleum jelly • ½″ or 1″ hypoallergenic tape • water-soluble lubricant • gloves • pH test strip • linen-saver pad • optional: emesis basin

Preparation of equipment

● Make sure the suction equipment works properly.

● When using a Salem sump tube with suction, connect the larger, primary lumen (for drainage and suction) to the suction equipment and select the appropriate setting, as ordered (usually low, constant suction).

● If the physician doesn't specify the setting, follow the manufacturer's directions. **MFR**

● A Levin tube usually calls for intermittent low suction. (See *Common gastric suction devices*.)

Implementation

- Confirm the patient's identity using two patient identifiers according to facility policy. **JCAHO**
- Explain the procedure to the patient and provide privacy. **PCP**
- Wash your hands, and put on gloves. **CDC**

Irrigating an NG tube

- Review the irrigation schedule (usually every 4 hours), if the physician orders this procedure. **AGA**
- Assess tube placement by looking for discrepancies in tube markings or by measuring the external tube length and comparing it with the length documented in the chart. Have the patient open his mouth so that you can check to see if the tube is coiled.
- Aspirate stomach contents *to check correct positioning in the stomach and to prevent the patient from aspirating the irrigant.* **AGA**
- Examine the aspirate and place a small amount on the pH test strip. The probability of gastric placement is increased if the aspirate has a typical gastric fluid appearance (grassy-green, clear and colorless with mucus shreds, or brown with a pH of less than or equal to 5.0). **EB**
- If the tube is used for gastric suction, the aspirate will be green or clear and colorless with off-white or tan mucus.
- Measure the amount of irrigant in the bulb syringe or in the 60-ml catheter-tip syringe (usually 10 to 20 ml) *to maintain an accurate intake and output record.* **Science**
- When using suction with a Salem sump tube or a Levin tube, unclamp and disconnect the tube from the suction equipment while holding it over a linen-saver pad or an emesis basin *to collect any drainage.*
- Slowly instill the irrigant into the NG tube. (When irrigating the Salem sump tube, you may instill small amounts of solution into the vent lumen without interrupting suction; however, you should instill greater amounts into the larger, primary lumen.) **Science**
- Gently aspirate the solution with the bulb syringe or 60-ml catheter-tip syringe or connect the tube to the suction equipment, as ordered. *Gentle aspiration prevents excessive pressure on a suture line and on delicate gastric mucosa.* Report any bleeding. **Science**
- Reconnect the tube to suction after completing irrigation.

Instilling solution through an NG tube

- If the physician orders *instillation,* inject the solution, and don't aspirate it. Note the amount of instilled solution as "intake" on the intake and output record.
- Reattach the tube to suction as ordered.
- After attaching the Salem sump tube's primary lumen to suction, instill 10 to 20 cc of air into the vent lumen *to verify patency.* Listen for a soft hiss in the vent. If you don't hear this sound, suspect a clogged tube; recheck patency by instilling 10 ml of normal saline solution and 10 to 20 cc of air in the vent. **AGA**

Monitoring patient comfort and condition

- Provide mouth care once per shift or as needed. Depending on the patient's condition, use sponge-tipped swabs to clean his teeth or assist him to brush them with toothbrush and toothpaste. Coat the patient's lips with petroleum jelly *to prevent dryness from mouth breathing.* (See "Mouth care," page 419.) **Science**
- Change the tape securing the tube as needed or at least daily. Clean the skin, apply fresh tape, and dab water-soluble lubricant on the nostrils as needed.
- Regularly check the tape that secures the tube *because sweat and nasal secretions may loosen the tape.*
- Assess bowel sounds regularly (every 4 to 8 hours) *to verify GI function.* **AGA** **Science**
- Measure the drainage amount and update the intake and output record every 8 hours. Be alert for electrolyte imbalances with excessive gastric output. **Science**
- Inspect gastric drainage and note its color, consistency, odor, and amount. Normal gastric secretions have no color or appear yellow-green from bile and have a mucoid consistency. Immediately report any drainage with a coffee-bean color *because it may indicate bleeding.* If you suspect that the drainage contains blood, use a screening test (such as Hematest) for occult blood according to your facility's policy. **Science**

Special considerations

- Irrigate the NG tube with 30 ml of irrigant before and after instilling medication. Wait about 30 minutes, or as ordered, after instillation before reconnecting the suction equipment *to allow sufficient time for the medication to be absorbed.*

● When no drainage appears, check the suction equipment for proper function. Then, holding the NG tube over a linen-saver pad or an emesis basin, separate the tube and the suction source. Check the suction equipment by placing the suction tubing in an irrigant container. If the apparatus draws the water, check the NG tube for proper function. Be sure to note the amount of water drawn into the suction container on the intake and output record.

● A dysfunctional NG tube may be clogged or incorrectly positioned. Attempt to irrigate the tube, reposition the patient, or rotate and reposition the tube. However, if the tube was inserted during surgery, avoid this maneuver *to ensure that the movement doesn't interfere with gastric or esophageal sutures.* Notify the physician.

● If you can ambulate the patient and interrupt suction, disconnect the NG tube from the suction equipment. Clamp the tube *to prevent stomach contents from draining out of the tube.*

● If the patient has a Salem sump tube, watch for gastric reflux in the vent lumen when pressure in the stomach exceeds atmospheric pressure. This problem may result from a clogged primary lumen or from a suction system that's set up improperly. Assess the suction equipment for proper functioning. Then irrigate the NG tube and instill 30 cc of air into the vent tube *to maintain patency.* Don't attempt to stop reflux by clamping the vent tube. Unless contraindicated, elevate the patient's torso more than 30 degrees, and keep the vent tube above his midline *to prevent a siphoning effect.*

Nursing diagnoses
● Acute pain
● Deficient fluid volume

Expected outcomes
The patient will:
● express relief from discomfort and pain
● have electrolytes that remain within normal limits and a fluid volume that remains adequate.

Complications
● Epigastric pain and vomiting may result from a clogged or improperly placed tube.

● Any NG tube (the Levin tube in particular) may move and aggravate esophagitis, ulcers, or esophageal varices, causing hemorrhage.

● Perforation may result from aggressive intubation.

● Dehydration and electrolyte imbalances may result from removing body fluids and electrolytes by suctioning.

● Pain, swelling, and salivary dysfunction may signal parotitis, which occurs in dehydrated, debilitated patients. Intubation can cause nasal skin breakdown and discomfort and increased mucus secretions.

● Aspiration pneumonia may result from gastric reflux.

● Vigorous suction may damage the gastric mucosa and cause significant bleeding, possibly interfering with endoscopic assessment and diagnosis.

Documentation
Regularly record tube placement confirmation (usually every 4 to 8 hours). Keep a precise record of fluid intake and output, including the instilled irrigant in fluid input. Track the irrigation schedule and note the actual time of each irrigation. Describe drainage color, consistency, odor, and amount. Note tape change times and condition of the nares.

Supportive references
Craven, R., and Hirnle, C. *Fundamentals of Nursing: Human Health and Function,* 4th ed. Philadelphia: Lippincott Williams & Wilkins, 2002.

Guenter, P., and Silkroski, M. *Tube Feeding: Practical Guidelines and Nursing Protocols.* Gaithersburg, Md.: Aspen Pubs., Inc., 2001.

Sweeney, J. "How Do I Verify NG Tube Placement," *Nursing2005* 35(8):25, August 2005. **EB**

Nasogastric tube insertion and removal

Usually inserted to decompress the stomach, a nasogastric (NG) tube can prevent vomiting after major surgery. An NG tube is typically in place for 48 to 72 hours after surgery, by which time peristalsis usually resumes. It may remain in place for shorter or longer periods, however, depending on its use. **AGA**

The NG tube has other diagnostic and therapeutic applications, especially in assessing and treating upper GI bleeding, collecting gastric contents for analy-

Types of NG tubes

The physician will choose the type and diameter of nasogastric (NG) tube that best suits the patient's needs, including lavage, aspiration, enteral therapy, or stomach decompression. Choices may include the Levin, Salem sump, and Moss tubes.

Levin tube

The Levin tube is a rubber or plastic tube that has a single lumen, a length of 42" to 50" (106.5 to 127" cm), and holes at the tip and along the side.

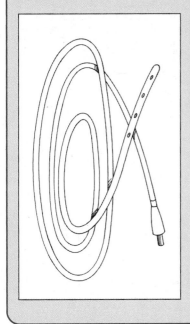

Salem sump tube

The Salem sump tube is a double-lumen tube made of clear plastic and has a blue sump port (pigtail) that allows atmospheric air to enter the patient's stomach. Thus, the tube floats freely and doesn't adhere to or damage gastric mucosa. The larger port of this 48" (121.9-cm) tube serves as the main suction conduit. The tube has openings at 17¾" (45 cm), 21⅝" (55 cm), 25⅝" (65 cm), and 29½" (75 cm) as well as a radiopaque line to verify placement.

Moss tube

The Moss tube has a radiopaque tip and three lumens. The first, positioned and inflated in the cardia, serves as a balloon inflation port. The second is an esophageal aspiration port. The third is a duodenal feeding port.

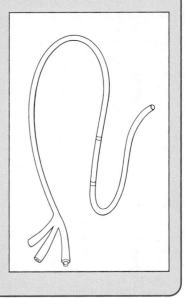

---

sis, performing gastric lavage, aspirating gastric secretions, and administering medications and nutrients. **AGA**

Inserting an NG tube requires close observation of the patient and verification of proper placement. Removing the tube requires careful handling *to prevent injury or aspiration.* The tube must be inserted with extra care in a pregnant patient and in one with an increased risk of complications. For example, the physician will order an NG tube for a patient with aortic aneurysm, myocardial infarction, gastric hemorrhage, or esophageal varices only if he believes that the benefits outweigh the risks of intubation.

Most NG tubes have a radiopaque marker or strip at the distal end so that tube position can be verified by X-ray. If the position can't be confirmed, the physician may order fluoroscopy to verify placement.

The most common NG tubes are the Levin tube, which has one lumen, and the Salem sump tube, which has two lumens, one for suction and drainage and a smaller one for ventilation. Air flows through the vent lumen continuously. This protects the delicate gastric mucosa by preventing a vacuum from forming should the tube adhere to the stomach lining. The Moss tube, which has a triple lumen, is usually inserted during surgery. (See *Types of NG tubes.*)

Equipment

Insertion of NG tube

Tube (usually #12, #14, #16, or #18 French for a normal adult) • towel or linen-saver pad • facial tissues • emesis basin • penlight • 1″ or 2″ hypoallergenic tape • gloves • water-soluble lubricant • cup or glass of water with straw (if appropriate) • pH test strip • tongue blade • catheter-tip or bulb syringe or irrigation set • safety pin • ordered suction equipment • optional: metal clamp, alcohol pad, warm water, large basin or plastic container, rubber band

Removal of NG tube

Gloves • catheter-tip syringe • normal saline solution • towel or linen-saver pad • adhesive remover • facial tissues • optional: clamp

Preparation of equipment

● Inspect the NG tube for defects, such as rough edges or partially closed lumens.
● Then check the tube's patency by flushing it with water.
● *To ease insertion,* increase a stiff tube's flexibility by coiling it around your gloved fingers for a few seconds or by dipping it into warm water.
● Stiffen a limp rubber tube by briefly chilling it in ice.

Implementation

● Whether you're inserting or removing an NG tube, be sure to provide privacy, wash your hands, and put on gloves before inserting the tube. Check the physician's order to determine the type of tube that should be inserted.

Inserting an NG tube

● Confirm the patient's identity using two patient identifiers according to facility policy. **JCAHO**
● Explain the procedure to the patient *to ease anxiety and promote cooperation.* Inform her that she may experience some nasal discomfort, that she may gag, and that her eyes may water. Emphasize that swallowing will ease the tube's advancement. **PCP**
● Agree on a signal that the patient can use if she wants you to stop briefly during the procedure.
● Gather and prepare all necessary equipment.
● Help the patient into high Fowler's position unless contraindicated.

● Stand at the patient's right side if you're right-handed or at her left side if you're left-handed *to ease insertion.*
● Drape the towel or linen-saver pad over the patient's chest *to protect her gown and bed linens from spills.*
● Have the patient gently blow her nose *to clear her nostrils.*
● Place the facial tissues and emesis basin well within the patient's reach.
● Help the patient face forward with her neck in a neutral position.
● *To determine how long the NG tube must be to reach the stomach,* hold the end of the tube at the tip of the patient's nose. Extend the tube to the patient's earlobe and then down to the xiphoid process (as shown below). **Science**

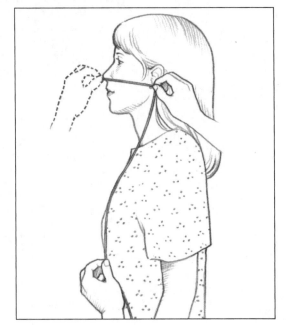

● Mark this distance on the tubing with tape, or note the marking already on the tube. (Average measurements for an adult range from 22″ to 26″ [56 to 66 cm].) It may be necessary to add 2″ (5.1 cm) to this measurement in tall individuals *to ensure entry into the stomach.*
● *To determine which nostril will allow easier access,* use a penlight and inspect for a deviated septum or other abnormalities. Ask the patient if she ever had

nasal surgery or a nasal injury. Assess airflow in both nostrils by occluding one nostril at a time while the patient breathes through her nose. Choose the nostril with the better airflow. **Science**

● Lubricate the first 3″ (7.6 cm) of the tube with a water-soluble gel *to minimize injury to the nasal passages. Using a water-soluble lubricant prevents lipoid pneumonia,* which may result from aspiration of an oil-based lubricant or from accidental slippage of the tube into the trachea.

● Instruct the patient to hold her head straight and upright.

● Grasp the tube with the end pointing downward, curve it if necessary, and carefully insert it into the more patent nostril (as shown below). **Science**

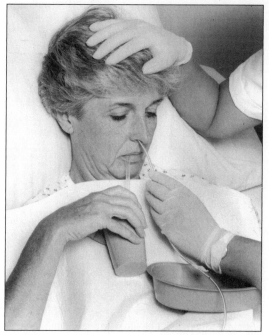

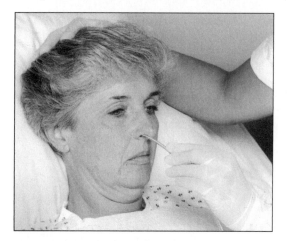

● Aim the tube downward and toward the ear closer to the chosen nostril. Advance it slowly *to avoid pressure on the turbinates and resultant pain and bleeding.* **Science**

● When the tube reaches the nasopharynx, you'll feel resistance. Instruct the patient to lower her head slightly *to close the trachea and open the esophagus.* Then rotate the tube 180 degrees toward the opposite nostril *to redirect it so that the tube won't enter the patient's mouth.* **Science**

● Unless contraindicated, offer the patient a cup or glass of water with a straw. Direct her to sip and swallow as you slowly advance the tube (as shown at top of next column). *This helps the tube pass to the esophagus.* (If you aren't using water, ask the patient to swallow.)

Ensuring proper tube placement

● Use a tongue blade and penlight to examine the patient's mouth and throat for signs of a coiled section of tubing (especially in an unconscious patient). *Coiling indicates an obstruction.* **Science**

● Keep an emesis basin and facial tissues readily available for the patient.

● As you carefully advance the tube and the patient swallows, watch for respiratory distress signs, *which may mean the tube is in the bronchus and must be removed immediately.*

● Stop advancing the tube when the tape mark or the tube marking reaches the patient's nostril.

● Attach a catheter-tip or bulb syringe to the tube and try to aspirate stomach contents (as shown at top of next page). If you don't obtain stomach contents, position the patient on her left side to move the contents into the stomach's greater curvature, and aspirate again. When confirming tube placement, never place the tube's end in a container of water. *If the tube is positioned incorrectly in the trachea, the patient may aspirate water.* Gently aspirate stomach contents. Examine the aspirate and place a small amount on the pH test strip. Probability of gastric placement is increased if the aspirate has a typical gastric fluid appearance (grassy-green, clear and colorless with mucus shreds, or brown) and the pH is less than or equal to 5.0. **AGA** **EB** **Science**

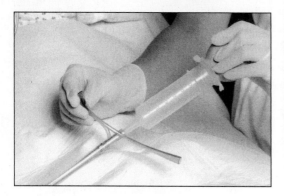

● Ideally, proper tube placement should be confirmed by X-ray. **AGA**
● Secure the NG tube to the patient's nose with hypoallergenic tape (or other designated tube holder). If the patient's skin is oily, wipe the bridge of the nose with an alcohol pad and allow it to dry. You'll need about 4″ (10 cm) of 1″ tape. Split one end of the tape up the center about 1½″ (4 cm). Make tabs on the split ends (by folding sticky sides together). Stick the uncut tape end on the patient's nose so that the split in the tape starts about ½″ (1.5 cm) to 1½″ from the tip of her nose. Crisscross the tabbed ends around the tube (as shown below). Then apply another piece of tape over the bridge of the nose to secure the tube.

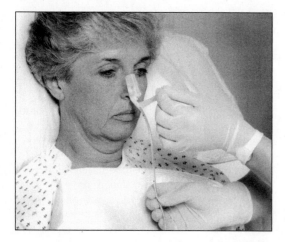

● Alternatively, stabilize the tube with a prepackaged product that secures and cushions it at the nose (as shown below).

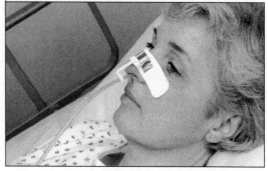

● *To reduce discomfort from the weight of the tube,* tie a slipknot around the tube with a rubber band, and then secure the rubber band to the patient's gown with a safety pin, or wrap another piece of tape around the end of the tube and leave a tab. Then fasten the tape tab to the patient's gown.
● Attach the tube to suction equipment, if ordered, and set the designated suction pressure.
● Provide frequent nose and mouth care while the tube is in place. (See "Mouth care," page 419.) **Science**

Removing an NG tube
● Confirm the patient's identity using two patient identifiers according to facility policy. **JCAHO**
● Explain the procedure to the patient, informing her that it may cause some nasal discomfort and sneezing or gagging.
● Assess bowel function by auscultating for peristalsis or flatus. **Science**
● Help the patient into semi-Fowler's position. Then drape a towel or linen-saver pad across her chest *to protect her gown and bed linens from spills.* **Science**
● Wash your hands, and put on gloves. **CDC**
● Using a catheter-tip syringe, flush the tube with 10 ml of normal saline solution *to ensure that the tube doesn't contain stomach contents that could irritate tissues during tube removal.*
● Untape the tube from the patient's nose, and then unpin it from her gown.
● Clamp the tube by folding it in your hand.
● Ask the patient to hold her breath *to close the epiglottis.* Then withdraw the tube gently and steadi-

ly. (When the distal end of the tube reaches the nasopharynx, you can pull it quickly.) Science

● When possible, immediately cover and remove the tube *because its sight and odor may nauseate the patient.*

● Assist the patient with thorough mouth care, and clean the tape residue from her nose with adhesive remover. (See "Mouth care," page 419.)

● For the next 48 hours, monitor the patient for signs of GI dysfunction, including nausea, vomiting, abdominal distention, and food intolerance. GI dysfunction may necessitate reinsertion of the tube.

Special considerations

● Ross-Hanson tape is a helpful device for calculating the correct tube length. Place the narrow end of this measuring tape at the tip of the patient's nose. Extend the tape to the patient's earlobe and down to the tip of the xiphoid process. Mark this distance on the edge of the tape labeled "nose to ear to xiphoid." The corresponding measurement on the opposite edge of the tape is the proper insertion length.

● If the patient has a deviated septum or other nasal condition that prevents nasal insertion, pass the tube orally after removing any dentures, if necessary. Sliding the tube over the tongue, proceed as you would for nasal insertion.

● When using the oral route, remember to coil the end of the tube around your hand. *This helps curve and direct the tube downward at the pharynx.*

● If your patient is unconscious, tilt her chin toward her chest *to close the trachea.* Then advance the tube between respirations *to ensure that it doesn't enter the trachea.*

● While advancing the tube in an unconscious patient (or in a patient who can't swallow), stroke the patient's neck *to encourage the swallowing reflex and to facilitate passage down the esophagus.*

● While advancing the tube, observe for signs that it has entered the trachea, such as choking or breathing difficulties in a conscious patient and cyanosis in an unconscious patient or a patient without a cough reflex. If these signs occur, remove the tube immediately. Allow the patient time to rest; then try to reinsert the tube.

● After tube placement, vomiting suggests tubal obstruction or incorrect position. Assess immediately to determine the cause.

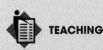

TEACHING

Using an NG tube at home

If your patient will need to have a nasogastric (NG) tube in place at home — for short-term feeding or gastric decompression, for example — find out who will insert the tube. If he'll have a home care nurse, identify her and, if possible, tell the patient when to expect her.

If the patient or a family member will perform the procedure, you'll need to provide additional instruction and supervision. Use this checklist to prepare your teaching topics:

● how and where to obtain equipment needed for home intubation

● how to insert the tube

● how to verify tube placement by aspirating stomach contents

● how to correct tube misplacement

● how to prepare formula for tube feeding

● how to store formula, if appropriate

● how to administer formula through the tube

● how to remove and dispose of an NG tube

● how to clean and store a reusable NG tube

● how to use the NG tube for gastric decompression, if appropriate

● how to set up and operate suctioning equipment

● how to troubleshoot suctioning equipment

● how to perform mouth care and other hygienic procedures.

TEACHING *An NG tube may be inserted or removed at home. Indications for insertion include gastric decompression and short-term feeding. A home care nurse or the patient may insert the tube, deliver the feeding, and remove the tube. (See* Using an NG tube at home.*)*

Nursing diagnoses

● Anxiety

● Deficient knowledge (procedure)

Expected outcomes

The patient will:

- cope with NG tube placement without severe anxiety
- express an understanding of the need for NG tube placement.

Complications
- Potential complications of prolonged intubation with an NG tube include skin erosion at the nostril, sinusitis, esophagitis, esophagotracheal fistula, gastric ulceration, and pulmonary and oral infection.
- Additional complications that may result from suction include electrolyte imbalances and dehydration.

Documentation
Record the type and size of the NG tube and the date, time, and route of insertion. Note the type and amount of suction, if used, and describe the drainage, including the amount, color, character, consistency, and odor. Note the patient's tolerance of the procedure, especially any signs or symptoms that signal complications, such as nausea, vomiting, or abdominal distention. Document any subsequent irrigation procedures and continuing problems after irrigation. When you remove the tube, be sure to record the date and time. Describe the color, consistency, and amount of gastric drainage. Note the patient's tolerance of the procedure, especially any unusual events such as nausea, vomiting, abdominal distention, or food intolerance.

Supportive references
Craven, R., and Hirnle, C. *Fundamentals of Nursing: Human Health and Function,* 4th ed. Philadelphia: Lippincott Williams & Wilkins, 2002.

Guenter, P., and Silkroski, M. *Tube Feeding: Practical Guidelines and Nursing Protocols.* Gaithersburg, Md.: Aspen Pubs., Inc., 2001.

Sweeney, J. "How Do I Verify NG Tube Placement," *Nursing2005* 35(8):25, August 2005. **EB**

Transabdominal tube feeding and care

To access the stomach, duodenum, or jejunum, the physician may place a tube through the patient's abdominal wall. This may be done surgically or percutaneously. A gastrostomy or jejunostomy tube is usually inserted during intra-abdominal surgery. The tube may be used for feeding during the immediate postoperative period or it may provide long-term enteral access, depending on the type of surgery. Typically, the physician will suture the tube in place to prevent gastric contents from leaking.

In contrast, a percutaneous endoscopic gastrostomy (PEG) or jejunostomy (PEJ) tube can be inserted endoscopically without the need for laparotomy or general anesthesia. Typically, the insertion is done in the endoscopy suite or at the patient's bedside. **AGA** A PEG or PEJ tube may be used for nutrition, drainage, and decompression. **AGA** Contraindications to endoscopic placement include obstruction (such as an esophageal stricture or duodenal blockage), previous gastric surgery, morbid obesity, and ascites. These conditions would necessitate surgical placement.

With either type of tube placement, feedings may begin after 24 hours (or when peristalsis resumes).

After a time, the tube may need replacement, and the physician may recommend a similar tube, such as an indwelling urinary catheter or a mushroom catheter, or a gastrostomy button — a skin-level feeding tube. (See "Gastrostomy feeding button care," page 417.)

Nursing care includes providing skin care at the tube site, maintaining the feeding tube, administering feeding, monitoring the patient's response to feeding, adjusting the feeding schedule, and preparing the patient for self-care after discharge.

Equipment
Feeding
Feeding formula • large-bulb or catheter-tip syringe • 120 ml of water • 4″ × 4″ gauze pads • soap • skin protectant • hypoallergenic tape • gravity-drip administration bags • mouthwash, toothpaste, or mild salt solution • stethoscope • gloves • optional: enteral infusion pump

Decompression
Suction apparatus with tubing and straight drainage collection set

Preparation of equipment
- Always check the expiration date on commercially prepared feeding formulas.
- If the formula has been prepared by the dietitian or pharmacist, check the preparation time and date.

• Discard any opened formula that's more than 1 day old.

• Commercially-prepared administration sets and enteral pumps allow continuous formula administration.

• Place the desired amount of formula into the gavage container and purge air from the tubing.

• *To avoid contamination,* hang only a 4- to 6-hour supply of formula at a time.

Implementation

• Provide privacy, and wash your hands. **CDC**

• Confirm the patient's identity using two patient identifiers according to facility policy. **JCAHO**

• Explain the procedure to the patient. Tell him, for example, that feedings usually start at a slow rate and increase as tolerated. After he tolerates continuous feedings, he may progress to intermittent feedings, as ordered.

• Assess for bowel sounds with a stethoscope before feeding, and monitor for abdominal distention. **Science**

• Ask the patient to sit, or assist him into semi-Fowler's position, for the entire feeding. *This helps to prevent esophageal reflux and pulmonary aspiration of the formula.* For an intermittent feeding, have him maintain this position throughout the feeding and for 1 hour afterward. **AGA**

• Put on gloves. Before starting the feeding, measure residual gastric contents. Attach the syringe to the feeding tube and aspirate. If the contents measure more than twice the amount infused, hold the feeding and recheck in 1 hour. If residual contents remain too high, notify the physician. *Chances are the formula isn't being absorbed properly.* Keep in mind that residual contents will be minimal with PEJ tube feedings. **AGA** **CDC**

• Allow 30 ml of water to flow into the feeding tube *to establish patency.*

• Be sure to administer formula at room temperature. *Cold formula may cause cramping.*

Intermittent feedings

• Allow gravity to help the formula flow over 30 to 45 minutes. *Faster infusions may cause bloating, cramps, or diarrhea.* **AGA**

• Begin intermittent feeding with a low volume (200 ml) daily. According to the patient's tolerance, increase the volume per feeding, as needed, *to reach the desired calorie intake.* **AGA**

• When the feeding finishes, flush the feeding tube with 30 to 60 ml of water *to maintain patency and provide hydration.* **Science**

• Cap the tube *to prevent leakage.*

• Rinse the feeding administration set thoroughly with hot water *to avoid contaminating subsequent feedings.* Allow it to dry between feedings.

Continuous feedings

• Measure residual gastric contents every 4 hours. **AGA**

• To administer the feeding with a pump, set up the equipment according to the manufacturer's guidelines, and fill the feeding bag. To administer the feeding by gravity, fill the container with formula and purge air from the tubing.

• Monitor the gravity drip rate or pump infusion rate frequently *to ensure accurate delivery of formula.*

• Flush the feeding tube with 30 to 60 ml of water every 4 hours *to maintain patency and to provide hydration.* **Science**

• Monitor intake and output *to anticipate and detect fluid or electrolyte imbalances.* **Science**

Decompression

• To decompress the stomach, connect the PEG port to the suction device with tubing or straight gravity drainage tubing. Jejunostomy feeding may be given simultaneously via the PEJ port of the dual-lumen tube.

Tube exit site care

• Provide daily skin care.

• Gently remove the dressing by hand. Never cut away the dressing over the catheter *because you might cut the tube or the sutures holding the tube in place.*

• At least daily and as needed, clean the skin around the tube's exit site using a 4″ × 4″ gauze pad soaked in the prescribed cleaning solution. When healed, wash the skin around the exit site daily with soap. Rinse the area with water and pat dry. Apply skin protectant if necessary. **EB** **Science**

• Anchor a gastrostomy or jejunostomy tube to the skin with hypoallergenic tape *to prevent peristaltic migration of the tube.* This also prevents tension on the suture anchoring the tube in place. **Science**

Caring for a PEG or PEJ site

The exit site of a percutaneous endoscopic gastrostomy (PEG) tube or percutaneous endoscopic jejunostomy (PEJ) tube requires routine observation and care. Follow these care guidelines:
- Change the dressing daily while the tube is in place.
- After removing the dressing, carefully slide the tube's outer bumper away from the skin (as shown below) about ½″ (1.5 cm).

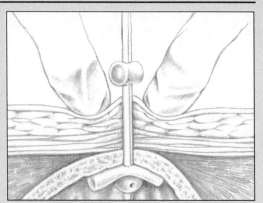

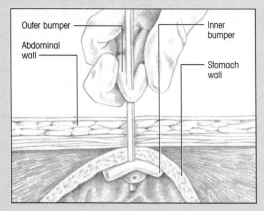

- Examine the skin around the tube. Look for redness and other signs of infection or erosion.
- Gently depress the skin surrounding the tube and inspect for drainage (as shown top right). Expect minimal wound drainage initially after implantation. This should subside in about 1 week.

- Inspect the tube for wear and tear. (A tube that wears out will need replacement.)
- Clean the site with the prescribed cleaning solution. Then apply povidone-iodine ointment over the exit site, according to facility guidelines.
- Rotate the outer bumper 90 degrees *to avoid repeating the same tension on the same skin area,* and slide the outer bumper back over the exit site.
- If leakage appears at the PEG site, or if the patient risks dislodging the tube, apply a sterile gauze dressing over the site. Don't put sterile gauze underneath the outer bumper. Loosening the anchor this way allows the feeding tube free play, which could lead to wound abscess.
- Write the date and time of the dressing change on the tape.

- Coil the tube, if necessary, and tape it to the abdomen *to prevent pulling and contamination of the tube.* PEG and PEJ tubes have toggle-bolt-like internal and external bumpers that make tape anchors unnecessary. (See *Caring for a PEG or PEJ site.*)

Special considerations
- If the patient vomits or complains of nausea, feeling too full, or regurgitation, stop the feeding immediately and assess his condition. Flush the feeding tube and attempt to restart the feeding again in 1 hour (measure residual gastric contents first). You may have to decrease the volume or rate of feedings. If the patient develops dumping syndrome, which includes nausea, vomiting, cramps, pallor, and diarrhea, the feedings may have been given too quickly.

- Provide mouth care frequently. Brush all surfaces of the teeth, gums, and tongue at least twice daily using mouthwash, toothpaste, or mild salt solution. (See "Mouth care," page 419.)
- You can administer most tablets and pills through the tube by crushing them and diluting as necessary. (However, don't crush enteric-coated or sustained-release drugs, which lose their effectiveness when crushed.) Medications should be in liquid form for administration.
- Control diarrhea resulting from dumping syndrome by using continuous pump or gravity-drip infusions, diluting the feeding formula, or adding antidiarrheal medications.

Syringe feeding instructions

If your patient plans to feed himself by syringe when he returns home, you'll need to teach him how to do so before he's discharged. Here are some points to emphasize.

Initial instructions

First, show the patient how to clamp the feeding tube, remove the syringe's bulb or plunger, and place the tip of the syringe into the feeding tube (as shown below). Then have him instill between 30 and 60 ml of water into the feeding tube *to make sure it stays open and patent.*

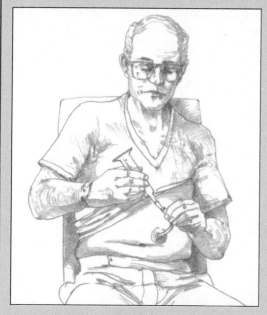

Next, tell him to pour the feeding solution into the syringe and begin the feeding (as shown top right). As the solution flows into the stomach, show him how to tilt the syringe *to allow air bubbles to escape.* Describe the discomfort that air bubbles may cause.

Tips for free flow

When about one-fourth of the feeding solution remains, direct the patient to refill the syringe. Caution him to avoid letting the syringe empty completely. *Doing so may result in abdominal cramping and gas.*

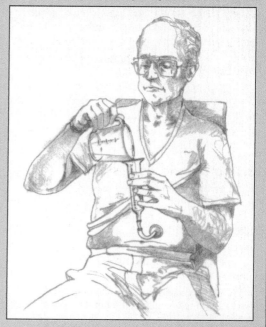

Demonstrate how to increase and decrease the solution's flow rate by raising or lowering the syringe. Explain also that he may need to dilute a thick solution *to promote free flow.*

Finishing up

Inform the patient that the feeding infusion process should take about 15 minutes or more. If the process takes less than 15 minutes, dumping syndrome may result.

Show the patient the steps needed to finish the feeding, including how to flush the tube with water, clamp the tube, and clean the equipment for later use. Naturally, if he's using disposable gear, urge him to discard it properly. Review how to store unused feeding solution as appropriate.

TEACHING *Instruct the patient and family members or other caregivers in all aspects of enteral feedings, including tube maintenance and site care.*

Specify signs and symptoms to report to the physician, define emergency situations, and review actions to take.

When the tube needs replacement, advise the patient that the physician may insert a replacement gastrostomy button or a latex, indwelling, or mushroom catheter after removing the initial feeding tube. The procedure may be done in the physician's office or the hospital's endoscopy suite.

As the patient's tolerance to tube feeding improves, he may wish to try syringe feedings rather than intermittent feedings. If appropriate, teach him how to feed himself by this method. (See Syringe feeding instructions, *page 435.)*

Nursing diagnoses
- Effective therapeutic regimen management
- Imbalanced nutrition: Less than body requirements

Expected outcomes
The patient (and family) will:
- be able to effectively manage care of tube and tube feeding
- maintain adequate nutritional and fluid needs as measured through weight and laboratory tests.

Complications
- Common complications related to transabdominal tubes include GI or other systemic problems, mechanical malfunction, and metabolic disturbances.
- Cramping, nausea, vomiting, bloating, and diarrhea may be related to medication, too-rapid infusion rate, formula contamination, osmolarity, or temperature (too cold or too warm), fat malabsorption, or intestinal atrophy from malnutrition.
- Constipation may result from inadequate hydration or insufficient exercise.
- Systemic problems may be caused by pulmonary aspiration, infection at the tube exit site, or contaminated formula. Proper positioning during feeding, verification of tube placement, meticulous skin care, and sterile formula preparation are ways to prevent these complications.
- Typical mechanical problems include tube dislodgment, obstruction, or impairment. For example, a

PEG or PEJ tube may migrate if the external bumper loosens. Occlusion may result from incompletely crushed and liquefied medication particles or inadequate tube flushing. Further, the tube may rupture or crack from age, drying, or frequent manipulation.
- Monitor the patient for vitamin and mineral deficiencies, glucose tolerance, and fluid and electrolyte imbalances, which may follow bouts of diarrhea or constipation.

Documentation
On the intake and output record, note the date, time, and amount of each feeding and the water volume instilled. Maintain total volumes for nutrients and water separately to allow calculation of nutrient intake. In your notes, document the type of formula, the infusion method and rate, the patient's tolerance of the procedure and formula, and the amount of residual gastric contents. Record complications and abdominal assessment findings. Note patient-teaching topics covered, and note the patient's progress in self-care.

Supportive references
Bowers, S. "All About Tubes: Your Guide to Enteral Feeding Devices," *Nursing2000* 30(12):41-47, December 2000. **EB**

Craven, R., and Hirnle, C. *Fundamentals of Nursing: Human Health and Function,* 4th ed. Philadelphia: Lippincott Williams & Wilkins, 2002.

Guenter, P., and Silkroski, M. *Tube Feeding: Practical Guidelines and Nursing Protocols.* Gaithersburg, Md.: Aspen Pubs., Inc., 2001.

Stone, S.J., et al. "Bedside Placement of Postpyloric Feeding Tubes," *AACN Clinical Issues* 11(4):517-30, November 2000.

Tube feeding

Tube feeding is delivery of a liquid feeding formula directly to the stomach (known as *gastric gavage*), duodenum, or jejunum. Gastric gavage typically is indicated for a patient who can't eat normally because of dysphagia, or oral or esophageal obstruction or injury. Gastric feedings may also be given to an unconscious or intubated patient, or to a patient recovering from GI tract surgery who can't ingest food orally.

According to the American Gastroenterological Association, nutrition support should be initiated after 1 to 2 weeks without nutrient intake. Enteral feeding is preferable to parenteral therapy provided there are no contraindications, access can be safely attained, and oral intake isn't possible. For short-term (less than 30-day) feeding, nasogastric (NG) or nasoenteric tubes are preferable to gastrostomy or jejunostomy tubes. Tube feeding is contraindicated in patients who have no bowel sounds or a suspected intestinal obstruction. **AGA**

Duodenal or jejunal feedings decrease the risk of aspiration because the formula bypasses the pylorus. Jejunal feedings result in reduced pancreatic stimulation; thus, patients may require an elemental diet. Patients usually receive gastric feedings on an intermittent schedule. For duodenal or jejunal feedings, however, most patients seem to better tolerate a continuous slow drip.

Liquid nutrient solutions come in various formulas for administration through an NG tube, a small-bore feeding tube, gastrostomy or jejunostomy tube, percutaneous endoscopic gastrostomy or jejunostomy tube, or gastrostomy feeding button. (See "Transabdominal tube feeding and care," page 432, and "Gastrostomy feeding button care," page 417.)

Equipment
Gastric feedings
Feeding formula • graduated container • bulb syringe • 120 ml of water • gavage bag with tubing and flow regulator clamp • towel or linen-saver pad • 60-ml syringe • pH test strip • optional: infusion controller and tubing set (for continuous administration), adapter to connect gavage tubing to feeding tube

Duodenal or jejunal feedings
Feeding formula • enteral administration set containing a gavage container, drip chamber, roller clamp or flow regulator, and tube connector • I.V. pole • 60-ml syringe with adapter tip • water • optional: pump administration set (for an enteral infusion pump), Y-connector

Nasal and oral care
Cotton-tipped applicators • water-soluble lubricant • sponge-tipped swabs • petroleum jelly

A bulb syringe or large catheter-tip syringe may be substituted for a gavage bag after the patient demonstrates tolerance for a gravity drip infusion. The physician may order an infusion pump to ensure accurate delivery of the prescribed formula.

Preparation of equipment
● Be sure to refrigerate formulas prepared in the dietary department or pharmacy.
● Refrigerate commercial formulas only after opening them.
● Check the dates on all formula containers and discard expired commercial formulas.
● Use powdered formulas within 24 hours of mixing.
● Always shake the container well to mix the solution thoroughly.
● Allow the formula to warm to room temperature before administration. *Cold formula can increase the chance of diarrhea.*
● Never warm formula over direct heat or in a microwave *because heat may curdle the formula or change its chemical composition, and hot formula may injure the patient.*
● Pour 60 ml of water into the graduated container.
● After closing the flow clamp on the administration set, pour the appropriate amount of formula into the gavage bag.
● Hang no more than a 4- to 6-hour supply at one time *to prevent bacterial growth.*
● Open the flow clamp on the administration set to remove air from the lines. *This keeps air from entering the patient's stomach and causing distention and discomfort.*

Implementation
● Confirm the patient's identity using two patient identifiers according to facility policy. **JCAHO**
● Provide privacy, and wash your hands. **CDC**
● Inform the patient that he'll receive nourishment through the tube, and explain the procedure to him. If possible, give him a schedule of subsequent feedings. **PCP**
● If the patient has a nasal or oral tube, cover his chest with a towel or linen-saver pad *to protect him and the bed linens from spills.*
● Assess the patient's abdomen for bowel sounds and distention. **Science**

Delivering a gastric feeding
● *To limit the risk of aspiration and reflux,* raise the head of the patient's bed 30 to 45 degrees during feeding and for 1 hour after feeding. Use intermittent or continuous feeding regimens rather than the rapid bolus method. **AGA**

● Check placement of the feeding tube *to make sure it hasn't slipped out since the last feeding.* **AGA**

⚠ ALERT *Never administer a tube feeding until you're sure the tube is properly positioned in the patient's stomach. Administering a feeding through a misplaced tube can cause formula to enter the patient's lungs.*

● To check tube patency and position, remove the cap or plug from the feeding tube, and use the syringe to aspirate stomach contents. Examine the aspirate and place a small amount on the pH test strip. The probability of gastric placement is increased if the aspirate has a gastric fluid appearance (grassy-green, clear and colorless with mucus shreds, or brown) and has a pH of less than or equal to 5.0. **EB1**

● If there's no gastric secretion return, the tube may be in the esophagus. You'll need to advance the tube and recheck placement before proceeding.

● To assess gastric emptying, aspirate and measure residual gastric contents. Hold feedings if residual volume is greater than the predetermined amount specified in the physician's order (usually 50 to 100 ml). Reinstill any aspirate obtained. **AGA** The guidelines by the American Society for Parenteral and Enteral Nutrition specify that feedings should be held if residual is greater than 200 ml on two successive assessments. **ASPEN**

● Connect the gavage bag tubing to the feeding tube. Depending on the type of tube used, you may need to use an adapter to connect the two.

● If you're using a bulb or catheter-tip syringe, remove the bulb or plunger and attach the syringe to the pinched-off feeding tube *to prevent excess air from entering the patient's stomach, causing distention.* If you're using an infusion controller, thread the tube from the formula container through the controller according to the manufacturer's directions. Blue food dye can be added to food *to quickly identify aspiration.* Purge the tubing of air and attach it to the feeding tube.

● Open the regulator clamp on the gavage bag tubing and adjust the flow rate appropriately. When using a bulb syringe, fill the syringe with formula and release the feeding tube *to allow formula to flow through it.* The height at which you hold the syringe will determine flow rate. When the syringe is three-quarters empty, pour more formula into it.

● *To prevent air from entering the tube and the patient's stomach,* never allow the syringe to empty

completely. If you're using an infusion controller, set the flow rate according to the manufacturer's directions. **MFR** Always administer a tube feeding slowly — typically 200 to 350 ml over 15 to 30 minutes, depending on the patient's tolerance and the physician's order — *to prevent sudden stomach distention, which can cause nausea, vomiting, cramps, and diarrhea.* **AGA**

● After administering the appropriate amount of formula, flush the tubing by adding about 60 ml of water to the gavage bag or bulb syringe, or manually flush it using a barrel syringe. *This maintains the tube's patency by removing excess formula, which could occlude the tube.*

● If you're administering a continuous feeding, flush the feeding tube every 4 hours *to help prevent tube occlusion.* Monitor gastric emptying every 4 hours. **EB2** **Science**

● To discontinue gastric feeding (depending on the equipment you're using), close the regulator clamp on the gavage bag tubing, disconnect the syringe from the feeding tube, or turn off the infusion controller.

● Cover the end of the feeding tube with its plug or cap *to prevent leakage and contamination of the tube.*

● Leave the patient in semi-Fowler's or high-Fowler's position for at least 1 hour. **AGA**

● Rinse all reusable equipment with warm water.

● Dry it and store it in a convenient place for the next feeding. Change equipment every 24 hours or according to your facility's policy.

Delivering a duodenal or jejunal feeding

● Elevate the head of the bed and place the patient in low Fowler's position. **AGA**

● Open the enteral administration set and hang the gavage container on the I.V. pole.

● If you're using a nasoduodenal tube, measure its length *to check tube placement.* Remember that you may not get any residual when you aspirate the tube.

● Open the flow clamp and regulate the flow to the desired rate. To regulate the rate using a volumetric infusion pump, follow the manufacturer's directions for setting up the equipment. Most patients receive small amounts initially, with volumes increasing gradually when tolerance is established.

● Flush the tube every 4 hours with water *to maintain patency and provide hydration.* A needle catheter jejunostomy tube may require flushing every 2 hours *to prevent formula buildup inside the tube.* A Y-connector may be useful for frequent flushing. Attach the continuous feeding to the main port, and use the side port for flushes.

● Change equipment every 24 hours or according to your facility's policy.

Special considerations

● If the feeding solution doesn't initially flow through a bulb syringe, attach the bulb and squeeze it gently to start the flow. Then remove the bulb. Never use the bulb to force the formula through the tube.

● If the patient becomes nauseated or vomits, stop the feeding immediately. The patient may vomit if the stomach becomes distended from overfeeding or delayed gastric emptying.

● *To reduce oropharyngeal discomfort from the tube,* allow the patient to brush his teeth or care for his dentures regularly, and encourage frequent gargling. If the patient is unconscious, administer oral care with wet sponge-tipped swabs every 4 hours. Use petroleum jelly on dry, cracked lips. Dry mucous membranes may indicate dehydration, which requires increased fluid intake. Clean the patient's nostrils with cotton-tipped applicators, apply lubricant along the mucosa, and assess the skin for signs of breakdown. **Science**

● During continuous feedings, assess the patient frequently for abdominal distention. Flush the tubing by adding about 50 ml of water to the gavage bag or bulb syringe. *This maintains the tube's patency by removing excess formula, which could occlude the tube.*

● If the patient develops diarrhea, administer small, frequent, less concentrated feedings, or administer bolus feedings over a longer time. Make sure the formula isn't cold and that proper storage and sanitation practices have been followed. The loose stools associated with tube feedings make extra perineal and skin care necessary. Changing to a formula with more fiber may eliminate liquid stools.

● If the patient becomes constipated, the physician may increase the fruit, vegetable, or sugar content of the formula. Assess the patient's hydration status *because dehydration may produce constipation.* Increase fluid intake as necessary. If the condition persists, administer an appropriate drug or enema, as ordered. **Science**

● Drugs can be administered through the feeding tube. Except for enteric-coated drugs or timed-release medications, crush tablets or open and dilute capsules in water before administering them. Be sure to flush the tubing afterward *to ensure full instillation of medication.* Keep in mind that some drugs may change the osmolarity of the feeding formula and cause diarrhea.

● Small-bore feeding tubes may kink, making instillation impossible. If you suspect this problem, try changing the patient's position, or withdraw the tube a few inches and restart. Never use a guide wire to reposition the tube. **EB3**

● Constantly monitor the flow rate of a blended or high-residue formula *to determine if the formula is clogging the tubing as it settles. To prevent such clogging,* squeeze the bag frequently to agitate the solution.

● Collect blood samples as ordered. *Glycosuria, hyperglycemia, and diuresis can indicate an excessive carbohydrate level, leading to hyperosmotic dehydration, which can be fatal.* Monitor blood glucose levels *to assess glucose tolerance.* (A patient with a serum glucose level of less than 200 mg/dl is considered stable.) Monitor serum electrolytes, blood urea nitrogen, serum glucose, serum osmolality, and other pertinent findings *to determine the patient's response to therapy and assess his hydration status.*

● Check the flow rate hourly *to ensure correct infusion.* (With an improvised administration set, use a time tape to record the rate *because it's difficult to get precise readings from an irrigation container or enema bag.*)

● For duodenal or jejunal feeding, most patients tolerate a continuous drip better than bolus feedings. *Bolus feedings can cause such complications as hyperglycemia and diarrhea.* **AGA**

● Until the patient acquires a tolerance for the formula, you may need to dilute it to one-half or three-quarters strength to start, and increase it gradually. A patient under stress or receiving steroids may experience a pseudodiabetic state. Assess him frequently to determine the need for insulin.

TEACHING *Patient education for home tube feeding includes instructions on an infusion control device to maintain accuracy, use of the syringe or bag and tubing, care of the tube and insertion site, and formula mixing. Formula may be mixed in an electric blender according to package* *directions. Formula not used within 24 hours must be discarded. If the formula must hang for more than 8 hours, advise the patient to use a gavage or pump administration set with an ice pouch to decrease the incidence of bacterial growth. Tell him to use a new bag daily.*

Teach family members signs and symptoms to report to the physician or home care nurse as well as measures to take in an emergency.

Nursing diagnoses
- Feeding self-care deficit
- Imbalanced nutrition: Less than body requirements

Expected outcomes
The patient (and family) will:
- demonstrate correct use of home tube feeding equipment
- maintain adequate nutrition and fluid intake as evidenced by weight increase or maintenance and laboratory tests.

Complications
- Erosion of esophageal, tracheal, nasal, and oropharyngeal mucosa can result if tubes are left in place for a long time. If possible, use smaller-lumen tubes *to prevent such irritation.* Check your facility's policy regarding the frequency of changing feeding tubes *to prevent complications.*
- When using the gastric route, frequent or large-volume feedings can cause bloating and retention. Dehydration, diarrhea, and vomiting can cause metabolic disturbances. Cramping and abdominal distention usually indicate intolerance.
- When using the duodenal or jejunal route, clogging of the feeding tube is common. The patient may experience metabolic, fluid, and electrolyte abnormalities including hyperglycemia, hyperosmolar dehydration, coma, edema, hypernatremia, and essential fatty acid deficiency.
- The patient may also experience dumping syndrome, in which a large amount of hyperosmotic solution in the duodenum causes excessive diffusion of fluid through the semipermeable membrane and results in diarrhea. In a patient with low serum albumin levels, these symptoms may result from low oncotic pressure in the duodenal mucosa. (See *Managing tube feeding problems,* page 413.)

Documentation
On the intake and output sheet, record the date, volume of formula, and volume of water. In your notes, include abdominal assessment (including tube exit site, if appropriate), amount of residual gastric contents, verification of tube placement, tube patency, and amount, type, and time of feeding. Document the patient's tolerance to the feeding, including nausea, vomiting, cramping, diarrhea, and distention. Note the result of blood and urine tests, hydration status, and any drugs given through the tube. Include the date and time of administration set changes, oral and nasal hygiene, and results of specimen collections.

Supportive references
American Gastroenterological Association. "AGA Medical Position Statement: Guidelines for the Use of Enteral Nutrition," *Gastroenterology* 108(4):1280-81, April 1995. Available at: *www.harcourthealth.com/gastro/policy/v108n4p1280.html.*

American Society for Parenteral and Enteral Nutrition. "Access for Administration of Nutrition Support," *Journal of Parenteral Enteral Nutrition* 26(Suppl 1):335A-415A, January-February 2002. Available at: *www.guideline.gov.*

Bowers, S. "All About Tubes: Your Guide to Enteral Feeding Devices," *Nursing2000* 30(12):41-47, December 2000. **EB2**

Craven, R., and Hirnle, C. *Fundamentals of Nursing: Human Health and Function,* 4th ed. Philadelphia: Lippincott Williams & Wilkins, 2002.

Guenter, P., and Silkroski, M. *Tube Feeding: Practical Guidelines and Nursing Protocols.* Gaithersburg, Md.: Aspen Pubs., Inc., 2001.

Metheny, N.A., and Titler, M.G. "Assessing Placement of Feeding Tubes," *AJN* 101(5):36-45, May 2001. **EB3**

Stone, S.J., et al. "Bedside Placement of Postpyloric Feeding Tubes," *AACN Clinical Issues* 11(4):517-30, November 2000.

Sweeney, J. "How Do I Verify NG Tube Placement," *Nursing2005* 35(8):25, August 2005. **EB1**

9

Renal and urologic care

Renal and urologic systems produce, transport, collect, and excrete urine. It's vital that they function properly to maintain fluid, electrolyte, and acid-base balance and to eliminate the body's waste products. To restore or facilitate effective function of these systems, treatment of renal and urologic disorders typically involves temporary or permanent insertion of a urinary, peritoneal, or vascular catheter or tube. Catheterization also allows for monitoring of renal and urologic systems, and aids in diagnosing dysfunction.

In this chapter, you'll find the information you need to provide the best care for patients with renal and urologic disorders. The chapter offers up-to-date management tips, discussions about innovative practices and disputed treatment issues, and creative solutions to problems that occur every day. It includes evidence-based **EB** best practice recommendations and best practices that derive from fundamental principles of science **Science**. In addition, you'll find suggested techniques from such organizations as the American Nephrology Nurses Association **ANNA**, the National Institute on Aging **NIA**, the National Kidney Foundation **NKF**, the Joint Commission on Accreditation of Healthcare Organizations **JCAHO**, and the International Foundation for Gastrointestinal Disorders **IFFGD** as well as the Agency for Health Care Research and Quality **AHRQ**, the Centers for Disease Control and Prevention **CDC**, and the American Hospital Association's Patient Care Partnership **PCP**. Equipment manufacturers **MFR** may have specific guidelines or recommendations for the use of their equipment.

Helping the patient cope

One goal in caring for a patient with a renal or urologic disorder is helping him accept an invasive procedure or adjust to a new body image. You can begin to meet this goal by assessing the amount and kind of information he needs and can absorb about the procedure. Present or reinforce this information — especially by letting him know what to expect — and provide comfort and support.

Managing procedures

Performing procedures skillfully is only one aspect of successfully managing renal and urologic disorders. You must understand the purpose of each step and be aware of the best practice for the procedure, the physiologic and scientific principles and evidence-based research that support its use, and the associated indications, contraindications, and clinical ramifications. You must also accurately assess the patient's status, plan the appropriate approach to the procedure, implement the procedure, and evaluate its overall effect on the patient.

Based on the results of continued patient assessment, you can make valid clinical decisions and establish priorities that will contribute to a positive outcome. Your ability to assess a situation, analyze it critically, and establish priorities has the greatest impact on the success of the nursing process.

Arteriovenous fistula and graft care

An arteriovenous (AV) fistula is created by connecting a vein to an arterial wall, using the patient's vessels. This type of access is preferred for a patient expected to be on long-term dialysis.

The National Kidney Foundation (NKF) recommends the wrist or elbow for AV fistulas because a fistula in those spots has a lower risk of complications, such as clotting, and will remain patent. If it isn't possible to establish either of these types of fistula, access may be established using an AV graft of synthetic material or a transposed brachial basilic vein fistula. Cuffed, tunneled central venous catheters should be discouraged as permanent vascular access because they have more complications than AV access and a shorter life. **NKF**

Because it takes 1 to 4 months for the fistula to mature, the patient needs temporary access for dialysis, such as a tunneled cuffed catheter. Use of the fistula before it matures increases the risk of early venous stenosis.

To enhance maturation of the graft site, the NKF recommends the following:
● Exercise the hand and arm with the fistula (squeezing a rubber ball) *to increase blood flow.*
● Selective obliteration of major venous side branches will speed maturation in an AV fistula that's maturing slowly.
● If the new AV fistula is infiltrated, it should be rested until the swelling subsides. **NKF**

> **ALERT** *According to the NKF, if the patient still has swelling at the AV fistula after 2 weeks, a venogram or some other contrast study should be performed on the AV access site to evaluate the central veins.* **NKF**

Placing a prosthetic graft or bridge between a vein and artery creates an AV graft. Grafts are typically used in patients who are also expected to be on long-term dialysis and have unsuitable vessels for a native AV fistula, or those patients whose native AV fistula has failed. The synthetic graft can be used within 2 to 6 weeks of placement. After insertion, the fistula and graft require regular assessment for patency and examination of the surrounding skin for signs of infection.

AV fistula and graft care also includes aseptically cleaning the arterial and venous exit sites, applying antiseptic ointment, and dressing the sites with sterile bandages. When done just before hemodialysis, this procedure prolongs the life of the fistula or graft, helps prevent infection, and allows for the early detection of clotting. Care needs to be done more often if the dressing becomes wet or nonocclusive.

Equipment
Drape ● stethoscope ● sterile gloves ● sterile 4″ × 4″ gauze pads ● sterile cotton-tipped applicators ● antiseptic (chlorhexidine or povidone-iodine solution) ● bulldog clamps ● plasticized or hypoallergenic tape ● optional: swab specimen kit, prescribed antimicrobial ointment (povidone-iodine), sterile elastic gauze bandage, 2″ × 2″ gauze pads, hydrogen peroxide

Kits containing the necessary equipment can be prepackaged and stored for use.

Implementation
● Confirm the patient's identity using two patient identifiers according to facility policy. **JCAHO**
● Explain the procedure to the patient. Provide privacy and wash your hands. **CDC** **PCP**
● Place the drape on a stable surface, such as a bedside table, *to reduce the risk of traumatic injury to the fistula or graft site.* Place the extremity on the draped surface.
● Remove the two bulldog clamps from the elastic gauze bandage, and unwrap the bandage from the fistula or graft area.
● Carefully remove the gauze dressing covering the shunt and the 4″ × 4″ gauze pad under the fistula or graft.
● Assess the arterial and venous exit sites for signs and symptoms of infection, such as erythema, swelling, excessive tenderness, or drainage. Obtain a swab specimen of any purulent drainage, and notify the practitioner immediately of any signs of infection. **Science**
● Check blood flow through the fistula by inspecting the color of the blood and comparing the warmth of the fistula with that of the surrounding skin. The blood should be bright red; the fistula should feel as warm as the skin.

> **ALERT** *If the blood is dark purple or black and the temperature of the fistula or graft is lower than the surrounding skin, clotting has occurred. Notify the practitioner immediately.*
● Use the stethoscope to auscultate the fistula between the arterial and venous exit sites. A bruit confirms normal blood flow. Palpate the fistula for a thrill (by lightly placing your fingertips over the access site and feeling for vibration), which also indicates normal blood flow. **NKF**
● Open a few packages of 4″ × 4″ gauze pads and cotton-tipped applicators, and soak them with the antiseptic. Put on the sterile gloves.
● Using a soaked 4″ × 4″ gauze pad, start cleaning the skin at one of the exit sites. Wipe away from the site to *remove bacteria and reduce the chance of contaminating the fistula.* **Science**
● Use the soaked cotton-tipped applicators to remove crusted material from the exit site *because the encrustations provide a medium for bacterial growth.*

- Clean the other exit site, using fresh, soaked 4″ × 4″ gauze pads and cotton-tipped applicators.
- Clean the rest of the skin that was covered by the gauze dressing with fresh, soaked 4″ × 4″ gauze pads.
- If ordered, apply antimicrobial ointment to the exit sites *to help prevent infection.*
- Cover the exit sites with a dry, sterile 4″ × 4″ gauze pad, and tape it securely *to keep the exit sites clean and protected.*
- For routine daily care, wrap the fistula or graft lightly with an elastic gauze bandage.

Special considerations

- Blood pressure measurement and venipuncture should be avoided in the affected arm *to prevent fistula or graft occlusion.* **Science**
- Always handle the arm with the fistula or graft and dressings carefully. Don't use scissors or other sharp instruments to remove the dressing *because you may accidentally cut into the fistula.* **EB**
- When cleaning the fistula exit sites, use each 4″ × 4″ gauze pad only once and avoid wiping the area more than once *to minimize the risk of contamination.* When re-dressing the site, make sure that the tape doesn't kink or occlude the fistula. If the exit sites are heavily encrusted, place a 2″ × 2″ hydrogen peroxide-soaked gauze pad on the area for about 1 hour *to loosen the crust.* Make sure that the patient isn't allergic to iodine before using povidone-iodine.

TEACHING *Teach the patient and his caregivers proper home care of his fistula or graft.*

Nursing diagnoses

- Risk for infection

Expected outcomes

The patient will:
- have a fistula site that remains free from signs and symptoms of infection
- maintain vital signs and laboratory values within normal limits.

Complications

Possible complications of AV fistula include clotting, hemorrhage, and infection.

Documentation

Record that graft or fistula care was administered, the condition of the graft or fistula and surrounding skin, any ointment used, and any instructions given to the patient.

Supportive references

Hayes, D.D. "Caring for Your Patient with a Permanent Hemodialysis Access," *Nursing2000* 30(3):41-46, March 2000. **EB**

National Kidney Foundation. "Clinical Practice Guidelines for Vascular Access. Guideline #3: Selection of Permanent Vascular Access and Order of Preference for Placement of AV Fistulae," 2000. *www.kidney.org/professionals/KDOQI/guidelines.cfm.*

National Kidney Foundation. "Clinical Practice Guidelines for Vascular Access. Guideline #9: "Access Maturation," 2000. *www.kidney.org/professionals/KDOQI/ guidelines. _updates/doqi_uptoc.html#va.*

National Kidney Foundation. "Clinical Practice Guidelines for Vascular Access. Guideline #10: Definition of Terms," 2000. *www.kidney.org/professionals/KDOQI/ guidelines.cfm.*

Stark, J. "The Renal System," in *Core Curriculum for Critical Care Nursing,* 6th ed. Edited by Alspach, J.G. Philadelphia: W.B. Saunders Co., 2006.

Bladder irrigation, continuous

Continuous bladder irrigation can help prevent urinary tract obstruction by flushing out small blood clots that form after prostate or bladder surgery. It may also be used to treat an irritated, inflamed, or infected bladder lining.

This procedure requires placement of a triple-lumen catheter: one lumen controls balloon inflation, one allows irrigant inflow, and one allows irrigant outflow. The continuous flow of irrigating solution through the bladder also creates a mild tamponade that may help prevent venous hemorrhage. Although the patient typically receives the catheter while he's in the operating room after prostate or bladder surgery, he may have it inserted at his bedside if he isn't a surgical patient.

Setup for continuous bladder irrigation

During continuous bladder irrigation, a triple-lumen catheter allows irrigating solution to flow into the bladder through one lumen and to flow out through another, as shown here. The third lumen is used to inflate the balloon that holds the catheter in place.

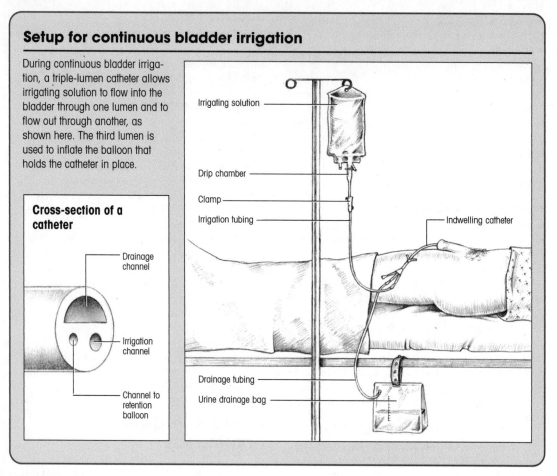

Cross-section of a catheter

Drainage channel

Irrigation channel

Channel to retention balloon

Irrigating solution

Drip chamber

Clamp

Irrigation tubing

Indwelling catheter

Drainage tubing

Urine drainage bag

Equipment

One 4,000-ml container or two 2,000-ml containers of irrigating solution (usually normal saline solution) or the prescribed amount of medicated solution • Y-type tubing made specifically for bladder irrigation • alcohol or a povidone-iodine pad • I.V. pole or bedside pole attachment • drainage bag and tubing

Implementation

• Before starting continuous bladder irrigation, double-check the irrigating solution against the practitioner's order. If the solution contains an antibiotic, check the patient's chart to make sure that he isn't allergic to the drug. Unless specified otherwise, the patient should remain on bed rest throughout continuous bladder irrigation.

• Confirm the patient's identity using two patient identifiers according to facility policy. **JCAHO**

• Wash your hands. Assemble all equipment at the patient's bedside. Explain the procedure to the patient and provide privacy. **PCP**

• Insert the spike of the Y-type tubing into the container of irrigating solution. (If you have a two-container system, insert one spike into each container.) (See *Setup for continuous bladder irrigation.*)

• Squeeze the drip chamber on the spike of the tubing.

• Open the flow clamp and flush the tubing to remove air, which could cause bladder distention. Then close the clamp.

• To begin, hang the irrigating solution on the I.V. pole.

• Clean the opening to the inflow lumen of the catheter with the alcohol or povidone-iodine pad.

• Insert the distal end of the Y-type tubing securely into the inflow lumen (third port) of the catheter.

- Make sure that the catheter's outflow lumen is securely attached to the drainage bag tubing.
- Open the flow clamp under the container of irrigating solution, and set the drip rate as ordered.
- To prevent air from entering the system, don't let the primary container empty completely before replacing it.
- If you have a two-container system, simultaneously close the flow clamp under the nearly empty container and open the flow clamp under the reserve container. This prevents reflux of irrigating solution from the reserve container into the nearly empty one. Hang a new reserve container on the I.V. pole and insert the tubing, maintaining asepsis.
- Empty the drainage bag about every 4 hours or as often as needed. Use sterile technique to avoid the risk of contamination.
- Monitor the patient's vital signs at least every 4 hours during irrigation; increase the frequency if his condition becomes unstable.

Special considerations

- Check the inflow and the outflow lines periodically for kinks to make sure that the solution is running freely. If the solution flows rapidly, check the lines frequently.
- Measure the outflow volume accurately. It should — allowing for urine production — exceed inflow volume. If inflow volume exceeds outflow volume postoperatively, suspect bladder rupture at the suture lines or renal damage, and notify the practitioner immediately.
- Assess outflow for changes in appearance and for blood clots, especially if irrigation is being performed postoperatively to control bleeding. If drainage is bright red, irrigating solution is usually infused rapidly with the clamp wide open until drainage clears. Notify the practitioner at once if you suspect hemorrhage. If drainage is clear, the solution is usually given at a rate of 40 to 60 gtt/minute. The practitioner typically specifies the rate for antibiotic solutions.
- Encourage oral fluid intake of 2 to 3 qt/day (2 to 3 L/day), unless contraindicated by another medical condition.
- Watch for interruptions in the continuous irrigation system.
- Check frequently for an obstruction in the catheter's outflow lumen.

Nursing diagnoses

- Risk for infection

Expected outcomes

The patient will:
- maintain stable vital signs
- remain free from infection.

Complications

Interruptions of the continuous irrigation system can predispose the patient to infection. Obstruction in the catheter's outflow lumen can cause bladder distention.

Documentation

Each time you finish a container of solution, record the date, time, and amount of fluid given on the intake and output record. Also, record the time and amount of fluid each time you empty the drainage bag. Note the appearance of the drainage and any complaints the patient has.

Supportive references

Ng, C. "Assessment and Intervention Knowledge of Nurses in Managing Catheter Patency in Continuous Bladder Irrigation Following TURP," *Urology Nursing* 21(2):97, April 2001.

Portable RN 2005. Philadelphia: Lippincott Williams & Wilkins, 2005.

Catheter (indwelling) care and removal

Intended to prevent infection and other complications by keeping the catheter site clean, routine catheter care is typically performed daily after the patient's morning bath and immediately after perineal care. (Bedtime catheter care may have to be performed before perineal care.)

Studies suggest that catheter care should include daily cleaning of the meatal-catheter area. The use of topical antibiotics is discouraged because it hasn't been proven to be effective in decreasing infection. **EB** The equipment and the patient's genitalia require inspection twice daily.

Experts agree that catheter surfaces and balloons that are exposed to urine will develop encrustations, and patients whose catheters develop a blockage have urine that's alkaline and high in concentrations of mucin, protein, and calcium salts. For this reason, it's recommended that catheterized patients drink lots of fluids to ensure increased urine output so that microorganisms are flushed out of the bladder.

🔺 **ALERT** *Be sure to assess the catheter every day for crystals or encrustations by palpating it between your fingers and assessing for sandy or granular materials. Be careful not to break off any crystals. If encrustations are present on the catheter, it should be removed and replaced.*

An indwelling urinary catheter should be removed when bladder decompression is no longer necessary, when the patient can resume voiding, or when the catheter is obstructed. Depending on the length of the catheterization, the practitioner may order bladder retraining before catheter removal.

Equipment

Catheter care: Soap and water • sterile gloves • eight sterile 4″ × 4″ gauze pads • basin • washcloth • leg bag • collection bag • adhesive tape or leg band • waste receptacle • optional: safety pin, rubber band, gooseneck lamp or flashlight, adhesive remover, specimen container

Perineal cleaning: Washcloth • additional basin • gloves • soap and water

Catheter removal: Gloves • alcohol pad • 10-ml syringe with a luer-lock • bedpan • linen-saver pad • optional: clamp for bladder retraining

Implementation

● Confirm the patient's identity using two patient identifiers according to facility policy. **JCAHO**
● Explain the procedure and its purpose to the patient. **PCP**
● Provide the patient with the necessary equipment for self-cleaning, if possible.
● Provide privacy.

Catheter care

● Make sure that the lighting is adequate *so you can see the perineum and catheter tubing clearly.* Place a gooseneck lamp or flashlight at the bedside if needed.
● Inspect the catheter for problems and check the urine drainage for mucus, blood clots, sediment, and turbidity. Pinch the catheter between two fingers *to determine if the lumen contains any material.* If you notice any of these conditions (or if your facility's policy requires it), obtain a urine specimen from the specimen collection port using a sterile needle and syringe. Collect at least 3 ml of urine, but don't fill the specimen cup more than halfway. Notify the practitioner about your findings. **Science**

🔺 **ALERT** *Be sure to clean the port with povidone-iodine solution before collecting the urine specimen.*

● Inspect the outside of the catheter where it enters the urinary meatus for encrusted material and suppurative drainage. Inspect the tissue around the meatus for irritation or swelling.
● Remove the leg band, or if adhesive tape was used to secure the catheter, remove the adhesive tape. Inspect the area for signs and symptoms of adhesive burns — redness, tenderness, or blisters.
● Put on the gloves. Clean the outside of the catheter and the tissue around the meatus, using soap and water. *To avoid contaminating the urinary tract,* always clean by wiping away from — *never* toward — the urinary meatus. Use a dry gauze pad to remove encrusted material. **Science**

🔺 **ALERT** *Don't pull on the catheter while you're cleaning it. This can injure the urethra and the bladder wall. It can also expose a section of the catheter that was inside the urethra, so that when you release the catheter, the newly contaminated section will reenter the urethra, introducing potentially infectious organisms.*

● Remove your gloves, reapply the leg band, and reattach the catheter to the leg band. If a leg band isn't available, tear a piece of adhesive tape from the roll.
● *To prevent skin hypersensitivity or irritation,* retape the catheter on the opposite side.

🔺 **ALERT** *Provide enough slack before securing the catheter to prevent tension on the tubing, which could injure the urethral lumen or bladder wall.*

● Most drainage bags have a plastic clamp on the tubing to attach them to the sheet. If this isn't available, wrap a rubber band around the drainage tubing, insert the safety pin through a loop of the rubber band, and pin the tubing to the sheet below bladder level. Attach the collection bag, below bladder level, to the bed frame.
● If necessary, use an adhesive remover to clean residue from the previous tape site. Dispose of used supplies in a waste receptacle.

Catheter removal

- Wash your hands. **CDC**
- Assemble the equipment at the patient's bedside. Explain the procedure and tell him that he may feel slight discomfort. Tell him that you'll check him periodically during the first 6 to 24 hours after catheter removal *to make sure he resumes voiding.* **PCP**
- Put on gloves. Place a linen-saver pad under the patient's buttocks. Attach the syringe to the luer-lock mechanism on the catheter. **CDC**
- Pull back on the plunger of the syringe. *This deflates the balloon by aspirating the injected fluid.* The amount of fluid injected is usually indicated on the tip of the catheter's balloon lumen and in the patient's chart.
- *Because urine may leak as the catheter is removed,* offer the patient a bedpan. Grasp the catheter, and pinch it firmly with your thumb and index finger *to prevent urine from flowing back into the urethra.* Gently pull the catheter from the urethra. If you meet resistance, don't apply force; instead, notify the practitioner. Remove the bedpan. **Science**
- Measure and record the amount of urine in the collection bag before discarding it. Remove and discard gloves, and wash your hands. For the first 24 hours after catheter removal, note the time and amount of each voiding.

Special considerations

- Your facility may require the use of specific cleaning agents for catheter care, so check the policy manual before beginning this procedure.
- Use a closed drainage system whenever possible to decrease the chance of the patient getting a urinary tract infection (UTI).
- Avoid raising the drainage bag above bladder level *to prevent reflux of urine. To avoid damaging the urethral lumen or bladder wall,* always disconnect the drainage bag and tubing from the bed linen and bed frame before helping the patient out of bed. **Science** Also, avoid contact with the floor.
- When possible, attach a leg bag *to allow the patient greater mobility.* If the patient will be discharged with an indwelling catheter, teach him how to use a leg bag. (See *Teaching about leg bags,* page 448.)
- Encourage patients with unrestricted fluid intake to increase intake to at least 3 qt (3 L)/day. *This helps flush the urinary system and reduces sediment formation. To prevent urinary sediment and calculi from ob-*structing the drainage tube, some patients are placed on an acid-ash diet to acidify urine.
- Although cranberry juice has been widely used to help prevent UTIs, research doesn't support its use for prevention or treatment. **EB**
- After catheter removal, assess the patient for incontinence, urgency, persistent dysuria or bladder spasms, fever, chills, or palpable bladder distention. The patient should void within 6 to 8 hours after catheter removal. **Science**
- When changing catheters after long-term use (usually 30 days), you may need a larger size catheter because the meatus enlarges, causing urine to leak around the catheter.

TEACHING *Instruct patients discharged with indwelling catheters to wash the urinary meatus and perineal area with soap and water twice daily, from front to back, and the anal area after each bowel movement.*

Nursing diagnoses

- Risk for infection

Expected outcomes

The patient will:
- not develop a UTI
- maintain vital signs and laboratory values within normal limits.

Complications

Sediment buildup can occur anywhere in a catheterization system, especially in a bedridden or dehydrated patient. To prevent this, keep the patient well hydrated if he isn't on fluid restriction. Change the indwelling catheter as ordered or when malfunction, obstruction, or contamination occurs.

Acute renal failure may result from a catheter obstructed by sediment. Stay alert for sharply reduced urine flow from the catheter. Assess for bladder discomfort or distention.

A UTI can result from catheter insertion or from intraluminal or extraluminal migration of bacteria up the catheter. Signs and symptoms may include cloudy urine, foul-smelling urine, hematuria, fever, malaise, tenderness over the bladder, and flank pain.

Major complications in removing an indwelling catheter are failure of the balloon to deflate and rupture of the balloon. If the balloon ruptures, cystoscopy is usually performed to ensure removal of balloon fragments.

Teaching about leg bags

A urine drainage bag attached to the leg provides the catheterized patient with greater mobility. Because the bag is hidden under clothing, it may also help him feel more comfortable about catheterization. Leg bags are usually worn during the day and are replaced at night with a standard collection device.

If the patient will be discharged with an indwelling catheter, teach him how to attach and remove a leg bag. To demonstrate, you'll need a bag with a short drainage tube, two straps, an alcohol pad, adhesive tape, and a screw clamp or hemostat.

Attaching the leg bag

● Provide privacy, and explain the procedure. Describe the advantages of a leg bag, but caution the patient that a leg bag is smaller than a standard collection device and may have to be emptied more frequently.

● Remove the protective covering from the tip of the drainage tube. Then show the patient how to clean the tip with an alcohol pad, wiping away from the opening *to avoid contaminating the tube.* Show him how to attach the tube to the catheter.

● Place the drainage bag on the patient's calf or thigh. Have him fasten the straps securely (as shown), and then show him how to tape the catheter to his leg. Emphasize that he must leave slack in the catheter to minimize pressure on the bladder, urethra, and related structures. *Excessive pressure or tension can lead to tissue breakdown.*

● Also tell the patient not to fasten the straps too tightly *to avoid interfering with his circulation.*

Avoiding complications

● Although most leg bags have a valve in the drainage tube that prevents urine reflux into the bladder, urge the patient to keep the drainage bag lower than his bladder at all times *because urine in the bag is a perfect growth medium for bacteria.* Caution him also not to go to bed or take long naps while wearing the leg bag.

● *To prevent a full leg bag from damaging the bladder wall and urethra,* encourage the patient to empty the bag when it's half full. He should also inspect the catheter and drainage tube periodically for compression or kinking, *which could obstruct urine flow and result in bladder distention.*

● Tell the patient to wash the leg bag with soap and water or a bacteriostatic solution before each use *to prevent infection.*

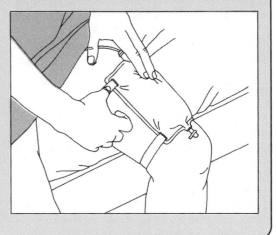

Documentation

Record the care you performed, any modifications, patient complaints, and the condition of the perineum and urinary meatus. Note the character of the urine in the drainage bag, any sediment buildup, and whether a specimen was sent for laboratory analysis. Record fluid intake and output. An hourly record is usually necessary for critically ill patients and those with renal insufficiency who are hemodynamically unstable.

Supportive references

Joanna Briggs Institute for Evidence Based Nursing and Midwifery. "Best Practice: Management of Short Term Indwelling Urethral Catheters to Prevent Urinary Tract Infections," 4(1), 2000. *www.joannabriggs.edu.au/bpmenu.html.*

Madigan, E., and Neff, D.F. "Care of Patients with Long-Term Indwelling Urinary Catheters," *Online Journal of Issues in Nursing* 8(3), June 2003. *www.nursingworld.org/ojin.* **EB**

Potter, P.A., and Perry, A.G. *Fundamentals of Nursing,* 6th ed. St. Louis: Mosby–Year Book, Inc., 2004.

Catheter (indwelling) insertion

An indwelling urinary catheter (Foley catheter) remains in the bladder to provide continuous urine drainage. A balloon inflated at the catheter's distal end prevents it from slipping out of the bladder after insertion. Indwelling catheters are used most commonly to relieve bladder distention caused by urine retention and to allow continuous urine drainage when the urinary meatus is swollen from childbirth, surgery, or local trauma. Other indications for an indwelling catheter include urinary tract obstruction (by a tumor or enlarged prostate), urine retention or infection from neurogenic bladder paralysis caused by spinal cord injury or disease, and an illness in which the patient's urine output must be monitored.

An indwelling catheter is inserted using sterile technique and only when absolutely necessary. Insertion should be performed with extreme care *to prevent injury and infection. To avoid trauma to the urethra and decrease the risk of infection,* always use the smallest size catheter with the smallest balloon. (See *Catheterization technique.*)

 CLINICAL IMPACT *Research has indicated that the most common complications of long-term indwelling urinary catheters are bacteriuria, encrustation, and blockage. Bacteriuria is more prevalent in female patients, older patients, and those with long-term use of indwelling urinary catheters. Research has also shown that silicone catheters and catheters with large lumens are less likely to develop encrustation.* **EB2**

Equipment

Sterile indwelling catheter (latex or silicone #10 to #22 French [average adult sizes are #14 to #16 French]) • syringe filled with 10 ml of sterile water (normal saline solution is sometimes used) • washcloth • towel • soap and water • two linen-saver pads • sterile gloves • sterile drape • sterile fenestrated drape • sterile cotton-tipped applicators (or cotton balls and plastic forceps) • povidone-iodine or other antiseptic cleaning agent • urine receptacle • sterile water-soluble lubricant • sterile drainage collection bag • intake and output sheet • adhesive tape • op-

CONTROVERSIAL ISSUE

Catheterization technique

Although strict sterile technique is believed to reduce the risk of urinary tract infections (UTIs) in catheterized patients, one study found that using nonsterile (clean) vs. sterile technique didn't make a difference in the rates of UTIs. The study (involving 156 patients) compared sterile catheterization, which includes a surgical scrub, sterile gloves, strict sterile no-touch technique, savlon solution, sterile catheter pack, lidocaine, and sterile water to inflate the balloon, to the clean technique, which includes handwashing, nonsterile gloves, and tap water for perineal cleaning and to fill the balloon.

Results showed no statistical difference in the incidence of UTIs between the patients catheterized using sterile technique and those catheterized using clean technique. There is, however, a considerable cost difference with the sterile method — it's more than twice as expensive as the clean method. The study concluded that strict sterility isn't necessary in preoperative short-term catheterization and that it's time consuming and more expensive. **EB1**

tional: urine-specimen container and laboratory request form, leg band with Velcro closure, gooseneck lamp or flashlight, pillows or rolled blankets

Prepackaged sterile disposable kits that usually contain all the necessary equipment are available. The syringes in these kits are prefilled with 10 ml of normal saline solution.

Preparation of equipment

Check the order on the patient's chart to determine if a catheter size or type has been specified. Wash your hands, select the appropriate equipment, and assemble it at the patient's bedside.

Implementation

● Confirm the patient's identity using two patient identifiers according to facility policy. **JCAHO**
● Explain the procedure to the patient and provide privacy. Check his chart and ask when he voided last. Percuss and palpate the bladder *to establish baseline data.* Ask if he feels the urge to void. **PCP** **Science**

● Have a coworker hold a flashlight or place a goose-neck lamp next to the patient's bed *so that you can see the urinary meatus clearly*.

● Place the female patient in the supine position, with her knees flexed and separated and her feet flat on the bed, about 2′ (61 cm) apart. If she finds this position uncomfortable, have her flex one knee and keep the other leg flat on the bed. **Science**

● Place the male patient in the supine position with his legs extended and flat on the bed. Ask the patient to hold the position *to give you a clear view of the urinary meatus and to prevent contamination*.

● If necessary, ask an assistant to help the patient stay in position or to direct the light.

ALERT *The elderly patient may need pillows or rolled towels or blankets to help with positioning.*

● Wash your hands, and put on gloves. Use a washcloth to clean the patient's genital area and perineum thoroughly with soap and water. Dry the area with the towel. **CDC**

● Place the linen-saver pads on the bed between the patient's legs and under the hips. *To create the sterile field*, open the prepackaged kit or equipment tray and place it between the female patient's legs or next to the male patient's hip. If the sterile gloves are the first item on the top of the tray, put them on. Place the sterile drape under the patient's hips. Drape the patient's lower abdomen with the sterile fenestrated drape so that only the genital area remains exposed. Take care not to contaminate your gloves. **Science**

● Open the rest of the kit or tray. Put on the sterile gloves if you haven't already done so.

● Make sure that the patient isn't allergic to iodine solution; if he *is* allergic, another antiseptic cleaning agent must be used.

● Tear open the packet of povidone-iodine or other antiseptic cleaning agent, and use it to saturate the sterile cotton balls or applicators. Be careful not to spill the solution on the equipment.

● Open the packet of water-soluble lubricant and apply it to the catheter tip; attach the drainage bag to the other end of the catheter. (If you're using a commercial kit, the drainage bag may be attached.) Make sure that all tubing ends remain sterile, and make sure that the clamp at the emptying port of the drainage bag is closed *to prevent urine leakage from the bag*. Some drainage systems have an air-lock chamber *to prevent bacteria from traveling to the bladder*

from urine in the drainage bag. Note: Some urologists and nurses use a syringe prefilled with water-soluble lubricant and instill the lubricant directly into the male urethra, instead of on the catheter tip. *This method helps prevent trauma to the urethral lining and, possibly, a urinary tract infection (UTI)*. Check your facility's policy.

● Before inserting the catheter, inflate the balloon with sterile water or normal saline solution *to inspect it for leaks*. To do this, attach the prefilled syringe to the luer-lock, and then push the plunger and check for seepage as the balloon expands. Aspirate the solution *to deflate the balloon*. Inspect the catheter for resiliency. *Rough, cracked catheters can injure the urethral mucosa during insertion, which can predispose the patient to infection*. **Science**

● For the female patient, separate the labia majora and labia minora as widely as possible with the thumb, middle, and index fingers of your nondominant hand *so you have a full view of the urinary meatus*. Keep the labia well separated throughout the procedure (as shown below) *so they don't obscure the urinary meatus or contaminate the area after it's cleaned.*

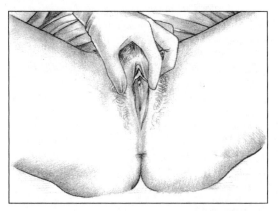

● With your dominant hand, use a sterile, cotton-tipped applicator (or pick up a sterile cotton ball with the plastic forceps) and wipe one side of the urinary meatus with a single downward motion (as shown at top of next page). Wipe the other side with another sterile applicator or cotton ball in the same way. Wipe directly over the meatus with still another sterile applicator or cotton ball. Take care not to contaminate your sterile glove. **Science**

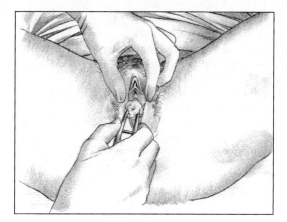

- For the male patient, hold the penis with your non-dominant hand. If he's uncircumcised, retract the foreskin. Gently lift and stretch the penis to a 60- to 90-degree angle. Hold the penis this way throughout the procedure *to straighten the urethra and maintain a sterile field* (as shown below).

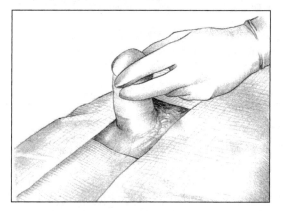

- Use your dominant hand to clean the glans with a sterile cotton-tipped applicator or a sterile cotton ball held in forceps. Clean in a circular motion, starting at the urinary meatus and working outward. **Science**
- Repeat the procedure using another sterile applicator or cotton ball and taking care not to contaminate your sterile glove.
- Pick up the catheter with your dominant hand and prepare to insert the lubricated tip into the urinary meatus. *To facilitate insertion by relaxing the sphincter,* ask the patient to cough as you insert the catheter. Tell the patient to breathe deeply and slowly *to further relax the sphincter.* Hold the catheter close to

its tip *to ease insertion and control its direction.* **Science**

ALERT *Never force a catheter during insertion. Maneuver it gently as the patient bears down or coughs. If you still meet resistance, stop and notify the practitioner. Sphincter spasms, strictures, misplacement in the vagina (in females), or an enlarged prostate (in males) may cause resistance.*

- For the female patient, advance the catheter about 2″ to 3″ (5 to 7.5 cm) — while continuing to hold the labia apart — until urine begins to flow (as shown below). If the catheter is inadvertently inserted into the vagina, leave it there as a landmark. Begin the procedure over again using new supplies. **Science**

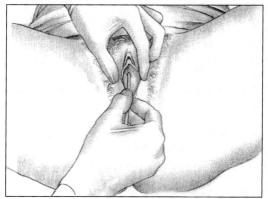

- For the male patient, advance the catheter to the bifurcation 5″ to 7½″ (12.5 to 19 cm) and check for urine flow (as shown below). If the foreskin was retracted, replace it *to prevent compromised circulation and painful swelling.* **Science**

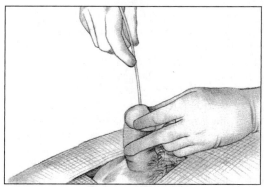

● When urine stops flowing, attach the prefilled syringe to the luer-lock. Push the plunger and inflate the balloon *to keep the catheter in place in the bladder* (as shown below).

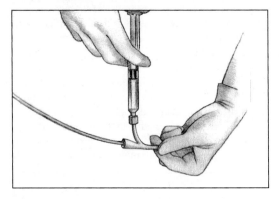

⚠ ALERT *Never inflate a balloon without first establishing urine flow, which assures you that the catheter is in the bladder.*

● Hang the collection bag below bladder level *to prevent urine reflux into the bladder,* which can cause infection, and *to facilitate gravity drainage of the bladder.* Make sure that the tubing doesn't get tangled in the bed's side rails. **Science**

● Tape the catheter to the female patient's thigh (as shown below) *to prevent possible tension on the urogenital trigone.*

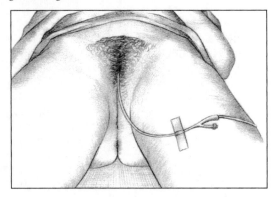

● Tape the catheter to the male patient's abdomen (with penis directed toward chest) or anterior thigh *to prevent pressure on the urethra at the penoscrotal junction,* which can lead to the formation of urethrocutaneous fistulas. **EB3** Taping also prevents traction

on the bladder and alterations in the normal direction of urine flow in males.

● As an alternative, secure the catheter to the patient's thigh using a leg band with a Velcro closure (as shown below). This decreases skin irritation, especially in patients with long-term indwelling catheters.

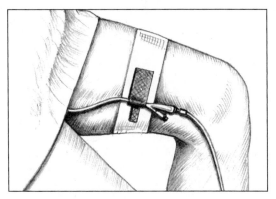

● Dispose of used supplies properly. **CDC**

Special considerations

● Indwelling urinary catheters should be used only after all other means of management have been considered.

● The patient's need for a catheter should be reviewed regularly, and it should be removed as soon as possible.

● Several types of catheters are available with balloons of various sizes. Each type has its own method of inflation and closure. For example, in one type of catheter, sterile solution or air is injected through the inflation lumen, and then the end of the injection port is folded over itself and fastened with a clamp or rubber band. *Note:* Injecting a catheter with air makes identifying leaks difficult and doesn't guarantee deflation of the balloon for removal.

● A similar catheter is inflated when a seal in the end of the inflation lumen is penetrated with a needle or the tip of the solution-filled syringe. Another type of balloon catheter self-inflates when a prepositioned clamp is loosened. The balloon size determines the amount of solution needed for inflation, and the exact amount is usually printed on the distal extension of the catheter used for inflating the balloon.

• If necessary, ask the female patient to lie on her side with her knees drawn up to her chest during the catheterization procedure (as shown below). *This position may be especially helpful for elderly or disabled patients such as those with severe contractures.*

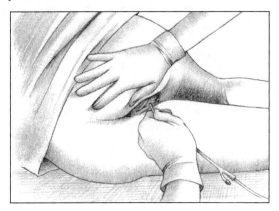

• If the practitioner orders a urine specimen for laboratory analysis, obtain it from the urine receptacle with a specimen collection container at the time of catheterization, and send it to the laboratory with the appropriate laboratory request form. Connect the drainage bag when urine stops flowing.
• Inspect the catheter and tubing periodically while they're in place *to detect compression or kinking that could obstruct urine flow.* Explain the basic principles of gravity drainage *so the patient realizes the importance of keeping the drainage tubing and collection bag lower than his bladder at all times.* If necessary, provide the patient with detailed instructions for performing clean intermittent self-catheterization. (See "Self-catheterization," page 481.)
• For monitoring purposes, empty the collection bag at least every 8 hours. Excessive fluid volume may require more frequent emptying *to prevent traction on the catheter,* which would cause the patient discomfort, and *to prevent injury to the urethra and bladder wall.* Some facilities encourage changing catheters at regular intervals, such as every 30 days, if the patient will have long-term continuous drainage.

⚠ **ALERT** *Observe the patient carefully for adverse reactions, such as hypovolemic shock, caused by removing excessive volumes of residual urine. Check your facility's policy beforehand to determine the maximum amount of urine that may*

be drained at one time (some facilities limit the amount to 700 to 1,000 ml). There's some controversy about whether to limit the amount of urine drained. Clamp the catheter at the first sign of an adverse reaction, and notify the practitioner.

🔖 **TEACHING** *If the patient will be discharged with a long-term indwelling catheter, teach him and his family all aspects of daily catheter maintenance, including care of the skin and urinary meatus, signs and symptoms of a UTI or obstruction, how to irrigate the catheter (if appropriate), and the importance of adequate fluid intake to maintain patency. Explain that a home care nurse should visit every 4 to 6 weeks — or more often if needed — to change the catheter.*

Nursing diagnoses
• Impaired urinary elimination
• Risk for infection

Expected outcomes
The patient will:
• have few complications
• maintain fluid balance
• remain free from infection
• maintain vital signs and laboratory values within normal limits.

Complications
A UTI can result from the introduction of bacteria into the bladder. Improper insertion can cause traumatic injury to the urethral and bladder mucosa. Bladder atony or spasms can result from rapid decompression of a severely distended bladder.

Documentation
Record the date, time, and size and type of indwelling catheter used. Describe the amount, color, and other characteristics of urine emptied from the bladder. Your facility may require only the intake and output sheet for fluid-balance data. If large volumes of urine have been emptied, describe the patient's tolerance for the procedure. Note whether a urine specimen was sent for laboratory analysis.

Supportive references
Carapeti, E.A., et al. "Randomised Study of Sterile Versus Non-sterile Urethral Catheterization," *Annals of the*

Royal College of Surgeons of England 78(1):59-60, January 1996. **EB1**

Hanchett, M. "Techniques for Stabilizing Urinary Catheters: Tape May be the Oldest Method, but it's not the Only One," *AJN* 102(3):44-48, March 2002. **EB3**

Joanna Briggs Institute for Evidence Based Nursing and Midwifery. "Best Practice: Management of Short Term Indwelling Urethral Catheters to Prevent Urinary Tract Infections," 4(1), 2000. *www.joannabriggs.edu.au/bpmenu.html.*

Madigan, E., and Neff, D.F. "Care of Patients with Long-Term Indwelling Urinary Catheters," *Online Journal of Issues in Nursing* 8(3), June 2003. *www.nursingworld.org/ojin.* **EB2**

National Collaborating Centre for Nursing and Supportive Care. "Infection Control. Prevention of Health-Care Associated Infections in Primary and Community Care," London (UK): National Institute for Clinical Excellence: 26 June, 2003. *www.nice.org.*

Potter, P.A., and Perry, A.G. *Fundamentals of Nursing,* 6th ed. St. Louis: Mosby–Year Book, Inc., 2004.

Catheter irrigation

Catheter irrigation may be performed to maintain or restore the catheter's patency; for example, to remove pus or blood clots that may block the catheter and prevent proper drainage.

The closed method is preferred when performing bladder or catheter irrigation *because it's associated with a lower risk of infection.* **EB** Closed catheter irrigations may be intermittent or continuous. Generally a triple-lumen catheter is used for closed irrigations. The irrigating solution is infused through the irrigating port of the catheter and into the bladder and then is drained out through the catheter's drainage lumen.

Occasionally, the open method of irrigation may be used to restore catheter patency. In this method, the risk of injecting a microorganism into the bladder is higher because the connection between the indwelling catheter and the drainage tube is broken. Sterile technique should be used to maintain the sterility of the drainage tubing connector and interior of the indwelling catheter *to minimize the risk of infection.* **Science**

The open method of catheter or bladder irrigation is performed with a double-lumen indwelling catheter and may be necessary for patients who develop blood clots or mucus plugs that occlude the catheter and when it's undesirable to change the catheter.

Equipment

Ordered irrigating solution (such as normal saline solution) • sterile graduated receptacle or emesis basin • sterile bulb syringe or 50-ml catheter tip syringe • two alcohol pads • sterile gloves • linen-saver pad • intake-output sheet • optional: basin of warm water

Commercially packaged sterile irrigating solution, a graduated receptacle, and a bulb or 50-ml catheter tip syringe is available. If the volume of irrigating solution instilled must be measured, use a graduated syringe instead of a noncalibrated bulb syringe.

Preparation of equipment

Check the expiration date on the irrigating solution. To prevent vesical spasms during instillation of solution, warm it to room temperature. If necessary, place the container in a basin of warm water. Never heat the solution on a burner or in a microwave oven because hot irrigating solution can injure the patient's bladder.

Implementation

● Confirm the patient's identity using two patient identifiers according to facility policy. **JCAHO**
● Wash your hands, and assemble the equipment at the bedside. Explain the procedure to the patient, and provide privacy. **CDC** **PCP**
● Place the patient in the dorsal recumbent position. Place a linen-saver pad under the patient's buttocks *to protect the bed linens.*
● Create a sterile field at the patient's bedside by opening the sterile equipment tray or commercial kit. Using sterile technique, clean the lip of the solution bottle by pouring a small amount into a sink or waste receptacle. Pour the prescribed amount of solution into the graduated receptacle or emesis basin. **Science**
● Place the tip of the syringe into the solution. Squeeze the bulb or pull back the plunger (depending on the type of syringe), and fill the syringe with the appropriate amount of solution (usually 30 ml).
● Open the package of alcohol pads, and then put on sterile gloves. Clean the juncture of the catheter and drainage tube with an alcohol pad *to remove as many bacterial contaminants as possible.*

- Disconnect the catheter and drainage tube by twisting them in opposite directions and carefully pulling them apart without creating tension on the catheter. Don't let go of the catheter — hold it in your nondominant hand. Place the end of the drainage tube on the sterile field, being sure not to contaminate the tube. Keep the end of the drainage tube sterile by placing a sterile gauze over it and securing the gauze with a piece of tape. **Science**
- Twist the bulb syringe or catheter-tip syringe onto the catheter's distal end.
- Squeeze the bulb or slowly push the plunger of the syringe *to instill the irrigating solution through the catheter.* If necessary, refill the syringe and repeat this step until you've instilled the prescribed amount of irrigating solution.
- Remove the syringe and direct the return flow from the catheter into a sterile receptacle.
- Wipe the end of the drainage tube and catheter with the remaining alcohol pad.
- Wait a few seconds until the alcohol evaporates, and then reattach the drainage tubing to the catheter.
- Dispose of used supplies properly.

Special considerations

- Catheter irrigation requires strict sterile technique *to prevent bacteria from entering the bladder.* The ends of the catheter and drainage tube and the tip of the syringe must be sterile throughout the procedure.
- If you encounter resistance during instillation of the irrigating solution, don't try to force the solution into the bladder. Instead, stop the procedure and notify the practitioner. If an indwelling catheter becomes totally obstructed, obtain an order to remove it and replace it with a new one *to prevent bladder distention, acute renal failure, urinary stasis, and subsequent infection.* **Science**
- The practitioner may order a continuous irrigation system. *This decreases the risk of infection by eliminating the need to disconnect the catheter and drainage tube repeatedly.*
- Encourage the catheterized patient not on restricted fluid intake to increase his intake to 3 qt (3 L) per day *to help flush the urinary system.*

Nursing diagnoses

- Acute pain
- Risk for infection
- Urinary retention

Expected outcomes

The patient will:
- be free from pain
- not develop a urinary tract infection or kidney infection
- maintain equal intake and output.

Documentation

Note the amount, color, and consistency of return urine flow, and document the patient's tolerance of the procedure. Note any resistance during instillation of the solution. If the return flow volume is less than the amount of solution instilled, note this on the intake and output balance sheets and in your notes.

Supportive references

Joanna Briggs Institute for Evidence Based Nursing and Midwifery. "Best Practice: Management of Short Term Indwelling Urethral Catheters to Prevent Urinary Tract Infections," 4(1), 2000. *www.joannabriggs.edu.au/ bpmenu.html.*

Madigan, E., and Neff, D.F. "Care of Patients with Long-Term Indwelling Urinary Catheters," *Online Journal of Issues in Nursing* 8(3), June 2003. *www.nursingworld. org/ojin.*

Potter, P.A., and Perry, A.G. *Fundamentals of Nursing,* 6th ed. St. Louis: Mosby–Year Book, Inc., 2004. **EB**

Continuous renal replacement therapy

Continuous renal replacement therapy (CRRT) is used to treat patients who suffer from acute renal failure. Unlike the more traditional intermittent hemodialysis (IHD), CRRT is administered around the clock, providing patients with continuous therapy and sparing them the destabilizing hemodynamic and electrolyte changes characteristic of IHD. CRRT is used for such patients as those who have hypotension, who can't tolerate traditional hemodialysis. For such patients, CRRT is usually the only choice of treatment; however, it can also be used on many patients who can tolerate IHD. CRRT methods vary in complexity. The techniques include the following:
- Slow continuous ultrafiltration (SCUF) uses arteriovenous (AV) access and the patient's blood pressure to circulate blood through a hemofilter. Because this

therapy's goal is the removal of fluids, the patient doesn't receive replacement fluids.

● Continuous arteriovenous hemofiltration (CAVH) uses the patient's blood pressure and AV access to circulate blood through a flow resistance hemofilter. However, to maintain the patency of the filter and systemic blood pressure, the patient receives replacement fluids.

● Continuous venovenous hemofiltration (CVVH) fuses SCUF and CAVH. A double-lumen catheter is used to provide access to a vein, and a pump moves blood through the hemofilter.

● Continuous arteriovenous hemodialysis (CAVH-D) combines hemofiltration with hemodialysis. In this technique, the infusion pump moves dialysate solution concurrent to blood flow, adding the ability to continuously remove solute while removing fluid. Like CAVH, it can also be performed in patients with hypotension and fluid overload.

● Continuous venovenous hemodialysis (CVVH-D) is similar to CAVH-D, except that a vein provides the access while a pump is used to move dialysate solution concurrent with blood flow.

✔ **CLINICAL IMPACT** *CVVH or CVVH-D is used instead of CAVH or CAVH-D in many facilities to treat critically ill patients. CVVH has several advantages over CAVH: It doesn't require arterial access, can be performed in patients with low mean arterial pressures, and has a better solute clearance than CAVH.*

Equipment

CRRT equipment ● heparin flush solution ● occlusive dressings for catheter insertion sites ● sterile gloves ● sterile mask ● antiseptic solution ● sterile 4″ × 4″ gauze pads ● tape ● filtration replacement fluid (FRF) as ordered ● infusion pump

Preparation of equipment

Prime the hemofilter and tubing according to the manufacturer's instructions.

Implementation

● Confirm the patient's identity using two patient identifiers according to facility policy. **JCAHO**

● Wash your hands. Assemble the equipment at the patient's bedside, and explain the procedure. (See *CAVH setup.*) **CDC**

● If necessary, assist with inserting the catheters into the femoral artery and vein, using strict sterile technique. (In some cases, an internal AV fistula or external AV shunt may be used instead of the femoral route.) If ordered, flush both catheters with heparin flush solution *to prevent clotting.*

● Apply occlusive dressings to the insertion sites, and mark the dressings with the date and time. Secure the tubing and connections with tape.

● Before starting therapy, weigh the patient, take his baseline vital signs, make sure that necessary laboratory studies have been done (usually, electrolyte levels, coagulation factors, complete blood count, blood urea nitrogen, and creatinine studies), and assess the patient's risk of bleeding.

● Monitor the patient's vital signs, cardiac rhythm and rate, level of consciousness, intravascular and extravascular volume status, respiratory status, biochemical profile, and coagulation and hematologic status throughout CRRT. **ANNA**

● Assess the patient for disequilibrium, including headache, nausea and vomiting, hypertension, decreased sensorium, seizures, and coma. **ANNA**

● Assess the patient for hyperglycemia. **ANNA**

● Put on the sterile gloves and mask. Prepare the connection sites by cleaning them with gauze pads soaked in antiseptic solution, and then connect them to the exit port of each catheter.

● Using sterile technique, connect the arterial and venous lines to the hemofilter.

● Turn on the hemofilter and monitor the blood flow rate through the circuit. The flow rate is usually kept between 500 and 900 ml/hour.

● Inspect the ultrafiltrate during the procedure. It should remain clear yellow, with no gross blood. Pink-tinged or bloody ultrafiltrate may signal a blood leak in the hemofilter, which permits bacterial contamination. If a leak occurs, follow your facility's policy for termination of treatment. **ANNA**

● Assess the affected leg for signs of obstructed blood flow, such as coolness, pallor, and a weak pulse. Check the groin area on the affected side *for signs of hematoma.* Ask the patient if he has pain at the insertion sites.

● Calculate the amount of FRF every hour, or as ordered, according to your facility's policy. Infuse the prescribed amount and type of FRF through the infusion pump into the arterial side of the circuit.

CAVH setup

During continuous arteri-ovenous hemofiltration (CAVH), the patient's arterial blood pressure serves as a natural pump, driving blood through the arterial line. A hemofilter removes water and toxic solutes (ultrafiltrate) from the blood. Filter replacement fluid is infused into a port on the arterial side; this same port can be used to infuse heparin. The venous line carries the replacement fluid, along with purified blood, to the patient. The illustration shows one of several CAVH setups.

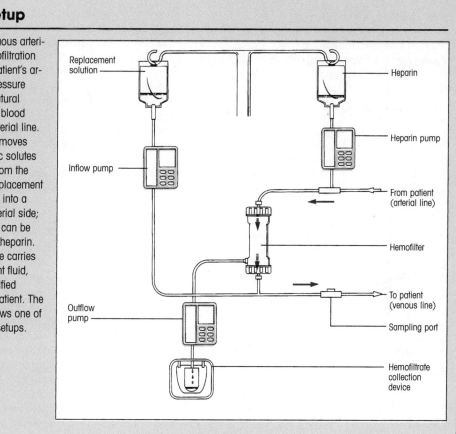

Replacement solution
Heparin
Heparin pump
Inflow pump
From patient (arterial line)
Hemofilter
To patient (venous line)
Sampling port
Outflow pump
Hemofiltrate collection device

Special considerations

● *Because blood flows through an extracorporeal circuit during CAVH and CVVH,* blood in the hemofilter may need to be anticoagulated. To do this, infuse heparin in low doses (starting at 500 units/hour) into an infusion port on the arterial side of the setup. Measure thrombin clotting time or the activated clotting time (ACT). *This ensures that the circuit, not the patient, is anticoagulated.* A normal ACT is 100 seconds; during CRRT, keep it between 100 and 300 seconds, depending on the patient's clotting times. If the ACT is too high or too low, the practitioner will adjust the heparin dose. **EB**

● Another way to prevent clotting in the hemofilter is to infuse medications or blood through another line.

● A third way to help prevent clots in the hemofilter, and also to prevent kinks in the catheter, is to make sure that the patient doesn't bend the affected leg more than 30 degrees at the hip.

● *To prevent infection,* perform skin care at the catheter insertion sites every 48 hours using sterile technique. Cover the sites with an occlusive dressing.

● If the ultrafiltrate flow rate decreases, raise the bed *to increase the distance between the collection device and the hemofilter.* Lower the bed *to decrease the flow rate.*

⚠ **ALERT** *Clamping the ultrafiltrate line is contraindicated with some types of hemofilters because pressure may build up in the filter, clotting it and collapsing the blood compartment.*

Preventing complications

Listed here are some possible complications of continuous renal replacement therapy and measures to prevent them from occurring.

Complication	Interventions
Hypotension	• Monitor blood pressure. • Decrease the speed of the blood pump temporarily for transient hypotension. • Increase the vasopressor support.
Hypothermia	• Use an inline fluid warmer placed on the blood return line to the patient or an external warming blanket.
Fluid and electrolyte imbalances	• Monitor fluid levels every 4 to 6 hours. • Monitor sodium, lactate, potassium, and calcium levels and replace as necessary.
Acid-base imbalances	• Monitor bicarbonate levels and arterial blood gas values.
Air embolism	• Observe for air in the system. • Use luer-lock devices on catheter openings.
Hemorrhage	• Keep all connections tight and the dialysis lines visible.
Infection	• Perform sterile dressing changes.

Nursing diagnoses
• Risk for imbalanced fluid volume
• Risk for infection

Expected outcomes
The patient will:
• maintain electrolyte levels within normal limits
• maintain equal fluid intake and output
• maintain stable vital signs
• remain free from infection.

Complications
Possible complications include hypotension, hemorrhage, hypothermia, infection, fluid and electrolyte imbalances, acid-base imbalances, air embolism, and thrombosis. (See *Preventing complications*.)

Documentation
Record the time the treatment began and ended, fluid balance information, times of dressing changes, complications, medications given, and the patient's tolerance.

Supportive references

American Nephrology Nurses Association. *Standards and Guidelines of Practice for Continuous Renal Replacement Therapy* (Revised 2005 edition). Pitman, N.J.

Dirkes, S.M. "Continuous Renal Replacement Therapy: Dialytic Therapy for Acute Renal Failure in Intensive Care," *Nephrology Nursing Journal* 27(6):581-90, December 2000. **EB**

Giuliano, K.K., and Pysznik, E.E. "Renal Replacement Therapy in Critical Care: Implementation of a Unit-Based Continuous Venovenous Hemodialysis Program," *Critical Care Nurse* 18(1):40-51, February 1998.

Higley, R. "Continuous Arteriovenous Hemofiltration: A Case Study," *Critical Care Nurse* 16(5):37-40, 43, October 1996.

Stark, J. "The Renal System," in *Core Curriculum for Critical Care Nursing*, 6th ed. Edited by Alspach, J.G. Philadelphia: W.B. Saunders Co., 2006.

Hemodialysis

Hemodialysis is performed to remove toxic wastes from the blood of patients in renal failure. This potentially life-saving procedure removes blood from the body, circulates it through a purifying dialyzer, and then returns it to the body. Various access sites can be used for this procedure. (See *Hemodialysis access sites*.) The most common access device for long-term treatment is an arteriovenous (AV) fistula. (See "Arteriovenous fistula and graft care," page 441.)

The underlying mechanism in hemodialysis is differential diffusion across a semipermeable membrane, which extracts by-products of protein metabolism, such as urea and uric acid as well as creatinine and excess body water. This process restores or maintains the balance of the body's buffer system and elec-

Hemodialysis access sites

Hemodialysis requires vascular access. The site and type of access may vary, depending on the expected duration of dialysis, the surgeon's preference, and the patient's condition.

Subclavian vein catheterization

Using the Seldinger technique, the practitioner or surgeon inserts an introducer needle into the subclavian vein. He then inserts a guide wire through the introducer needle and removes the needle. Using the guide wire, he threads a 5″ to 12″ (12.5 to 30.5 cm) plastic or Teflon catheter (with a Y hub) into the patient's vein.

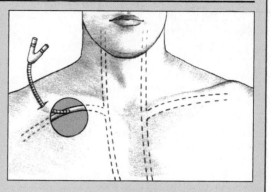

Femoral vein catheterization

Using the Seldinger technique, the practitioner or surgeon inserts an introducer needle into the left or right femoral vein. He then inserts a guide wire through the introducer needle and removes the needle.

Using the guide wire, he threads a 5″ to 12″ plastic or Teflon catheter with a Y hub or two catheters, one for inflow and another placed about ½″ (1 cm) distal to the first for outflow.

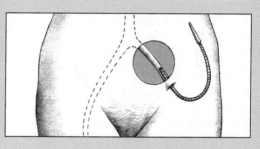

Arteriovenous fistula

To create a fistula, the surgeon makes an incision into the patient's wrist or lower forearm, then a small incision in the side of an artery and another in the side of a vein. He sutures the edges of the incisions together to make a common opening 3 to 7 mm long.

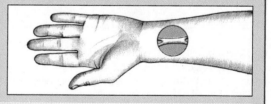

Arteriovenous shunt

To create a shunt, the surgeon makes an incision in the patient's wrist, lower forearm, or (rarely) an ankle. He then inserts a 6″ to 10″ (15 to 25.5 cm) transparent Silastic cannula into an artery and another into a vein. Finally, he tunnels the cannulas out through stab wounds and joins them with a piece of Teflon tubing.

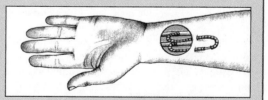

Arteriovenous graft

To create a graft, the surgeon makes an incision in the patient's forearm, upper arm, or thigh. He then tunnels a natural or synthetic graft under the skin and sutures the distal end to an artery and the proximal end to a vein.

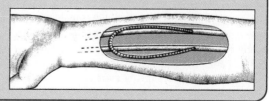

How hemodialysis works

In hemodialysis, blood flows from the patient to an external dialyzer (or artificial kidney) through an arterial access site. Inside the dialyzer, blood and dialysate flow countercurrently, divided by a semipermeable membrane. The dialysate's composition resembles normal extracellular fluid. The blood contains an excess of specific solutes (metabolic waste products and some electrolytes), and the dialysate contains electrolytes that may be at abnormal levels in the patient's bloodstream. The dialysate's electrolyte composition can be modified to raise or lower electrolyte levels, according to the patient's need.

Excretory function and electrolyte homeostasis are achieved by *diffusion,* the movement of a molecule across the dialyzer's semipermeable membrane, from an area of higher solute concentration to an area of lower concentration. Water (solvent) crosses the membrane from the blood into the dialysate by *ultrafiltration.* This process removes excess water, waste products, and other metabolites through *osmotic pressure* and *hydrostatic pressure.* Osmotic pressure is the movement of water across the semipermeable membrane from an area of lesser solute concentration to one of greater solute concentration. Hydrostatic pressure forces water from the blood compartment into the dialysate compartment. Cleaned of impurities

and excess water, the blood returns to the body through a venous site.

Types of dialyzers

There are three types of dialyzers: the hollow-fiber, the flat-plate or parallel flow-plate, and the coil.

The *hollow-fiber dialyzer,* the most common type, contains fine capillaries, with a semipermeable membrane enclosed in a plastic cylinder. Blood flows through these capillaries as the system pumps dialysate in the opposite direction on the outside of the capillaries.

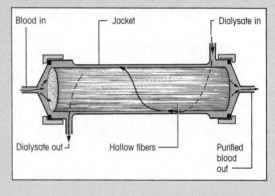

trolyte level. Hemodialysis thus promotes a rapid return to normal serum values and helps prevent complications associated with uremia. (See *How hemodialysis works.*)

Hemodialysis provides temporary support for patients with acute reversible renal failure. It's also used for regular long-term treatment of patients with chronic end-stage renal disease. A less common indication for hemodialysis is acute poisoning, such as barbiturate or analgesic overdose. The patient's condition (rate of creatinine accumulation, weight gain) determines the number and duration of hemodialysis treatments.

According to the National Kidney Foundation (NKF), the delivered dose of hemodialysis solution should be reevaluated in adult and pediatric hemodialysis patients at least once per month. There are four instances in which the measurement of the de-

livered dose of hemodialysis should occur more often:
● Patients are noncompliant with their hemodialysis prescriptions (missed treatments, late for treatments).
● Frequent problems are noted in delivering the prescribed dose of hemodialysis, such as treatment interruptions because of hypotension or angina pectoris.
● Wide variability in urea kinetic modeling results is observed in the absence of prescription changes.
● The hemodialysis prescription is modified. NKF

Specially trained personnel usually perform this procedure in a hemodialysis unit. However, if the patient is acutely ill and unstable, hemodialysis can be done at the bedside in the intensive care unit.

Equipment

Preparing the hemodialysis machine: Hemodialysis machine with appropriate dialyzer ● I.V. solution, administration sets, lines, and related equipment ●

The *flat-plate* or *parallel flow-plate dialyzer* has two or more layers of semipermeable membrane, bound by a semirigid or rigid structure. Blood ports are located at both ends, between the membranes. Blood flows between the membranes, and dialysate flows in the opposite direction along the outside of the membranes.

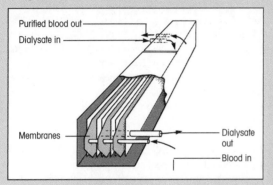

The *coil dialyzer* (no longer widely used) consists of one or more semipermeable membrane tubes supported by mesh and wrapped concentrically around a central core. Blood passes through the coils as dialysate circulates at high speed around the coils and meshwork.

The flat-plate and hollow-fiber dialyzers may be used several times on each patient. Heparin is used *to prevent clot formation during hemodialysis.* Three system types can be used to deliver dialysate. The *batch system* uses a reservoir for recirculating dialysate. The *regenerative system* uses sorbents to purify and regenerate recirculating dialysate. The *proportioning system* (the most common) mixes concentrate with water to form dialysate, which then circulates through the dialyzer and goes down a drain after a single pass, followed by fresh dialysate.

dialysate • optional: heparin, 3-ml syringe with needle, medication label, hemostats

Hemodialysis with a double-lumen catheter: Povidone-iodine pads • two sterile 4″ × 4″ gauze pads • two 3-ml and two 5-ml syringes • tape • heparin bolus syringe • clean gloves • sterile labels • sterile marker

Hemodialysis with an arteriovenous (AV) fistula: Two winged fistula needles (each attached to a 10-ml syringe filled with heparin flush solution) • linen-saver pad • povidone-iodine pads • sterile 4″ × 4″ gauze pads • tourniquet • clean gloves • adhesive tape • sterile labels • sterile marker

Hemodialysis with an AV shunt: Alcohol pads • povidone-iodine pads • sterile gloves • two sterile shunt adapters • sterile Teflon connector • two bulldog clamps • two 10-ml syringes • normal saline solution • four short strips of adhesive tape • optional: sterile shunt spreader, sterile labels, sterile marker

Discontinuing hemodialysis with a double-lumen catheter: Sterile 4″ × 4″ gauze pads • povidone-iodine pads • precut gauze dressing • clean and sterile gloves • normal saline solution • alcohol pads • heparin flush solution • luer-lock injection caps • optional: transparent occlusive dressing, skin barrier preparation, tape, materials for culturing drainage, sterile labels, sterile marker

Discontinuing hemodialysis with an AV fistula: Clean gloves • sterile 4″ × 4″ gauze pads • two adhesive bandages • hemostats • optional: sterile absorbable gelatin sponges (Gelfoam)

Discontinuing hemodialysis with an AV shunt: Sterile gloves • two bulldog clamps • two hemostats • povidone-iodine solution • sterile 4″ × 4″ gauze pads • alcohol pads • elastic gauze bandages • plasticized or hypoallergenic tape

Preparation of equipment

Prepare the hemodialysis equipment following the manufacturer's instructions **MFR** and your facility's protocol. Maintain strict sterile technique to prevent introducing pathogens into the patient's bloodstream during dialysis. Be sure to test the dialyzer and dialysis machine for residual disinfectant after rinsing, and to test all the alarms.

Implementation

- Confirm the patient's identity using two patient identifiers according to facility policy. **JCAHO**
- Weigh the patient. *To determine ultrafiltration requirements,* compare his present weight to his weight after the last dialysis and his target weight. Record his baseline vital signs, taking his blood pressure while he's sitting and standing. Auscultate his heart for rate, rhythm, and abnormalities. Observe respiratory rate, rhythm, and quality. Assess for edema. Check his mental status and the condition and patency of the access site. Check for problems since the last dialysis, and evaluate previous laboratory data. **Science**
- Help the patient into a comfortable position (supine or sitting in recliner chair with feet elevated). Make sure that the access site is well supported and resting on a clean drape.
- If the patient is undergoing hemodialysis for the first time, explain the procedure in detail.
- Use standard precautions in all cases *to prevent transmission of infection.* Wash your hands before beginning. **CDC**
- Label all medications, medication containers, and other solutions on and off the sterile field. **JCAHO**

Beginning hemodialysis with a double+lumen catheter

- Prepare venous access. If extension tubing isn't already clamped, clamp it *to prevent air from entering the catheter.* Clean each catheter extension tube, clamp, and luer-lock injection cap with povidone-iodine pads *to remove contaminants.* Next, place a sterile 4″ × 4″ gauze pad under the extension tubing, and place two 5-ml syringes and two sterile gauze pads on the drape.
- Prepare the anticoagulant regimen as ordered.
- Identify arterial and venous blood lines, and place them near the drape.

- *To remove clots and ensure catheter patency,* remove catheter caps, attach syringes to each catheter port, open one clamp, and aspirate 1.5 to 3 ml of blood. Close the clamp and repeat the procedure with the other port. Flush each port with 5 ml of heparin flush solution.
- Attach blood lines to patient access. First, remove the syringe from the arterial port, and attach the line to the arterial port. Administer the heparin according to protocol. *This prevents clotting in the extracorporeal circuit.*
- Grasp the venous blood line and attach it to the venous port. Open the clamps on the extension tubing, and secure the tubing to the patient's extremity with tape *to reduce tension on the tube and minimize trauma to the insertion site.*
- Begin hemodialysis according to your facility's policy.

Beginning hemodialysis with an AV fistula

- Flush the fistula needles, using attached syringes containing heparinized normal saline solution, and set them aside.
- Place a linen-saver pad under the patient's arm.
- Using sterile technique, clean a 3″ × 10″ (7.5 × 25 cm) area of skin over the fistula with povidone-iodine pads. Discard each pad after one wipe. (If the patient is sensitive to iodine, use chlorhexidine gluconate [Hibiclens] or alcohol.)
- Apply a tourniquet above the fistula *to distend the veins and facilitate venipuncture.* Be sure to avoid occluding the fistula. **Science**
- Put on clean gloves. Perform the venipuncture with a fistula needle. Remove the needle guard and squeeze the wing tips firmly together. Insert the arterial needle at least 1″ (2.5 cm) above the anastomosis, being careful not to puncture the fistula.
- Release the tourniquet and flush the needle with heparin flush solution *to prevent clotting.* Clamp the arterial needle tubing with a hemostat, and secure the wing tips of the needle to the skin with adhesive tape *to prevent it from dislodging within the vein.*
- Perform another venipuncture with the venous needle a few inches above the arterial needle. Flush the needle with heparin flush solution. Clamp the venous needle tubing, and secure the wing tips of the venous needle as you did the arterial needle.
- Remove the syringe from the end of the arterial tubing, uncap the arterial line from the hemodialysis

machine, and connect the two lines. Tape the connection securely *to prevent it from separating during the procedure.* Repeat these two steps for the venous line.
- Release the hemostats and start hemodialysis.

Beginning hemodialysis with an AV shunt
- Remove the bulldog clamps and place them within easy reach of the sterile field. Remove the shunt dressing, and clean the shunt, using sterile technique, as you would for daily care. (See "Arteriovenous fistula and graft care," page 441.) Clean the bulldog clamps with an alcohol pad.
- Assemble the shunt adapters according to the manufacturer's directions.
- Clean the arterial and venous shunt connection with povidone-iodine pads *to remove contaminants.* Use a separate pad for each tube, and wipe in one direction only, from the insertion site to the connection sites. Allow the tubing to air-dry.
- Put on sterile gloves. **CDC**
- Clamp the arterial side of the shunt with a bulldog clamp *to prevent blood from flowing through it.* Clamp the venous side *to prevent leakage when the shunt is opened.*
- Open the shunt by separating its sides with your fingers or with a sterile shunt spreader, if available. Both sides of the shunt should be exposed. Always inspect the Teflon connector on one side of the shunt *to see if it's damaged or bent.* If necessary, replace it before proceeding. Note which side contains the connector *so you can use the new one to close the shunt after treatment.*
- *To adapt the shunt to the lines of the machine,* attach a shunt adapter and 10-ml syringe filled with about 8 ml of normal saline solution to the side of the shunt containing the Teflon connector. Attach the new Teflon connector to the other side of the shunt with the second adapter. Attach the second 10-ml syringe filled with about 8 ml of normal saline solution to the same side.
- Flush the shunt's arterial tubing by releasing its clamp and gently aspirating it with the normal saline solution-filled syringe. Flush the tubing slowly, observing it for signs of fibrin buildup. Repeat the procedure on the venous side of the shunt.
- Secure the shunt to the adapter connection with adhesive tape *to prevent separation during treatment.*
- Connect the arterial and venous lines to the adapters and secure the connections with tape. Tape each line to the patient's arm *to prevent unnecessary strain on the shunt during treatment.*
- Begin hemodialysis according to facility policy.

Discontinuing hemodialysis with a double-lumen catheter
- Wash your hands. **CDC**
- Clamp the extension tubing *to prevent air from entering the catheter.* Clean all connection points on the catheter and blood lines as well as the clamps *to reduce the risk of systemic or local infection.* **Science**
- Place a clean drape under the catheter, and place two sterile 4" × 4" gauze pads on the drape beneath the catheter lines. Soak the pads with povidone-iodine solution. Prepare the catheter flush solution with normal saline or heparin flush solution as ordered.
- Put on clean gloves. Grasp each blood line with a gauze pad and disconnect each line from the catheter.
- Flush each port with normal saline solution *to clean the extension tubing and catheter of blood.* Administer additional heparin flush solution as ordered *to ensure catheter patency.* Attach luer-lock injection caps *to prevent air entry or blood loss.* Clamp the extension tubing.
- When hemodialysis is complete, re-dress the catheter insertion site; also re-dress it if it's occluded, soiled, or wet. Position the patient supine with his face turned away from the insertion site *so that he doesn't contaminate the site by breathing on it.*
- Wash your hands and remove the outer occlusive dressing. Put on sterile gloves, remove the old inner dressing, and discard the gloves and the inner dressing. **CDC**
- Set up a sterile field, and observe the site for drainage. Obtain a drainage sample for culture if necessary. Notify the practitioner if the suture is missing.
- Put on sterile gloves and clean the insertion site with an alcohol pad *to remove skin oils.* Clean the site with a povidone-iodine pad and allow it to air-dry.
- Place a precut gauze dressing under the catheter, and place another gauze dressing over the catheter.
- Apply a skin barrier preparation to the skin surrounding the gauze dressing. Cover the gauze and catheter with a transparent occlusive dressing.
- Apply a 4" to 5" (10 to 12.5 cm) piece of 2" tape over the cut edge of the dressing *to reinforce the lower edge.*

Discontinuing hemodialysis with an AV fistula

● Wash your hands. Turn the blood pump on the hemodialysis machine to 50 to 100 ml/minute.
● Put on clean gloves and remove the tape from the connection site of the arterial lines. Clamp the needle tubing with the hemostat and disconnect the lines. The blood in the machine's arterial line will continue to flow toward the dialyzer, followed by a column of air. Just before the blood reaches the point where the normal saline solution enters the line, clamp the blood line with another hemostat.
● Unclamp the normal saline solution *to allow a small amount to flow through the line.* Unclamp the hemostat on the machine line. *This allows all blood to flow into the dialyzer where it passes through the filter and back to the patient through the venous line.*
● After blood is retransfused, clamp the venous needle tubing and the machine's venous line with hemostats. Turn off the blood pump.
● Remove the tape from the connection site of the venous lines and disconnect the lines.
● Remove the venipuncture needle and apply pressure to the site with a folded 4″ × 4″ gauze pad until all bleeding stops, usually within 10 minutes. Apply an adhesive bandage. Repeat the procedure on the arterial line.
● When hemodialysis is complete, assess the patient's weight, vital signs (including standing blood pressure), and mental status. Compare your findings with your predialysis assessment data. Document your findings.
● Disinfect and rinse the delivery system according to the manufacturer's instructions.

Discontinuing hemodialysis with an AV shunt

● Wash your hands. Turn the blood pump on the hemodialysis machine to 50 to 100 ml/minute.
● Put on the sterile gloves and remove the tape from the connection site of the arterial lines. Clamp the arterial cannula with a bulldog clamp, and then disconnect the lines. The blood in the machine's arterial line will continue to flow toward the dialyzer, followed by a column of air. Just before the blood reaches the point where the normal saline solution enters the line, clamp the blood line with a hemostat. **CDC**
● Unclamp the normal saline solution *to allow a small amount to flow through the line.* Reclamp the

normal saline solution line and unclamp the hemostat on the machine line. *This allows all blood to flow into the dialyzer where it's circulated through the filter and back to the patient through the venous line.*
● Just before the last volume of blood enters the patient, clamp the venous cannula with a bulldog clamp and the machine's venous line with a hemostat.
● Remove the tape from the connection site of the venous lines. Turn off the blood pump and disconnect the lines.
● Reconnect the shunt cannula. Remove the older of the two Teflon connectors and discard it. Connect the shunt, taking care to position the Teflon connector equally between the two cannulas. Remove the bulldog clamps.
● Secure the shunt connection with plasticized or hypoallergenic tape *to prevent accidental disconnection.*
● Clean the shunt and its site with the gauze pads soaked with povidone-iodine solution. When the cleaning procedure is finished, remove the povidone-iodine with alcohol pads.
● Make sure that blood flows through the shunt adequately.
● Apply a dressing to the shunt site and wrap it securely (but not too tightly) with elastic gauze bandages. Attach the bulldog clamps to the outside dressing.
● When hemodialysis is complete, assess the patient's weight, vital signs, and mental status. Compare your findings with your predialysis assessment data. Document your findings.
● Disinfect and rinse the delivery system according to the manufacturer's instructions.

Special considerations

● Obtain blood samples from the patient as ordered. Samples are usually drawn before beginning hemodialysis.

△ **ALERT** *To avoid pyrogenic reactions and bacteremia with septicemia resulting from contamination, use strict sterile technique during preparation of the machine. Discard equipment that has fallen on the floor or that has been disconnected and exposed to the air.*
● Immediately report a machine malfunction or equipment defect.
● Avoid unnecessary handling of shunt tubing. However, be sure to inspect the shunt carefully for patency by observing its color. Look for clots and serum

and cell separation, and check the temperature of the Silastic tubing. Assess the shunt insertion site for signs of infection, such as purulent drainage, inflammation, and tenderness, *which may indicate the body's rejection of the shunt.* Check to see if the shunt insertion tips are exposed.

ALERT *Make sure that you complete each step in this procedure correctly. Overlooking a single step or performing it incorrectly can cause unnecessary blood loss or inefficient treatment from poor clearances or inadequate fluid removal. For example, never allow a normal saline solution bag to run dry while priming and soaking the dialyzer. This can cause air to enter the patient portion of the dialysate system. Ultimately, failure to perform accurate hemodialysis therapy can lead to patient injury and even death.*

● If bleeding continues after you remove an AV fistula needle, apply pressure with a sterile, absorbable gelatin sponge. If bleeding persists, apply a similar sponge soaked in topical thrombin solution.

● Throughout hemodialysis, carefully monitor the patient's vital signs. Read blood pressure at least hourly or as often as every 15 minutes, if necessary. Monitor the patient's weight before and after the procedure *to ensure adequate ultrafiltration during treatment.* (Many dialysis units are now equipped with bed scales.)

● Perform periodic tests for clotting time on the patient's blood samples and samples from the dialyzer. If the patient receives meals during treatment, make sure that they're light.

● Continue necessary drug administration during dialysis unless the drug would be removed in the dialysate; if so, administer the drug after dialysis.

TEACHING *Before the patient leaves the facility, teach him how to care for his vascular access site. Instruct him to keep the incision clean and dry to prevent infection, and to clean it daily until it heals completely and the sutures are removed (usually 10 to 14 days after surgery). He should notify the practitioner of pain, swelling, redness, or drainage in the affected arm. Teach him how to use a stethoscope to auscultate for bruits and how to palpate a thrill.*

Explain that after the access site heals, he may use the arm freely. In fact, exercise is beneficial because it helps stimulate vein enlargement. *Remind him not to allow any treatments or procedures on the accessed*
arm, including blood pressure monitoring or needle punctures. Tell him to avoid putting excessive pressure on the arm. He shouldn't sleep on it, wear constricting clothing on it, or lift heavy objects or strain with it. He also should avoid getting wet for several hours after dialysis.

Teach the patient exercises for the affected arm to promote vascular dilation and enhance blood flow. He may start by squeezing a small rubber ball or other soft object for 15 minutes, when advised by the practitioner.

If the patient will be performing hemodialysis at home, thoroughly review all aspects of the procedure with the patient and his family. Give them the phone number of the dialysis center. Emphasize that training for home hemodialysis is a complex process requiring 2 to 3 months to ensure that the patient or family member performs it safely and competently. *Keep in mind that this procedure is stressful.*

Nursing diagnoses
● Deficient knowledge (procedure)
● Risk for infection

Expected outcomes
The patient will:
● state or demonstrate an understanding of what has been taught
● maintain stable vital signs and exhibit normal laboratory values.

Complications
Bacterial endotoxins in the dialysate may cause fever. Rapid fluid removal and electrolyte changes during hemodialysis can cause early dialysis disequilibrium syndrome. Signs and symptoms include headache, nausea, vomiting, restlessness, hypertension, muscle cramps, backache, and seizures.

Excessive removal of fluid during ultrafiltration can cause hypovolemia and hypotension. Diffusion of the sugar and sodium content of the dialysate solution into the blood can cause hyperglycemia and hypernatremia. These conditions, in turn, can cause hyperosmolarity.

Cardiac arrhythmias can occur during hemodialysis as a result of electrolyte and pH changes in the blood. They can also develop in patients taking antiarrhythmic drugs because the dialysate removes these drugs during treatment. Angina may develop in patients with anemia or preexisting arteriosclerotic cardiovascular disease because of the physiologic stress on the blood during purification and ultrafiltration. Reduced oxygen levels resulting from extracorporeal blood flow or membrane sensitivity may require increasing oxygen administration during hemodialysis.

Some complications of hemodialysis can be fatal. For example, an air embolism can result if the dialyzer retains air, if tubing connections become loose, or if the normal saline solution container empties. Symptoms include chest pain, dyspnea, coughing, and cyanosis.

Hemolysis can result from obstructed flow of the dialysate concentrate or from incorrect setting of the conductivity alarm limits. Symptoms include chest pain, dyspnea, cherry red blood, arrhythmias, acute decrease in hematocrit, and hyperkalemia.

Hyperthermia, another potentially fatal complication, can result if the dialysate becomes overheated. Exsanguination can result from separations of the blood lines or from rupture of the blood lines or dialyzer membrane.

Documentation

Record the time treatment began and any problems with it. Note the patient's vital signs and weight before and during treatment. Note the time blood samples were taken for testing, the test results, and treatment for complications. Record the time the treatment was completed and the patient's response to it.

Supportive references

American Nephrology Nurses'Association. Position Statement: Daily Hemodialysis/Nocturnal Hemodialysis, 2005. *www.annanurse.org.*

Morgan, L. "A Decade Review: Methods to Improve Adherence to the Treatment Regimen among Hemodialysis Patients," *Nephrology Nursing Journal* 27(3):299-304, June 2000.

National Kidney Foundation. "Clinical Practice Guidelines for Hemodialysis Adequacy: Update 2000." *www.kidney.org/professionals/kdoqi/guidelines_updates/doqi. html.*

Pfettscher, S.A. "Chronic Renal Failure and Renal Transplant," in *Critical Care Nursing.* Edited by Bucher, L., and Melander, S. Philadelphia: W.B. Saunders Co., 1999.

Stark, J. "The Renal System," in *Core Curriculum for Critical Care Nursing,* 6th ed. Edited by Alspach, J.G. Philadelphia: W.B. Saunders Co., 2006

Incontinence management

Urinary incontinence (UI) plagues approximately 10 million adults, including 1.5 million nursing home residents, in the United States. Studies have found that fecal incontinence affects up to 47% of the patients in such facilities. **IFFGD** Because of the social stigma of UI, many patients never report the problem to their practitioner.

Contrary to popular opinion, UI is neither a disease nor a part of normal aging. Incontinence may be caused by confusion, dehydration, fecal impaction, or restricted mobility. It's also a sign of various disorders, such as prostatic hyperplasia, bladder calculus, bladder cancer, urinary tract infection (UTI), stroke, diabetic neuropathy, Guillain-Barré syndrome, multiple sclerosis (MS), prostate cancer, prostatitis, spinal cord injury, and urethral stricture. It may also result from urethral sphincter damage after prostatectomy. In addition, certain drugs, including diuretics, hypnotics, sedatives, anticholinergics, antihypertensives, and alpha antagonists, may trigger UI.

According to the National Institute on Aging, UI has four distinct types: urge, stress, overflow, and functional.

● *Urge incontinence* is the involuntary loss of urine associated with a strong desire to void (urgency). It can occur in healthy people, but also in people with diabetes, Alzheimer's disease, Parkinson's disease, stroke, and MS. It can also be a sign of bladder cancer.

● *Stress incontinence* usually presents clinically as the involuntary loss of urine from sudden physical strain, such as a sneeze, cough, quick movement, or during exercise. It's the most common type that occurs in younger and middle-aged women.

● *Overflow incontinence* results in the involuntary loss of urine due to overdistention of the bladder, which causes dribbling because the distended bladder can't contract strongly enough to force a urine stream. This can occur in men with enlarged prostate or patients with diabetes or spinal cord injuries.

Bladder retraining

The incontinent patient typically feels frustrated, embarrassed, and hopeless. Fortunately, his problem can usually be corrected by bladder retraining — a program that aims to establish a regular voiding pattern. Follow these guidelines.

Assess elimination patterns

First, assess the patient's intake and voiding patterns and reason for each accidental voiding such as a coughing spell. Use an incontinence monitoring record.

Establish a voiding schedule

Encourage the patient to void regularly — for example, every 2 hours. When he can stay dry for 2 hours, increase the interval by 30 minutes every day until he achieves a 3- to 4-hour voiding schedule. Teach the patient to practice relaxation techniques such as deep breathing, which help decrease the sense of urgency.

Record results and remain positive

Keep a record of continence and incontinence for about 5 days. *This may reinforce the patient's efforts to remain continent.* Remember, your own and the patient's positive attitudes are crucial to his successful bladder retraining.

Take steps for success

Here are some tips to boost the patient's success:
● Situate the patient's bed near a bathroom or portable toilet. Leave a light on at night. If the patient needs assistance getting out of bed or a chair, promptly answer the call for help.

● Teach the patient measures to prevent urinary tract infections, such as adequate fluid intake (at least 2 qt [2 L]/day unless contraindicated), drinking cranberry juice to help acidify urine, wearing cotton underpants, and bathing with nonirritating soaps.
● Encourage the patient to empty his bladder completely before and after meals and at bedtime.
● Advise the patient to urinate whenever the urge arises and never to ignore it.
● Instruct the patient to take prescribed diuretics on rising in the morning.
● Advise the patient to limit the use of sleeping aids, sedatives, and alcohol; they decrease the urge to urinate and can increase incontinence, especially at night.
● If the patient is overweight, encourage weight loss.
● Suggest exercises to strengthen pelvic muscles.
● Instruct the patient to increase dietary fiber *to decrease constipation and incontinence*.
● Monitor the patient for signs and symptoms of anxiety and depression.
● Reassure the patient that periodic incontinent episodes don't mean that the program has failed. Encourage persistence, tolerance, and a positive attitude.

● *Functional incontinence* results in urine leakage even though the bladder and urethra function normally. This condition is usually related to cognitive or environmental factors, such as mental impairment or the inability to get to the toilet in time because of arthritis or other disorders.

Care of persons with UI should include attention to toileting schedules, monitoring of fluid and dietary intake, strategies to decrease urine loss at night, use of the most absorbent and skin-friendly protective garments possible, and prevention and early treatment of skin breakdown.

Treatment for UI includes bladder control training. Pelvic (Kegel) exercises are taught to patients with stress and urge incontinence to improve their muscle strength and, therefore, allow them to hold urine longer. Biofeedback, timed voiding, and bladder training are also used. (See *Bladder retraining*.)

Pharmacologic treatment for UI includes medications that prevent bladder contractions, relax muscles to help the bladder fully empty, or contract muscles to cut down on leakage. Surgical treatment for UI includes transurethral resection of the prostate in men, repair of the anterior vaginal wall or retropelvic suspension of the bladder in women, urethral sling, and bladder augmentation. (See *Artificial urinary sphincter impant*, page 468.)

Fecal incontinence, the involuntary passage of feces, may occur gradually (as in dementia) or suddenly (as in spinal cord injury), but most commonly oc-

Artificial urinary sphincter implant

An artificial urinary sphincter implant can help restore continence to a patient with a neurogenic bladder. Criteria for inserting an implant include:
- incontinence associated with a weak urinary sphincter
- incoordination between the detrusor muscle and the urinary sphincter (if drug therapy fails)
- inadequate bladder storage (if intermittent catheterization and drug therapy are unsuccessful).

Configuration and placement
An implant consists of a control pump, an occlusive cuff, and a pressure-regulating balloon. The cuff is placed around the bladder neck, and the balloon is placed under the rectus muscle in the abdomen. The balloon holds fluid that inflates the cuff. In men, the surgeon places the control pump in the scrotum; in women, the surgeon places the pump in the labium.

Using the implant
To void, the patient squeezes the bulb to deflate the cuff, which opens the urethra by returning fluid to the balloon. After voiding, the cuff reinflates automatically, sealing the urethra until the patient needs to void again.

Complications and care
If complications develop, the implant may need to be repaired or removed. Possible complications include cuff leakage (uncommon), trapped blood or other fluid contaminants (which can cause control pump problems), skin erosion around the bulb or erosion in the bladder neck or the urethra, infection, inadequate occlusion pressures, and kinked tubing. If the bladder holds residual urine, intermittent self-catheterization may be needed.

Care includes avoiding strenuous activity for about 6 months after surgery and having regular checkups.

Implant position in a man

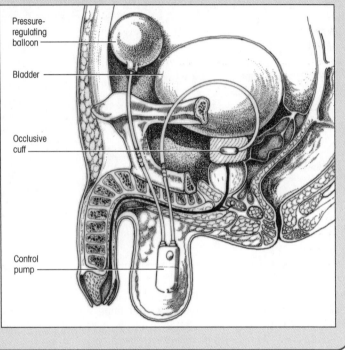

Pressure-regulating balloon

Bladder

Occlusive cuff

Control pump

---

curs as a result of diarrhea or constipation. It can also result from many factors, such as fecal stasis and impaction secondary to reduced activity; inappropriate diet; untreated painful anal conditions; chronic laxative use; reduced fluid intake; neurologic deficit; pelvic, prostatic, or rectal surgery; or the use of certain medications, including antihistamines, psychotropics, and iron preparations. Not usually a sign of serious illness, fecal incontinence can seriously impair an individual's physical and psychological well being.

Management of fecal incontinence includes managing the patient's diet, bowel retraining, and biofeedback to improve sensation and control. Surgery, such as a sphincteroplasty to repair the anal sphincter muscles or to transpose muscle from another part of the body, can also be done if appropriate. **IFFGD**

Patients with urinary or fecal incontinence should be carefully assessed for underlying disorders. Most can be treated; some can even be cured.

Equipment

Bladder retraining record sheet • gloves • stethoscope (to assess bowel sounds) • lubricant • moisture barrier cream • incontinence pads • bedpan • specimen container • laboratory request form • optional: stool collection kit, urinary catheter

Implementation

● Whether the patient reports urinary or fecal incontinence or both, you'll need to perform initial and continuing assessments to plan effective interventions.

Urinary incontinence

● Ask the patient when he first noticed urine leakage and whether it began suddenly or gradually. Have him describe his typical urinary pattern: Does incontinence usually occur during the day or at night? Ask him to rate his urinary control: Does he have moderate control, or is he completely incontinent? If he sometimes urinates with control, ask him to identify when and how much he usually urinates.

● Evaluate related problems, such as urinary hesitancy, frequency, urgency, nocturia, and decreased force or an interrupted urine stream. Ask the patient to describe previous treatment he has had for incontinence or measures he has performed by himself. Ask about medications, including nonprescription drugs.

● Assess the patient's environment. Is a toilet or commode readily available, and how long does the patient take to reach it? After the patient is in the bathroom, assess his manual dexterity; for example, how easily does he manipulate his clothes?

● Evaluate the patient's mental status and cognitive function.

● Quantify the patient's normal daily fluid intake.

● Review the patient's medication and diet history for drugs and foods that affect digestion and elimination.

● Review or obtain the patient's medical history, noting especially the number and route of births (in women) and incidence of UTIs, prostate disorders, spinal injury or tumor, stroke, and bladder, prostate, or pelvic surgery. Assess for such disorders as deliri-

um, dehydration, urine retention, restricted mobility, fecal impaction, infection, inflammation, or polyuria.

● Inspect the urethral meatus for obvious inflammation or anatomic defects. Have the female patient bear down while you note any urine leakage. Gently palpate the abdomen for bladder distention, which signals urine retention. If possible, have the patient examined by a urologist.

● Obtain specimens for appropriate laboratory tests as ordered. Label each specimen container and send it to the laboratory with a request form.

● Begin incontinence management by implementing an appropriate bladder retraining program.

● To manage stress incontinence, begin an exercise program to help strengthen the pelvic floor muscles. (See *Strengthening pelvic floor muscles,* page 470.)

● To manage functional incontinence, frequently assess the patient's mental and functional status. Regularly remind him to void. Respond to his calls promptly, and help him get to the bathroom quickly. Provide positive reinforcement.

● *To ensure healthful hydration and to prevent a UTI,* make sure that the patient maintains adequate daily fluid intake (six to eight 8-oz glasses of fluid). Restrict fluid intake after 6 p.m. **Science**

Fecal incontinence

● Ask the patient with fecal incontinence to identify its onset, duration, severity, and pattern (for instance, determine whether it occurs at night or with diarrhea). Focus the history on GI, neurologic, and psychological disorders.

● Note the frequency, consistency, and volume of stool passed in the previous 24 hours. Obtain a stool specimen, if ordered. Protect the patient's bed with an incontinence pad.

● Assess for chronic constipation, GI and neurologic disorders, and laxative abuse. Inspect the abdomen for distention, and auscultate for bowel sounds. If not contraindicated, put on gloves, apply lubricant, and check for fecal impaction (a factor in overflow incontinence). Remove gloves when finished. Checking for fecal impaction may stimulate a bowel movement, so keep a bedpan readily available. **Science**

● Assess the patient's medication regimen. Check for drugs that affect bowel activity, such as aspirin, anticholinergics, anti-Parkinson drugs, aluminum hydroxide, calcium carbonate antacids, diuretics, iron

Strengthening pelvic floor muscles

Stress incontinence, the most common kind of urinary incontinence in women, usually results from weakening of the urethral sphincter. In men, it may sometimes occur after a radical prostatectomy.

You can help a patient prevent or minimize stress incontinence by teaching her pelvic floor (Kegel) exercises to strengthen the pubococcygeal muscles. Here's how.

Learning Kegel exercises

First, explain how to locate the muscles of the pelvic floor. Instruct the patient to tense the muscles around the anus, as if to retain stool.

Next, teach the patient to tighten the muscles of the pelvic floor to stop the flow of urine while urinating and then to release the muscles to restart the flow. Once learned, these exercises can be done anywhere at any time.

Establishing a regimen

Explain to the patient that contraction and relaxation exercises are essential to muscle retraining. Suggest that she start out by contracting the pelvic floor muscles for 10 seconds, then relax for 10 seconds before slowly tightening the muscles and then releasing them.

Typically, the patient starts with 15 contractions in the morning and afternoon and 20 at night. Or she may exercise for 10 minutes three times per day, working up to 25 contractions at a time as strength improves.

Advise the patient not to use stomach, leg, or buttock muscles. Also discourage leg crossing or breath holding during these exercises.

---

preparations, opiates, tranquilizers, tricyclic antidepressants, and phenothiazines.

● For the neurologically capable patient with chronic incontinence, provide bowel retraining. (See *Steps in bowel training.*) **IFFGD**

● Advise the patient to consume a fiber-rich diet, with raw, leafy vegetables (such as carrots and lettuce), unpeeled fruits (such as apples), and whole grains (such as wheat or rye breads and cereals). If the patient has a lactose deficiency, suggest calcium supplements to replace calcium lost by eliminating dairy products from the diet. **Science**

● Encourage adequate fluid intake. **Science**

● Teach the elderly patient to gradually eliminate laxative use. Point out that using laxative agents to promote regular bowel movement may have the opposite effect, producing either constipation or incontinence over time. Suggest natural laxatives, such as prunes and prune juice, instead. **Science**

● Promote regular exercise by explaining how it helps to regulate bowel motility. Even a nonambulatory patient can perform some exercises while sitting or lying in bed. **Science**

Special considerations

● To rid the bladder of residual urine, teach the patient to perform Valsalva's or Credé's maneuver, or institute clean intermittent catheterization. Use an indwelling urinary catheter only as a last resort *because of the risk of UTI.*

● For fecal incontinence, maintain effective hygienic care *to increase the patient's comfort and prevent skin breakdown and infection.* Clean the perineal area frequently, and apply a moisture barrier cream. Control foul odors as well.

● Schedule extra time to provide encouragement and support for the patient, who may feel shame, embarrassment, and powerlessness from loss of control.

Nursing diagnoses

● Bowel incontinence
● Functional urinary incontinence
● Stress urinary incontinence
● Total urinary incontinence
● Urge urinary incontinence

Expected outcomes

The patient will:
● establish and maintain a regular pattern of bowel care
● state an understanding of the bowel care routine
● void at appropriate intervals
● achieve urinary continence.

Complications

Skin breakdown and infection may result from incontinence. Psychological problems resulting from incontinence include social isolation, loss of independence, lowered self-esteem, and depression.

Documentation

Record all bladder and bowel retraining efforts, noting scheduled bathroom times, food and fluid intake, elimination amounts, and the patient's response to training efforts, as appropriate. Record the duration of continent periods.

Supportive references

Doughty, D.B. *Urinary and Fecal Incontinence: Nursing Management,* 2nd ed. St. Louis: Mosby–Year Book, Inc., 2000. **EB**

International Foundation for Gastrointestinal Disorders (IFFGD). "Prevalence of Bowel Incontinence," updated: March 2003. *www.aboutincontinence.org/prevalence.html.*

International Foundation for Gastrointestinal Disorders (IFFGD). "Treatment for Bowel Incontinence," updated: August 2005. *www.aboutincontinence.org/treatment.html.*

National Institutes of Health, National Institute on Aging. "Age Page: Urinary Incontinence." updated: December 2005. *www.niapublications.org/agepages/urinary.asp.*

Smeltzer, S.C., and Bare, B.G. *Brunner and Suddarth's Textbook of Medical-Surgical Nursing,* 10th ed. Philadelphia: Lippincott Williams & Wilkins, 2003.

Peritoneal dialysis

Peritoneal dialysis is indicated for patients with chronic renal failure who have cardiovascular instability, vascular access problems that prevent hemodialysis, fluid overload, or electrolyte imbalances. In this procedure, dialysate — the solution instilled into the peritoneal cavity by a catheter — draws waste products, excess fluid, and electrolytes from the blood across the semipermeable peritoneal membrane. (See *Principles of peritoneal dialysis,* page 472.) After a prescribed period, the dialysate is drained from the peritoneal cavity, removing impurities with it. The dialysis procedure is then repeated, using a new dialysate each time, until waste removal is complete and fluid, electrolyte, and acid-base balance has been restored. **NKF**

The catheter is inserted in the operating room or at the patient's bedside with a nurse assisting. With special preparation, the nurse may perform dialysis, either manually or using an automatic or semiautomatic cycle machine.

Steps in bowel training **EB**

These are the essential steps to include in a bowel management program.
- Make sure that the patient has easy access to a toilet or commode.
- Remove impacted stool and clean the distal colon.
- Instruct the patient to take stool softeners *to help normalize stool consistency.*
- Have the patient establish a regular schedule for defecation and reserve enough time to defecate.
- Advise the patient to adhere to the schedule; attempts at defecation should occur after meals, and he should use stimuli (for example, coffee or hot water) to induce peristalsis.
- Teach the patient with intact sphincter and sensory function to respond appropriately to the "urge to go," in addition to attempting defecation on schedule.
- For a patient with loss of sensory awareness and sphincter control: Use additional stimuli to stimulate peristalsis and to induce rectal filling and evacuation (for example, digital stimulation, suppository, mini-enema). Tell the patient to time the stimulus to coincide with scheduled defecation. For instance, a suppository may be given just before a meal, with defecation scheduled just after the meal.
- Monitor the patient's progress and modify the program as needed.

Equipment

Catheter placement and dialysis: Prescribed dialysate (in 1- or 2-L bottles or bags as ordered) • warmer, heating pad, or water bath • at least three face masks • medication, such as heparin, if ordered • dialysis administration set with drainage bag • two pairs of sterile gloves • I.V. pole • fenestrated sterile drape • vial of 1% or 2% lidocaine • povidone-iodine pads • 3-ml syringe with 25G 1″ needle scalpel (with #11 blade) • ordered type of multi-eyed, nylon, peritoneal catheter (see *Comparing peritoneal dialysis catheters,* page 473) • peritoneal stylet • sutures or hypoallergenic tape • povidone-iodine solution (to prepare abdomen) • precut drain dressings • protective cap for catheter • small, sterile plastic clamp • 4″ × 4″ gauze pads • sterile labels • sterile marker • optional: 10-ml syringe with 22G 1½″ needle, protein

Principles of peritoneal dialysis

Peritoneal dialysis works through a combination of diffusion and osmosis.

Diffusion

In diffusion, particles move through a semipermeable membrane from an area of high-solute concentration to an area of low-solute concentration.

In peritoneal dialysis, the water-based dialysate being infused contains glucose, sodium chloride, calcium, magnesium, acetate or lactate, and no waste products. Therefore, the waste products and excess electrolytes in the blood cross through the semipermeable peritoneal membrane into the dialysate. Removing the waste-filled dialysate and replacing it with fresh solution keeps the waste concentration low and encourages further diffusion.

Osmosis

In osmosis, fluids move through a semipermeable membrane from an area of low-solute concentration to an area of high-solute concentration. In peritoneal dialysis, dextrose is added to the dialysate to give it a higher solute concentration than the blood, creating a high osmotic gradient. Water migrates from the blood through the membrane at the beginning of each infusion, when the osmotic gradient is highest.

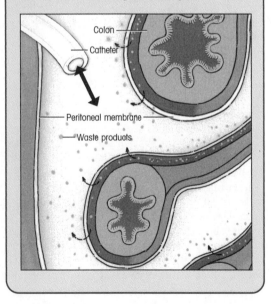

Colon
Catheter
Peritoneal membrane
Waste products

or potassium supplement, specimen container, label, laboratory request form

Dressing changes: One pair of sterile gloves • 10 sterile cotton-tipped applicators or sterile 2″ × 2″ gauze pads • povidone-iodine ointment • two precut drain dressings • adhesive tape • povidone-iodine solution or normal saline solution • two sterile 4″ × 4″ gauze pads

All equipment must be sterile. Commercially packaged dialysis kits or trays are available.

Preparation of equipment

Bring all equipment to the patient's bedside. Make sure that the dialysate is at body temperature. This decreases patient discomfort during the procedure and reduces vasoconstriction of the peritoneal capillaries. Dilated capillaries enhance blood flow to the peritoneal membrane surface, increasing waste clearance into the peritoneal cavity. Place the container in a warmer or water bath, or wrap it in a heating pad set at 98.6° F (37° C) for 30 to 60 minutes to warm the solution. **Science**

Implementation

● Confirm the patient's identity using two patient identifiers according to facility policy. **JCAHO**
● Explain the procedure to the patient. Assess and record his vital signs and weight *to establish baseline levels.* **PCP** **Science**
● Review recent laboratory values (blood urea nitrogen [BUN], serum creatinine, sodium, potassium, and complete blood count).
● Identify the patient's hepatitis B virus and human immunodeficiency virus status, if known. **CDC**

Catheter placement and dialysis

● Have the patient try to urinate. *This reduces the risk of bladder perforation during the insertion of the peritoneal catheter.* If he can't urinate and you suspect that his bladder isn't empty, obtain an order for straight catheterization *to empty his bladder.* **Science**
● Place the patient in the supine position, and have him put on one of the sterile face masks.
● Wash your hands. **CDC**
● Inspect the warmed dialysate, which should appear clear and colorless.
● Put on a sterile face mask. Prepare to add any prescribed medication to the dialysate, using strict sterile technique *to avoid contaminating the solution.* Label

Comparing peritoneal dialysis catheters

The first step in any type of peritoneal dialysis is the insertion of a catheter to allow instillation of dialyzing solution. The surgeon may insert one of three different catheters described here.

Tenckhoff catheter

To implant a Tenckhoff catheter, the surgeon inserts the first 6¾" (17 cm) of the catheter into the patient's abdomen. The next 2¾" (7 cm) segment, which may have a Dacron cuff at one or both ends, is imbedded subcutaneously. Within a few days after insertion, the patient's tissues grow around the cuffs, forming a tight barrier against bacterial infiltration. The remaining 3⅞" (10 cm) of the catheter extends outside of the abdomen and is equipped with a metal adapter at the tip that connects to dialyzer tubing.

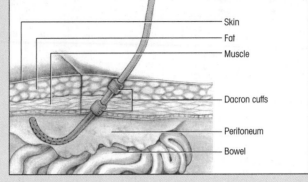

Flanged-collar catheter

To insert this type of catheter, the surgeon positions its flanged collar just below the dermis so that the device extends through the abdominal wall. He keeps the cuff's distal end from extending into the peritoneum, *where it could cause adhesions.*

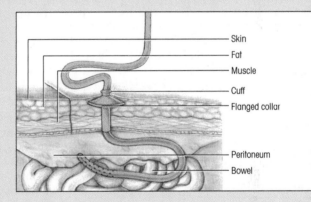

Column-disk peritoneal catheter

To insert a column-disk peritoneal catheter (CDPC), the surgeon rolls up the flexible disk section of the implant, inserts it into the peritoneal cavity, and retracts it against the abdominal wall. The implant's first cuff rests just outside the peritoneal membrane, while its second cuff rests just underneath the skin. Because the CDPC doesn't float freely in the peritoneal cavity, it keeps inflowing dialyzing solution from being directed at the sensitive organs, *which increases patient comfort during dialysis.*

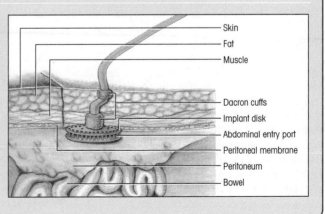

Setup for peritoneal dialysis

This illustration shows the proper setup for peritoneal dialysis.

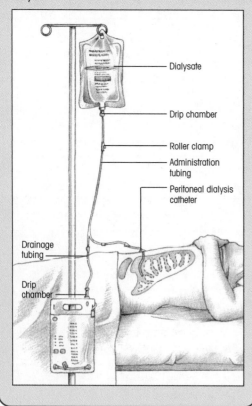

- Dialysate
- Drip chamber
- Roller clamp
- Administration tubing
- Peritoneal dialysis catheter
- Drainage tubing
- Drip chamber

infusion lines and allow the solution to flow until all lines are primed. Close all clamps.

- At this point, the practitioner puts on a mask and a pair of sterile gloves. He cleans the patient's abdomen with povidone-iodine solution and drapes it with a sterile drape.
- Wipe the stopper of the lidocaine vial with povidone-iodine and allow it to dry. Invert the vial and hand it to the practitioner so he can withdraw the lidocaine, using the 3-ml syringe with the 25G 1" needle.
- The practitioner anesthetizes a small area of the patient's abdomen below the umbilicus. He then makes a small incision with the scalpel, inserts the catheter into the peritoneal cavity — using the stylet to guide the catheter — and sutures or tapes the catheter in place.
- If the catheter is already in place, clean the site with povidone-iodine solution in a circular outward motion, according to your facility's policy, before each dialysis treatment.
- Connect the catheter to the administration set, using strict sterile technique *to prevent contamination of the catheter and the solution, which could cause peritonitis.* **Science**
- Open the drain dressing and the 4" × 4" gauze pad packages. Put on the other pair of sterile gloves. Apply the precut drain dressings around the catheter. Cover them with the gauze pads and tape them securely.
- Unclamp the lines to the patient. Rapidly instill 500 ml of dialysate into the peritoneal cavity *to test the catheter's patency.*
- Clamp the lines to the patient. Immediately unclamp the lines to the drainage bag *to allow fluid to drain into the bag.* Outflow should be brisk.
- Having established the catheter's patency, clamp the lines to the drainage bag and unclamp the lines to the patient *to infuse the prescribed volume of solution over a period of 5 to 10 minutes.* As soon as the dialysate container empties, clamp the lines to the patient *to prevent air from entering the tubing.*
- Allow the solution to dwell in the peritoneal cavity for the prescribed time (4 to 6 hours). *This lets excess fluid, electrolytes, and accumulated wastes move from the blood through the peritoneal membrane and into the dialysate.* **NKF**
- Warm the solution for the next infusion.

all medications, medication containers, and other solutions on and off the sterile field. **JCAHO** Medications should be added immediately before the solution will be hung and used. Disinfect multiple-dose vials by soaking them in povidone-iodine solution for 5 minutes. Heparin is typically added to the dialysate *to prevent fibrin accumulation in the catheter.*

- Prepare the dialysis administration set as shown. (See *Setup for peritoneal dialysis.*)
- Close the clamps on all lines. Place the drainage bag below the patient *to facilitate gravity drainage,* and connect the drainage line to it. Connect the dialysate infusion lines to the bottles or bags of dialysate. Hang the bottles or bags on the I.V. pole at the patient's bedside. To prime the tubing, open the

● At the end of the prescribed dwell time, unclamp the line to the drainage bag and allow the solution to drain from the peritoneal cavity into the drainage bag (normally 30 to 40 minutes). **NKF**

● Repeat the infusion-dwell-drain cycle immediately after outflow until the prescribed number of fluid exchanges have been completed.

● If the practitioner or your facility's policy requires a dialysate specimen, you'll usually collect one after every 10 infusion-dwell-drain cycles (*always* during the drain phase), after every 24-hour period, or as ordered. To do this, attach the 10-ml syringe to the 22G $1/2''$ needle and insert it into the injection port on the drainage line, using strict sterile technique, and aspirate the drainage sample. Transfer the sample to the specimen container, label it appropriately, and send it to the laboratory with a laboratory request form.

● After completing the prescribed number of exchanges, clamp the catheter, and put on sterile gloves. Disconnect the administration set from the peritoneal catheter. Place the sterile protective cap over the catheter's distal end.

● Dispose of used equipment appropriately.

Dressing changes

● Explain the procedure to the patient and wash your hands. **CDC** **PCP**

● If necessary, carefully remove the old dressings *to avoid putting tension on the catheter and accidentally dislodging it and to avoid introducing bacteria into the tract through the catheter's movement.*

● Put on the sterile gloves. **CDC**

● Saturate the sterile applicators or the $4'' \times 4''$ gauze pads with povidone-iodine, and clean the skin around the catheter, moving in concentric circles from the catheter site outward. Remove any crusted material carefully. **Science**

● Inspect the catheter site for drainage and the tissue around the site for redness and swelling.

● Apply povidone-iodine ointment to the catheter site with a sterile gauze pad.

● Place two precut drain dressings around the catheter site. Tape the $4'' \times 4''$ gauze pads over them *to secure the dressing.*

Special considerations

● During and after dialysis, monitor the patient and his response to treatment. Peritoneal dialysis is usually contraindicated in the patient who has had exten-

sive abdominal or bowel surgery or extensive abdominal trauma or who has severe vascular disease, obesity, or respiratory distress. **NKF**

● According to the National Kidney Foundation, the decision to switch a patient from peritoneal dialysis to hemodialysis should be based on three factors: the clinical assessment, the patient's ability to reach hemodialysis goals, and his willingness to go onto hemodialysis. Signs that suggest a patient should be switched to hemodialysis include:

– failure to achieve target BUN and creatinine levels consistently

– recurrent peritonitis or other peritoneal dialysis-related complications

– inadequate solute transport or fluid removal; high transporters may have poor ultrafiltration or excessive protein losses

– severely high triglyceride levels in the blood

– development of technical or mechanical problems

– acute malnutrition even with aggressive management. **NKF**

● Monitor the patient's vital signs every 10 to 15 minutes for the first 1 to 2 hours of exchanges, then every 2 to 4 hours, or more frequently if necessary. Notify the practitioner of abrupt changes in the patient's condition.

● *To reduce the risk of peritonitis,* use strict sterile technique during catheter insertion, dialysis, and dressing changes. All personnel in the room should wear masks whenever the dialysis system is opened or entered. Change the dressing at least every 24 hours or whenever it becomes wet or soiled. *Frequent dressing changes will also help prevent skin excoriation from any leakage.*

● *To prevent respiratory distress,* position the patient for maximal lung expansion. Promote lung expansion through turning and deep-breathing exercises.

ALERT *If the patient suffers severe respiratory distress during the dwell phase of dialysis, drain the peritoneal cavity and notify the practitioner. Monitor the patient on peritoneal dialysis who's being weaned from a ventilator.*

● *To prevent protein depletion,* the practitioner may order a high-protein diet or protein supplement. He'll also monitor serum albumin levels.

● Dialysate is available in three concentrations — 4.25% dextrose, 2.5% dextrose, and 1.5% dextrose. The 4.25% solution usually removes the largest amount of fluid from the blood because its glucose concentration is highest. If the patient receives this concentrated solution, monitor him carefully *to prevent excess fluid loss.* Some of the glucose in the 4.25% solution may enter the patient's bloodstream, causing hyperglycemia severe enough to require an insulin injection or an insulin addition to the dialysate.

● Patients with low serum potassium levels may require the addition of potassium to the dialysate solution *to prevent further losses.*

● Monitor fluid volume balance, blood pressure, and pulse *to help prevent fluid imbalance.* Assess fluid balance at the end of each infusion-dwell-drain cycle. Fluid balance is positive if less than the amount infused was recovered; it's negative if more than the amount infused was recovered. Notify the practitioner if the patient retains 500 ml or more of fluid for three consecutive cycles or if he loses at least 1 L of fluid for three consecutive cycles. **Science**

● Weigh the patient daily *to help determine how much fluid is being removed during dialysis treatment.* Note the time and any variations in the weighing technique next to his weight on his chart. **Science**

● If inflow and outflow are slow or absent, check the tubing for kinks. You can also try raising the I.V. pole or repositioning the patient *to increase the inflow rate.* **Science** Repositioning the patient or applying manual pressure to the lateral aspects of the patient's abdomen may also help increase drainage. If these maneuvers fail, notify the practitioner. Improper positioning of the catheter or an accumulation of fibrin may obstruct the catheter.

● Always examine outflow fluid (effluent) for color and clarity. Normally it's clear or pale yellow, but pink-tinged effluent may appear during the first three or four cycles. If the effluent remains pink-tinged or if it's grossly bloody, suspect bleeding into the peritoneal cavity and notify the practitioner. Notify the practitioner if the outflow contains feces, which suggests bowel perforation, or if it's cloudy, which suggests peritonitis. Obtain a sample for culture and Gram stain. Send the sample in a labeled specimen container to the laboratory with a laboratory request form.

● Patient discomfort at the start of the procedure is normal. If the patient experiences pain during the procedure, determine when it occurs, its quality and duration, and whether it radiates to other body parts. Notify the practitioner. Pain during infusion usually results from a dialysate that's too cool or acidic. Pain may also result from rapid inflow; *slowing the inflow rate may reduce the pain.* Severe, diffuse pain with rebound tenderness and cloudy effluent may indicate peritoneal infection. Pain that radiates to the shoulder commonly results from air accumulation under the diaphragm. Severe, persistent perineal or rectal pain can result from improper catheter placement.

● The patient undergoing peritoneal dialysis will require a great deal of assistance in his daily care. *To minimize his discomfort,* perform daily care during a drain phase in the cycle, when the patient's abdomen is less distended.

TEACHING *Teach the patient and his family how to use sterile technique throughout the procedure, especially for cleaning and dressing changes, to prevent complications such as peritonitis. Also teach them the signs and symptoms of peritonitis (cloudy fluid, fever, and abdominal pain and tenderness) and infection (redness and drainage). Stress the importance of notifying the practitioner immediately if such signs or symptoms arise.*

Inform the patient about the advantages of an automated continuous cycler for home use. Instruct the patient to record his weight and blood pressure daily and to check regularly for swelling of the extremities. Teach him to keep an accurate record of intake and output.

Nursing diagnoses
● Deficient knowledge (procedure)
● Risk for imbalanced fluid volume

Expected outcomes
The patient (or caregiver) will:
● state and demonstrate an understanding of the procedure
● measure and record weight, blood pressure, and intake and output
● maintain normal weight and blood pressure.

Complications
Peritonitis, the most common complication, usually follows contamination of the dialysate, but it may develop if solution leaks from the catheter exit site and flows back into the catheter tract.

Protein depletion may result from the diffusion of protein in the blood into the dialysate solution through the peritoneal membrane. As much as ½ oz (14.2 g) of protein may be lost daily — more in patients with peritonitis.

Respiratory distress may result when dialysate in the peritoneal cavity increases pressure on the diaphragm, which decreases lung expansion.

Constipation is a major cause of inflow-outflow problems; therefore, *to ensure regular bowel movements,* give a laxative or stool softener as needed.

Excessive fluid loss from the use of 4.25% solution may cause hypovolemia, hypotension, and shock. Excessive fluid retention may lead to blood volume expansion, hypertension, peripheral edema, and even pulmonary edema and heart failure.

Other possible complications include electrolyte imbalance and hyperglycemia, which can be identified by frequent blood tests.

Documentation

Record the amount of dialysate infused and drained, any medications added to the solution, and the color and character of effluent. Record the patient's daily weight and fluid balance.

Use a peritoneal dialysis flowchart to compute total fluid balance after each exchange. Note the patient's vital signs and tolerance of the treatment and other pertinent observations. (See *Documenting peritoneal dialysis.*)

Supportive references

National Kidney Foundation. "Clinical Practice Guidelines for Peritoneal Dialysis Adequacy," 2000. *www.kidney. org/professionals/doqi/guidelines/doqi_uptoc.html#pd.*

National Kidney and Urologic Diseases Information Clearinghouse. "Peritoneal Dialysis Dose and Adequacy," NIH Publication No. 04-4578. May 2004. *http://kidney.niddk.nih.gov/kudiseases/pubs/ peritonealdose/index.htm.*

National Kidney and Urologic Disease Information Clearinghouse. "Treatment Methods for Kidney Failure: Peritoneal Dialysis," NIH Publication No. 01-4688. May 2001. *http://kidney.niddk.nih.gov/kudiseases/pubs/ peritoneal/index.htm.*

Stark, J. "The Renal System," in *Core Curriculum for Critical Care Nursing,* 6th ed. Edited by Alspach, J.G. Philadelphia: W.B. Saunders Co., 2006.

Documenting peritoneal dialysis

● During and after dialysis, monitor and document the patient's response to treatment.
● Be aware of any abrupt changes in the patient's condition, notify the practitioner, and document doing so.
● Record each time you notify the practitioner of an abnormality.
● Document the amount of dialysate infused and drained and any medications added.
● Complete a peritoneal dialysis flowchart every 24 hours.
● Note the condition of the patient's skin at the dialysis catheter site, the patient's reports of unusual discomfort or pain, and your interventions.

Peritoneal dialysis, continuous ambulatory

Continuous ambulatory peritoneal dialysis (CAPD) requires insertion of a permanent peritoneal catheter, such as a Tenckhoff catheter, to circulate dialysate in the peritoneal cavity constantly. Inserted under local anesthetic, the catheter is sutured in place and its distal portion tunneled subcutaneously to the skin surface. There it serves as a port for the dialysate, which flows in and out of the peritoneal cavity by gravity. (See *Continuous ambulatory peritoneal dialysis: Three major steps,* page 478.)

CAPD is used most commonly for patients with end-stage renal disease. CAPD can be a welcome alternative to hemodialysis because it gives the patient more independence and requires less travel for treatments. It also provides more stable fluid and electrolyte levels than conventional hemodialysis.

✔ **CLINICAL IMPACT** *Renal function has been shown to decline over months or years on dialysis. Therefore, the number or volume of exchanges will likely increase for the patient on CAPD to maintain control over waste products.*

Patients or family members can usually learn to perform CAPD after only 2 weeks of training. Also, because the patient can resume normal daily activities between solution changes, CAPD helps promote

Continuous ambulatory peritoneal dialysis: Three major steps

A bag of dialysate is attached to the tube entering the patient's abdominal area *so the fluid flows into the peritoneal cavity.*

While the dialysate remains in the peritoneal cavity, the patient can roll up the bag, place it under his shirt, and go about his normal activities.

Unrolling the bag and suspending it below the pelvis allows the dialysate to drain from the peritoneal cavity back into the bag.

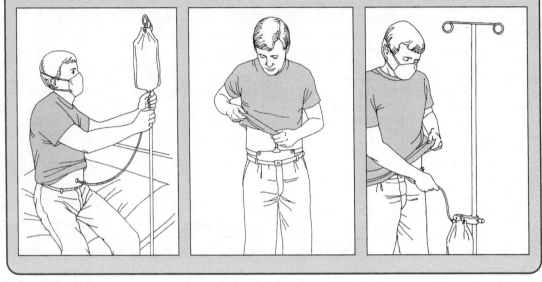

independence and a return to a near-normal lifestyle. It also costs less than hemodialysis.

Conditions that may prohibit CAPD include recent abdominal surgery, abdominal adhesions, an infected abdominal wall, diaphragmatic tears, ileus, and respiratory insufficiency.

Equipment

To infuse dialysate: Prescribed amount of dialysate (usually in 2-L bags) • heating pad or commercial warmer • three face masks • 42" (106.5-cm) connective tubing with drain clamp • six to eight packages of sterile 4" × 4" gauze pads • medication, if ordered • povidone-iodine pads • hypoallergenic tape • plastic snap-top container • povidone-iodine solution • sterile basin • container of alcohol • sterile gloves • belt or fabric pouch • two sterile waterproof paper drapes (one fenestrated) • optional: syringes, labeled specimen container

To discontinue dialysis temporarily: Three sterile waterproof paper barriers (two fenestrated) • 4" × 4" gauze pads (for cleaning and dressing the catheter) •

two face masks • sterile basin • hypoallergenic tape • povidone-iodine solution • sterile gloves • sterile rubber catheter cap

All equipment for infusing the dialysate and discontinuing the procedure must be sterile. **Science**

Commercially prepared sterile CAPD kits are available.

Preparation of equipment

Check the concentration of the dialysate and compare it to the practitioner's order. Check the expiration date and appearance of the solution — it should be clear, not cloudy. Warm the solution to body temperature with a heating pad or a commercial warmer if one is available. Don't warm the solution in a microwave oven because the temperature is unpredictable.

To minimize the risk of contaminating the bag's port, leave the dialysate container's wrapper in place. This also keeps the bag dry, which makes examining it for leakage easier after you remove the wrapper.

Wash your hands and put on a surgical mask. Remove the dialysate container from the warming setup, and remove its protective wrapper. Squeeze the bag firmly to check for leaks.

If ordered, use a syringe to add prescribed medication to the dialysate, using sterile technique *to avoid contamination.* (The ideal approach is to add medication under a laminar flow hood.) Disinfect multiple-dose vials in a 5-minute povidone-iodine soak. Insert the connective tubing into the dialysate container. Open the drain clamp to prime the tube. Close the clamp.

Place a povidone-iodine pad on the dialysate container's port. Cover the port with a dry gauze pad, and secure the pad with tape. Remove and discard the surgical mask. Tear the tape so it will be ready to secure the new dressing. Commercial devices with povidone-iodine pads are available for covering the dialysate container and tubing connection.

Implementation

● Confirm the patient's identity using two patient identifiers according to facility policy. **JCAHO**
● Weigh the patient *to establish a baseline level.* Weigh him at the same time every day *to help monitor fluid balance.*

Infusing dialysate

● Assemble all equipment at the patient's bedside, and explain the procedure to him. **PCP** Prepare the sterile field by placing a waterproof, sterile paper drape on a dry surface near the patient. Take care to maintain the drape's sterility.
● Fill the snap-top container with povidone-iodine solution, and place it on the sterile field. Place the basin on the sterile field. Place four pairs of sterile gauze pads in the sterile basin, and saturate them with the povidone-iodine solution. Drop the remaining gauze pads on the sterile field. Loosen the cap on the alcohol container, and place the cap next to the sterile field.
● Put on a clean surgical mask and provide one for the patient.
● Carefully remove the dressing covering the peritoneal catheter and discard it. Be careful not to touch the catheter or skin. Check skin integrity at the catheter site, and look for signs of infection such as purulent drainage. If drainage is present, obtain a

swab specimen, put it in a labeled specimen container, and notify the practitioner. **CDC**
● Put on the sterile gloves and palpate the insertion site and subcutaneous tunnel route for tenderness or pain. If these symptoms occur, notify the practitioner.
● Wrap one gauze pad saturated with povidone-iodine solution around the distal end of the catheter, and leave it in place for 5 minutes. Clean the catheter and insertion site with the rest of the gauze pads, moving in concentric circles away from the insertion site. Use straight strokes to clean the catheter, beginning at the insertion site and moving outward. Use a clean area of the pad for each stroke. Loosen the catheter cap one notch and clean the exposed area. Place each used pad at the base of the catheter *to help support it.* After using the third pair of pads, place the fenestrated paper drape around the base of the catheter. Continue cleaning the catheter for another minute with one of the remaining pads soaked with povidone-iodine. **Science**
● Remove the povidone-iodine pad on the catheter cap, remove the cap, and use the remaining povidone-iodine pad to clean the end of the catheter hub. Attach the connective tubing from the dialysate container to the catheter. Be sure to secure the luer-lock connector tightly.
● Open the drain clamp on the dialysate container *to allow solution to enter the peritoneal cavity by gravity* over a period of 5 to 10 minutes. Leave a small amount of fluid in the bag *to make folding it easier.* Close the drain clamp.
● Fold the bag and secure it with a belt, or tuck it in the patient's clothing or a small fabric pouch.
● After the prescribed dwell time (usually 4 to 6 hours), unfold the bag, open the clamp, and allow peritoneal fluid to drain back into the bag by gravity.
● When drainage is complete, attach a new bag of dialysate and repeat the infusion.
● Discard used supplies appropriately.

Discontinuing dialysis temporarily

● Wash your hands, put on a surgical mask, and provide one for the patient. Explain the procedure to him. **CDC** **PCP**
● Using sterile gloves, remove and discard the dressing over the peritoneal catheter.
● Set up a sterile field next to the patient by covering a clean, dry surface with a waterproof drape. Be sure to maintain the drape's sterility. Place all equipment

Continuous-cycle peritoneal dialysis

Continuous ambulatory peritoneal dialysis is easier for the patient who uses an automated continuous cycler system. When set up, the system runs the dialysis treatment automatically until all the dialysate is infused. The system remains closed throughout the treatment, *which reduces the risk of contamination.* Continuous-cycle peritoneal dialysis (CCPD) can be performed while the patient is awake or asleep. The system's alarms warn about general system, dialysate, and patient problems.

The cycler can be set to an intermittent or continuous dialysate schedule at home or in a health care facility. The patient typically initiates CCPD at bedtime and undergoes three to seven exchanges, according to his prescription. On awakening, the patient infuses the prescribed dialysis volume, disconnects himself from the unit, and carries the dialysate in his peritoneal cavity during the day.

The continuous cycler follows the same sterile care and maintenance procedures as the manual method.

on the sterile field, and place the 4″ × 4″ gauze pads in the basin. Saturate them with the povidone-iodine solution. Open the 4″ × 4″ gauze pads to be used as the dressing, and drop them onto the sterile field. Tear pieces of tape as needed.

● Tape the dialysate tubing to the side rail of the bed *to keep the catheter and tubing off the patient's abdomen.*

● Change to another pair of sterile gloves. Place one of the fenestrated drapes around the base of the catheter.

● Use a pair of povidone-iodine pads to clean about 6″ (15 cm) of the dialysis tubing. Clean for 1 minute, moving in one direction only, away from the catheter. Clean the catheter, moving from the insertion site to the junction of the catheter and dialysis tubing. Place used pads at the base of the catheter *to prop it up.* Use two more pairs of pads to clean the junction for a total of 3 minutes. **Science**

● Place the second fenestrated paper drape over the first at the base of the catheter. With the fourth pair of sponges, clean the junction of the catheter and 6″ of the dialysate tubing for another minute.

● Disconnect the dialysate tubing from the catheter. Pick up the catheter cap and fasten it to the catheter, making sure that it fits securely over both notches of the hard plastic catheter tip.

● Clean the insertion site and a 2″ (5 cm) radius around it with povidone-iodine pads, working from the insertion site outward. Let the skin air-dry before applying the dressing.

● Remove tape and discard used supplies appropriately.

Special considerations

● Absolute contraindications for CAPD include:
– documented loss of peritoneal function or extensive abdominal adhesions that limit dialysate flow
– physical or mental incapacity to perform peritoneal dialysis and no assistance available at home
– mechanical defects that prevent effective dialysis, which can't be corrected, or increase the risk of infection (such as surgically irreparable hernia, omphalocele, gastroschisis, diaphragmatic hernia, and bladder extrophy). **NKF**

● *Relative* contraindications for CAPD include:
– fresh intra-abdominal foreign bodies (for example, 4-month wait after abdominal vascular prostheses, recent ventricular-peritoneal shunt)
– peritoneal leaks or infection, or infection of the abdominal wall or skin
– body size limitations — either a patient who's too small to tolerate adequate dialysate, or a patient who's too large to be effectively dialyzed
– inability to tolerate the necessary volumes of dialysate for peritoneal dialysis to be successful
– inflammatory or ischemic bowel disease, or recurrent episodes of diverticulitis
– morbid obesity in short individuals, or patients suffering from severe malnutrition. **NKF**

● If inflow and outflow are slow or absent, check the tubing for kinks. You can also try raising the solution or repositioning (turning from side to side) the patient *to increase the inflow rate.* Repositioning the patient or applying manual pressure to the lateral aspects of the patient's abdomen *may also help increase drainage.*

TEACHING *Discuss the importance of compliance with therapy. Inform the patient that skipping treatments has been shown to increase the risk of hospitalization and death. Assist the patient with setting up and adjusting his CAPD schedule.*

Teach the patient and his family how to use sterile technique throughout the procedure, especially for cleaning and dressing changes, to prevent complications such as peritonitis.

Inform the patient about the advantages of an automated continuous cycler system for home use. (See Continuous-cycle peritoneal dialysis.*)*

Teach the patient and his family the signs and symptoms of peritonitis — cloudy fluid, fever, and abdominal pain and tenderness — and stress the importance of notifying the practitioner immediately if such signs or symptoms arise. Tell them to call the practitioner if redness and drainage occur; these are also signs of infection.

Instruct the patient to record his weight and blood pressure daily and to check regularly for swelling of the extremities. Teach him to keep an accurate record of intake and output.

Nursing diagnoses

● Deficient knowledge (procedure)
● Risk for imbalanced fluid volume

Expected outcomes

The patient will:
● state and demonstrate an understanding of the procedure
● measure and record weight, blood pressure, and intake and output
● maintain normal weight and blood pressure.

Complications

Peritonitis is the most common complication of CAPD. Although treatable, it can permanently scar the peritoneal membrane, decreasing its permeability and reducing the efficiency of dialysis. Untreated peritonitis can cause septicemia and death.

Excessive fluid loss may result from a concentrated (4.25%) dialysate solution, improper or inaccurate monitoring of inflow and outflow, or inadequate oral fluid intake. Excessive fluid retention may result from improper or inaccurate monitoring of inflow and outflow, or excessive salt or oral fluid intake.

Documentation

Record the type and amount of fluid instilled and returned for each exchange, the time and duration of the exchange, and medications added to the dialysate. Note the color and clarity of the returned exchange fluid and check it for mucus, pus, and blood. Note any discrepancy in the balance of fluid intake and output as well as signs of fluid imbalance, such as weight changes, decreased breath sounds, peripheral edema, ascites, and changes in skin turgor. Record the patient's weight, blood pressure, and pulse rate after his last fluid exchange for the day.

Supportive references

National Kidney Foundation. "Clinical Practice Guidelines for Peritoneal Dialysis Adequacy Update," 2000. *www.kidney.org/professionals/doqi/guidelines/ doqi_uptoc.html#pd.*

National Kidney and Urologic Diseases Information Clearinghouse. "Peritoneal Dialysis Dose and Adequacy." NIH Publication No. 04-4578. May 2004. *http://kidney.niddk.nih.gov/kudiseases/pubs/ peritonealdose/index.htm.*

Pfettscher, S.A. "Chronic Renal Failure and Renal Transplant," in *Critical Care Nursing.* Edited by Bucher, L., and Melander, S. Philadelphia: W.B. Saunders Co., 1999.

Stark, J. "The Renal System," in *Core Curriculum for Critical Care Nursing,* 6th ed. Edited by Alspach, J.G. Philadelphia: W.B. Saunders Co., 2006.

Self-catheterization

Self-catheterization is performed by many patients who have some form of impaired or absent bladder function.

CLINICAL IMPACT *Clean intermittent catheterization is safer than an indwelling catheter to prevent urinary tract infections (UTIs), and is a recommended alternative by the Centers for Disease Control and Prevention for the patient requiring urinary catheterization.* **CDC**

The two major advantages of self-catheterization are that patient independence is maintained and bladder control is regained. In addition, self-catheterization allows normal sexual intimacy without the fear of incontinence, decreases the chance of urinary reflux, reduces the use of aids and appliances and, in many cases, allows the patient to return to work.

Self-catheterization requires thorough and careful teaching by the nurse. At home the patient will use clean technique for self-catheterization, but if the patient is hospitalized he must use sterile technique because of the increased risk of acquiring a nosocomial UTI.

Equipment

Rubber catheter • washcloth, soap, and water • small packet of water-soluble lubricant • plastic storage bag • optional: drainage container, paper towels, cornstarch, rubber or plastic sheets, gooseneck lamp, catheterization record, mirror

Preparation of equipment

Instruct the patient to keep a supply of catheters at home and to use each catheter only once before cleaning it. Advise him to wash the used catheter in warm, soapy water, rinse it inside and out, then dry it with a clean towel and store it in a plastic bag until the next time it's needed. Because catheters become brittle with repeated use, tell the patient to check them often and to order a new supply well in advance.

Implementation

• Tell the patient to begin by trying to urinate into the toilet or, if a toilet isn't available or if he needs to measure urine quantity, into a drainage container. He should wash his hands thoroughly with soap and water and dry them.
• Demonstrate how the patient should perform the catheterization, explaining each step clearly and carefully. Position a gooseneck lamp nearby if room lighting is inadequate *to make the urinary meatus clearly visible*. Arrange the patient's clothing so that it's out of the way.

Teaching the female patient

• Demonstrate and explain to the female patient that she should separate the vaginal folds as widely as possible with the fingers of her nondominant hand *to obtain a full view of the urinary meatus*. She may need to use a mirror to visualize the meatus. Ask if she's right- or left-handed and then tell her which is her nondominant hand. While holding her labia open with the nondominant hand, she should use the dominant hand to wash the perineal area thoroughly with a soapy washcloth, using downward strokes. Tell her to rinse the area with the washcloth, using downward strokes as well. **Science**

• Show her how to squeeze the lubricant onto the first 3″ (7.5 cm) of the catheter and then how to insert the catheter. (See *Teaching self-catheterization*.)
• When the urine stops draining, tell her to remove the catheter slowly, get dressed, and wash the catheter with warm, soapy water. She should rinse it inside and out and dry it with a paper towel. **Science**

Teaching the male patient

• Instruct the male patient to wash and rinse the end of his penis thoroughly with soap and water, pulling back the foreskin if appropriate. He should keep the foreskin pulled back during the procedure. **Science**
• Show him how to squeeze lubricant onto a paper towel and have him roll the first 7″ to 10″ (17.5 to 25 cm) of the catheter in the lubricant. Tell him that copious lubricant will make the procedure more comfortable for him. Show him how to insert the catheter.
• When the urine stops draining, tell him to remove the catheter slowly and, if necessary, pull the foreskin forward again. Have him get dressed and wash and dry the catheter as described above.

Special considerations

• Impress upon the patient that the timing of catheterization is critical *to prevent overdistention of the bladder, which can lead to infection*. Self-catheterization usually occurs every 4 to 6 hours around the clock (or more often at first). **Science**
• Female patients should be able to identify the body parts involved in self-catheterization: labia majora, labia minora, vagina, and urinary meatus.
• Keep in mind the difference between boiling and sterilization. Boiling kills bacteria, viruses, and fungi, but doesn't kill spores, whereas sterilization does. However, because catheter cleaning will be done in the patient's home, boiling provides sufficient safeguard against spreading infections.
• Advise the patient to hold off storing the cleaned catheters in a plastic bag until after they're completely dry *to prevent growth of gram-negative organisms*.
• Stress the importance of regulating fluid intake, as ordered, *to prevent incontinence while maintaining adequate hydration*. However, explain that incontinent episodes may occur occasionally. For managing incontinence, the practitioner or a home health care nurse can help develop a plan such as more frequent catheterizations. After an incontinent episode, tell the

patient to wash with soap and water, pat himself dry with a towel, and expose the skin to the air for as long as possible. Bedding and furniture can be protected by covering them with rubber or plastic sheets and then covering the rubber or plastic with fabric.

Science

● Stress the importance of taking medications as ordered *to increase urine retention and help prevent incontinence.* Advise the patient to avoid calcium-rich and phosphorus-rich foods, as ordered, *to reduce the chance of renal calculus formation.*

Nursing diagnoses
● Urinary retention

Expected outcomes
The patient will:
● maintain equal intake and output
● not develop complications, such as an infection or bladder distention.

Complications
Overdistention of the bladder can lead to a UTI and urine leakage. Improper hand washing or equipment cleaning can also cause a UTI. Incorrect catheter insertion can injure the urethral or bladder mucosa.

Documentation
Record the date and times of catheterization, character of urine (color, odor, clarity, presence of particles or blood), the amount of urine (increase, decrease, no change), and any problems encountered during the procedure. Note whether the patient has difficulty performing a return demonstration.

Supportive references
Joanna Briggs Institute for Evidence Based Nursing and Midwifery. "Best Practice: Management of Short Term Indwelling Urethral Catheters to Prevent Urinary Tract Infections," 4(1), 2000. *www.joannabriggs.edu.au/pmenu.html.*

Madigan, E., and Neff, D.F. "Care of Patients with Long-Term Indwelling Urinary Catheters," *Online Journal of Issues in Nursing* 8(3), June 2003. *www.nursingworld.org/ojin.*

Potter, P.A., and Perry, A.G. *Fundamentals of Nursing,* 6th ed. St. Louis: Mosby–Year Book, Inc., 2004.

 TEACHING

Teaching self-catheterization

Female patient
Instruct the female patient to hold the catheter in her dominant hand as if it were a pencil or a dart, about ½" (1 cm) from its tip. Keeping the vaginal folds separated, she should slowly insert the lubricated catheter about 3" (7.5 cm) into the urethra. Tell her to press down with her abdominal muscles to empty the bladder, allowing all urine to drain through the catheter and into the toilet or drainage container.

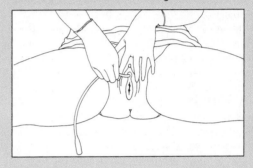

Male patient
Teach the male patient to hold his penis in his non-dominant hand, at a right angle to his body. He should hold the catheter in his dominant hand as if it were a pencil or a dart and slowly insert it 7" to 10" (17.5 to 25 cm) into the urethra—until urine begins flowing. Then he should gently advance the catheter about 1" (2.5 cm) farther, allowing all urine to drain into the toilet or drainage container.

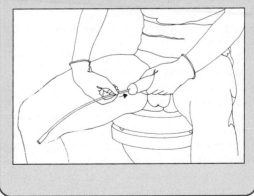

10

Orthopedic care

Orthopedics began as a specialty for the prevention and treatment of children's musculoskeletal deformities. However, this branch of medicine has expanded dramatically to include prevention, treatment, and care of musculoskeletal conditions affecting patients of all ages.

The American Nurses Association defines orthopedic nursing as the diagnosis and treatment of human responses to actual and potential health problems related to musculoskeletal function. More specifically, orthopedic nursing focuses on promoting wellness and self-care and on preventing further injury and illness in patients with degenerative, traumatic, inflammatory, neuromuscular, congenital, metabolic, and oncologic disorders.

Traditionally, orthopedic nurses have needed to operate special mechanical and traction equipment. Today, they need to understand principles of internal and external fixation, prosthetics, orthotics, immobilization, and implantation.

Despite the evolution of complex surgical procedures and mechanical devices that characterize modern orthopedic care, some things remain the same. A patient hospitalized for an orthopedic procedure — whether it's cast application, traction, or arthroplasty — is vulnerable to similar complications, such as:
- joint stiffness and skin breakdown from impaired physical mobility
- dislocations and fractures from mishandling osteoporotic extremities
- pain management issues and adverse reactions
- neurovascular compromise from pressure on major blood vessels and nerves caused by immobilization devices or compartmental edema
- infection of surgical wounds or skeletal pin tracts
- prolonged healing from failure to observe sound principles of immobilization.

In addition, the patient's level of understanding and effectiveness of coping skills must be assessed.

In this chapter, you'll find recommendations that will allow you to provide the best nursing care for your patients with orthopedic disorders or injuries. Some recommendations are evidence-based **EB**, grounded in current research; others are based on fundamental principles of science **Science**. Numerous best practices have the support of organizations, such as the American Pain Society **APS**, the Agency for Healthcare Research and Quality **AHRQ**, the National Association of Orthopedic Nurses **NAON**, the Joint Commission on Accreditation of Health Care Organizations **JCAHO**, the National Institute for Neurologic Disorders and Stroke **NINDS**, the Arthritis Foundation **AF**, the National Institutes of Health **NIH**, and the American Hospital Association's Patient Care Parnership **PCP** Equipment manufacturers **MFR** may have specific guidelines or recommendations for the use of their equipment.

Consistent care

Without exception, orthopedic complications can be prevented or minimized by appropriate and consistent assessment, monitoring, and therapy. For example, the orthopedic patient's neurovascular status must be assessed at regular intervals; otherwise, signs and symptoms of neurovascular compromise may go undetected until irreversible damage occurs. Consistent orthopedic care remains the surest way to promote rapid healing and successful rehabilitation.

Ready for an emergency

Orthopedic nursing care is characterized by the high incidence of emergency procedures you're likely to perform. The first step in administering emergency care at the scene of an accident is to immediately assess the patient for a life-threatening condition. Don't move him before completing an assessment unless danger is imminent *because this might worsen the injury and increase pain.* If the patient must be moved, assess him for possible spinal injury so that the appropriate transfer techniques can be used. After determining that no life-threatening injury exists, conduct an initial head-to-toe assessment, comparing bilaterally where applicable.

Always evaluate the patient's neurovascular status. Check the five P's: pain, pallor, pulse, paresthesia, and paralysis. Assess the injury thoroughly, and use strict sterile technique when caring for open wounds *to prevent infection.* If you suspect a bone injury, apply a splint *to reduce injury and immobilize the bone.*

In nonemergencies, performing orthopedic procedures correctly can ease pain, prevent further injury, and encourage proper healing.

Arthroplasty care

Arthroplasty involves surgical replacement of all or part of the joint. Joint arthroplasty is done *to decrease or eliminate pain and improve functional status.* Two of the most commonly replaced joints are the hip and the knee. Hip replacement may be total, replacing the femoral head and acetabulum, or partial, replacing only one joint component. (See *Total hip replacement.*) Knee replacement may also be partial, replacing either the medial or lateral compartment of the knee joint, or total, replacing the entire knee joint. Total knee replacement is commonly used to treat severe pain, joint contractures, and deterioration of joint surfaces — conditions that prohibit full extension or flexion.

According to the National Institutes of Health (NIH), to be considered for total hip replacement (THR), a patient should have some radiographic evidence of joint damage and moderate to severe pain or disability (or both) that isn't relieved by nonsurgical measures. The measures should include use of assistive devices (walkers), nonsteroidal anti-inflammatory drugs, physical therapy, and a reduction in physical activity. NIH statistics show that THR is most commonly used for patients with osteoarthritis. Other indications include:
- rheumatoid arthritis
- avascular necrosis
- traumatic arthritis
- certain hip fractures
- benign and malignant bone tumors

Total hip replacement

To form a totally artificial hip, the surgeon cements a femoral head prosthesis in place to articulate with a cup, which he then cements into the deepened acetabulum. He may avoid using cement by implanting a prosthesis with a porous coating that promotes bony ingrowth.

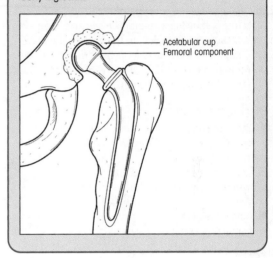

Acetabular cup
Femoral component

- arthritis associated with Paget's disease
- ankylosing spondylitis
- juvenile rheumatoid arthritis. **NIH**

Arthroplasty care includes maintaining alignment of the affected joint, assisting with exercises, and providing routine postoperative care.

Nursing responsibilities include teaching the patient safe mobility while performing activities of daily living, home care, and exercises that may continue for several years, depending on the type of arthroplasty performed and the patient's conditioning.

Equipment

Traction frame with trapeze • comfort device (such as static air mattress overlay, low-air-loss bed, or sheepskin) • bed sheets • incentive spirometer • continuous passive motion (CPM) machine (total knee replacement) • compression stocking • sterile dressings • hypoallergenic tape • ice bag • skin lotion • warm water • crutches or walker • pain medications • closed-wound drainage system • I.V. antibiotics • pillow •

abduction splint • anticoagulants • optional: closed drainage system, slings

After total knee replacement, a knee immobilizer may be applied in the operating room, or the leg may be placed in CPM.

Preparation of equipment

After the patient goes to the operating room, make a Balkan frame with a trapeze on his bed frame. *This will allow him some mobility after the operation.* Make the bed, using a comfort device and clean sheets. Have the bed taken to the operating room. *This enables immediate placement of the patient on his hospital bed after surgery and eliminates the need for an additional move from his recovery room bed.*

Implementation

● Check the patient's vital signs every 15 minutes twice, every 30 minutes until they stabilize, and then every 2 to 4 hours and routinely thereafter, according to facility protocol. Report changes in his vital signs *because they may indicate infection, hemorrhage, or postoperative complications.* **NAON**

● Encourage the patient to perform deep-breathing and coughing exercises. Assist with incentive spirometry as ordered *to prevent respiratory complications.* **Science**

● Assess the patient's neurovascular status every 2 hours for the first 48 hours and then every 4 hours *for signs of complications.* Check the affected leg for color, temperature, toe movement, sensation, edema, capillary refill, and pedal pulse. Investigate complaints of pain, burning, numbness, or tingling. **NAON**

● Apply the compression stocking to the unaffected leg, as ordered, *to promote venous return and prevent phlebitis and pulmonary emboli.* Once every 8 hours, remove it, inspect the leg — especially the heel — for pressure ulcers, and reapply it. **Science**

● Administer pain medication, as ordered. **APS**

● For 24 hours after surgery, administer I.V. antibiotics, as ordered, *to minimize the risk of wound infection.*

● Administer anticoagulant therapy, as ordered, *to minimize the risk of thrombophlebitis and embolus formation.* Observe for bleeding. Observe the leg for signs and symptoms of phlebitis, such as warmth, swelling, tenderness, redness, and a positive Homans' sign. **NAON** **Science**

● Check dressings for excessive bleeding. Circle any drainage on the dressing and mark it with your initials, the date, and the time. As needed, apply more sterile dressings, using hypoallergenic tape. Report excessive bleeding to the practitioner.

● Observe the closed-wound drainage system for discharge color and amount. *Proper drainage prevents hematoma. Purulent discharge and fever may indicate infection.* Empty and measure drainage as ordered, using clean technique.

● Monitor fluid intake and output every shift; include wound drainage in the output measurement.

● Apply an ice bag, as ordered, to the affected site for the first 48 hours *to reduce swelling, relieve pain, and control bleeding.* **APS** **Science**

● Reposition the patient every 2 hours. *These position changes enhance comfort, prevent pressure ulcers, and help prevent respiratory complications.* **Science**

● Help the patient use the trapeze to reposition himself every 2 hours. Provide skin care for the back and buttocks, using warm water and lotion, as indicated.

● Instruct the patient to perform muscle-strengthening exercises for affected and unaffected extremities, as ordered, *to help maintain muscle strength and range of motion and to help prevent phlebitis.* **NAON**

● Before ambulation, give an analgesic as ordered, 30 minutes before activity, *because movement is very painful.* Encourage the patient during exercise. **APS**

● Help the patient with progressive ambulation, using adjustable crutches or a walker when needed.

After hip arthroplasty

● Keep the affected leg in abduction and in the neutral position *to stabilize the hip and keep the cup and femur head in the acetabulum.* Place a pillow between the patient's legs *to maintain hip abduction.* **NAON** **Science**

CLINICAL IMPACT *Positioning of the patient after hip surgery varies, based on the surgical approach used and the surgeon's preference. For the anterior approach:*
● *No adduction past midline*
● *No flexion greater than 90 degrees*
● *No external rotation past midline*
For the posterior approach:
● *No adduction past midline*
● *No flexion greater than 60 to 90 degrees*
● *No internal rotation past midline*
● *No extension past neutral*

● Keep the patient in the supine position, with the affected hip in full extension, for 1 hour three times per day and at night. *This will help prevent hip flexion contracture.* **NAON** **Science**

● On the day after surgery, have the patient begin plantar flexion and dorsiflexion exercises of the foot on the affected leg. When ordered, instruct him to begin quadriceps exercises. Progressive ambulation protocols vary. In most cases, the patient is permitted to begin transfer and progressive ambulation with assistive devices on the first day.

After total knee replacement

● Elevate the affected leg, as ordered, *to reduce swelling.* **Science**

● Instruct the patient to begin quadriceps exercises and straight leg-raising, when ordered (usually on the first postoperative day). Encourage flexion-extension exercises, when ordered (usually after the first dressing change).

● If the practitioner orders use of the CPM machine, he'll adjust the machine daily *to gradually increase the degree of flexion of the affected leg.* Typically, patients can dangle their feet on the first day after surgery and begin ambulation with partial weight bearing as tolerated (cemented knee) or toe-touch ambulation only (uncemented knee) by the second day. The patient may need to wear a knee immobilizer for support when walking; otherwise, he should be in CPM for most of the day and night or during waking hours only. Check your facility's protocol.

● The degree of flexion, extension, and weight bearing status will depend on the practitioner's specific orders, surgical approach used, and the surgeon's preference.

Special considerations

● Before surgery, explain the procedure to the patient. Emphasize that frequent assessment — including monitoring his vital signs, neurovascular integrity, and wound drainage — is normal after the operation.

● Inform the patient that he'll receive I.V. antibiotics for about 2 days. Make sure that he understands that he'll receive medication around the clock for pain control. Explain the need for immobilizing the affected leg and exercising the unaffected one.

● Before discharge, instruct the patient regarding home care and exercises.

Nursing diagnoses

● Acute pain
● Impaired physical mobility

Expected outcomes

The patient will:
● express feelings of comfort and pain relief
● maximize mobility and ambulate safely.

Complications

Immobility after arthroplasty may result in such complications as pulmonary embolism, pneumonia, phlebitis, paralytic ileus, urine retention, and bowel impaction. A deep wound or infection at the prosthesis site is a serious complication that may force the removal of the prosthesis. Although these are the most common complications, the incidence of occurrence has been significantly reduced because of the use of prophylactic antibiotics and anticoagulants and early mobilization.

Dislocation of a total hip prosthesis may occur after violent hip flexion or adduction or during internal rotation. Signs and symptoms of dislocation include the inability to rotate the hip or bear weight, shortening of the leg, and increased pain.

Fat embolism, a potentially fatal complication resulting from release of fat molecules in response to increased intermedullary canal pressure from the prosthesis, may develop within 72 hours after surgery. Watch for such signs and symptoms as apprehension, diaphoresis, fever, dyspnea, pulmonary effusion, tachycardia, cyanosis, seizures, decreased level of consciousness, and a petechial rash on the chest and shoulders.

Documentation

Record the patient's neurovascular status. Describe his position (especially the position of the affected leg), skin care and condition, respiratory care and condition, and the use of compression stockings. Document all exercises performed and their effect, and record ambulatory efforts and the type of support used.

On the appropriate flowchart, record the patient's vital signs and fluid intake and output. Record discharge instructions and how well the patient seems to understand them.

Electrical bone growth stimulation

Electrical bone growth stimulation may be invasive or noninvasive.

Invasive system

An invasive system involves placing a spiral cathode inside the bone at the fracture site. A wire leads from the cathode to a battery-powered generator, also implanted in local tissues. The patient's body completes the circuit.

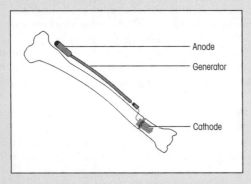

Noninvasive system

A noninvasive system may include a cuff-like transducer or fitted ring that wraps around the patient's limb at the level of the injury. Electric current penetrates the limb.

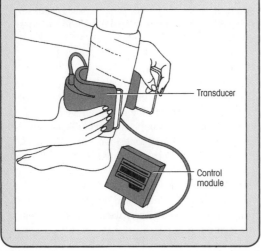

Supportive references

Geerts, W.H., et al. Seventh ACCP Conference on Antithrombotic and Thrombolytic Therapy. "Prevention of Venous Thromboembolism," *Chest* 126(3 Suppl):338S-400S, September 2004.

Maher, A., et al. *Orthopaedic Nursing*, 3rd ed. Philadelphia: W.B. Saunders Co., 2002.

National Institutes of Health Consensus Development Conference on Total Hip Replacement. *NIH Consensus Statement* 12(5):1-31, September 1994.

Bone growth stimulation, electrical

The use of electricity as an aid in bone healing was first acknowledged in 1812. However, full realization of the process didn't occur until 1953. Indications for the use of bone stimulators include augmentation of open reduction with internal and external fixation, promotion of bone growth, treatment of infected nonunions and failed arthrodesis and, most recently, treatment of disuse osteoporosis. By limiting the body's natural electrical forces, this procedure initiates or accelerates the healing process.

Three basic electrical bone stimulation techniques are available: fully implantable direct current stimulation, semi-invasive percutaneous stimulation, and noninvasive electromagnetic coil stimulation. (See *Electrical bone growth stimulation.*) Choice of technique depends on the fracture type and location, the practitioner's preference, and the patient's ability and willingness to comply. The invasive device requires little or no patient involvement. With the other two methods, however, the patient must manage his own treatment schedule and maintain the equipment. Treatment time averages 3 to 6 months.

Equipment

Direct current stimulation: The equipment set consists of a small generator and leadwires that connect to a titanium cathode wire surgically implanted into the nonunited bone site.

Percutaneous stimulation: The set consists of an external anode skin pad with a leadwire, lithium battery pack, and one to four Teflon-coated stainless steel cathode wires that are surgically implanted.

Electromagnetic stimulation: The set consists of a generator that plugs into a standard 110-volt outlet and two strong electromagnetic coils placed on either side of the injured area. The coils can be incorporated into a cast, cuff, or orthotic device. (See *Using an external bone growth stimulator,* page 490.)

Preparation of equipment

All equipment comes in sets with instructions provided by the manufacturer. Follow the instructions carefully. **MFR** Make sure that all parts are included and are sterilized according to facility policy and procedure.

Implementation

● Confirm the patient's identity using two patient identifiers according to facility policy. **JCAHO**
● Tell the patient whether he'll have an anesthetic and, if possible, which kind. **PCP**

Direct current stimulation

● Implantation is performed with the patient under general anesthesia. Afterward, the practitioner may apply a cast or external fixator *to immobilize the limb.* The patient is usually hospitalized for 2 to 3 days after implantation. Weight bearing may be ordered as tolerated.
● After the bone fragments join, the generator and leadwire can be removed under local anesthesia. The titanium cathode remains implanted.

Percutaneous stimulation

● Remove excessive body hair from the injured site before applying the anode pad. Avoid stressing or pulling on the anode wire. Instruct the patient to change the anode pad every 48 hours. Tell him to report local pain to his practitioner and not to bear weight for the duration of treatment.

Electromagnetic stimulation

● Show the patient where to place the coils, and tell him to apply them for 3 to 10 hours each day as ordered by his practitioner.
● Urge the patient not to interrupt the treatments for more than 10 minutes at a time.
● Teach the patient how to use and care for the generator.
● Relay the practitioner's instructions for weight bearing. Usually, the practitioner will advise against bearing weight until evidence of healing appears on X-rays.

Special considerations

● A patient with direct current electrical bone stimulation shouldn't undergo electrocauterization, diathermy, or magnetic resonance imaging (MRI). *Electrocautery may "short" the system; diathermy may potentiate the electrical current, possibly causing tissue damage; and MRI will interfere with or stop the current.*
● Percutaneous electrical bone stimulation is contraindicated if the patient has any kind of inflammatory process. Ask the patient if he's sensitive to nickel or chromium *because both are present in the electrical bone stimulation system.*
● Electromagnetic coils are contraindicated for a pregnant patient, a patient with a tumor, or a patient with an arm fracture or a pacemaker.

> **TEACHING** *Teach the patient how to care for his cast or external fixation devices. Tell him how to care for the electrical generator. Urge him to follow treatment instructions faithfully.*

Nursing diagnoses

● Impaired physical mobility

Expected outcomes

The patient will:
● maximize mobility and ambulate safely
● maintain muscle strength and joint mobility.

Complications

Complications associated with any surgical procedure, including increased risk of infection, may occur with direct current electrical bone stimulation equipment. Local irritation or skin ulceration may occur around cathode pin sites with percutaneous devices. No complications are associated with the use of electromagnetic coils.

Documentation

Record the type of electrical bone stimulation equipment provided, including the date, time, and location, as appropriate. Note the patient's skin condition and tolerance of the procedure. Record instructions given to the patient and his family as well as their ability to understand and act on those instructions.

Using an external bone growth stimulator

An external bone growth stimulator (EBGS) is a noninvasive and painless alternative to surgical bone grafting to promote healing. To use it, first gather the necessary equipment and familiarize the patient with the components of the EBGS system.

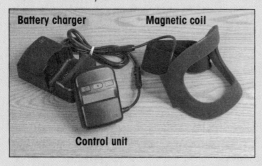

Battery charger   **Magnetic coil**

Control unit

Teach the patient where and how to place the coil. Inform her that she may place the coil over her cast or against her skin. A layer of clothing between the coil and her skin will provide adequate protection against skin irritation. Show her how to secure the coil with the strap and connect the control unit to the coil.

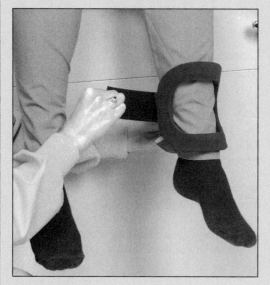

Pressing the button will start the unit, which will begin transmitting and recording. Be sure to show the patient when the battery needs changing. Depending on the type of unit, she may need to do this after each use or when the words "recharge battery" appear on the light-emitting diode (LED) screen. To charge the unit, tell her to plug it into an outlet at home and leave it plugged in for at least 2 hours.

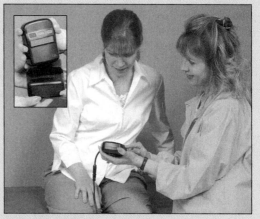

On the patient's return visits, turn on the control unit. The LED screen should display the hourly use per day and the number of days used and not used. Use these data to determine if she has used the EBGS according to her prescribed regimen. Be sure to document the usage times in her medical record.

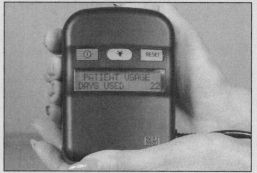

Adapted with permission from Patterson, M. "What's the Buzz on External Bone Growth Stimulators?" *Nursing2000* 30(6):44-45, June 2000.

Supportive references

LeeEvans, R.D., et al. "Electrical Stimulation with Bone and Wound Healing," *Clinics in Podiatric Medicine and Surgery* 18(1):79-95, January 2001.

Patterson, M. "What's the Buzz on External Bone Growth Stimulators?" *Nursing2000* 30(6):44-45, June 2000.

Ryaby, J. "Clinical Effects of Electromagnetic and Electric Fields on Fracture Healing," *Clinical Orthopaedics and Related Research* (355 Suppl):S205-15, October 1998.

External fixation

External fixation is a system of percutaneous pins and wires that are inserted through the skin and muscle into the bone and affixed to an adjustable external frame, which maintains the bones in proper alignment. Specialized types of external fixators may be used to lengthen leg bones or immobilize the cervical spine. (See *External fixation devices*.)

An advantage of external fixation over other immobilization techniques is that it *stabilizes the fracture while allowing full visualization and access to open wounds.* It also facilitates early ambulation, *thus reducing the risk of complications from immobilization.*

The Ilizarov Fixator is a special type of external fixation device. This device is a combination of rings and tensioned transosseous wires used primarily in limb lengthening, bone transport, and limb salvage. Highly complex, it provides gradual distraction resulting in good-quality bone formation with a minimum of complications.

Equipment

Sterile cotton-tipped applicators • prescribed antiseptic cleaning solution • ice bag • sterile gauze pads • analgesic or opioid • antimicrobial solution and ointment

Equipment varies with the type of fixator and the type and location of the fracture. Typically, sets of pins, stabilizing rods, and clips are available from manufacturers. Don't reuse pins.

Preparation of equipment

Make sure that the external fixation set includes all the equipment it's supposed to include and that the equipment has been sterilized according to your facility's policy.

External fixation devices

The practitioner's selection of an external fixation device depends on the severity of the patient's fracture and on the type of bone alignment needed.

Universal day frame

A universal day frame is used to manage tibial fractures. The frame allows the practitioner to readjust the position of bony fragments by angulation and rotation. The compression-distraction device allows compression and distraction of bony fragments.

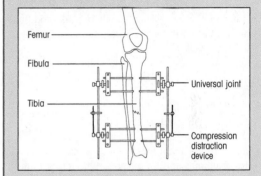

Portsmouth external fixation bar

A Portsmouth external fixation bar is used to manage complicated tibial fractures. The locking nut adjustment on the mobile carriage only allows bone compression, so the practitioner must accurately reduce bony fragments before applying the device.

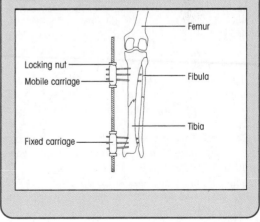

Implementation

● Confirm the patient's identity using two patient identifiers according to facility policy. **JCAHO**

● Explain the procedure to the patient *to reduce his anxiety.* Emphasize that he'll feel little pain after the fixation device is in place. Assure him that his feelings of anxiety are normal. **PCP**

● Tell the patient that he'll be able to move with the apparatus in place, which may help him resume normal activities more quickly.

● After the fixation device is in place, perform neurovascular checks every 2 to 4 hours for 24 hours and then every 4 to 8 hours, as appropriate, *to assess for possible neurologic damage.* Assess color, sensation, warmth, movement, edema, capillary refill, and pulses of the affected extremity. Compare with the unaffected side. **NAON**

● Apply an ice bag to the surgical site, as ordered, *to reduce swelling, relieve pain, and lessen bleeding.* **Science**

● Administer analgesics or opioids, as ordered, 30 minutes to 1 hour before exercising or mobilizing the affected extremity *to promote comfort.* **APS** **Science**

● Monitor the patient for pain not relieved by analgesics or opioids and for burning, tingling, or numbness, *which may indicate nerve damage, circulatory impairment, or compartment syndrome.* **Science**

● Elevate the affected extremity, if appropriate, *to minimize edema.* **Science**

● Perform pin-site care, as ordered, *to prevent infection.* Pin-site care varies, but you'll usually follow guidelines such as these: Use sterile technique; avoid digging at pin sites with the cotton-tipped applicator; if ordered, clean the pin site and surrounding skin with a cotton-tipped applicator dipped in ordered antiseptic solution; if ordered, apply antimicrobial ointment to pin sites; and apply a loose sterile dressing, or dress with sterile gauze pads with antimicrobial solution as ordered. Perform pin-site care as often as necessary, depending on the amount of drainage. **NAON**

● Check for redness, tenting of the skin, prolonged or purulent drainage from the pin site, swelling, elevated body or pin-site temperature, and any bowing or bending of pins, which may stress the skin.

✓ **CLINICAL IMPACT** *The National Association of Orthopedic Nurses (NAON) Pin-Site Care Expert Panel found that chlorhexidine 2-mg/ml so-*

lution may be the most effective cleaning solution for pin sites. Because of limited studies, the NAON recommends its use with a call for further research. Additional research is needed to fully establish which solutions are most effective in preventing infection and whether pin-site care or no pin-site care at all is more effective in preventing infection. **EB**

Special considerations
Patient with an Ilizarov Fixator

● When the device has been placed and preliminary calluses have begun to form at the insertion sites (in 5 to 7 days), gentle distraction is initiated by turning the appropriate screws one-quarter turn (1 mm) every 4 to 6 hours as ordered.

● Teach the patient that he must be consistent in turning the screws every 4 to 6 hours around the clock. Make sure that he understands that he must be strongly committed to compliance with the protocol for the procedure to be successful. Because the treatment period may be prolonged (4 to 10 months), discuss with the patient and his family the psychological effects of long-term care.

● Don't administer nonsteroidal anti-inflammatory drugs (NSAIDs) to patients being treated with the Ilizarov Fixator. *NSAIDs may decrease the necessary inflammation caused by the distraction, resulting in delayed bone formation.*

● Encourage the patient to stop smoking and provide smoking-cessation materials because smoking delays bone healing.

All patients

● Before discharge, teach the patient and his family how to provide pin-site care. This is a sterile procedure in the hospital, but the patient can use clean technique at home. Also, provide him with written instructions and have him demonstrate the procedure before leaving the hospital. **NAON** Teach him to recognize signs of pin-site infection. Tell him to keep the affected limb elevated when sitting or lying down.

Nursing diagnoses

● Risk for infection
● Risk for peripheral neurovascular dysfunction

Expected outcomes

The patient will:

- remain free from infection
- maintain circulation in the extremity
- not experience disability related to peripheral neurovascular dysfunction.

Complications

Complications of external fixation include loosening of pins and loss of fracture stabilization, infection of the pin tract or wound, skin breakdown, nerve damage, and muscle impingement.

Ilizarov Fixator pin sites are more prone to infection because of the extended treatment period and because of the pins' movement to accomplish distraction. The pins are also more likely to break because of their small diameter. The large number of pins used increases the patient's risk of neurovascular compromise.

Documentation

Record the patient's reaction to the apparatus. Assess and document the condition of the pin sites and skin. Document the patient's reaction to ambulation and his understanding of teaching instructions.

Supportive references

Holmes, S.B., and Brown, S.J. "Skeletal Pin Site Care: NAON Guidelines for Orthopaedic Nursing," *Orthopaedic Nursing* 24(2):99-107, March-April 2005. **EB**

Maher, A., et al. *Orthopaedic Nursing,* 3rd ed. Philadelphia: W.B. Saunders Co., 2002.

Schoen, D.C. *Core Curriculum for Orthopaedic Nursing,* 4th ed. Pitman, N.J.: National Association of Orthopaedic Nurses, 2001.

Sims, M., and Whiting, J. "Pin Site Care," *Nursing Times* 96(48):46, November-December 2000.

Internal fixation

Open reduction is a surgical procedure to realign a fracture; internal fixation is the addition of devices to stabilize the fracture. Internal fixation devices include nails, screws, pins, wires, and rods. They can be used individually or in combination with metal plates to attain stabilization. (See *Internal fixation devices,* page 494.)

Typically, internal fixation is used to treat fractures of the face and jaw, spine, bones of the arms and legs, and fractures involving a joint (most commonly, the hip). Internal fixation *permits earlier mobilization and can shorten hospitalization,* particularly in elderly patients with hip fractures.

Equipment

Ice bag • pain medication (analgesic or opioid) • incentive spirometer • compression stockings

Patients with leg fractures may also need the following: overhead frame with trapeze • pressure-relief mattress • crutches or walker • pillow (hip fractures may require abductor pillows).

Preparation of equipment

Equipment is collected and prepared in the operating room.

Implementation

- Explain the procedure to the patient *to alleviate his fears.* Tell him what to expect during postoperative assessment and monitoring, teach him how to use an incentive spirometer, and prepare him for proposed exercise and progressive ambulation regimens if necessary. **PCP**
- After the procedure, monitor the patient's vital signs every 2 to 4 hours for 24 hours, then every 4 to 8 hours, according to your facility's protocol. *Changes in the patient's vital signs may indicate hemorrhage or infection.* **NAON**
- Monitor fluid intake and output every 4 to 8 hours.
- Perform neurovascular checks every 2 to 4 hours for 24 hours, then every 4 to 8 hours as appropriate. Assess color, warmth, sensation, movement, edema, capillary refill, and pulses of the affected area. Compare findings with the unaffected side. **NAON**
- Apply an ice bag to the operative site, as ordered, *to reduce swelling, relieve pain, and lessen bleeding.* **APS** **Science**
- Administer opioids, as ordered, before exercising or mobilizing the affected area *to promote comfort.* If the patient is using patient-controlled analgesia, instruct him to administer a dose before exercising or mobilizing. **APS**
- Monitor the patient for pain unrelieved by opioids and for burning, tingling, or numbness, *which may indicate infection, impaired circulation, or compartment syndrome.* **Science**
- Elevate the affected limb on a pillow, if appropriate, *to minimize edema.* **APS** **Science**

Internal fixation devices

The choice of a specific internal fixation device depends on the location, type, and configuration of the fracture.

In trochanteric or subtrochanteric fractures, the surgeon may use a hip pin or nail, with or without a screw plate. A pin or plate with extra nails stabilizes the fracture by impacting the bone ends at the fracture site.

In an uncomplicated fracture of the femoral shaft, the surgeon may use an intramedullary rod. This device permits early ambulation with partial weight bearing.

Another choice for fixation of a long-bone fracture is a screw plate, shown below on the tibia.

In an arm fracture, the surgeon may fix the involved bones with a plate, rod, or nail. Most radial and ulnar fractures may be fixed with plates, whereas humeral fractures are commonly fixed with rods

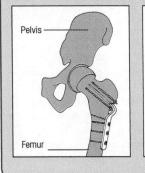

Pelvis
Femur

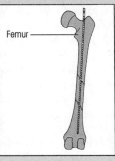

Femur

Fibula
Tibia

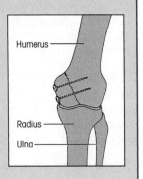

Humerus
Radius
Ulna

● Check surgical dressings for excessive drainage or bleeding. Check the incision site for signs of infection, such as erythema, drainage, edema, and unusual pain. **NAON**

● Assist and encourage the patient to perform range-of-motion and other muscle strengthening exercises, as ordered, *to promote circulation, improve muscle tone, and maintain joint function.* **Science**

● Teach the patient to perform progressive ambulation and mobilization using an overhead frame with trapeze, or crutches or a walker, as appropriate.

● Continue anticoagulation therapy as ordered by the practitioner.

● Teach the patient signs and symptoms of venous thromboembolism.

Special considerations

● *To avoid the complications of immobility after surgery,* have the patient use an incentive spirometer. Apply compression stockings and a sequential compression device, as appropriate. The patient may also require a pressure-relief mattress.

TEACHING *Before discharge, instruct the patient and his family how to care for the incisional site and recognize signs and symptoms of infection.*

Teach the patient and his family about administering pain medication, practicing an exercise regimen (if any), and using assistive ambulation devices (such as crutches or a walker), if appropriate.

Nursing diagnoses

● Acute pain
● Risk for infection

Expected outcomes

The patient will:
● report pain relief
● remain free from infection.

Complications

Wound infection and, more critically, infection involving metal fixation devices may require reopening the incision, draining the suture line and, possibly, removing the fixation device. Any such infection would require wound dressings and antibiotic therapy. Other complications may include malunion, nonunion, fat or pulmonary embolism, neurovascular impairment, and chronic pain.

Documentation

In the patient record, document perioperative findings on cardiovascular, respiratory, and neurovascular status. Name pain management techniques used. Describe incision appearance and alignment of the affected bone. Document the patient's response to teaching about appropriate exercise, care of the incision site, use of assistive devices (if appropriate), and symptoms that should be reported to the practitioner.

Supportive references

Geerts, W.H., et al. Seventh ACCP Conference on Antithrombotic and Thrombolytic Therapy. "Prevention of Venous Thromboembolism," *Chest* 126(3 Suppl):338S-400S, September 2004.

Maher, A., et al. *Orthopaedic Nursing,* 3rd ed. Philadelphia: W.B. Saunders Co., 2002.

Schoen, D.C. *Core Curriculum for Orthopaedic Nursing,* 4th ed. Pitman, N.J.: National Association of Orthopaedic Nurses, 2001.

Smith, S., ed. *Orthopaedic Nursing Care Competencies: Adult Acute Care.* Pitman, N.J.: National Association of Orthopaedic Nurses, 1999.

Low back pain prevention

In the United States, low back pain affects 60% to 80% of adults at some time during their lives, and up to 50% of adults have back pain within a given year. Back pain symptoms are among the 10 leading reasons for patient visits to emergency departments, hospital outpatient departments, and practitioners' offices. Although symptoms are usually acute and self-limiting, low back pain typically recurs and, in some cases, becomes a chronic disability. Back symptoms are the most common cause of disability for persons under age 45. Treatment is expensive; annual costs for back pain increase from approximately $35 to $56 billion when disability costs are included. Back pain can arise from many causes. It can range from a dull ache to absolute agony. Many cases of back pain are caused by stress on the muscles and ligaments that support the spine.

Many back injuries are occupational in nature. Occupational back injury is clearly related to lifting and repeated activities. Persons in occupations that require repetitive lifting, such as nursing and heavy industry, are especially at risk.

Managing acute low back pain

By advising your patient about the following guidelines, you can help him manage low back pain and prevent recurrence.

TEACHING *Sitting. When in acute pain, sit for as little as possible and only for short periods. Place a supportive roll in the small of the back, especially when sitting in a car or lounge chair. Avoid sitting on a soft chair or couch; instead, choose a high chair with a straight back.* Sitting in a chair or couch with a deep seat will force your knees to be higher than your hips.

To maintain good positioning when rising from sitting, move to the front of the seat, stand up by straightening the legs, and avoid bending forward at the waist.

Driving a car
If you're in pain, try not to drive, or drive as little as possible. If driving, position your seat close enough to the steering wheel to allow you to maintain the lordosis. If your hips are lower than your knees, you may be able to raise yourself by sitting on a pillow.

Bending forward
When in acute pain, avoid activities that require bending forward or stooping because you'll be forced to lose the lordosis.

Lifting
When in acute pain, avoid heavy lifting altogether for the first 6 weeks. (For correct lifting techniques, see "Body mechanics," page 32.)

Sleeping
When sleeping on your side, try curling up into a fetal position with a pillow between your legs.

When sleeping on your back, place a pillow under your knees to relieve pressure. Use a pillow under your head that provides enough support to maintain spinal alignment without pushing your head too far forward.

When rising from lying, you must retain the lordosis: Turn on one side, draw both knees up and drop your feet over the edge of the bed. Sit up by pushing yourself up with the hands, and avoid bending forward at the waist.

Exercising NIH

Avoid jogging, contact sports, golf, ballet, weight lifting, stretching, situps with straight legs, and leg lifts when lying on your stomach during your initial recovery. Light cardiovascular training, such as walking, stationary bicycling, and swimming, can help promote healing by helping blood flow to your back and strengthen your stomach and back muscles.

Preventing low back injury

According to the Agency for Health Care Research and Quality (AHRQ), there's minimal evidence to support interventions that prevent low back pain. The following clinical considerations have been recommended by the AHRQ with caution that further research is needed.

● Although there's no good evidence to support regular exercise, back strengthening exercise and regular physical activity have other health benefits.
● The use of lumbar supports or back belts hasn't been shown to prevent back pain and may actually increase the risk.
● Educational sessions in work settings aren't effective in decreasing the incidence of low back pain, but may prevent further back injury in people with recurrent or chronic low back pain. AHRQ

The following activity instructions can be followed when the patient resumes normal activities to help alleviate further pain and injury.

TEACHING *Sitting. At work, sit close to your desk or work table to avoid bending over. Keep your feet firmly on the floor.*

If sitting for a prolonged period, maintaining proper positioning is vital. If you can't maintain lordosis with your own muscles, use a supportive roll placed in the small of your back to keep proper alignment.

Interrupt prolonged sitting at regular intervals. On long car trips, get out of the car every 1 or 2 hours,

stand upright, bend backward 5 to 6 times, and walk around for a few minutes.

Bending forward

When engaged in activities that require prolonged forward bending or stooping, such as gardening or vacuuming, stand upright to restore the lordosis and bend backward 5 to 6 times before pain begins.

Frequent interruption of prolonged bending by reversing the curve in the low back should enable you to continue with most activities. Science

Lifting

When lifting an object, maintain a wide support base. Lift with your legs, not your back, and keep a close center of gravity. (For correct lifting techniques, see "Body mechanics," page 32.)

Special considerations

According to the National Institute for Neurologic Disorders and Stroke, treatment of back pain includes the use of over-the-counter pain relievers and anti-inflammatory medications.

Although hot and cold compresses haven't been proven to resolve back pain, an ice bag or hot water bottle applied to the back may help alleviate pain. Prolonged bed rest isn't beneficial because it weakens muscles; therefore, it's only recommended for 1 or 2 days. The patient should resume normal activities as soon as possible and use exercise to strengthen back and abdominal muscles. NINDS

Nursing diagnoses
● Acute pain

Expected outcomes
The patient will:
● report pain relief.

Documentation
● Document the patient's efforts to perform proper body mechanics.
● Document patient teaching and the patient's ability to verbalize an understanding of what was taught.

Supportive references

National Institute of Neurological Disorders and Stroke. "NINDS Back Pain Information Page," January 2006. *www.ninds.nih.gov/disorders/backpain/backpain.htm.*

Owen, B. "Preventing Injuries Using an Ergonomic Approach," *AORN Journal* 72(6):1031-1036, December 2000.

U.S. National Library of Medicine and National Institutes of Health. "Medline Plus: Back Pain — Low," July 2005. *www.nlm.nih.gov/medlineplus/ency/article/003108.htm.*

U.S. Preventative Service Task Force. (USPSTF) "Primary Care Interventions to Prevent Low Back Pain in Adults: Recommendation Statement." Rockville, MD: Agency for Healthcare Research and Quality, February 2004.

Mechanical traction

Mechanical traction is used to reduce fractures, treat dislocations, correct or prevent deformities, improve or correct contractures, or decrease muscle spasms. It works by exerting a pulling force on an injured or diseased part of the body — usually the spine, pelvis, or bones of the arms or legs, while countertraction pulls in the opposite direction. **Science**

The three types of traction are manual, skin, and skeletal. Manual traction involves placing hands on the affected body part and applying a steady pull, usually during a procedure such as cast application, fracture reduction, or halo application.

Skin traction is ordered when a light, temporary, or noncontinuous pulling force is required. Contraindications for skin traction include a severe injury with open wounds, an allergy to tape or other skin traction equipment, circulatory disturbances, dermatitis, and varicose veins.

In skeletal traction, an orthopedist inserts a pin or wire through the bone and attaches the traction equipment to the pin or wire to exert a direct, constant, longitudinal pulling force. Indications for skeletal traction include fractures of the tibia, femur, and humerus. Infections, such as osteomyelitis, contraindicate skeletal traction.

Nursing responsibilities for this procedure include supervising the setup of the traction frame. (See *Traction frames,* page 498.) The design of the patient's bed usually dictates whether to use a claw clamp or I.V.-post-type frame. (However, the claw-type Balkan frame is rarely used.) A nurse with special skills, an orthopedic technician, or the practitioner can set up the specific traction. Instructions for setting up these traction units usually accompany the equipment.

After the patient is placed in the specific type of traction ordered by the orthopedist, the nurse is responsible for preventing complications from immobility; for routinely inspecting the equipment; for adding traction weights as ordered; and, in patients with skeletal traction, for monitoring the pin insertion sites for signs of infection. (See *Comparing types of traction,* page 499.) **NAON**

Equipment

Claw-type basic frame: 102″ (259-cm) plain bar • two 66″ (167.5-cm) swivel-clamp bars • two upper-panel clamps • two lower-panel clamps

I.V.-type basic frame: 102″ plain bar • 27″ (68.5-cm) double-clamp bar • 48″ (122-cm) swivel-clamp bar • two 36″ (91.5-cm) plain bars • four 4″ (10-cm) I.V. posts with clamps • cross clamp

I.V.-type Balkan frame: Two 102″ plain bars • two 27″ double-clamp bars • two 48″ swivel-clamp bars • five 36″ plain bars • four 4″ I.V. posts with clamps • eight cross clamps

All frame types: Trapeze with clamp • wall bumper or roller

Skeletal traction care: Sterile cotton-tipped applicators • prescribed antiseptic solution • sterile gauze pads • povidone-iodine solution • optional: antimicrobial ointment

Preparation of equipment

Arrange with central supply or the appropriate department to have the traction equipment transported to the patient's room on a traction cart. If appropriate, gather the equipment for pin-site care at the patient's bedside. Pin-site care protocols may vary with each facility or practitioner.

Implementation

● Confirm the patient's identity using two patient identifiers according to facility policy. **JCAHO**

● Explain the purpose of traction to the patient. Emphasize the importance of maintaining proper body alignment after the traction equipment is set up. **PCP**

✓ **CLINICAL IMPACT** *Regardless of the type of traction used, several principles should be maintained:*

Traction frames

You may encounter three types of traction frames, as described here.

Claw-type basic frame

With a claw-type frame, claw attachments secure the uprights to the footboard and headboard.

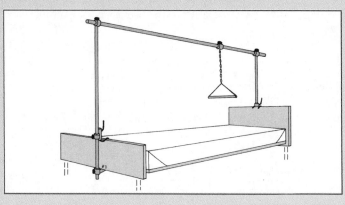

I.V.-type basic frame

With an I.V.-type basic frame, I.V. posts, placed in I.V. holders, support the horizontal bars across the foot and head of the bed. These horizontal bars then support the two uprights.

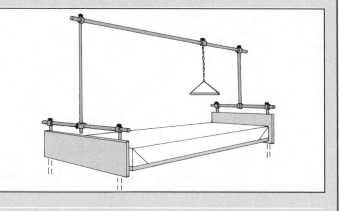

I.V.-type Balkan frame

The I.V.-type Balkan frame features I.V. posts and horizontal bars (secured in the same manner as those for the I.V.-type basic frame) that support four uprights.

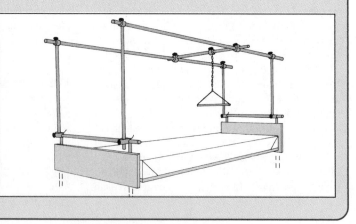

• *Countertraction must always be provided by the patient's body weight, pull of weights in the opposite direction, or elevation of the bed.*
• *The line of the pull should be maintained at all times.*
• *The weights should hang freely at all times.*
• *Friction should be prevented on the traction apparatus.* **EB**

Setting up a claw-type basic frame

• Attach one lower-panel and one upper-panel clamp to each 66″ swivel-clamp bar.
• Fasten one bar to the footboard and one to the headboard by turning the clamp knobs clockwise until they're tight and then pulling back on the upper clamp's rubberized bar until it's tight.
• Secure the 102″ horizontal plain bar atop the two vertical bars, making sure that the clamp knobs point up.
• Using the appropriate clamp, attach the trapeze to the horizontal bar about 2′ (61 cm) from the head of the bed.

Setting up an I.V.-type basic frame

• Attach one 4″ I.V. post with clamp to each end of both 36″ horizontal plain bars.
• Secure an I.V. post in each I.V. holder at the bed corners. Using a cross clamp, fasten the 48″ vertical swivel-clamp bar to the middle of the horizontal plain bar at the foot of the bed.
• Fasten the 27″ vertical double-clamp bar to the middle of the horizontal plain bar at the head of the bed.
• Attach the 102″ horizontal plain bar to the tops of the two vertical bars, making sure that the clamp knobs point up.
• Using the appropriate clamp, attach the trapeze to the horizontal bar about 2′ from the head of the bed.

Setting up an I.V.-type Balkan frame

• Attach one 4″ I.V. post with clamp to each end of two 36″ horizontal plain bars.
• Secure an I.V. post in each I.V. holder at the bed corners.
• Attach a 48″ vertical swivel-clamp bar, using a cross clamp, to each I.V. post clamp on the horizontal plain bar at the foot of the bed.

Comparing types of traction

Traction therapy applies a pulling force to an injured or diseased limb. For traction to be effective, it must be combined with an equal mix of countertraction. Weights provide the pulling force. Countertraction is produced by positioning the patient's body weight against the traction pull.

Skin traction

Skin traction immobilizes a body part intermittently over an extended period through direct application of a pulling force on the patient's skin. The force may be applied using adhesive or nonadhesive traction tape or other skin traction devices, such as a boot, belt, or halter.

This traction exerts a light pull and uses up to 8 lb (3.6 kg) per extremity for an adult.

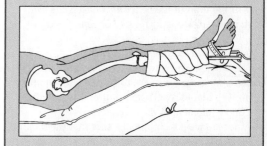

Skeletal traction

Skeletal traction immobilizes a body part for prolonged periods by attaching weighted equipment directly to the patient's bones. This may be accomplished with pins, screws, wires, or tongs. The amount of weight applied is determined by body size and the extent of the injury.

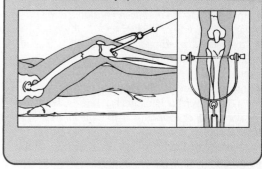

- Fasten one 36″ horizontal plain bar across the midpoints of the two 48″ swivel-clamp bars, using two cross clamps.
- Attach a 27″ vertical double-clamp bar to each I.V. post clamp on the horizontal bar at the head of the bed.
- Using two cross clamps, fasten a 36″ horizontal plain bar across the midpoints of two 27″ double-clamp bars.
- Clamp a 102″ horizontal plain bar onto the vertical bars on each side of the bed, making sure that the clamp knobs point up.
- Use two cross clamps to attach a 36″ horizontal plain bar across the two overhead bars, about 2′ from the head of the bed.
- Attach the trapeze to this 36″ horizontal bar.

After setting up any frame
- Attach a wall bumper or roller to the vertical bar or bars at the head of the bed. *This protects the walls from damage caused by the bed or equipment.*

Caring for the traction patient
- Show the patient how much movement he's allowed and instruct him not to readjust the equipment. Tell him to report pain or pressure from the traction equipment. **PCP**
- At least once per shift, make sure that the traction equipment connections are tight. Check for impingements such as ropes rubbing on the footboard or getting caught between pulleys. *Friction and impingement reduce the effectiveness of traction.* **EB**
- Inspect the traction equipment *to ensure the correct alignment.* **EB**
- Inspect the ropes for fraying, *which can eventually cause a rope to break.*
- Make sure that the ropes are positioned properly in the pulley track. *An improperly positioned rope changes the degree of traction.*
- *To prevent tampering and aid stability and security,* make sure that all rope ends are taped above the knot.
- Inspect the equipment regularly to make sure that the traction weights hang freely. *Weights that touch the floor, bed, or each other reduce the amount of traction.* **EB**
- About every 2 hours, check the patient for proper body alignment, and reposition the patient as necessary. *Misalignment causes ineffective traction and*

may keep the fracture from healing properly. **NAON** **Science**
- *To prevent complications from immobility,* assess the patient's neurovascular integrity routinely. His condition, the hospital routine, and the practitioner's orders determine the frequency of neurovascular assessments. **NAON**
- Provide skin care, encourage coughing and deep-breathing exercises, and assist with ordered range-of-motion exercises for unaffected extremities. Typically, an order for compression stockings is written. Check elimination patterns and provide laxatives as ordered. **Science**
- For the patient with skeletal traction, make sure that the protruding pin or wire ends are covered with cork *to prevent them from tearing the bedding or injuring the patient and staff.*
- Check the pin site and surrounding skin regularly for signs of infection.
- If ordered, clean the pin site and surrounding skin. Pin-site care varies. Check your facility's policy, or follow orders prescribed by the practitioner. (See "External fixation," page 491, for how to perform pin-site care.)

Special considerations
- When using skin traction, apply ordered weights slowly and carefully *to avoid jerking the affected extremity. To avoid injury in case the ropes break,* arrange the weights so they don't hang over the patient.
- When applying Buck's traction, make sure that the line of pull is always parallel to the bed and not angled downward *to prevent pressure on the heel.* Placing a flat pillow under the extremity may be helpful as long as it doesn't alter the line of pull.

Nursing diagnoses
- Impaired physical mobility
- Risk for infection

Expected outcomes
The patient will:
- maximize mobility while on bed rest
- maintain muscle strength and joint range of motion
- not develop complications, such as contractures, venous stasis, skin breakdown, or pneumonia
- remain free from infection.

Complications

Immobility during traction may result in pressure ulcers; muscle atrophy, weakness, or contractures; and osteoporosis. Immobility can also cause GI disturbances, such as constipation; urinary problems, including stasis and calculi; respiratory problems, such as stasis of secretions and hypostatic pneumonia; and circulatory disturbances, including stasis and thrombophlebitis. Prolonged immobility, especially after traumatic injury, may promote depression or other emotional disturbances. Skeletal traction may cause osteomyelitis originating at the pin or wire sites.

Documentation

In the patient record, document the amount of traction weight used daily, noting the application of additional weights and the patient's tolerance. Document equipment inspections and patient care, including routine checks of neurovascular integrity, skin condition, respiratory status, and elimination patterns. If applicable, note the condition of the pin site and any care given.

Supportive references

Maher, A.B., et al. *Orthopaedic Nursing,* 3rd ed. Philadelphia: W.B. Saunders Co., 2002. **EB**

Osteoarthritis treatment

Osteoarthritis (OA), or degenerative joint disease, is one of the most common types of arthritis. It's characterized by the breakdown of the joint's cartilage — the part of the joint that cushions the ends of bones. Cartilage breakdown causes bones to rub against each other, causing pain and loss of movement.

Most commonly affecting middle-aged people or the elderly, OA can occur at any age and occurs equally in both sexes. Its earliest symptoms typically begin after age 40 and may progress with advancing age.

Disability depends on the site of involvement and can range from minor limitation of dexterity of the fingers to severe disability in persons with hip or knee involvement. The rate of progression varies, and joints may remain stable for years in an early stage of deterioration.

There are many factors that can cause OA. Although age is a risk factor, research has shown that OA isn't an inevitable part of aging. Obesity may lead to OA of the knees. In addition, people with joint injuries due to sports, work-related activity, or accidents may be at increased risk for developing OA.

Genetics has a role in the development of OA, particularly in the hands. Some people may be born with defective cartilage or with slight defects in the way that joints fit together. As a person ages, these defects may cause early cartilage breakdown in the joint. In the process of cartilage breakdown, there may be some inflammation, with enzymes released and more cartilage damage.

A thorough physical examination confirms typical symptoms, and absence of systemic symptoms rules out an inflammatory joint disorder. X-rays of the affected joint help confirm the diagnosis of OA but may be normal in the early stages. X-rays may require many views and typically show:
- narrowing of the joint space or margin
- cystlike bony deposits in the joint space and margins and sclerosis of the subchondral space
- joint deformity because of degeneration or articular damage
- bony growths at weight-bearing areas
- fusion of joints. **EB1**

Implementation

According to the Arthritis Foundation, treatment of OA focuses on decreasing pain, improving joint movement, and minimizing disability and may include:
- exercises to keep joints flexible and improve muscle strength
- medications, such as COX-2 inhibitors and nonsteroidal anti-inflammatory drugs, for pain control (For mild pain without inflammation, analgesics may be used.)
- joint protection to prevent strain or stress on painful joints
- surgery (sometimes) to relieve chronic pain in damaged joints (see *Surgery for osteoarthritis,* page 502)
- weight control to prevent extra stress on weight-bearing joints. **AF**

Effective treatment also reduces stress by supporting or stabilizing the joint with crutches, braces, a cane, a walker, a cervical collar, or traction. Other supportive measures include massage, moist heat, paraffin dips for the hands, protective techniques for preventing undue stress on the joints, and adequate rest (particularly after activity).

Surgery for osteoarthritis

Surgical treatment for osteoarthritis is reserved for patients who have severe disability or uncontrollable pain and may include:

- arthroplasty (partial or total) — replacement of the deteriorated part of the joint with a prosthetic appliance
- arthrodesis — surgical fusion of bones, used primarily in the spine (laminectomy)
- osteoplasty — scraping and lavage of deteriorated bone from joint
- osteotomy — change in alignment of bone to relieve stress by excision of wedge of bone or cutting of bone.

Specific patient care **EB2**

- *Hand:* Apply hot soaks and paraffin dips to relieve the pain as ordered. **Science**
- *Spine:* Recommend that the patient sleep on a firm mattress or bed board to reduce morning pain.
- *Cervical spine:* Check the cervical collar for fit and constriction. Watch for signs of redness with prolonged use.
- *Hip:* Use moist heating pads to relieve pain and administer antispasmodic drugs, as ordered. Assist patient with range-of-motion (ROM) exercises and make sure that he gets adequate rest afterward. Check cane, crutches, braces, and walkers for the proper fit and teach the patient to use them correctly.
- *Knee:* Twice daily, assist the patient with ROM exercises, exercises to maintain muscle tone, and progressive resistance exercises to increase muscle strength. Provide elastic support braces if needed.

> **TEACHING** *Tell the patient to maintain proper body alignment, especially when stooping or picking up objects.* **Science** *Tell the patient to wear proper fitting shoes and not to allow the heels to become worn down.*

Special considerations

Other interventions for managing osteoarthritis include:

- planning rest periods during the day, and providing for adequate sleep at night (Moderation is the key; teach the patient to pace activities.)

- assisting with physical therapy, and encouraging the patient to perform gentle, isometric ROM exercises
- providing appropriate preoperative and postoperative care (if the patient needs surgery)
- providing emotional support and helping the patient cope with limited mobility. (Inform the patient that OA isn't a systemic disease.) **EB2**

Nursing diagnoses

- Acute pain
- Chronic pain

Expected outcomes

The patient will:

- report pain relief after taking prescribed medications
- develop a pain management program that includes activity and exercise, rest, and a medication regimen.

Supportive references

Arthritis Foundation. "Osteoarthritis." *www.arthritis.org/conditions/DiseaseCenter/default.asp.*

Hanter, D.J., et al. "The Association of Meniscal Pathologic Changes with Cartilage Loss in Symptomatic Knee Osteoarthritis," *Arthritis and Rheumatism* 54(3):795-802, March 2006.

Maher, A.B., et al. *Orthopaedic Nursing,* 3rd ed. Philadelphia: W.B. Saunders Co., 2002. **EB2**

Ross, C. "A Comparison of Osteoarthritis and Rheumatoid Arthritis: Diagnosis and Treatment," *Nurse Practitioner* 22(9):20, September 1997. **EB1**

Osteoporosis prevention

Osteoporosis is a metabolic bone disorder in which the rate of bone reabsorption accelerates while the rate of bone formation slows down, causing a loss of bone mass, or bone density. Bones affected by this disease lose calcium and phosphate salts and thus become porous, brittle, and abnormally vulnerable to fractures. Osteoporosis may be primary or secondary to an underlying disease. Primary osteoporosis is typically called postmenopausal osteoporosis because it most commonly develops in postmenopausal women.

The exact cause of osteoporosis is unknown. Two major factors contribute to bone mass: the peak bone mass achieved during young adulthood and the rate of bone loss that occurs after menopause or during late adulthood. Achievement of 100% optimal peak bone mass occurs by age 35 and is influenced by genetic factors and enhanced by adequate calcium intake, weight-bearing exercise, and the absence of risk factors. The rate of bone loss is strongly influenced by genetics, estrogen level, and risk factors. (See *Assessing risk of osteoporosis.*)

The first evidence of osteoporosis is typically a painful fracture. The annual incidence of osteoporotic fractures in the United States exceeds 1.5 million, including more than 300,000 femoral fractures and more than 500,000 vertebral fractures.

Prevention guidelines NIH

There are several factors to consider in the prevention of osteoporosis, including dietary measures, exercise, and lifestyle changes. Teach your patient the following.

Calcium

An inadequate supply of calcium over a person's lifetime is thought to play a significant role in contributing to the development of osteoporosis. Studies show that low calcium intake appears to be associated with low bone mass and high fracture rates. Foods high in calcium include low-fat dairy products, such as milk, cheese, yogurt, and ice cream, and dark green leafy vegetables, such as spinach, broccoli, collard greens, and bok choy. Other foods high in calcium include sardines and salmon (with the bones), tofu, and almonds. Foods fortified with calcium should also be included in the diet, such as orange juice, cereals, and breads. Depending on how much calcium you get every day, you may need to take a supplement. (See *Recommended calcium intake,* page 504.)

Vitamin D

Vitamin D plays a major role in calcium reabsorption and in bone health. It's synthesized in the skin through exposure to sunlight. Most people can acquire enough vitamin D naturally; however, studies show that vitamin D production decreases in elderly people, during the winter, and in people who are homebound. A supplement may be required for these individuals to ensure a daily intake of 400 to 800 international units.

Assessing risk of osteoporosis

Estrogen deficiency increases the risk of osteoporosis in women. Factors that may contribute to estrogen deficiency include early menopause, surgically induced menopause, and amenorrhea in the premenopausal woman. Other factors that increase the risk of osteoporosis include race, diet, glucocorticoid use, and certain aspects of lifestyle.

To help you determine your patient's risk of developing osteoporosis, assess her for the following points:

- White or Asian?
- Small body frame?
- Amenorrhea (if premenopausal)?
- Early menopause or surgically induced menopause?
- Postmenopausal?
- Smoking or excessive alcohol consumption?
- Diet low in calcium or dairy products?
- Sedentary lifestyle, lacking in exercise?
- Use of glucocorticoids or cortisone-like drugs for arthritis, asthma, or cancer?

Exercise

Like muscle, bone gets stronger with exercise. The best exercises for the bones are those that are weight bearing and force you to work against gravity. These exercises include walking, running, hiking, weight training, stair climbing, tennis, and dancing. Exercise at least three times per week for 30 to 60 minutes per day.

Smoking and alcohol

Smoking is bad for your bones as well as the rest of your body. Studies have shown that women who smoke have lower estrogen levels and go through menopause earlier. Smokers also absorb less calcium from their diet. Alcohol consumption of 2 to 3 oz per day may damage the skeleton, even in young women and men. Those who drink heavily are prone to bone loss and fractures because of poor nutrition and increased risk for falling.

Recommended calcium intake
EB

Here's the recommended daily calcium intake.

Age (years)	Recommended amount (mg/day)
1 to 3	500
4 to 8	800
9 to 18	1,300
19 to 50	1,000 to 1,200
51 and over	1,500
Pregnant/lactating women	1,200

Medications
Long-term use of glucocorticoids can lead to loss of bone density. Other drug therapies that can cause bone loss include long-term treatment with certain anti-seizure drugs, certain cancer treatments, gonadotropin-releasing hormone, analogs to treat endometriosis, and excessive thyroid hormones. It's important for a patient who requires these drug therapies to talk to her practitioner about the use of these drugs and not to stop or alter her medication dose on her own.

Nursing diagnoses
● Effective therapeutic regimen management

Expected outcomes
The patient will:
● work toward increasing calcium intake
● make plans to incorporate lifestyle changes into the daily regimen.

Supportive references
Burke, S. "Boning Up on Osteoporosis," *Nursing2001* 31(10 part 1):38, October 2001. **EB**

Maher, A., et al. *Orthopaedic Nursing,* 3rd ed. Philadelphia: W.B. Saunders Co., 2002.

National Institutes of Health. Osteoporosis and Related Bone Diseases National Resource Center. *Osteoporosis Overview 2005. www.osteo.org/osteolinks.asp#gen.*

Stump and prosthesis care

Patient care immediately after limb amputation includes wound healing, pain control, reducing edema, and stump shaping and conditioning. Postoperative care of the stump will vary slightly, depending on the amputation site (arm or leg) and the type of dressing applied to the stump (elastic bandage or plaster cast).

After the stump heals, it requires only routine daily care, such as proper hygiene and continued muscle-strengthening exercises. The prosthesis — when in use — also requires daily care. Typically, a plastic prosthesis, the most common type, must be cleaned and lubricated and checked for proper fit. As the patient recovers from the physical and psychological trauma of amputation, he'll need to learn correct procedures for routine daily care of the stump and the prosthesis. **EB**

Equipment
Postoperative stump care: Pressure dressing ● abdominal (ABD) pad ● suction equipment, if ordered ● overhead trapeze ● 1″ adhesive tape, bandage clips or safety pins ● sandbags or trochanter roll (for a leg) ● elastic stump shrinker or 4″ elastic bandage ● optional: tourniquet (as last resort *to control bleeding*)

Stump and prosthesis care: Mild soap or alcohol pads ● stump socks or athletic tube socks ● two washcloths ● two towels ● appropriate lubricating oil

Implementation
● Confirm the patient's identity using two patient identifiers according to facility policy. **JCAHO**
● Perform routine postoperative care. Frequently assess the patient's respiratory status and level of consciousness, monitor his vital signs and I.V. infusions, check tube patency, and provide for his comfort and safety. **Science**

Monitoring stump drainage
● *Because gravity causes fluid to accumulate at the stump,* frequently check the amount of blood and

drainage on the dressing. Notify the practitioner if accumulations of drainage or blood increase rapidly. If excessive bleeding occurs, notify the practitioner immediately, and apply a pressure dressing or compress the appropriate pressure points. If this doesn't control bleeding, use a tourniquet only as a last resort. Keep a tourniquet available. **EB**

● Tape the ABD pad over the moist part of the dressing as necessary. *This provides a dry area to help prevent bacterial infection.*

● Monitor the suction drainage equipment, and note the amount and type of drainage.

Positioning the extremity

● Elevate the extremity for the first 24 hours *to reduce swelling and promote venous return.* **EB**

● *To prevent contractures,* position an arm with the elbow extended and the shoulder abducted. **EB**

● To correctly position a leg, elevate the foot of the bed slightly and place sandbags or a trochanter roll against the hip *to prevent external rotation.* **EB**

  CLINICAL IMPACT *Don't place a pillow under the stump for an extended period because this may lead to the development of contractures.*

● After a below-the-knee amputation, maintain knee extension *to prevent hamstring muscle contractures.*

● After a leg amputation, place the patient on a firm surface in the prone position for at least 2 hours per day, with his legs close together and without pillows under his stomach, hips, knees, or stump, unless this position is contraindicated. *This position helps prevent hip flexion, contractures, and abduction; it also stretches the flexor muscles.* **EB**

Assisting with prescribed exercises

● After arm amputation, encourage the patient to exercise the remaining arm *to prevent muscle contractures.* Help the patient perform isometric and range-of-motion (ROM) exercises for both shoulders, as prescribed by the physical therapist, *because use of the prosthesis requires both shoulders.* **Science**

● After leg amputation, stand behind the patient and, if necessary, support him with your hands at his waist during balancing exercises.

  CONTROVERSIAL ISSUE *Most patients recovering from a leg amputation spend time in an acute rehabilitation setting. Debate exists over whether learning how to walk again with a prosthesis takes precedence over wound healing, strengthening, balance, and limb shaping.*

● Instruct the patient to exercise the affected and unaffected limbs *to maintain muscle tone and increase muscle strength.* The patient with a leg amputation may perform push-ups as ordered (in the sitting position, arms at his sides), or pull-ups on the overhead trapeze *to strengthen his arms, shoulders, and back in preparation for using crutches.*

Wrapping and conditioning the stump

● If the patient doesn't have a rigid cast, apply an elastic stump shrinker *to prevent edema and shape the limb in preparation for the prosthesis.* Wrap the stump so that it narrows toward the distal end. *This helps to ensure comfort when the patient wears the prosthesis.* **EB**

● If an elastic stump shrinker isn't available, you can wrap the stump in a 4″ elastic bandage. To do this, stretch the bandage to about two-thirds its maximum length as you wrap it diagonally around the stump, with the greatest pressure distally. (Depending on the size of the leg, you may need to use two 4″ bandages.) Secure the bandage with clips, safety pins, or adhesive tape. Make sure that the bandage covers all portions of the stump smoothly *because wrinkles or exposed areas encourage skin breakdown.* (See *Wrapping a stump,* page 506.) **EB**

● The use of an immediate postoperative prosthesis has proved effective in decreasing the time until final prosthetic fitting. **EB**

● If the patient experiences throbbing after the stump is wrapped, the bandage may be too tight; remove the bandage immediately and reapply it less tightly. *Throbbing indicates impaired circulation.* **Science**

● Check the bandage regularly. Rewrap it when it begins to bunch up at the end (usually about every 12 hours for a moderately active patient) or as necessary.

● After removing the bandage to rewrap it, massage the stump gently, always pushing toward the suture line rather than away from it. *This stimulates circulation and prevents scar tissue from adhering to the bone.*

● When healing begins, instruct the patient to push the stump against a pillow. Have him progress gradually to pushing against harder surfaces, such as a

Wrapping a stump

Proper stump care *helps protect the limb, reduces swelling, and prepares the limb for a prosthesis.* As you perform the procedure, teach it to the patient.

Start by obtaining two 4″ elastic bandages. Center the end of the first 4″ bandage at the top of the patient's thigh. Unroll the bandage downward over the stump and to the back of the leg (as shown below).

Make three figure-eight turns to adequately cover the ends of the stump. As you wrap, be sure to include the roll of flesh in the groin area. Use enough pressure to ensure that the stump narrows toward the end *so that it fits comfortably into the prosthesis.*

Use the second 4″ bandage to anchor the first bandage around the waist. For a below-the-knee amputation, use the knee to anchor the bandage in place. Secure the bandage with clips, safety pins, or adhesive tape. Check the stump bandage regularly, and rewrap it if it bunches at the end.

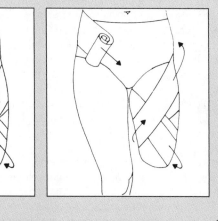

padded chair and then a hard chair. *These conditioning exercises will help the patient adjust to experiencing pressure and sensation in the stump.*

✓ **CLINICAL IMPACT** *Avoid applying lotion to the residual stump because it may clog follicles, increasing the risk of infection. In addition, it's a desired goal of the healing process to toughen the area to tolerate the prosthesis.*

Caring for the healed stump

● Bathe the stump but never shave it *to prevent infection.* If possible, bathe the stump at the end of the day *because the warm water may cause swelling, making reapplication of the prosthesis difficult.* Don't soak the stump for long periods. **Science**

● Rub the stump with alcohol daily *to toughen the skin, reducing the risk of skin breakdown.* (Avoid using powders or lotions *because they can soften or irri-*

tate the skin.) Because alcohol may cause severe irritation in some patients, instruct the patient to watch for and report this sign.

● Inspect the stump for redness, swelling, irritation, and calluses. Report any of these to the practitioner. Following the first cast change, many surgeons will have the patient begin partial weight bearing, if the wound appears stable. **EB**

● Continue muscle-strengthening exercises *so that the patient can build the strength he'll need to control the prosthesis.*

● Change and wash the patient's elastic bandages every day *to avoid exposing the skin to excessive perspiration, which can be irritating.* Wash the elastic bandages in warm water and gentle nondetergent soap; lay them flat on a towel to dry. *Machine washing or drying may shrink the elastic bandages. To*

Caring for a severed body part

After traumatic amputation, a surgeon may be able to reimplant the severed body part through microsurgery. The chance of successful reimplantation is much greater if the amputated part has received proper care.

If a patient arrives at the hospital with a severed body part, first make sure that bleeding at the amputation site has been controlled. Then follow these guidelines for preserving the body part.

● Put on sterile gloves. Place several sterile gauze pads and an appropriate amount of sterile roller gauze in a sterile basin, and pour sterile normal saline or sterile lactated Ringer's solution over them. *Never* use another solution, and don't try to scrub or debride the part.

● Holding the body part in one gloved hand, carefully pat it dry with sterile gauze. Place saline-soaked gauze pads over the stump, and then wrap the whole body part with saline-soaked roller gauze. Wrap the gauze with a sterile towel, if available. Then put this package in a watertight container or bag and seal it.

● Fill another plastic bag with ice and place the part, still in its watertight container, inside. Seal the outer bag. (Always protect the part from direct contact with ice and — *never* use dry ice — *to prevent irreversible tissue damage, which would make the part unsuitable for reimplantation.*) Keep this bag ice-cold until the surgeon is ready to do the reimplantation surgery.

● Label the bag with the patient's name, identification number, identification of the amputated part, the hospital identification number, and the date and time when cooling began.

Note: The body part must be wrapped and cooled quickly. *Irreversible tissue damage occurs after only 6 hours at ambient temperature.* However, hypothermic management seldom preserves tissues for more than 24 hours.

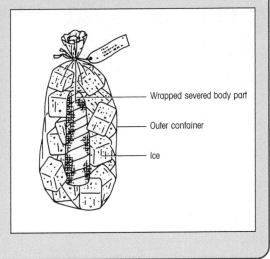

Wrapped severed body part

Outer container

Ice

---

shape the stump, have the patient wear an elastic bandage 24 hours per day except while bathing. **EB**

Caring for the plastic prosthesis **EB**

● Wipe the plastic socket of the prosthesis with a damp cloth and mild soap or alcohol *to prevent bacterial accumulation.*

● Wipe the insert (if the prosthesis has one) with a dry cloth.

● Dry the prosthesis thoroughly; if possible, allow it to dry overnight.

● Maintain and lubricate the prosthesis, as instructed by the manufacturer.

● Check for malfunctions and adjust or repair the prosthesis as necessary *to prevent further damage.*

● Check the condition of the shoe on a foot prosthesis frequently, and change it as necessary.

Applying the prosthesis

● Apply a stump sock. Keep the seams away from bony prominences.

● If the prosthesis has an insert, remove it from the socket, place it over the stump, and insert the stump into the prosthesis.

● If it has no insert, merely slide the prosthesis over the stump. Secure the prosthesis onto the stump according to the manufacturer's directions.

Special considerations

● If a patient arrives at the hospital with a traumatic amputation, the amputated part may be saved for possible reimplantation. (See *Caring for a severed body part.*) **EB**

● For a below-the-knee amputation, you may substitute an athletic tube sock for a stump sock by cutting off the elastic band. If the patient has a rigid plaster of Paris dressing, perform normal cast care. Check the cast frequently to make sure that it doesn't slip off. If it does, apply an elastic bandage immediately and notify the practitioner *because edema will develop rapidly.*

TEACHING *Emphasize to the patient that proper care of his stump can speed healing. Tell him to inspect his stump carefully every day, using a mirror, and to continue proper daily stump care. Instruct him to call the practitioner if the incision appears to be opening, looks red or swollen, feels warm, is painful to touch, or is seeping drainage.*

Explain to the patient that a 10-lb (4.5-kg) change in body weight will alter his stump size and require a new prosthesis socket to ensure a correct fit.

Tell the patient to massage the stump toward the suture line to mobilize the scar and prevent its adherence to bone. *Advise him to avoid exposing the skin around the stump to excessive perspiration, which can be irritating. Tell him to change his elastic bandages or stump socks daily to avoid this.*

Tell the patient that he may experience twitching, spasms, or phantom limb pain as his stump muscles adjust to amputation. Advise him that he can decrease these symptoms with heat, massage, or gentle pressure. If his stump is sensitive to touch, tell him to rub it with a dry washcloth for 4 minutes three times per day.

Inform the patient that exercising the remaining muscles in an amputated limb must begin the day after surgery. A physical therapist will direct these exercises. For example, arm exercises progress from isometrics to assisted ROM to active ROM. Leg exercises include rising from a chair, balancing on one leg, and ROM exercises of the knees and hips.

Stress the importance of performing prescribed exercises to help minimize complications, maintain muscle strength and tone, prevent contractures, and promote independence. *Stress the importance of positioning* to prevent contractures and edema.

Nursing diagnoses
- Disturbed body image
- Impaired skin integrity

Expected outcomes
The patient will:
- acknowledge the change in his body image

- communicate feelings about his body image
- exhibit no skin breakdown
- exhibit healing from the surgical wound.

Complications
The most common postoperative complications include hemorrhage, stump infection, contractures, and a swollen or flabby stump. Complications that may develop at any time after an amputation include skin breakdown or irritation from lack of ventilation; friction from an irritant in the prosthesis; a sebaceous cyst or boil from tight socks; psychological problems, such as denial, depression, or withdrawal; and phantom limb pain caused by stimulation of nerves that once carried sensations from the distal part of the extremity.

Documentation
Record the date, time, and specific procedures of postoperative care, including amount and type of drainage, condition of the dressing, need for dressing reinforcement, and appearance of the suture line and surrounding tissue. Note signs of skin irritation or infection, complications and the interventions taken, the patient's tolerance of exercises, and his psychological reaction to the amputation.

During routine daily care, document the date, time, type of care given, and condition of the skin and suture line, noting signs of irritation, such as redness or tenderness. Record the patient's progress in caring for the stump or prosthesis.

Supportive references
Bryant, G. "Stump Care," *AJN* 101(2):67, February 2001.
Goldberg, T., et al. "Postoperative Management of Lower Extremity Amputation," *Physical Medicine and Rehabilitation Clinics of North America* 11(3):559-68, August 2000.
Maher, A.B., et al. *Orthopaedic Nursing,* 3rd ed. Philadelphia: W.B. Saunders Co., 2002. **EB**
Skinner, H. *Current Diagnosis and Treatment in Orthopedics,* 2nd ed. New York: Lange Medical Books, McGraw-Hill, 2000.

Walkers

Walkers are used for patients who don't have sufficient strength and balance to use crutches or a cane.

A walker provides the maximum support for the patient; however, use of a walker requires a slow gait.

A walker consists of a metal frame with handgrips and four legs that buttresses the patient on three sides. Attachments for standard walkers and modified walkers help meet special needs. For example, a walker may have a platform added to support an injured arm.

Before a patient starts using a walker, the correct height must be determined. *To check for the correct height,* have the patient stand inside the walker frame with arms at his sides. The walker handles should be at wrist level so that the patient's elbows are flexed 15 to 30 degrees when holding the walker. **EB1**

Equipment

Walker • platform or wheel attachments, as necessary
    Various types of walkers are available. The standard walker is used by the patient with unilateral or bilateral weakness or an inability to bear weight on one leg. It requires arm strength and balance. Platform attachments may be added to a standard walker for the patient with arthritic arms or a casted arm, who can't bear weight directly on his hand, wrist, or forearm. With the practitioner's approval, wheels may be placed on the front legs of the standard walker to allow the extremely weak or poorly coordinated patient to roll the device forward, instead of lifting it. However, wheels are applied infrequently *because they may be a safety hazard.* Four-wheeled walkers are used by patients who require a larger base of support but don't rely on it to bear weight. They are used for patients who walk long distances and are at higher functioning.

The stair walker — used by the patient who must negotiate stairs without bilateral handrails — requires good arm strength and balance. Its extra set of handles extends toward the patient on the open side. The rolling walker — used by the patient with very weak legs — has four wheels and a seat. The reciprocal walker — used by the patient with very weak arms — allows one side to be advanced ahead of the other.

Preparation of equipment

Obtain the appropriate walker with the advice of a physical therapist, and adjust it to the patient's height: His elbows should be flexed at a 15- to 30-degree angle when standing comfortably within the walker with his hands on the grips. To adjust the walker, turn it upside down, and change the leg length by pushing in the button on each shaft and releasing it when the leg is in the correct position. Make sure that the walker is level before the patient attempts to use it.

Implementation

● Confirm the patient's identity using two patient identifiers according to facility policy. **JCAHO**
● Help the patient stand within the walker, and instruct him to hold the handgrips firmly and equally. Stand behind him, closer to the involved leg. **EB2**
● If the patient has one-sided leg weakness, tell him to advance the walker 6″ to 8″ (15 to 20 cm) and to step forward with the involved leg and follow with the uninvolved leg, supporting himself on his arms. Encourage him to take equal strides. If he has equal strength in both legs, instruct him to advance the walker 6″ to 8″ and to step forward with either leg. If he can't use one leg, tell him to advance the walker 6″ to 8″ and to swing onto it, supporting his weight on his arms. **EB1**
● If the patient is using a reciprocal walker, teach him the two-point gait. Instruct the patient to stand with his weight evenly distributed between his legs and the walker. Stand behind him, slightly to one side. Tell him to simultaneously advance the walker's right side and his left foot. Have the patient advance the walker's left side and his right foot.
● If the patient is using a reciprocal walker, you may also teach him the four-point gait. Instruct the patient to evenly distribute his weight between his legs and the walker. Stand behind him and slightly to one side. Have him move the right side of the walker forward. Have the patient move his left foot forward. Next, instruct him to move the left side of the walker forward. Have him move his right foot forward.
● If the patient is using a wheeled or stair walker, reinforce the physical therapist's instructions. Stress the need for caution when using a stair walker.
● Teach the patient how to use a chair safely. (See *Teaching safe use of a walker,* page 510.)

Special considerations

If the patient starts to fall, support his hips and shoulders *to help maintain an upright position if possible.*

Nursing diagnoses

● Impaired physical mobility

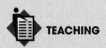 **TEACHING**

Teaching safe use of a walker

Sitting down

● First, tell the patient to stand with the back of his stronger leg against the front of the chair, his weaker leg slightly off the floor, and the walker directly in front.
● Tell him to grasp the armrests on the chair one arm at a time while supporting most of his weight on the stronger leg. (In the illustrations below, the patient has left leg weakness.)
● Tell the patient to lower himself into the chair and slide backward. After he's seated, he should place the walker beside the chair.

Getting up

● After bringing the walker to the front of his chair, tell the patient to slide forward in the chair. Placing the back of his stronger leg against the seat, he should then advance the weaker leg.
● Next, with both hands on the armrests, the patient can push himself to a standing position. Supporting himself with the stronger leg and the opposite hand, the patient should grasp the walker's handgrip with his free hand.
● Then have the patient grasp the free handgrip with his other hand.

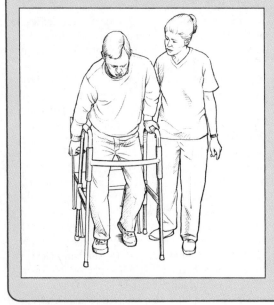

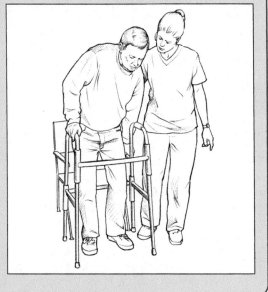

Expected outcomes

The patient will:
● maintain mobility and use the walker safely.

Documentation

Record the type of walker and attachments used, patient teaching, the degree of guarding required, the distance walked, and the patient's tolerance of ambulation.

Supportive references

Sloan, H., et al. "Teaching the Use of Walkers and Canes," *Home Healthcare Nurse* 19(4):241-46, April 2001. **EB2**

Stewart, K., and Murray, H. "How to Use a Walker Correctly," *Nursing98* 28(9):22-23, September 1998.

Van Hook, F.W., et al. "Ambulatory Devices for Chronic Gait Disorders in the Elderly," *American Family Physician* 67(8):1717-24, April 2003. **EB1**

The skin is the body's largest organ. Besides helping to shape a patient's self-image, the skin performs many physiologic functions. For example, it protects internal body structures from the environment and potential pathogens. It also regulates body temperature and homeostasis and serves as an organ of sensation and excretion. Meticulous skin care is essential to overall health because intact, healthy skin is the body's first line of defense. To ensure that a patient maintains healthy skin, you must make certain that all skin care measures prevent injury, control infection, promote skin growth, and control pain. Providing emotional support to a patient whose self-image may be affected by a skin disorder or injury is also an essential element to good nursing care.

To enhance natural healing, skin wounds need regular dressing changes (with extra changes for soiled dressings), thorough cleaning and, if necessary, debridement to remove debris, reduce bacterial growth, and encourage tissue repair.

To control pain, you'll need to assess the patient's pain and response to therapy. If he has minor pain or pruritus, a topical agent may be all that's needed. For moderate pain, such techniques as positioning and bed rest may help. A patient in severe pain may require a strong opioid analgesic for pain relief.

A patient who has a disfiguring or painful skin disorder may suffer from frustration, depression, and anger. Along with physical support, the patient will require emotional support as he develops coping mechanisms to deal with his altered self-image.

If you're working with a patient who has impaired skin integrity — for example, a patient with burns or pressure ulcers — your primary goal is to prevent or control infection because damage to skin integrity increases the risk of infection, which could delay healing, worsen pain, and possibly threaten the patient's life. To provide the best care, it's important that you're aware of the current recommendations from such organizations as the Agency for Healthcare Research and Quality **AHRQ**, the American Burn Association **ABA**, the American College of Surgeons Committee **ACSC**, the Centers for Disease Control and Prevention **CDC**, the Dermatology Nurses Association **DNA**, the Joint Commission on Accreditation of Healthcare Organizations **JCAHO**, the Wound Healing Society **WHS**, and the Wound, Ostomy and Continence Nurses Society **WOCN**. In this chapter, many practices are evidence-based **EB**. You'll find additional practices that are grounded in basic principles of science **Science** and the American Hospital Association's Patient Care Partnership **PCP**.

Arterial ulcer care

Arterial ulcers can result from arterial insufficiency caused by arterial vessel compression or obstruction or from trauma to an ischemic limb. Usually, these ulcers occur on the leg or foot. Consider your patient at risk for an arterial ulcer if he has these conditions: atherosclerosis (most common cause of arterial problems), absence of a lowerextremity pulses, claudication (muscle pain that occurs after exercise), or pain that occurs when the patient is resting, which is a symptom of severe arterial insufficiency.

Assessment of an arterial ulcer should include a comprehensive clinical history and specific information related to the history of the arterial ulcer. Patients with arterial ulcers are typically older; have peripheral vascular disease, diabetes, hypertension, or hyperlipidemia; and are smokers. Assess the intact skin surrounding the ulcer for temperature changes and capillary refill, which mostly likely will be longer than 3 seconds. Obtain ankle brachial indices (ABI; the ankle pressure divided by the brachial pressure) using Doppler blood pressure measurements. The test compares blood pressure in the brachial artery to that in the ankle. Arterial insufficiency is likely to be present if the ABI is 0.9 or less. Severe ischemia is present when the ABI is less than 0.5. **WOCN** Transcutaneous oxygen measurements ($TcPO_2$) can also be taken if the ulcer is not healing. A $TcPO_2$ of less than 40 mm Hg indicates poor wound healing. **WOCN**

When assessing the patient at risk for arterial insufficiency, be sure to inspect and palpate the skin for changes in color and temperature. Always compare one side of the body with the other, and apply the backs of both of your hands to the patient's legs at the same time to ensure that the temperature difference is the patient's and not your own. During palpation, be sure to assess all pulses in the lower extremities (femoral, dorsalis pedis, popliteal, and posterior tibial pulse). However, don't be surprised if you aren't able to feel the dorsalis pedis pulses, because some patients don't have them even if their arterial system is normal. The popliteal pulse can be hard to palpate, but don't skip this pulse even if you find the dorsalis pedis or posterior tibial pulse and know that blood is getting to the foot.

Also, assess the patient's level of pain. He may experience it in the form of intermittent claudication, resting pain, nocturnal pain, positional pain, or pain that hasn't responded to analgesia.

ALERT *A "bounding" popliteal pulse is usually an early indicator of a popliteal aneurysm. Be sure to immediately report this finding to the physician for further evaluation.*

Complete or partial arterial blockage may lead to tissue necrosis and ulceration. Signs and symptoms on the affected extremity include:
● pulselessness
● painful ulceration
● small, punctate ulcers that are usually well circumscribed
● cool or cold skin
● pallor on elevation or dependent rubor
● edema
● pale or necrotic wound base
● delayed capillary refill time (briefly push on the end of the toe and release; normal color should return to the toe in 3 seconds or less)
● skin that's shiny, thin, or dry
● loss of hair.

Use noninvasive vascular tests, such as Doppler, ABI, and $TcPO_2$ measurements, to aid in the diagnosis. Duplex scanning and arteriograms may also be performed, if indicated.

Treatment of an arterial ulcer has many goals, the primary one being to increase the circulation to the area in question. This can be done surgically or medically depending on the cause of the ulcer and the patient's overall medical condition. Bypass grafting is the standard surgical treatment. Percutaneous angioplasty and the placement of stents are also done. Keeping the tissue base moist and free from infection and necrotic debris are also concerns. Frequent assessment of the wound base for signs and symptoms of infection is vital because signs can be subtle as a result of reduced blood flow.

Pain control, another goal of treatment, can be managed in the patient with intermittent claudication by encouraging him to walk to the point of near-maximal pain three times per week. This has been shown to increase pain-free walking and total distance. **WOCN** L-arginine taken orally for 2 weeks has also been shown to improve symptoms of intermittent claudication. **WOCN** The Wound, Ostomy and Continence Nurses Society (WOCN) has established guidelines for treating arterial ulcers.

Other suggested treatments include hyperbaric oxygen therapy, topical autologous activated mononuclear cells (which have been shown to benefit ischemic ulcers), and intermittent pneumatic compression, which may help patients with intermittent claudication.

Equipment

Bedside table ● piston-type irrigating system ● two pairs of gloves ● normal saline solution, as ordered ● sterile 4″ × 4″ gauze pads ● sterile cotton swabs ● selected topical dressing ● linen-saver pads ● impervious plastic trash bag ● disposable wound-measuring device (a square, transparent card with concentric circles arranged in bull's-eye fashion and bordered with a straightedge ruler)

Implementation

● Confirm the patient's identity using two patient identifiers according to facility policy. **JCAHO**
● Wash your hands. **CDC**
● Explain the procedure to the patient. **PCP**
● If the patient has adequate circulation to heal an arterial ulcer, the objective is to keep the ulcer moist. Moist dressings should be applied only after vascular

supply is restored. Because of poor circulation, an arterial ulcer bed dries out fast; keeping the dressing moist will decrease the risk of tissue damage during dressing changes. **WOCN**

● Irrigate the arterial ulcer with normal saline solution, and be sure to blot the surrounding skin dry.

● Moisten the gauze dressing with saline solution.

● Gently place the dressing over the surface of the ulcer. *To separate surfaces within the wound,* gently place a dressing between opposing wound surfaces. *To avoid damage to tissues,* don't pack the gauze tightly.

● Change the dressing often enough *to keep the wound moist.*

● An occlusive dressing is contraindicated when peripheral pulses are absent. The typical choice for an arterial ulcer is a dressing that provides for frequent visualization and protects the surrounding skin. Choose a dressing that controls exudate, enhances autolytic debridement, and maintains a moist wound environment, which accelerates the healing process. Modern wound dressings haven't been shown to have a significant impact on wound healing. **EB**

● If debridement is going to be used to treat an arterial ulcer, it should occur only after vascular supply is restored. **WOCN**

TEACHING *Patients should be taught about arterial disease management. Include the following to help them avoid additional problems.*

● *Avoid chemical, thermal, or mechanical trauma.*

● *Seek out regular nail and foot care by a professional.*

● *Wear proper-fitting shoes with socks or hose.*

● *Avoid pressure on the toes and heels.*

● *Stop smoking to slow progression of arteriosclerosis.* **WOCN**

● *Increase calorie and protein intake.*

Nursing diagnoses

● Acute pain

● Impaired tissue integrity

Expected outcomes

The patient will:

● express pain relief

● voice intent to stop smoking and manage dressing change routine

● remain free from ulcers, color changes, and edema.

Complications

Infection, one of the most common complications of an ulcer, may cause foul-smelling drainage, persistent pain, severe erythema, induration, and elevated skin and body temperatures. Advancing infection or cellulitis can lead to septicemia. Severe erythema may signal worsening cellulitis, which indicates that the offending organisms have invaded the tissue and are no longer localized.

Documentation

Document the ulcer's location; its length, width, and depth; and any tunneling of the wound (using centimeters). Record the appearance of the wound bed and the date and time the dressing was changed. If your facility allows, photograph the wound to supplement your documentation.

Supportive references

Bouza et al. "Efficacy of Modern Dressings in the Treatment of Leg Ulcers," *Wound Repair and Regeneration* 13(3):218-29, May-June 2005. **EB**

Davis, J., and Gray, M. "Is the Unna's Boot Bandage as Effective as a Four-Layer Wrap for Managing Venous Leg Ulcers?" *Journal of Wound, Ostomy, & Continence Nursing* 32(3):153-56, May-June 2005.

McMullin, G.M. "Improving the Treatment of Leg Ulcers," *Medical Journal of Australia* 175(7):375-78, August 2001.

Sieggreen, M.Y., and Kline, R.A. "Arterial Insufficiency and Ulceration: Diagnosis and Treatment Options," *Nurse Practitioner* 29(9):46-52, September 2004.

WOCN. *Clinical Fact Sheet: Arterial Insufficiency.* Glenview, Ill.: WOCN; 2004. *www.wocn.org.*

WOCN. *Guideline for Management of Wounds in Patients with Lower-Extremity Arterial Disease.* Glenview, Ill.: WOCN; June 2002.

Wipke-Tevis, D., and Sae-Sia, W. "Management of Vascular Leg Ulcers," *Advances in Skin & Wound Care* 18(8):446-47, October 2005.

Zafar, A. "Management of Diabetic Foot—Two Years Experience," *Journal of Ayub Medical College, Abbottabad* 13(1):14-16, January-March 2001.

Burn care

The goals of burn care are to maintain the patient's physiologic stability, repair skin integrity, prevent infection, and promote maximal functioning and psy-

Burn care at the scene

By acting promptly when a burn injury occurs, you can improve the patient's chance of uncomplicated recovery. Emergency care at the scene should include steps to stop the burn from worsening; assessment of the patient's airway, breathing, and circulation (ABCs); a call for help from an emergency medical team; and emotional and physiologic support for the patient.

Stop the burning process

● If the victim is on fire, tell him to fall to the ground and roll to put out the flames. (*If he panics and runs, air will fuel the flames, worsening the burn and increasing the risk of inhalation injury.*) Or, if you can, wrap the victim in a blanket or other large covering *to smother the flames and protect the burned area from dirt.* Keep his head outside the blanket *so that he doesn't breathe in toxic fumes.* As soon as the flames are out, unwrap the patient *so that the heat can dissipate.*
● Cool the burned area with any nonflammable liquid. *This decreases pain and stops the burn from growing deeper or larger.*
● If possible, remove potential sources of heat, such as jewelry, belt buckles, and some types of clothing. *In addition to adding to the burning process, these items may cause constriction as edema develops.* If the patient's clothing adheres to his skin, don't try to remove it. Rather, cut around it.
● Cover the wound with a tablecloth, sheet, or other smooth, nonfuzzy material.

Assess the damage

● Call for help as quickly as possible. Send someone to contact the emergency medical service (EMS).
● Assess the patient's ABCs, and perform cardiopulmonary resuscitation, if necessary. Then check for other serious injuries, such as fractures, spinal cord injury, lacerations, blunt trauma, and head contusions.
● Estimate the extent and depth of the burns. If flames caused the burns and the injury occurred in a closed space, assess for signs of inhalation injury: singed nasal hairs, burns on the face or mouth, soot-stained sputum, coughing or hoarseness, wheezing, or respiratory distress.
● If the patient is conscious and alert, try to get a brief medical history as soon as possible.
● Reassure the patient that help is on the way. Provide emotional support by staying with him, answering questions, and explaining what's being done for him.
● When help arrives, give the EMS a report on the patient's status.

---

chosocial health. Competent care immediately after a burn occurs can dramatically improve the success of overall treatment. (See *Burn care at the scene.*)

Every burn victim should be evaluated initially as a trauma patient after the systematic approach developed by the American College of Surgeons Committee. The primary survey focuses mainly on maintaining the patient's airway, breathing, and circulation. When the burn is caused by a chemical agent, the priority is to remove the offending agent and irrigate the affected area with water. The secondary survey focuses on a head-to-toe assessment, followed by efforts to stop the burn and contain the injury. Specific elements of the survey should include burn severity, which is determined by the depth and extent of the burn; determination of a possible inhalation injury; and other factors, such as age, complications, coexisting illnesses, and the possibility of abuse. (See *Esti-mating burn surfaces.* Also see *Evaluating burn severity,* page 516.)

According to the American Burn Association, you'll need to carefully monitor your patient's respiratory status, especially if he has suffered smoke inhalation. Be aware that a patient with burns involving more than 20% of his total body surface area usually needs fluid resuscitation, which aims to support the body's compensatory mechanisms without overwhelming them. Expect to give fluids (such as lactated Ringer's solution) to keep the patient's urine output at 30 to 50 ml/hour, and expect to monitor blood pressure and heart rate. You'll also need to control body temperature *because skin loss interferes with temperature regulation.* Use warm fluids, heat lamps, and hyperthermia blankets, as appropriate, to keep the patient's temperature above 97° F (36.1° C), if possible. Additionally, you'll frequently review laboratory values,

Estimating burn surfaces

Different methods are required to assess body surface area (BSA) in children and adults because the proportion of BSA changes as the body grows.

Rule of nines

The "rule of nines" quantifies BSA in percentages, either in fractions of nine or multiples of nine. To use this method, mentally assess the patient's burns using the body chart shown below. Add the corresponding percentages for each body section burned. Use the total — a rough estimate of burn extent — to calculate initial fluid replacement needs.

Lund-Browder chart

The rule of nines isn't accurate for infants and children because their body proportions differ from those of adults. An infant's head, for example, accounts for about 17% of his total BSA, whereas an adult's head comprises 7% of his BSA. The Lund-Browder chart, as shown below, is based on human anatomic studies relating the proportion of a specific body area to the body as a whole and can be used for infants, children, and adults

Percentage of burned body surface by age

	At birth	0 to 1 year	1 to 4 years	5 to 9 years	10 to 15 years	Adult
A: Half of head	9½%	8½%	6½%	5½%	4½%	3½%
B: Half of one thigh	2¾%	3¼%	4%	4¼%	4½%	4¾%
C: Half of one leg	2½%	2½%	2¾%	3%	3½%	3½%

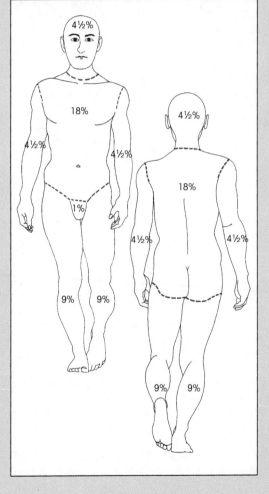

Evaluating burn severity

To judge a burn's severity, assess its depth and extent, color, and other factors, as shown below.

Superficial partial-thickness (first-degree) burn

Does the burned area appear pink or red with minimal edema? Is the area sensitive to touch and temperature changes? If so, the patient most likely has a superficial partial-thickness — or first-degree — burn affecting only the epidermal skin layer.

Deep partial-thickness (second-degree) burn

Does the burned area appear pink or red, with a mottled appearance? Do red areas blanch when you touch them? Does the skin have large, thick-walled blisters with subcutaneous edema? Does touching the burn cause severe pain? Is the hair still present? If so, the person most likely has a deep partial-thickness — or second-degree — burn affecting the epidermal and dermal layers.

Full-thickness (third-degree) burn

Does the burned area appear red, waxy white, brown, or black? Does red skin remain red with no blanching when you touch it? Is the skin leathery with extensive subcutaneous edema? Is the skin insensitive to touch? Does the hair fall out easily? If so, the patient most likely has a full-thickness — or third-degree — burn that affects all skin layers.

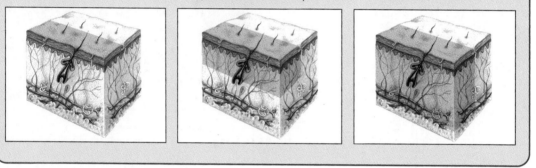

such as serum electrolyte levels, to detect early changes in the patient's condition. **ABA**

Infection can increase wound depth, cause rejection of skin grafts, slow healing, worsen pain, prolong hospitalization, and even lead to death. To help prevent infection, use strict aseptic technique during care, dress the burn site as ordered, monitor and rotate I.V. lines regularly, and carefully assess the extent of the burn as well as body system function and the patient's emotional status.

Early positioning after a burn is extremely important to prevent contractures. Careful positioning and regular exercise for burned extremities help maintain joint function and minimize deformity. When the extremities aren't being exercised, they should be maintained in maximal extension, using splints if necessary. Particular attention should be focused on the hands and neck because they're the most prone to rapid contracture. **ABA** (See *Positioning the burn patient to prevent deformity*.)

Skin integrity is repaired through aggressive wound debridement, followed by maintenance of a clean wound bed until the wound heals or is covered with a skin graft.

Early excision and debridement of the wound in the first 48 hours has been shown to decrease blood loss and reduce hospital stay; however, this procedure should be used only on wounds that are clearly full-thickness burns. **ABA** Surgery takes place as soon as possible after fluid resuscitation. Most wounds are managed with twice-daily dressing changes using a topical antibiotic. Burn dressings encourage healing by barring germ entry and by removing exudate, eschar, and other debris that host infection. After thorough wound cleaning, a topical antibacterial is applied and the wound is covered with absorptive, coarse mesh gauze. Roller gauze typically tops the dressing and is secured with elastic netting or tape.

Positioning the burn patient to prevent deformity

For each of the potential deformities listed below, you can use the corresponding positioning and interventions to help prevent the deformity.

Burned area	Potential deformity	Preventive positioning	Nursing interventions
Neck	• Flexion contracture of neck • Extensor contracture of neck	• Extension • Prone with head slightly raised	• Remove pillow from bed. • Place pillow or rolled towel under upper chest to flex cervical spine, or apply cervical collar.
Axilla	• Adduction and internal rotation • Adduction and external rotation	• Shoulder joint in external rotation and 100- to 130-degree abduction • Shoulder joint in forward flexion and 100- to 130-degree abduction	• Use an I.V. pole, bedside table, or sling to suspend arm. • Use an I.V. pole, bedside table, or sling to suspend arm.
Pectoral region	• Shoulder protraction	• Shoulders abducted and externally rotated	• Remove pillow from bed.
Chest or abdomen	• Kyphosis	• Same as for pectoral region, with hips neutral (not flexed)	• Use no pillow under head or legs.
Lateral trunk	• Scoliosis	• Supine; affected arm abducted	• Put pillows or blanket rolls at sides.
Elbow	• Flexion and pronation	• Arm extended and supinated	• Use an elbow splint, arm board, or bedside table.
Wrist	• Flexion • Extension	• Splint in 15-degree extension • Splint in 15-degree flexion	• Apply a hand splint. • Apply a hand splint.
Fingers	• Adhesions of the extensor tendons; loss of palmar grasp	• Metacarpophalangeal joints in maximum flexion; interphalangeal joints in slight flexion; thumb in maximum abduction	• Apply a hand splint; wrap fingers separately.
Hip	• Internal rotation, flexion, and adduction; possibly joint subluxation if contracture is severe	• Neutral rotation and abduction; maintain extension by prone position	• Put a pillow under buttocks (if supine) or use trochanter rolls or knee or long leg splints.
Knee	• Flexion	• Extension maintained	• Use a knee splint with no pillows under legs.
Ankle	• Plantar flexion if foot muscles are weak or their tendons are divided	• 90-degree dorsiflexion	• Use a footboard or ankle splint.

Equipment

Normal saline solution • bowl • blunt scissors • tissue forceps • ordered topical medication (for example, silver nitrate solution or silver sulfadiazine) • burn gauze • roller gauze • elastic netting or tape • fine-mesh gauze • elastic gauze • cotton-tipped applicators • ordered pain medication • three pairs of gloves • gown • mask • surgical cap • heat lamps • impervious plastic trash bag • cotton bath blanket • 4" × 4" gauze pads

A sterile field is required, so all equipment and supplies used to clean and dress the wound should be sterile.

Preparation of equipment

Warm the normal saline solution by immersing unopened bottles in warm water. Assemble equipment on the dressing table. Make sure the treatment area has adequate light *to allow accurate wound assessment.* Open equipment packages using sterile technique. Arrange supplies on a sterile field according to the order of use.

To prevent cross-contamination, plan to dress the cleanest areas first and the dirtiest or most contaminated areas last. *To help prevent excessive pain or cross-contamination,* you may need to dress the wounds in stages to avoid exposing all wounds at the same time.

Implementation

● Confirm the patient's identity using two patient identifiers according to facility policy. **JCAHO**
● Administer the ordered pain medication about 20 minutes before beginning wound care *to maximize patient comfort and cooperation.*
● Explain the procedure to the patient and provide privacy. **PCP**
● Turn on overhead heat lamps *to keep the patient warm.* Make sure they don't overheat the patient.
● Pour the warmed normal saline solution into the sterile bowl in the sterile field.
● Wash your hands. **CDC**

Removing a dressing without hydrotherapy

● Put on a gown, a mask, and sterile gloves. **CDC**
● Remove dressing layers down to the innermost layer by cutting the outer dressings with sterile blunt scissors. Lay open these dressings.

● If the inner layer appears dry, soak it with warmed normal saline solution *to ease removal.*
● Remove the inner dressing with sterile tissue forceps or your gloved hand.
● *Because soiled dressings harbor infectious microorganisms,* dispose of the dressings carefully in the impervious plastic trash bag according to facility policy. Dispose of your gloves, and wash your hands. **CDC**
● Put on a new pair of sterile gloves. Using gauze pads moistened with normal saline solution, gently remove exudate and old topical medication.
● Carefully remove all loose eschar with sterile forceps and scissors, if ordered. (See "Mechanical debridement," page 526.) **ABA**
● Assess the wound's condition. It should appear clean, with no debris, loose tissue, purulence, inflammation, or darkened margins.
● Before applying a new dressing, remove your gown, gloves, and mask. Discard of them properly, and put on a clean gown, gloves, mask, and surgical cap. **ABA** **CDC**

Applying a wet dressing

● Soak fine-mesh gauze and the elastic gauze dressing in a large, sterile basin containing the ordered topical medication (for example, silver nitrate solution). **ABA**
● Wring out the fine-mesh gauze until it's moist but not dripping, and apply it to the wound. Warn the patient that he may feel transient pain when you apply the dressing.
● Wring out the elastic gauze dressing, and position it to hold the fine-mesh gauze in place.
● Roll an elastic gauze dressing over the dressing *to keep dressings intact.*
● Cover the patient with a cotton bath blanket *to prevent chills.* Change the blanket if it becomes damp. Use an overhead heat lamp, if necessary.
● Change the dressings frequently, as ordered, *to keep the wound moist,* especially if you're using silver nitrate. *Silver nitrate becomes ineffective and the silver ions may damage tissue if the dressing becomes dry.* (To maintain moisture, some protocols call for irrigating the dressing with solution at least every 4 hours through small slits cut into the outer dressing.) **ABA**

Applying a dry dressing with a topical medication

● Remove old dressings, and clean the wound as described previously.

● Apply a thin layer (2 to 4 mm thick) of the ordered medication to the wound with your gloved hand. Apply several layers of burn gauze over the wound *to contain the medication but allow exudate to escape.*

● Remember to cut the dressing to fit only the wound areas; don't cover unburned areas.

● Cover the entire dressing with roller gauze, and secure it with elastic netting or tape.

Providing arm and leg care

● Apply the dressings from the distal to the proximal area *to stimulate circulation and prevent constriction.* Wrap the burn gauze once around the arm or leg so the edges overlap slightly. Continue wrapping in this way until the gauze covers the wound. **ABA** **Science**

● Apply dry roller gauze dressing *to hold the bottom layers in place.* Secure with elastic netting or tape.

Providing hand and foot care

● Wrap each finger separately with a single layer of a 4″ × 4″ gauze pad to allow the patient to use his hands and to prevent webbing contractures.

● Place the hand in a functional position, and secure this position using a dressing. Apply splints, if ordered. **Science**

● Put gauze between each toe as appropriate, to prevent webbing contractures.

Providing chest, abdomen, and back care

● Apply the ordered medication to the wound in a thin layer. Cover the entire burned area with sheets of burn gauze.

● Wrap with roller gauze or apply a specialty vest dressing *to hold the burn gauze in place.*

● Secure the dressing with elastic netting or tape. Make sure the dressing doesn't restrict respiratory motion, especially in very young or elderly patients or in those with circumferential injuries.

Providing facial care

● If the patient has scalp burns, clip or shave the hair around the burn, as ordered. Clip other hair until it's about 2″ (5 cm) long *to prevent contamination of burned scalp areas.*

● Shave facial hair if it comes in contact with burned areas. **ABA**

● Typically, facial burns are managed with milder topical medications (such as triple antibiotic ointment) and are left open to air. If dressings are required, make sure they don't cover the eyes, nostrils, or mouth.

Providing ear care

● Clip or shave the hair around the affected ear.

● Remove exudate and crusts with cotton-tipped applicators dipped in normal saline solution.

● Place a layer of 4″ × 4″ gauze behind the auricle *to prevent webbing.*

● Apply the ordered topical medication to 4″ × 4″ gauze pads, and place the pads over the burned area. Before securing the dressing with a roller bandage, position the patient's ears normally *to avoid damaging the auricular cartilage.* **ABA**

● Assess the patient's hearing ability. **ABA**

Providing eye care

● Clean the area around the eyes and eyelids with a cotton-tipped applicator and normal saline solution every 4 to 6 hours, or as needed, *to remove crusts and drainage.* **ABA**

● Administer ordered eye ointment or eyedrops.

● If the eyes can't be closed, apply lubricating ointment or drops, as ordered. **Science**

● Be sure to close the patient's eyes before applying eye pads *to prevent corneal abrasion.* Don't apply topical ointment near the eyes without a physician's order.

Providing nasal care

● Check the nostrils for inhalation injury, such as inflamed mucosa, singed vibrissae, and soot.

● Clean the nostrils with cotton-tipped applicators dipped in normal saline solution. Remove crusts.

● Apply the ordered ointment.

● If the patient has a nasogastric tube, use tracheostomy ties to secure the tube. Be sure to check ties frequently for tightness resulting from facial tissue swelling. Clean the area around the tube every 4 to 6 hours. **ABA**

Special considerations

● Thorough assessment and documentation of the wound's appearance are essential *to detect infection*

Successful burn care after discharge

Wound care

Instruct the patient or a family member to follow this procedure when changing dressings:

- Clean the bathtub, shower, or washbasin thoroughly, and then assemble the required equipment (topical medication, if ordered, and dressing supplies). Open the supplies aseptically on a clean surface.
- Wash your hands. Remove the old dressing and discard it.
- Using a clean washcloth and mild soap and water, wash the wound to remove all the old medication. Try to remove any loose skin as well. Pat the skin dry with a clean towel.
- Check the burned area for signs of infection: redness, heat, foul odor, increased pain, and difficulty moving the area. If any of these signs is present, notify the physician after completing the dressing change.
- Wash your hands. If ordered, apply a thin layer of topical medication to the burned area.
- Cover the burned area with thin layers of gauze, and wrap it with a roller gauze. Finally, secure the dressing with tape or elastic netting.

Self-care

To enhance healing, instruct the patient to eat well-balanced meals with adequate carbohydrates and proteins, to eat between-meal snacks, and to include at least one protein source in each meal and snack. Tell him to avoid tobacco, alcohol, and caffeine *because they constrict peripheral blood flow.*

Advise the patient to wash new skin with mild soap and water. *To prevent excessive skin dryness,* instruct him to use a lubricating lotion and to avoid lotions containing alcohol or perfume. Caution the patient to avoid bumping or scratching regenerated skin tissue.

Recommend nonrestrictive, nonabrasive clothing, which should be laundered in a mild detergent. (New clothing should be washed before it's worn.) Advise the patient to wear protective clothing during cold weather *to prevent frostbite.*

Warn the patient not to expose new skin to strong sunlight and to always use a sunblock with a sun protection factor of 20 or higher. Also, tell him not to expose new skin to irritants, such as paint, solvents, strong detergents, and antiperspirants. Recommend cool baths or ice packs *to relieve itching.*

To minimize scar formation, the patient may need to wear a pressure garment—usually for 23 hours a day for 6 months to 1 year. Instruct him to remove it only during daily hygiene. Advise him that the garment is too tight if it causes cold, numbness, or discoloration in the fingers or toes or if its seams and zippers leave deep, red impressions for more than 10 minutes after the garment is removed. If these signs or symptoms appear, he should consult his physician.

---

and other complications. A purulent wound or green-gray exudate indicates infection, an overly dry wound suggests dehydration, and a wound with a swollen, red edge suggests cellulitis. Suspect a fungal infection if the wound is white and powdery. Healthy granulation tissue appears clean, pinkish, faintly shiny, and free from exudate.

- *Blisters protect underlying tissue,* so leave them intact unless they impede joint motion, become infected, or cause the patient discomfort.
- Keep in mind that the patient with healing burns has increased nutritional needs. He'll require extra protein and carbohydrates *to accommodate an almost doubled basal metabolism.*
- If you must manage a burn with topical medications, exposure to air, and no dressing, you'll need to watch for such problems as wound adherence to bed linens, poor drainage control, and partial loss of topical medications.

TEACHING *Begin discharge planning as soon as the patient enters the facility to help him (and his family) make a smooth transition from facility to home. To encourage therapeutic compliance, prepare him to expect scarring, teach him wound management and pain control, and urge him to follow the prescribed exercise regimen.*

Provide encouragement and emotional support, and urge the patient to join a burn survivor support group. Teach the family or caregivers how to encourage, support, and provide care for the patient. (See Successful burn care after discharge.*)*

Nursing diagnoses

- Acute pain
- Impaired skin integrity

Expected outcomes

The patient will:

- express pain relief
- exhibit improved or healed wounds
- not develop complications, such as infection or deformities.

Complications

Infection is the most common burn complication. Others include disfigurement, pain, and emotional issues.

Documentation

Record the date and time of all care provided. Describe the wound's condition, special dressing-change techniques, topical medications administered, positioning of the burned area, and the patient's tolerance of the procedure.

Supportive references

ABA. *Practice Guidelines for Burn Care.* Supplement to *Journal of Burn Care and Rehabilitation* 22(3 Suppl), May-June 2001.

McCallon, S.K., and Browing, K. "Treatment of Partial Thickness Burns Using Balsam Peru, Castor Oil, Trypsin Ointment: A Case Study: 607," *Journal of Wound, Ostomy & Continence Nursing* 32(3S)(Suppl 2):S5, May-June 2005.

Mendez-Eastman, S. "Burn Injuries," *Plastic Surgical Nursing* 25(3):133-39, July-September 2005.

Diabetic ulcer care

Diabetic foot ulcers are usually caused by peripheral neuropathy, both sensory (lack of sensation) and motor (decreased function of the motor nerves in the foot), but they may also result from peripheral vascular disease. Arterial insufficiency can be another cause of a nonhealing ulcer in a patient with diabetes. An ulcer can also result from trauma or excess pressure undetected by the patient because of neuropathy. The border is undefined and may be small at the surface, although the wound may have a large subcutaneous abscess. Drainage usually is absent unless the ulcer is infected.

To assess the diabetic foot ulcer start by taking a complete history, which could help you to determine the patient's knowledge about the disease and see whether he's complying with his treatment regimen. Assess the patient's feet for ulcers on the plantar aspect of the toes, laterally to the foot, between the toes, and on the tips of the toes. Be sure to look at the surrounding intact skin for erythema, induration, and maceration. Assess the footwear usually worn by the patient. Does it protect the feet or does it promote rubbing that could lead to skin breakdown? Assess the wound for granulation tissue, necrotic tissue, anatomic structures, color of the wound bed and exudate, and odor. (See *Tailoring wound care to wound color,* page 522.)

Toe brachial index or ankle brachial index, taken with a Doppler and a specially sized pneumatic cuff, provide an objective indicator of arterial blood flow to the lower extremity.

Diabetic neuropathic ulcers should be treated like pressure ulcers, with debridement of necrotic tissue, moist wound healing, and off-loading of pressure.

Equipment

Bedside table • piston-type irrigating system • two pairs of gloves • normal saline solution, as ordered • sterile 4″ × 4″ gauze pads • sterile cotton swabs • selected topical dressing • linen-saver pads • impervious plastic trash bag • disposable wound-measuring device (a square, transparent card with concentric circles arranged in bull's-eye fashion and bordered with a straightedge ruler)

Preparation of equipment

Assemble equipment at the patient's bedside. Cut the tape into strips for securing the dressings. Loosen the lids on cleaning solutions and medications for easy removal. Loosen existing dressing edges and tape before putting on gloves. Attach an impervious plastic trash bag to the bedside table to hold used dressings and other refuse.

Implementation

- Confirm the patient's identity using two patient identifiers according to facility policy. **JCAHO**
- Explain the procedure to the patient. **PCP**
- Premedicate the patient, as needed, before changing the dressing.

Tailoring wound care to wound color

With any wound, promote healing by keeping it moist, clean, and free from debris. If your patient has an open wound, you can assess how well it's healing by inspecting its color, and then use wound color to guide the specific management approach.

Red wounds
Red, the color of healthy granulation tissue, indicates normal healing. When a wound begins to heal, a layer of pale pink granulation tissue covers the wound bed. As this layer thickens, it becomes beefy red. Cover a red wound, keep it moist and clean, and protect it from trauma. Use a transparent dressing, a hydrocolloidal dressing, or a gauze dressing moistened with sterile normal saline solution or impregnated with petroleum jelly or an antibiotic.

Yellow wounds
Yellow is the color of exudate produced by microorganisms in an open wound. When a wound heals without complications, the immune system removes microorganisms. But if there are too many microorganisms to remove, exudate accumulates and becomes visible. Exudate usually appears whitish yellow, creamy yellow, yellowish green, or beige. Water content influences the shade—dry exudate appears darker.

If your patient has a yellow wound, clean it and remove the exudate, using high-pressure irrigation, and then cover it with a moist dressing. Use absorptive products or a moist gauze dressing with or without an antibiotic. You may also use hydrotherapy with whirlpool or high-pressure irrigation.

Black wounds
Black, the least healthy color, signals necrosis. Dead, avascular tissue slows healing and provides a site for microorganisms to proliferate.

Black wounds should be debrided. After the dead tissue is removed, apply a dressing to keep the wound moist and guard against external contamination. As ordered, use enzyme products, surgical debridement, hydrotherapy with whirlpool or high-pressure irrigation, or a moist gauze dressing.

Multicolored wounds
You may note two or even all three colors in a wound. In this case, you would classify the wound according to the least healthy color present. For example, if your patient's wound is both red and yellow, classify it as a yellow wound.

- Wash your hands, and put on sterile gloves. Be sure to review your facility's policy on standard precautions. **CDC**
- Remove the existing dressing, and place it into the impervious trash bag. (If the dressing is dry, soak it with saline before removing it so that granulating tissue isn't removed when the dressing is pulled off.) **CDC**
- Inspect the wound. Note the location, pain, shape, size of the wound, wound base and edges, periwound skin and the color, amount, and odor of drainage or necrotic debris. Measure the wound perimeter with the disposable wound-measuring device.
- Irrigate the wound, using a piston-style syringe containing normal saline solution.
- Remove and discard your soiled gloves, wash your hands, and put on a pair of sterile gloves.

- Insert a cotton-tipped swab into the wound to assess for tunneling. Gauge the tunnel depth by how far you can insert your finger or cotton swab.
- Clean the ulcer with normal saline solution or a commercially prepared noncytotoxic cleanser. When applying the gauze, use a moist dressing to promote a moist wound environment. **WOCN**
- To apply a moist dressing, squeeze out the excess saline from the gauze layers. Place the layer of moist gauze into the wound. If there's tunneling, make sure the dressing is tucked loosely into the tunneled areas. Make sure that the moist dressing touches all the tissue in the wound, filling up all of the wound's dead space. Avoid overpacking the wound. (See "Pressure ulcer care," page 527, for more detailed instructions.) Your patient may need absorbent dressings if the ulcer has moderate to heavy drainage.

• Notify the practitioner of your assessment findings. The patient may need ulcer debridement or surgical intervention. Debridement helps ulcer healing by removing necrotic tissue that acts as a physical barrier to wound repair. If the ulcer is caused by arterial insufficiency, the patient may need surgery. **WOCN**

• If the patient's wound is infected, prepare him for a tissue biopsy — the gold standard to confirm the diagnosis of infection — and the possible need for a systemic antibiotic. **WOCN**

• Check the patient's laboratory test results, and notify the physician of any findings that fall outside the reference range.

• Prepare the patient for tests that may be performed to determine ulcer severity and the presence of complications. Radiographic imaging is used to help rule out gas formation, the presence of foreign objects, and bony abnormalities. Magnetic resonance imaging is used to help diagnose osteomyelitis. A transcutaneous oxygen tension measurement determines skin perfusion. If the ulcer is in an atypical location or doesn't respond to treatment, a biopsy may be performed.

• Apply growth factors, as ordered, after necrotic tissue and infection have been eliminated and perfusion to the wound is adequate. **WOCN**

• Assess the patient's level of pain, and refer him to a pain specialist if necessary.

TEACHING *Tell the patient to thoroughly inspect his feet daily, wear proper-fitting shoes and socks, avoid walking barefoot in the home, and not to test the temperature of bath water with his feet. Also, suggest that he see a podiatrist for his foot care needs.*

Instruct the patient to keep his legs elevated above the level of his heart while sitting or sleeping. Suggest that he place phone books in between his mattress and box spring so that his legs are elevated above his head.

Nursing diagnoses

• Deficient knowledge (procedure)
• Impaired skin integrity

Expected outcomes

The patient will:
• explain his skin care regimen
• verbalize an understanding of those behaviors he should follow to avoid complications
• exhibit improved or healed wounds.

Complications

Gangrene is a common complication of diabetic ulcers, especially those that occur on the feet. In many cases, amputation is necessary to control the spread of infection.

Documentation

Document the ulcer's anatomic location and its length, width, and depth. Record the extent of tunneling or undermining, if present. Reassess the wound at specified intervals, and document the date and time of dressing changes. If the wound is infected, its dimensions may change rapidly. Also document any ulcer-related pain, asking the patient if he feels pain, teaching him to use a pain-rating scale, and looking for nonverbal indicators. Photograph the wound to supplement your comprehensive wound care documentation.

Supportive references

Brooks, B., et al. "TBI or not TBI: That is the Question. Is it Better to Measure Toe Pressure than Ankle Pressure in Diabetic Patients?" *Diabetic Medicine* 18(7):528-32, July 2001.

McMullin, G.M. "Improving the Treatment of Leg Ulcers," *Medical Journal of Australia* 175(7):375-78, August 2001.

Wound, Ostomy and Continence Nurses Society (WOCN). *Guideline for Management of Wounds in Patients with Lower-Extremity Neuropathic Disease.* Glenview, Ill.: WOCN; 2004.

"Wound Snapshots: Diabetic Ulcers," *Advances in Skin & Wound Care* 16(5):224, September 2003.

Zafar, A. "Management of Diabetic Foot — Two Years Experience," *Journal of Ayub Medical College, Abbottabad* 13(1):14-16, January-March 2001.

Laser therapy

Using the highly focused, intense energy of a laser beam, a surgeon can treat various skin lesions. What's more, laser surgery has several advantages. As a surgical instrument, the laser offers precise control. It spares normal tissue, speeds healing, and deters infection by sterilizing the operative site. In addition, by sealing tiny blood vessels as it vaporizes tissue, the laser beam leaves a nearly bloodless operative field. The procedure can be performed on an outpatient basis. The lasers used most commonly to

Types of laser therapy

Laser therapy is now an essential tool for treating many types of skin lesions. The number of lasers used in dermatology is ever-growing, and each type is used for specific conditions. The term *laser* is an acronym for *light amplification by the stimulated emission of radiation*. When directed toward the skin, most of this light energy is absorbed by chromophores, substances that absorb specific wavelengths of light. This is the basis of selective photothermolysis, which has revolutionized cutaneous laser surgery. Melanin is the target chromophore in pigmented lesions, and oxyhemoglobin within microvessels is the target chromophore in vascular lesions.

It's important to be familiar with the various lasers and the indications for use of each.

Lasers for vascular lesions
The laser most commonly used for vascular lesions is the flashlamp-pumped dye laser. Other lasers used for vascular lesions include copper vapor, argon, KTP, krypton, frequency-doubled Q-switched neodymium:yttrium-aluminum-garnet (Nd:YAG), and Nd:YAG lasers. The choice of the laser depends on the specific vascular lesion. Port-wine stains, hemangiomas, venous lake, rosacea, telangiectasia, and Kaposi's sarcoma are examples of vascular lesions that are appropriate for laser therapy.

Lasers for pigmented lesions
Lasers that are effective in treating tattoos and dermal and epidermal pigmented lesions include Q-switched ruby, Q-switched Nd:YAG, Q-switched alexandrite, flashlamp-pumped pigmented lesion dye, copper vapor, krypton, and KTP. Pigmented lesions that are appropriate for laser treatment include tattoos, nevi of Ota, melasma, solar lentigo, café au lait spots, Becker's nevi, and epidermal nevi.

Carbon dioxide laser
The carbon dioxide laser is one of the oldest lasers, but it's less commonly used since the advent of lasers working on the principle of selective photothermolysis. This laser causes thermal injury, resulting in ablation in the defocused mode. It cuts tissue in the focused mode. It's used to treat actinic cheilitis, rhinophyma, warts, keloids, and other lesions.

Lasers for hair removal
Lasers used to eliminate unwanted hair include ruby, diode, alexandrite, and Nd:YAG. Laser treatment is effective in removing only dark-colored hair; it isn't effective for removing blonde, red, white, or gray hair.

---

treat skin lesions are vascular, pigment, and carbon dioxide (CO_2) lasers. (See *Types of laser therapy*.)

In general, laser surgery is safe, although bleeding and scarring can result. One pronounced hazard — to the patient and treatment staff alike — is eye damage or other injury caused by unintended laser beam reflection. For this reason, anyone in the surgical suite, including the patient, must wear special goggles to filter laser light. The surgeon must use special nonreflective instruments. Access to the room must be strictly controlled, and all windows must be covered.

Equipment
Laser • filtration face masks • protective eyewear • laser vacuum • extra vacuum filters • surgical drape • prescribed cleaning solution • sterile gauze • nonadherent dressings • surgical tape • cotton-tipped applicators • nonreflective surgical instruments • gowns • sterile gloves

Preparation of equipment
Before the procedure begins, prepare the tray. It should include a local anesthetic, as ordered, and dry and wet gauze. The gauze is used *to control bleeding, protect healthy tissue, and abrade and remove any eschar,* which would otherwise inhibit laser absorption. Prepare nonreflective surgical instruments, as needed.

Implementation
● Put on a gown, a filtration face mask, and protective eyewear. **CDC**
● Tell the patient how the laser works and what its benefits are. Point out the equipment, and outline the procedure *to help allay his concerns.* **PCP**

- Just before the surgeon begins, position the patient comfortably, drape him, and place protective gauze, if needed, around the operative site. Confirm that everyone in the room — including the patient — has protective eyewear on *to filter the laser light.*
- Lock the door to the surgical suite to keep unprotected persons from inadvertently entering the room.
- After the surgeon administers the anesthetic and it takes effect, activate the laser vacuum. The CO_2 laser has a vacuum hose attached to a separate apparatus. Use this apparatus *to clear the surgical site.* The vacuum has a filter that traps and collects most of the vaporized tissue. Change the filter whenever suction decreases, and follow facility guidelines for filter disposal.
- When the surgeon finishes the procedure, apply direct pressure with a sterile gauze pad to any bleeding wound for 20 minutes. (Wear sterile gloves.) If the wound continues to bleed, notify the physician. **Science**
- After the bleeding is controlled, use aseptic technique to clean the area with a cotton-tipped applicator dipped in the prescribed cleaning solution. Size and cut a nonadherent dressing. Secure the dressing with surgical tape. **Science**
- Vascular and pigment lasers won't result in a wound; only superficial skin changes will occur.

Special considerations

- The surgeon uses the laser beam much as he would a scalpel to excise the lesion. Explain to the patient that the laser causes a burnlike wound that can be deep, and will appear charred. Tell the patient that some of the eschar will be removed during the initial postoperative cleaning and that more will gradually dislodge at home. **PCP**
- Warn the patient to expect a burning odor and smoke during the procedure. A machine called a smoke evacuator, which sounds like a vacuum cleaner, will clear it away. Advise the patient that he may sense heat from the laser. Urge him to tell the physician immediately if pain develops. **PCP**
- The nurse must have thorough knowledge of how each laser operates and of laser safety considerations for the patient and health care providers.

   TEACHING *Teach the patient how to dress his wound or care for his skin daily, as ordered by the surgeon. Tell him that he can take showers but shouldn't immerse the wound site in*

water, to promote wound healing and prevent infection.

If the wound bleeds at home, demonstrate how to apply direct pressure on the site with clean gauze or a washcloth for 20 minutes. If pressure doesn't control the bleeding, tell the patient to call his physician. **Science**

If the patient's foot or leg was operated on, urge him to keep the extremity elevated and to use it as little as possible because pressure can inhibit healing. **Science**

Warn the patient to protect the treated area from exposure to the sun to avoid changes in pigmentation. Tell him to call the physician if a fever of 100° F (37.8° C) or higher persists longer than 1 day.

Nursing diagnoses

- Deficient knowledge (procedure)

Expected outcomes

The patient will:
- verbalize expectations of results of laser treatment
- verbalize an understanding of those behaviors he should follow after surgery.

Complications

Bleeding, scarring, and infection are rare complications of laser surgery.

Documentation

Most patients who have laser surgery for skin lesions are treated as outpatients. Note the patient's skin condition before and after the procedure. Document any bleeding, record the type of dressing applied, and list the patient's complaints of pain. Note whether the patient comprehends the home care instructions.

Supportive references

Franz, R. "Laser Therapy and Microdermabrasion Treat Acne Scars," *Dermatology Nursing* 13(5):396, October 2001.

Loo, W.J., and Lanigan, S.W. "Recent Advances in Laser Therapy for the Treatment of Cutaneous Vascular Disorders," *Lasers in Medical Science* 17(1):9-12, 2002.

McBurney, E. "Side Effects and Complications of Laser Therapy," *Dermatology Clinic* 20(1):165-76, January 2002.

Mechanical debridement

Debridement involves removing necrotic tissue by mechanical, chemical, or surgical means to allow underlying healthy tissue to regenerate. Removal of eschar allows the underlying healing tissue to regenerate, prevents or controls infection, and prepares the site to receive a graft, should it become the treatment of choice.

Mechanical debridement procedures include irrigation, hydrotherapy, and excision of dead tissue with forceps and scissors. The procedure may be done at the bedside or in a specially prepared room. Other debridement techniques include chemical debridement (with wound-cleaning beads or topical agents that absorb exudate and debris) or surgical excision and skin grafting (usually reserved for deep burns or ulcers). Typically, the patient receives a local or general anesthetic.

Ideally, the wound should be debrided daily during the dressing change. Frequent, regular debridement guards against possible hemorrhage resulting from more extensive and forceful debridement. It also reduces the need to conduct extensive debridement under anesthesia.

Equipment

Ordered pain medication • two pairs of sterile gloves • two gowns or aprons • mask • cap • sterile scissors • sterile forceps • sterile 4″ × 4″ gauze pads • sterile solutions and medications, as ordered • hemostatic agent, as ordered • pick-ups • knife • 15 blade (used for fine debriding) • 10 or 20 blade (used for thin slices of tissue)

Be sure to have the following equipment immediately available to control hemorrhage: needle holder • gut suture with needle • silver nitrate sticks.

Implementation

● Confirm the patient's identity using two patient identifiers according to facility policy. **JCAHO**
● Explain the procedure to the patient *to allay his fears and promote cooperation.* Teach him distraction and relaxation techniques, if possible, *to minimize his discomfort.* **PCP**
● Provide privacy. Administer an analgesic 20 minutes before debridement begins, or give an I.V. analgesic immediately before the procedure. **Science**

● Keep the patient warm. Expose only the area to be debrided *to prevent chilling and fluid and electrolyte loss.* **Science**
● Wash your hands and put on a cap, mask, gown or apron, and sterile gloves. **ABA** **CDC**
● Remove the burn dressings, and clean the wound. (For detailed directions, see "Burn care," page 513.)
● Remove your gown or apron and dirty gloves, and change to another gown or apron and sterile gloves. **ABA** **CDC**
● Lift loosened edges of eschar with forceps. Use the blunt edge of scissors or forceps to probe the eschar. Cut the dead tissue from the wound with the scissors. Leave a ¼″ (0.6 cm) edge on remaining eschar *to avoid cutting into viable tissue.*
● Because debridement removes only dead tissue, bleeding should be minimal. If bleeding occurs, apply gentle pressure on the wound with sterile 4″ × 4″ gauze pads. Apply the hemostatic agent. If bleeding persists, notify the physician and maintain pressure on the wound until the physician assesses the patient. Excessive bleeding or spurting vessels may require ligation.
● Perform additional procedures, such as application of topical medications and dressing replacements, as ordered.

Special considerations

● Work quickly, with an assistant if available, to complete this painful procedure as soon as possible. Limit the procedure time to 20 minutes, if possible.
● Acknowledge the patient's discomfort and provide emotional support.
● Debride no more than a 4″ (10.2 cm) square area at one time.

Nursing diagnoses

● Impaired skin integrity
● Risk for infection

Expected outcomes

The patient will:
● exhibit improved or healed wounds
● have no complications
● not develop infection at the wound site.

Complications

Infection may develop despite the use of aseptic technique and equipment. In addition, some blood loss may occur if debridement exposes an eroded blood vessel or if you inadvertently cut a vessel. Fluid and electrolyte imbalances may result from exudate lost during the procedure.

Documentation

Record the date and time of wound debridement, the area debrided, and solutions and medications used. Describe the wound's condition, noting signs of infection or skin breakdown. Record the patient's tolerance of and reaction to the procedure. Note indications for additional therapy.

Supportive references

Attinger, C.E., et al. "Surgical Debridement. The Key to Successful Wound Healing and Reconstruction," *Clinics in Podiatric Medicine and Surgery* 17(4):599-630, October 2000.

Ayello, E.A., and Cuddigan, J.E. "Debridement: Controlling the Necrotic/Cellular Burden," *Advances in Skin & Wound Care* 17(2):66-75, March 2004.

Pressure ulcer care

A pressure ulcer is a lesion caused by unrelieved pressure that results in damage to underlying tissues. Most pressure ulcers develop over bony prominences, where friction and shearing force combine with pressure to break down skin and underlying tissues. About 95% of pressure ulcers occur in the lower part of the body, with the sacrum and the heel being the two most common sites that experience skin breakdown.

Successful pressure ulcer treatment involves relieving pressure, restoring circulation and, if possible, resolving or managing related disorders. Typically, the effectiveness and duration of treatment depend on the pressure ulcer's characteristics. Ideally, prevention is the key to avoiding extensive therapy. Preventive strategies include recognizing the risk, decreasing the effects of pressure, assessing nutritional status, avoiding excessive bed rest, and preserving skin integrity. Although many systems have been developed to help classify, or "stage," wounds, the system that the Agency for Healthcare Research and Quality and the Wound, Ostomy and Continence Nurses Society (WOCN) recommend is a four-stage system based on the tissue layers involved. **AHRQ** **WOCN** (See *Assessing pressure ulcers,* page 528.) The Braden scale, on

the other hand, is the assessment tool of choice for determining the *risk* of developing pressure ulcers; it's also used to direct implementation of preventive strategies. (See *Braden scale: Predicting pressure ulcer risk,* pages 530 and 531.)

Treatment includes methods to decrease pressure, such as frequent repositioning to shorten pressure duration, and the use of special equipment to reduce pressure intensity. Treatment may involve special pressure-reducing devices, such as beds, mattresses, mattress overlays, and chair cushions. Other therapeutic measures include decreasing risk factors and use of topical treatments, wound cleaning, debridement, and the use of dressings to support moist wound healing. (See *Topical agents for pressure ulcers,* page 532.)

✔ **CLINICAL IMPACT** *The WOCN suggests using clean gloves for wound cleaning and routine dressing changes with or without mechanical or chemical enzymatic debridement, but sterile gloves for dressing changes with sharp, conservative bedside debridement. Also, wound irrigation solutions and equipment initially should be sterile and maintained as clean according to facility policy; however, when cleaning a wound that's deep and has sharp, conservative bedside debridement, the solution should be sterile.* **EB** **WOCN**

✔ **CLINICAL IMPACT** *Vacuum-assisted closure (VAC) is a treatment for wounds that are difficult to heal. Approved by the Food and Drug Administration in 1995, VAC aids wound healing by applying controlled levels of negative pressure to remove blood or serous drainage, accelerating debridement, and promoting wound healing.*

Nurses usually perform or coordinate treatments, according to facility policy. The procedures detailed below address cleaning and dressing the pressure ulcer. Always follow the standard precautions guidelines of the Centers for Disease Control and Prevention.

Equipment

Hypoallergenic tape or elastic netting • overbed table • piston-type irrigating system • two pairs of gloves • normal saline solution, as ordered • sterile 4″ × 4″ gauze pads • sterile cotton swabs • selected topical dressing • linen-saver pad • impervious plastic trash bag • disposable wound-measuring device (a square, transparent card with concentric circles arranged in

Assessing pressure ulcers

To select the most effective treatment for a pressure ulcer, you first need to assess its characteristics. The pressure ulcer stages described below, recommended by the Wound, Ostomy and Continence Nurses Society and the Agency for Health Care Research and Quality, reflect the anatomic depth of exposed tissue. Keep in mind that if the wound contains necrotic tissue, you won't be able to determine the stage until you can see the wound base.

Stage I

An ulcer at stage I is a nonblanchable erythema of intact skin. The heralding lesion of a pressure ulcer is persistent redness in lightly pigmented skin and persistent red, blue, or purple hues on darker skin. Other indicators include changes in temperature, consistency, or sensation.

Stage II

Stage II is marked by partial-thickness skin loss involving the epidermis, dermis, or both. The ulcer is superficial and appears as an abrasion, blister, or shallow crater.

Stage III

At stage III, the ulcer constitutes a full-thickness wound penetrating the subcutaneous tissue, which may extend to — but not through — underlying fascia. The ulcer resembles a deep crater and may or may not undermine adjacent tissue.

Stage IV

At stage IV, the ulcer extends through the skin, accompanied by extensive destruction, tissue necrosis, or damage to muscle, bone, or supporting structures (such as tendons and joint capsules).

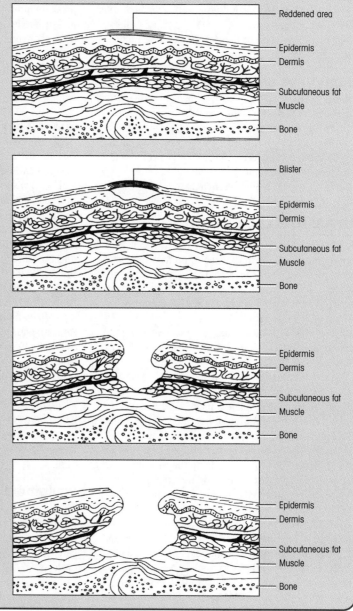

bull's-eye fashion and bordered with a straight-edge ruler)

Preparation of equipment

Assemble equipment at the patient's bedside. Cut the tape into strips for securing dressings. Loosen the lids on cleaning solutions and medications for easy removal. Loosen existing dressing edges and tape before putting on gloves. Attach an impervious plastic trash bag to the bedside table to hold used dressings and refuse.

Implementation

● Premedicate the patient if necessary.
● Before a dressing change, wash your hands, and review standard precautions. **CDC**

Cleaning the pressure ulcer

● Confirm the patient's identity using two patient identifiers according to facility policy. **JCAHO**
● Provide privacy, and explain the procedure to the patient *to allay his fears and promote cooperation.* **PCP**
● Position the patient to increase his comfort, but make sure his position allows easy access to the pressure ulcer site.
● Cover the bed linens with a linen-saver pad *to prevent soiling.*
● Open the normal saline solution container and the piston syringe. Carefully pour normal saline solution into an irrigation container *to avoid splashing.* (This container may be clean or sterile, depending on facility policy.) Put the piston syringe into the opening provided in the irrigation container.
● Open the packages of supplies.
● Put on gloves to remove the old dressing and expose the pressure ulcer. Discard the soiled dressing in the impervious plastic trash bag *to avoid contaminating the sterile field and spreading infection.* **CDC**
● Inspect the wound. Note the color, amount, and odor of drainage and necrotic debris. Measure the wound perimeter with the disposable wound-measuring device. **WOCN**
● Using the piston syringe, apply full force to irrigate the pressure ulcer *to remove necrotic debris.* **WOCN**
● Remove and discard your soiled gloves, and put on a fresh pair. **CDC**

● Insert a sterile cotton swab into the wound to assess wound tunneling or undermining. *Tunneling usually signals wound extension along fascial planes.*
● Next, reassess the condition of the skin and the ulcer. Note the character of the clean wound bed and the surrounding skin.
● If you observe adherent necrotic material, notify a wound care specialist or a physician *to ensure appropriate debridement.* (See *Understanding pressure ulcer debridement,* page 533.)
● Prepare to apply the appropriate topical dressing. Directions for typical moist saline gauze, hydrocolloid, transparent, alginate, foam, and hydrogel dressings follow. For other dressings or topical agents, follow facility policy or the supplier's instructions. (See *Choosing a pressure ulcer dressing,* page 534.)

CONTROVERSIAL ISSUE *The debate continues over who should be allowed to perform conservative sharp wound debridement. Conservative sharp wound debridement is defined as the removal of loose avascular tissue without pain or bleeding. This procedure doesn't require the administration of general anesthesia. The WOCN said in its 1996 position statement that an enterostomal (ET) nurse or nurse specializing in wound care may perform sharp, conservative wound debridement when certain criteria are met:*
● *The ET nurse and the wound care nurse confirm that their state nurse practice act recognizes debridement to be within the scope of nursing.*
● *A policy and procedure is in place within the facility, addressing educational requirements, certification, and a validation process for conservative sharp wound debridement.*
● *The debridement is done with the awareness of the patient's primary care provider.*
● *Collaboration between the nurse and practitioner (surgeon or dermatologist) exists to refine technical skills.* **WOCN**

Applying a moist saline gauze dressing

● Irrigate the pressure ulcer with normal saline solution. Blot the surrounding skin dry.
● Moisten the gauze dressing with normal saline solution.
● Gently place the dressing over the surface of the ulcer. *To separate surfaces within the wound,* gently

(Text continues on page 532.)

Braden scale: Predicting pressure ulcer risk

The Braden scale, shown below, is the most reliable of several instruments for assessing the older patient's risk of developing pressure ulcers. The numbers to the left of each description are the points to be tallied; the lower the score, the greater the risk.

Patient's name _____ **Evaluator's name** _____

Sensory perception Ability to respond meaningfully to pressure-related discomfort	**1 Completely limited** Patient is unresponsive (doesn't moan, flinch, or grasp in response) to painful stimuli due to diminished level of consciousness or sedation. OR Patient has limited ability to feel pain over most of body surface.	**2 Very limited** Patient responds only to painful stimuli; can't communicate discomfort except through moaning or restlessness. OR Patient has a sensory impairment that limits ability to feel pain or discomfort over half of his body.
Moisture Degree to which skin is exposed to moisture	**1 Constantly moist** Patient's skin is kept moist almost constantly by perspiration, urine, and so forth; dampness is detected every time he's moved or turned.	**2 Very moist** Patient's skin is often but not always moist; linen must be changed at least once per shift.
Activity Degree of physical activity	**1 Bedfast** Patient is confined to bed.	**2 Chairfast** Patient's ability to walk is severely limited or nonexistent; he can't bear his own weight and must be assisted into a chair or wheelchair.
Mobility Ability to change and control body position	**1 Completely immobile** Patient doesn't make even slight changes in body or extremity position without assistance.	**2 Very limited** Patient makes occasional slight changes in body or extremity position but can't make frequent or significant changes independently.
Nutrition Usual food intake pattern	**1 Very poor** Patient never eats a complete meal; he rarely eats more than one-third of food offered, eats two servings or less of protein (meat or dairy products) per day, takes fluids poorly, and doesn't take a liquid dietary supplement. OR Patient is given nothing by mouth or maintained on clear liquids or I.V. fluids for more than 5 days.	**2 Probably inadequate** Patient rarely eats a complete meal and generally eats only about half of food offered; his protein intake includes only three servings of meat or dairy products per day, but he'll occasionally take a dietary supplement. OR Patient receives less than optimum amount of liquid diet or tube feeding.
Friction and shear	**1 Problem** Patient requires moderate to maximum assistance in moving. Complete lifting without sliding against sheets is impossible; he often slides down in bed or chair, requiring frequent repositioning with maximum assistance. Spasticity, contractures, or agitation lead to almost constant friction.	**2 Potential problem** Patient moves feebly or requires minimum assistance during a move; his skin probably slides to some extent against sheets, chair, restraints, or other devices. He maintains relatively good position in chair or bed most of the time but occasionally slides down.

	Date of Assessment					

3 Slightly limited
Patient responds to verbal commands but can't always communicate discomfort or the need to be turned.
OR
Patient has some sensory impairment that limits ability to feel pain or discomfort in one or two extremities.

4 No impairment
Patient responds to verbal commands; he has no sensory deficit that would limit ability to feel or voice pain or discomfort.

3 Occasionally moist
Patient's skin is occasionally moist, requiring an extra linen change approximately once per day.

4 Rarely moist
Patient's skin is usually dry; linen requires changing only at routine intervals.

3 Walks occasionally
Patient walks occasionally during day, but for very short distances, with or without assistance; he spends majority of each shift in bed or chair.

4 Walks frequently
Patient walks outside room at least twice per day and inside room at least once every 2 hours during waking hours.

3 Slightly limited
Patient makes frequent though slight changes in body or extremity position independently.

4 No limitations
Patient makes major and frequent changes in position without assistance.

3 Adequate
Patient eats more than half of most meals, with four servings of protein (meat and dairy products) per day. He occasionally refuses a meal, but will usually take a supplement if it's offered.
OR
Patient is on a tube feeding or total parenteral nutrition regimen that probably meets most of his nutritional needs.

4 Excellent
Patient eats most of every meal and never refuses a meal. He usually eats four or more servings of meat and dairy products per day, occasionally eats between meals, and doesn't require supplementation.

3 No apparent problem
Patient moves in bed and in chair independently and has sufficient muscle strength to lift up completely during move; he maintains good position in bed or chair.

Total score: 6 to 23

Topical agents for pressure ulcers

Topical agents	Nursing considerations
Antibiotics Silver sulfadiazine, triple antibiotics	• Consider a 2-week trial of topical antibiotics for clean or exudated pressure ulcers that aren't responding to moist-wound healing therapy.
Circulatory stimulants (Granulex, Proderm)	• Use these agents to promote blood flow. Both contain balsam of Peru and castor oil, but Granulex also contains trypsin, an enzyme that facilitates debridement.
Enzymes Collagenase (Santyl)	• Apply collagenase in thin layers after cleaning the wound with normal saline solution. • Avoid concurrent use of collagenase with agents that decrease enzymatic activity, including detergents, hexachlorophene, antiseptics with heavy-metal ions, iodine, or such acid solutions as Burow's solution. • Use collagenase cautiously near the patient's eyes. If contact occurs, flush the eyes repeatedly with normal saline solution or sterile water.
Exudate absorbers Dextranomer beads (Debrisan)	• Use dextranomer beads on secreting ulcers. Discontinue use when secretions stop. • Clean — but don't dry — the ulcer before applying dextranomer beads. Don't use in tunneling ulcers. • Remove gray-yellow beads (which indicate saturation) by irrigating with sterile water or normal saline solution. • Use cautiously near the eyes. If contact occurs, flush the eyes repeatedly with normal saline solution or sterile water.
Isotonic solutions Normal saline solution	• This agent moisturizes tissue without injuring cells.

place a dressing between opposing wound surfaces. *To avoid damage to tissues,* don't pack the gauze tightly. **WOCN**

• Change the dressing often enough to keep the wound moist.

CONTROVERSIAL ISSUE *A wet-to-moist dressing is generally prepared in the same manner as a wet-to-dry dressing; however, it's intended to remain continuously moist until removal. Studies have shown that wet-to-dry dressings shouldn't be used for wound care for several reasons:*

• *Gauze dressings present no physical barrier to the entry of exogenous bacteria; therefore, patients whose wounds are dressed with gauze dressings are more susceptible to infection in those wounds.*

• *Removing a moist dressing from a wound disperses much bacteria into the air, and the risk of releasing airborne bacteria is greater after the dressing has been dried out.*

Applying a hydrocolloid dressing **WOCN**

• Irrigate the pressure ulcer with normal saline solution. Blot the surrounding skin dry.

• Choose a clean, dry, presized dressing, or cut one to overlap the pressure ulcer by about 1″ (2.5 cm). Remove the dressing from its package, pull the release paper from the adherent side of the dressing, and apply the dressing to the wound. *To minimize irritation,* carefully smooth out wrinkles as you apply the dressing.

• If the dressing's edges need to be secured with tape, apply a skin sealant to the intact skin around the ulcer. After the area dries, tape the dressing to the skin. *The sealant protects the skin and promotes tape adherence.* Avoid using tension or pressure when applying the tape.

• Remove your gloves, and discard them in the impervious plastic trash bag. Dispose of refuse according to facility policy, and wash your hands. **CDC**

Understanding pressure ulcer debridement

Because moist, necrotic tissue promotes the growth of pathologic organisms, removing such tissue aids pressure ulcer healing. A pressure ulcer can be debrided using various methods; the patient's condition and the goals of care determine which method to use. Sharp debridement is indicated for patients with an urgent need for debridement, such as those with sepsis or cellulitis; otherwise, another method — such as mechanical, enzymatic, or autolytic debridement — may be used. Sometimes several methods are used in combination.

Sharp debridement

The most rapid method, sharp debridement removes thick, adherent eschar and devitalized tissue through the use of a scalpel, scissors, or another sharp instrument. Small amounts of necrotic tissue can be debrided at the bedside; extensive amounts must be debrided in the operating room.

Mechanical debridement

Typically, mechanical debridement involves the use of wet-to-dry dressings. Gauze moistened with normal saline solution is applied to the wound and then removed after it dries and adheres to the wound bed. The goal is to debride the wound as the dressing is removed. Mechanical debridement has certain disadvantages; for example, it's often painful and may take a long time to completely debride the ulcer.

Enzymatic debridement

Enzymatic debridement removes necrotic tissue by breaking down tissue elements. Topical enzymatic debriding agents are placed on the necrotic tissue. If eschar is present, it must be crosshatched to allow the enzyme to penetrate the tissue.

Autolytic debridement

Autolytic debridement involves the use of moisture-retentive dressings to cover the wound bed. Necrotic tissue is then removed through self-digestion of enzymes in the wound fluid. Although this method takes longer than other debridement methods, it's appropriate for patients who can't tolerate other methods. If the ulcer is infected, autolytic debridement isn't the treatment of choice.

● Change a hydrocolloid dressing every 2 to 7 days, as needed — for example, if the patient complains of pain, the dressing no longer adheres, or leakage occurs.

Applying a transparent dressing
● Irrigate the pressure ulcer with normal saline solution. Blot the surrounding skin dry.
● Clean and dry the wound as described above.
● Select a dressing to overlap the ulcer by 2″ (5 cm).
● Gently lay the dressing over the ulcer. *To prevent shearing force,* don't stretch the dressing. Press firmly on the edges of the dressing *to promote adherence.* Although this type of dressing is self-adhesive, you may have to tape the edges *to prevent them from curling.*
● If necessary, aspirate accumulated fluid with a 21G needle and syringe. After aspirating the pocket of fluid, clean the aspiration site with an alcohol pad, and cover it with another strip of transparent dressing.
● Change the dressing every 3 to 7 days, depending on the amount of drainage.

Applying an alginate dressing
● Irrigate the pressure ulcer with normal saline solution. Blot the surrounding skin dry.
● Apply the alginate dressing to the ulcer surface. Cover the area with a second dressing (such as gauze pads), as ordered. Secure the dressing with tape or elastic netting.
● If the wound is draining heavily, change the dressing once or twice daily for the first 3 to 5 days. As drainage decreases, change the dressing less frequently — every 2 to 4 days or as ordered. When the drainage stops or the wound bed looks dry, stop using alginate dressing.

Applying a foam dressing
● Irrigate the pressure ulcer with normal saline solution. Blot the surrounding skin dry.
● Gently lay the foam dressing over the ulcer.
● Use tape, elastic netting, or gauze to hold the dressing in place.

Choosing a pressure ulcer dressing

Choosing the proper dressing for a wound can be guided by four basic questions:
- What does the wound need (for example, does it need to be drained, protected, or kept moist)?
- What does the dressing do?
- How well does the product do it? (For example, if the wound is draining a large amount, how absorptive is the dressing?)
- What is available and practical?

Gauze dressings

Made of absorptive cotton or synthetic fabric, gauze dressings are permeable to water, water vapor, and oxygen and may be impregnated with petroleum jelly or another agent. When uncertain about which dressing to use, you may apply a gauze dressing moistened in normal saline solution until a wound specialist recommends definitive treatment.

Hydrocolloid dressings

Hydrocolloid dressings are adhesive, moldable wafers made of a carbohydrate-based material and usually have waterproof backings. They're impermeable to oxygen, water, and water vapor, and most have some absorptive properties.

Transparent film dressings

Clear, adherent, and nonabsorptive, transparent film dressings are polymer-based dressings permeable to oxygen and water vapor but not to water. Their transparency allows visual inspection. Because they can't absorb drainage, transparent film dressings are used on partial-thickness wounds with minimal exudate.

Alginate dressings

Made from seaweed, alginate dressings are nonwoven, absorptive dressings available as soft, white sterile pads or ropes. They absorb excessive exudate and may be used on infected wounds. As these dressings absorb exudate, they turn into a gel that keeps the wound bed moist and promotes healing. When exudate is no longer excessive, switch to another type of dressing.

Foam dressings

Foam dressings are spongelike polymer dressings that may be impregnated or coated with other materials. Somewhat absorptive, they may be adherent. These dressings promote moist wound healing and are useful when a nonadherent surface is desired.

Hydrogel dressings

Water-based and nonadherent, hydrogel dressings are polymer-based and have some absorptive properties. They're available as a gel in a tube, as flexible sheets, and as saturated gauze packing strips. They may have a cooling effect, which eases pain.

- Change the dressing when the foam no longer absorbs the exudate.

Applying a hydrogel dressing
- Irrigate the pressure ulcer with normal saline solution. Blot the surrounding skin dry.
- Apply gel to the wound bed.
- Cover the area with a second dressing.
- Change the dressing daily, or as needed, *to keep the wound bed moist.*
- If the dressing you select comes in sheet form, cut the dressing to match the wound base; *otherwise, the intact surrounding skin can become macerated.*

- Hydrogel dressings also come in prepackaged, saturated gauze for wounds that require "dead space" to be filled. Follow the manufacturer's directions for use.

Preventing pressure ulcers Science
- Turn and reposition the patient every 1 to 2 hours, unless contraindicated. For a patient who can't turn himself or one who's turned on a schedule, use a pressure-reducing device, such as air, gel, or a 4″ (10.2 cm) foam mattress overlay. Low or high air-loss therapy may be indicated *to reduce excessive pressure and promote evaporation of excess moisture.* As ap-

propriate, implement active or passive range-of-motion exercises *to relieve pressure and promote circulation.* To save time, combine these exercises with bathing, if applicable.

• When turning the patient, lift him rather than slide him *because sliding increases friction and shear.* Use a turning sheet, and get help from coworkers if necessary.

• Use pillows *to position your patient and increase his comfort.* Be sure to eliminate sheet wrinkles that could increase pressure and cause discomfort.

• Post a turning schedule at the patient's bedside. Adapt position changes to his situation. Emphasize the importance of regular position changes to the patient and his family, and encourage their participation in treatment and prevention of pressure ulcers by having them perform a position change correctly after you've demonstrated how.

• Avoid placing the patient directly on the trochanter. Instead, position him on his side, at an angle of about 30 degrees.

• Except for brief periods, avoid raising the head of the bed more than 30 degrees *to prevent shearing pressure.*

• Direct the patient confined to a chair or wheelchair to shift his weight every 15 minutes *to promote blood flow to compressed tissues.* Show a paraplegic patient how to shift his weight by doing push-ups in the wheelchair. If the patient needs your help, sit next to him, and help him shift his weight to one buttock for 60 seconds, then repeat the procedure on the other side. Provide him with pressure-relieving cushions, as appropriate. However, avoid seating the patient on a rubber or plastic doughnut, *which can increase localized pressure at vulnerable points.*

• Adjust or pad appliances, casts, or splints, as needed, to ensure proper fit and avoid increased pressure and impaired circulation.

• Tell the patient to avoid heat lamps and harsh soaps *because they dry the skin.* Applying lotion after bathing will help keep his skin moist. Tell him to avoid vigorous massage *because it can damage capillaries.*

• If the patient's condition permits, recommend a diet that includes adequate calories, protein, and vitamins. Dietary therapy may involve nutritional consultation, food supplements, enteral feeding, or total parenteral nutrition.

• If diarrhea develops or if the patient is incontinent, clean and dry the soiled skin. Apply a protective moisture barrier *to prevent skin maceration.*

• Make sure the patient, family members, and caregivers learn strategies to prevent and treat pressure ulcers so that they understand the importance of care, the choices that are available, the rationales for treatments, and their role in selecting goals and shaping the care plan.

Special considerations

• Avoid using elbow and heel protectors that fasten with a single narrow strap. *The strap may impair neurovascular function in the involved hand or foot.*

• Avoid using artificial sheepskin. It doesn't reduce pressure and may create a false sense of security.

• Repair of stages 3 and 4 ulcers may require surgical intervention — such as direct closure, skin grafting, or flaps — depending on the patient's needs. They may also be treated with growth factors, electrical stimulation, heat therapy, or vacuum-assisted wound closure. **WOCN**

Nursing diagnoses

• Impaired skin integrity

Expected outcomes

The patient will:

• exhibit improved or healed wounds

• not develop infection

• report increased comfort.

Complications

Infection may cause foul-smelling drainage, persistent pain, severe erythema, induration, and elevated skin and body temperatures. Advancing infection or cellulitis can lead to septicemia. Severe erythema may signal worsening cellulitis, which indicates that the offending organisms have invaded the tissue and are no longer localized.

Documentation

Record the date and time of initial and subsequent treatments. Note the specific treatment given. Detail preventive strategies performed. Document the pressure ulcer's location and size (length, width, and depth); color and appearance of the wound bed; amount, odor, color, and consistency of drainage; and the condition of the surrounding skin. Reassess pressure ulcers at least weekly.

Update the care plan as required. Note on the clinical record changes in the condition or size of the pressure ulcer and any elevation of skin temperature. Document when the physician was notified of pertinent abnormal observations. Record the patient's temperature daily on the graphic sheet to allow easy assessment of body temperature patterns.

Supportive references

Ayello, E.A., and Baranoski, S. "Examining the Problem of Pressure Ulcers," *Advances in Skin & Wound Care* 18(4):192, May 2005.

Chua, P.C., et al. "Vacuum-Assisted Wound Closure," *AJN* 100(12):45-48, December 2000.

Ovington, L.G. "Hanging Wet-to-Dry Dressing Out to Dry," *Home Health Nurse* 19(8):477-83, August 2001.

Ovington, L.G., and Schaum, K.D. "Wound Care Products: How to Choose," *Home Healthcare Nurse* 19(4):224, April 2001.

Thomas, D.R. "Prevention and Treatment of Pressure Ulcers: What Works? What Doesn't?" *Cleveland Clinic Journal of Medicine* 68(8):704-22, August 2001.

Wound, Ostomy and Continence Nurses Society (WOCN). *Position Statement: Clean vs Sterile: Management of Chronic Wounds.* Glenview Ill.: WOCN; 2005. *www.wocn.org.* **EB**

Wound, Ostomy and Continence Nurses Society. *Position Statement: Conservative Sharp Wound Debridement for Registered Nurses.* Glenview Ill.: WOCN; 1996. *www.wocn.org.*

Wound, Ostomy and Continence Nurses Society. *Guidelines for Prevention and Management of Pressure Ulcers.* Glenview, Ill.: WOCN; 2003.

Understanding types of grafts

A burn patient may receive one or more of the graft types described below.

Split-thickness

The type used most commonly for covering open burns, a split-thickness graft includes the epidermis and part of the dermis. It may be applied as a sheet (usually on the face or neck *to preserve the cosmetic result*) or as a mesh. A mesh graft has tiny slits cut in it, which allow the graft to expand up to nine times its original size. Mesh grafts prevent fluids from collecting under the graft and typically are used over extensive full-thickness burns.

Full-thickness

This graft type includes the epidermis and the entire dermis. Consequently, the graft contains hair follicles, sweat glands, and sebaceous glands, which typically aren't included in split-thickness grafts. Full-thickness grafts usually are used for small burns that cause deep wounds.

Pedicle-flap

This full-thickness graft includes not only skin and subcutaneous tissue but also subcutaneous blood vessels, *to ensure a continued blood supply to the graft.* Pedicle-flap grafts may be used during reconstructive surgery *to cover previous defects.*

Skin graft care

A skin graft consists of healthy skin taken from either the patient (autograft) or a donor (allograft) and applied to an area of the patient's body damaged by burns, traumatic injury, or surgery. Care procedures for an autograft or an allograft are essentially the same. However, an autograft requires care for two sites on the patient: the graft site and the donor site.

Skin grafts are indicated where skin loss has occurred due to burns or, for reconstructive purposes, after trauma, infection (such as necrotizing fasciitis), malformation, deformity, congenitally deformed tissue, removal of malignant lesions, or plastic surgery in which direct closure by suturing isn't possible.

The graft itself may be one of several types: split thickness, full thickness, or pedicle flap. (See *Understanding types of grafts*.) Successful grafting depends on various factors, including clean wound granulation with adequate vascularization, complete contact of the graft with the wound bed, aseptic technique to prevent infection, adequate graft immobilization, and skilled care.

The size and depth of the patient's burns determine whether the burns require grafting. Grafting usually occurs at the completion of wound debridement. The goal is to cover all wounds with an autograft or allograft within 2 weeks. With enzymatic debridement, grafting may be performed 5 to 7 days after debride-

Caring for a donor graft site

Autografts are usually taken from another area of the patient's body with a dermatome, an instrument that cuts uniform, split-thickness skin portions — typically, about 0.013 to 0.05 cm thick. Autografting makes the donor site a partial-thickness wound, which may bleed, drain, and cause pain.

This site needs scrupulous care to prevent infection, which could convert the site to a full-thickness wound. Depending on the graft's thickness, tissue may be obtained from the donor site again in as few as 10 days.

Usually, Xeroflo gauze is applied postoperatively. The outer gauze dressing can be taken off on the first postoperative day; the Xeroflo will protect the new epithelial proliferation.

Care for the donor site as you care for the autograft, using dressing changes at the initial stages *to prevent infection and promote healing.* Follow the guidelines below.

Dressing the wound
- Wash your hands, and put on sterile gloves.
- Remove the outer gauze dressings within 24 hours. Inspect the Xeroflo for signs of infection; then leave it open to the air *to speed drying and healing.*
- Leave small amounts of fluid accumulation alone. Using aseptic technique, larger amounts may be aspirated through the dressing with a small-gauge needle and syringe.
- Apply a lanolin-based cream daily to completely healed donor sites *to keep skin tissue pliable and to remove crusts.*

Postoperative graft care

Both full-thickness and split-thickness skin grafts require compliance with a postoperative activity schedule to prevent complications.

Postoperative timetable	Instructions
1 to 6 days	Strict elevation, above the head
7 days	5 minutes dangling/hour
8 days	10 minutes dangling/hour
9 days	15 minutes dangling/hour
2 to 3 weeks	Physical therapy for range-of-motion exercises
4 to 6 weeks	Partial weight bearing as tolerated, with an assistive device
6 to 8 weeks	Full weight bearing

ment is complete; with surgical debridement, grafting can occur the same day as the surgery.

Depending on facility policy, a physician or specially trained nurse may change graft dressings. The dressings usually stay in place for 5 to 7 days after surgery *to avoid disturbing the graft site.* Meanwhile, the donor graft site needs diligent care. (See *Caring for a donor graft site* and *Postoperative graft care.*)

Equipment
Ordered analgesic • clean and sterile gloves • sterile gown • cap • mask • sterile forceps • sterile scissors • sterile scalpel • sterile 4″ × 4″ gauze pads • Xeroflo

Evacuating fluid from a sheet graft

When small pockets of fluid (called *blebs*) accumulate beneath a sheet graft, the fluid will be evacuated using a sterile scalpel and cotton-tipped applicators. First, the center of the bleb is perforated with the scalpel.

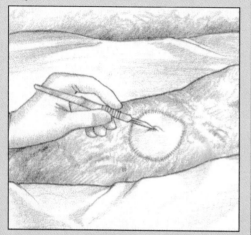

Then the fluid is gently expressed with the cotton-tipped applicators.

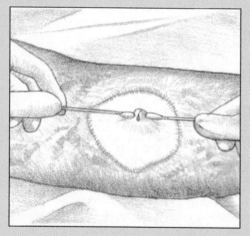

The fluid is never expressed by rolling the bleb to the edge of the graft. This disturbs healing in other areas.

gauze • elastic gauze dressing • warm normal saline solution • moisturizing cream • topical medication (such as micronized silver sulfadiazine cream) • optional: sterile cotton-tipped applicators

Preparation of equipment
Assemble the equipment on the dressing cart.

Implementation
- Confirm the patient's identity using two patient identifiers according to facility policy. **JCAHO**
- Explain the procedure to the patient, and provide privacy. **PCP**
- Administer an analgesic, as ordered, 20 to 30 minutes before beginning the procedure. Alternatively, give an I.V. analgesic immediately before the procedure. **Science**
- Wash your hands. **CDC**
- Put on the sterile gown and the clean mask, cap, and gloves. **CDC**
- Gently lift off all outer dressings. Soak the middle dressings with warm saline solution. Remove these carefully and slowly *to avoid disturbing the graft site.* Leave the Xeroflo intact *to avoid dislodging the graft.*
- Remove and discard the clean gloves, wash your hands, and put on the sterile gloves.
- Assess the condition of the graft. If you see purulent drainage, notify the physician.
- Remove the Xeroflo with sterile forceps, and clean the area gently. If necessary, soak the Xeroflo with warm saline solution *to ease removal.*
- Inspect an allograft for signs of rejection, such as infection and delayed healing. Inspect a sheet graft frequently for blebs. Notify the physician for evacuation if necessary. (See *Evacuating fluid from a sheet graft.*)
- Apply topical medication if ordered.
- Place fresh Xeroflo over the site *to promote wound healing and prevent infection.* Use sterile scissors to cut the appropriate size. Cover this with a 4″ × 4″ sterile gauze pad and elastic gauze dressing.
- Clean completely healed areas, and apply a moisturizing cream to them *to keep the skin pliable and to retard scarring.*

Special considerations
- *To avoid dislodging the graft,* hydrotherapy is usually discontinued, as ordered, 3 to 4 days after grafting. Avoid using a blood pressure cuff over the graft.

Don't tug or pull dressings during dressing changes. Keep the patient from lying on the graft.

● If the graft dislodges, apply sterile skin compresses *to keep the area moist until the surgeon reapplies the graft.* If the graft affects an arm or a leg, elevate the affected extremity *to reduce postoperative edema.* Check for bleeding and signs of neurovascular impairment — increasing pain, numbness or tingling, coolness, and pallor.

TEACHING *Teach the patient how to apply moisturizing cream.*

Stress the importance of using a sunscreen that has a sun protection factor of 20 or higher and contains titanium dioxide or oxybenzone on all grafted areas to avoid sunburn and discoloration.

Nursing diagnoses
● Disturbed body image
● Risk for infection

Expected outcomes
The patient will:
● acknowledge a change in body image
● not develop infection after the procedure.

Complications
The most common reason for graft failure is hematoma. Other reasons include traumatic injury, infection, an inadequate graft bed, rejection, or compromised nutritional status.

Documentation
Record the time and date of all dressing changes. Document all medications used, and note the patient's response to the medications. Describe the condition of the graft, and note signs of infection or rejection. Record additional treatment, and note the patient's reaction to the graft.

Supportive references
Donato, M., et al. "Skin Grafting: Historical and Practical Approaches," *Clinics in Podiatric Medicine and Surgery* 17(4):561-98, October 2000.

Mendez-Eastman, S. "Full-Thickness Skin Grafting: A Procedural Review," *Plastic Surgery Nursing* 24(2):41-45, April 2004.

Choosing a dressing

Wounds aren't static entities; their needs change as they progress or deteriorate. Ongoing assessment of the wound is critical for successful management. Use a general performance-based approach to choose a wound dressing, following these guidelines:

● Examine the wound and the periwound skin *to determine exactly what the wound needs.*
● Review product literature and examine the comparative clinical studies *to determine what the product does and how well it performs.*
● Assess the patient's medical and psychosocial status *to determine what the patient needs.*
● Evaluate what's available in your facility, what's covered by the patient's insurance, and what's practical, focusing on the goal of treatment.

Adapted with permission from Ovington, L.G., and Schaum, K.D. "Wound Care Products: How to Choose," *Home Healthcare Nurse* 19(4):224-32, 240, April 2001.

Surgical wound management

The primary goal of surgical wound management is to promote healing and prevent infection. The two primary methods used to manage a draining surgical wound are dressing and pouching. Dressing is preferred unless caustic or excessive drainage is compromising your patient's skin integrity. Usually, lightly seeping wounds with drains and wounds with minimal purulent drainage can be managed with packing and gauze dressings. Some wounds, such as those that become chronic, may require an occlusive dressing.

A wound with copious, excoriating drainage calls for pouching to protect the surrounding skin. If your patient has a surgical wound, you must monitor him and choose the appropriate dressing.

Dressing a wound calls for sterile technique and sterile supplies to prevent contamination. To choose a dressing, use a performance-based approach, focusing primarily on what the wound needs. (See *Choosing a dressing.*)

Be sure to change the dressing often enough to keep the skin dry. Always follow standard precautions set by the Centers for Disease Control and Prevention (CDC).

Equipment

Waterproof trash bag • clean gloves • sterile gloves • gown and face shield or goggles, if indicated • sterile 4″ × 4″ gauze pads • large absorbent dressings, if indicated • sterile cotton-tipped applicators • sterile dressing set • povidone-iodine swabs • topical medication, if ordered • adhesive or other tape • soap and water • optional: skin protectant, nonadherent pads, collodion spray or acetone-free adhesive remover, sterile normal saline solution, graduated container, Montgomery straps, a fishnet tube elasticized dressing support, or a T-binder

Wound with a drain

Sterile scissors • sterile 4″ × 4″ gauze pads without cotton lining • sump drain • ostomy pouch or another collection bag • sterile precut tracheostomy pads or drain dressings • adhesive tape (paper or silk tape if the patient is hypersensitive) • surgical mask

Pouching a wound

Collection pouch with drainage port • sterile gloves • skin protectant • sterile gauze pads

Preparation of equipment

- Ask the patient about allergies to tapes and dressings.
- Assemble all equipment in the patient's room.
- Check the expiration date on each sterile package, and inspect for tears.
- Open the waterproof trash bag, and place it near the patient's bed.
- Position the bag to avoid reaching across the sterile field or the wound when disposing of soiled articles. **Science**
- Form a cuff by turning down the top of the trash bag to provide a wide opening and to prevent contamination of instruments or gloves by touching the bag's edge.

Implementation

- Confirm the patient's identity using two patient identifiers according to facility policy. **JCAHO**
- Premedicate the patient for pain, if indicated, 20 minutes before a dressing change.
- Explain the procedure to the patient to allay his fears and ensure his cooperation. **PCP**

Removing the old dressing

- Check the physician's order for specific wound care and medication instructions. Be sure to note the location of surgical drains *to avoid dislodging them during the procedure.*
- Assess the patient's condition.
- Identify the patient's allergies, especially to adhesive tape, povidone-iodine or other topical solutions, or medications.
- Provide the patient with privacy, and position him as necessary. *To avoid chilling him,* expose only the wound site. **PCP** **Science**
- Wash your hands thoroughly. Put on a gown and face shield, if necessary. Put on clean gloves. **CDC**
- Loosen the soiled dressing by holding the patient's skin and pulling the tape or dressing toward the wound. *This protects the newly formed tissue and prevents stress on the incision.* Moisten the tape with acetone-free adhesive remover, if necessary, *to make the tape removal less painful (particularly if the skin is hairy).* Don't apply solvents to the incision *because they could contaminate the wound.*
- Slowly remove the soiled dressing. If the gauze adheres to the wound, loosen the gauze by moistening it with sterile normal saline solution.
- Observe the dressing for the amount, type, color, and odor of drainage.
- Discard the dressing and gloves in the waterproof trash bag.

Caring for the wound

- Wash your hands. Establish a sterile field with all the equipment and supplies you'll need for suture-line care and the dressing change, including a sterile dressing set and povidone-iodine swabs. **CDC** If the physician has ordered ointment, squeeze the needed amount onto the sterile field. If you're using an antiseptic from a nonsterile bottle, pour the antiseptic cleaning agent into a sterile container *so you won't contaminate your gloves.* Put on sterile gloves. (See *How to put on sterile gloves.*)
- Saturate the sterile gauze pads with the prescribed cleaning agent. Avoid using cotton balls *because they may shed fibers in the wound, causing irritation, infection, or adhesion.*
- If ordered, obtain a wound culture, and then proceed to clean the wound.
- Pick up the moistened gauze pad or swab, and squeeze out the excess solution.

How to put on sterile gloves

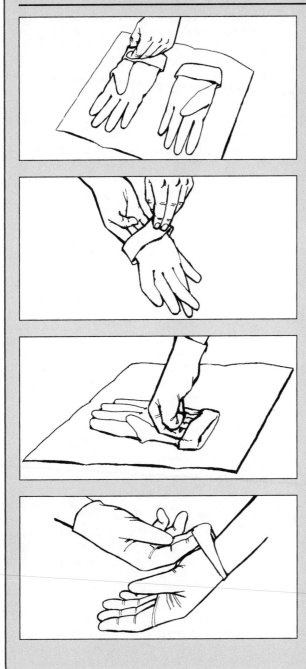

Using your nondominant hand, pick up the opposite glove by grasping the exposed inside of the cuff.

Pull the glove onto your dominant hand. Be sure to keep your thumb folded inward *to avoid touching the sterile part of the glove.* Allow the glove to come uncuffed as you finish inserting your hand, but don't touch the outside of the glove.

Slip the gloved fingers of your dominant hand under the cuff of the loose glove to pick it up.

Slide your nondominant hand into the glove, holding your dominant thumb as far away as possible *to avoid brushing against your arm.* Allow the glove to come uncuffed as you finish putting it on, but don't touch the skin side of the cuff with your other gloved hand.

● Working from the top of the incision, wipe once to the bottom, and then discard the gauze pad. With a second moistened pad, wipe from top to bottom in a vertical path next to the incision (as shown below). **Science**

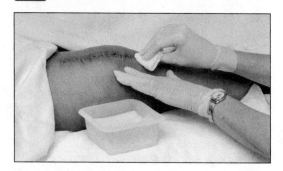

● Continue to work outward from the incision in lines running parallel to it. Always wipe from the clean area toward the less clean area (usually from top to bottom). Use each gauze pad or swab for only one stroke *to avoid tracking wound exudate and normal body flora from surrounding skin to the clean areas.* Remember that the suture line is cleaner than the adjacent skin and the top of the suture line is usually cleaner than the bottom *because more drainage collects at the bottom of the wound.* **Science**
● Use sterile cotton-tipped applicators for efficient cleaning of tight-fitting wire sutures, deep and narrow wounds, or wounds with pockets. *Because the cotton on the swab is tightly wrapped,* it's less likely than a cotton ball to leave fibers in the wound. Remember to wipe only once with each applicator.
● If the patient has a surgical drain, clean the drain's surface last. *Because moist drainage promotes bacterial growth,* the drain is considered the most contaminated area. Clean the skin around the drain by wiping in half or full circles from the drain site outward. **Science**
● Clean all areas of the wound to wash away debris, pus, blood, and necrotic material. Try not to disturb sutures or irritate the incision. Clean to at least 1″ (2.5 cm) beyond the end of the new dressing. If you aren't applying a new dressing, clean to at least 2″ (5 cm) beyond the incision.
● Check to make sure the edges of the incision are lined up properly, and check for signs of infection (heat, redness, swelling, induration, and odor), dehiscence, or evisceration. If you observe such signs or if

the patient reports pain at the wound site, notify the physician.
● Irrigate the wound, as ordered.
● Wash the skin surrounding the wound with soap and water, and pat dry using a sterile 4″ × 4″ gauze pad. Avoid oil-based soap *because it may interfere with pouch adherence.* Apply any prescribed topical medication.
● Apply a skin protectant, if needed.
● If ordered, pack the wound with gauze pads or strips folded to fit, using sterile forceps. Avoid using cotton-lined gauze pads *because cotton fibers can adhere to the wound surface and cause complications.* Pack the wound using the wet-to-damp method. Soaking the packing material in solution and wringing it out so that it's slightly moist provides a moist wound environment that absorbs debris and drainage, and removing the packing won't disrupt new tissue. Don't pack the wound tightly; doing so will exert pressure and may damage the wound.

Applying a fresh gauze dressing

● Gently place sterile 4″ × 4″ gauze pads at the center of the wound, and move progressively outward to the edges of the wound site. Extend the gauze at least 1″ (2.5 cm) beyond the incision in each direction, and cover the wound evenly with enough sterile dressings (usually two or three layers) to absorb all drainage until the next dressing change. Use large absorbent dressings to form outer layers, if needed, *to provide greater absorbency.*
● Secure the dressing's edges to the patient's skin with strips of tape to maintain the sterility of the wound site (as shown below).

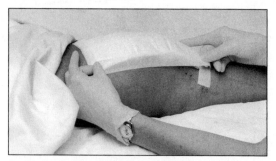

Or, secure the dressing with a T-binder or Montgomery straps *to prevent skin excoriation,* which may occur with repeated tape removal necessitated by frequent dressing changes. (See *How to make Mont-*

How to make Montgomery straps

An abdominal dressing requiring frequent changes can be secured with Montgomery straps to promote the patient's comfort. If ready-made straps aren't available, follow these steps to make your own:

● Cut four to six strips of 2″-to-3″-wide hypoallergenic tape of sufficient length, allowing the tape to extend about 6″ (15 cm) beyond the wound on each side. (The length of the tape varies, depending on the patient's size and the type and amount of dressing.)

● Fold one of each strip 2″ to 3″ back on itself (sticky sides together) *to form a nonadhesive tab.* Cut a small hole in the folded tab's center, close to its top edge. Make as many pairs of straps as you'll need to snugly secure the dressing.

● Clean the patient's skin *to prevent irritation.* After the skin dries, apply a skin protectant. Apply the sticky side of each tape to a skin barrier sheet composed of opaque hydrocolloidal

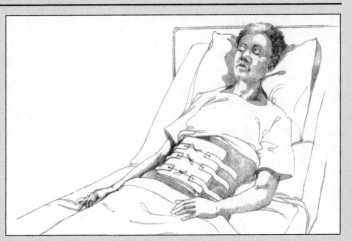

or nonhydrocolloidal materials, and apply the sheet directly to the skin near the dressing. Next, thread a separate piece of gauze tie, umbilical tape, or twill tape (about 12″ [30.5 cm]) through each pair of holes in the straps, and fasten each tie as you would a shoelace. Don't stress the surrounding skin by securing the ties too tightly.

● Repeat this procedure according to the number of Montgomery straps needed.

● Replace Montgomery straps whenever they become soiled (every 2 to 3 days). If skin maceration occurs, place new tapes about 1″ (2.5 cm) away from any irritation.

gomery straps.) If the wound is on a limb, secure the dressing with a fishnet tube elasticized dressing support.

● Make sure the patient is comfortable.

● Properly dispose of the solutions and trash bag, and clean or discard soiled equipment and supplies according to facility policy. If your patient's wound has purulent drainage, don't return unopened sterile supplies to the sterile supply cabinet *because this could cause cross-contamination of other equipment.* **CDC**

Dressing a wound with a drain

● Prepare a drain dressing by using sterile scissors to cut a slit in a sterile 4″ × 4″ gauze pad. Fold the pad in half; then cut inward from the center of the folded edge. Don't use a cotton-lined gauze pad *because cut-*

ting the gauze opens the lining and releases cotton fibers into the wound. Prepare a second pad the same way, or use commercially precut gauze.

● Gently press one folded pad close to the skin around the drain so that the tubing fits into the slit. Press the second folded pad around the drain from the opposite direction so that the two pads encircle the tubing.

● Layer as many uncut sterile 4″ × 4″ gauze pads or large absorbent dressings around the tubing as needed *to absorb expected drainage.* Tape the dressing in place, or use a T-binder or Montgomery straps.

Pouching a wound

● If your patient's wound is draining heavily or if drainage may damage surrounding skin, you'll need to apply a pouch.

● Measure the wound. Cut an opening $^3/_8''$ (1 cm) larger than the wound in the facing of the collection pouch (as shown below).

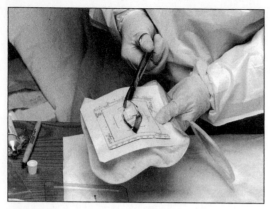

● Apply a skin protectant as needed. (Some protectants are incorporated within the collection pouch and also provide adhesion.)
● Before you apply the pouch, keep in mind the patient's usual position. Plan to position the pouch's drainage port so that gravity facilitates drainage.
● Make sure the drainage port at the bottom of the pouch is closed firmly *to prevent leaks.* Gently press the contoured pouch opening around the wound, starting at its lower edge, *to catch drainage* (as shown below).

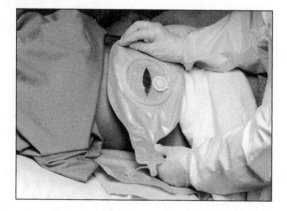

● To empty the pouch, put on gloves and a face shield or mask and goggles *to avoid splashing.* Insert the pouch's bottom half into a graduated biohazard container, and open the drainage port (as shown at top of next column).

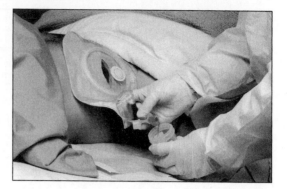

Note the color, consistency, odor, and amount of fluid. If ordered, obtain a culture specimen and send it to the laboratory immediately. Remember to follow the CDC's standard precautions when handling infectious drainage. **CDC**
● Wipe the bottom of the pouch and the drainage port with a gauze pad *to remove drainage that could irritate the patient's skin or cause an odor.* Reseal the port. Change the pouch only if it leaks or fails to adhere. *More frequent changes are unnecessary and only irritate the patient's skin.*

Special considerations

● If the patient has two wounds in the same area, cover each wound separately with layers of sterile 4″ × 4″ gauze pads. Cover each site with a large absorbent dressing secured to the patient's skin with tape. Avoid using a single large absorbent dressing to cover both sites *because drainage quickly saturates a pad, promoting cross-contamination.*
● When packing a wound, don't pack it too tightly *because this compresses adjacent capillaries and may prevent the wound edges from contracting.* Avoid overlapping damp packing onto surrounding skin *because this macerates the intact tissue.*
● To save time when dressing a wound with a drain, use precut tracheostomy pads or drain dressings instead of custom-cutting gauze pads to fit around the drain. If your patient is sensitive to adhesive tape, use paper or silk tape *because it's less likely to cause a skin reaction and will peel off more easily than adhesive tape.* Use a surgical mask to cradle a chin or jawline dressing; *this provides a secure dressing and avoids the need to shave the patient's hair.*
● If ordered, use a collodion spray or similar topical protectant instead of a gauze dressing. Moisture- and

contaminant-proof, this covering dries in a clear, impermeable film that leaves the wound visible for observation and avoids the friction caused by a dressing.
● If a sump drain isn't adequately collecting wound secretions, reinforce it with an ostomy pouch or another collection bag. Use waterproof tape to strengthen a spot on the front of the pouch near the adhesive opening; then cut a small "X" in the tape. Feed the drain catheter into the pouch through the "X" cut. Seal the cut around the tubing with more waterproof tape, and then connect the tubing to the suction pump. *This method frees the drainage port at the bottom of the pouch so that you don't have to remove the tubing to empty the pouch.* If you use more than one collection pouch for a wound or wounds, record drainage volume separately for each pouch. Avoid using waterproof material over the dressing *because it reduces air circulation and promotes infection from accumulated heat and moisture.*
● Because many physicians prefer to change the first postoperative dressing themselves to check the incision, don't change the first dressing unless you have specific instructions. If you have no such instructions and drainage comes through the dressing, reinforce it with fresh sterile gauze. Request an order to change the dressing, or ask the physician to change it as soon as possible. A reinforced dressing shouldn't remain in place longer than 24 hours *because it's an excellent medium for bacterial growth.*
● For the recent postoperative patient or a patient with complications, check the dressing every 15 to 30 minutes or as ordered. For the patient with a properly healing wound, check the dressing at least once every 8 hours.
● If the dressing becomes wet from the outside (for example, from spilled drinking water), replace it as soon as possible *to prevent wound contamination.*
● If your patient will need wound care after discharge, provide appropriate teaching.
● If he'll be caring for the wound himself, stress the importance of using aseptic technique, and teach him how to examine the wound for signs of infection and other complications. Show him how to change dressings, and give him written instructions for all procedures to be performed at home.

Nursing diagnoses
● Acute pain
● Impaired skin integrity

Documenting surgical incision care

Besides documenting vital signs and the level of consciousness when the patient returns from surgery, pay particular attention to maintaining records pertaining to the surgical incision and drains and the care you provide. Read the records that travel with the patient from the postanesthesia care unit. Look for a physician's order to determine whether you or the physician will perform the first dressing change. Be sure to document:

● date, time, and type of wound management procedure
● amount of spoiled dressing and packing removed
● wound appearance (including size, condition of margins, and presence of necrotic tissue) and odor (if present)
● type, color, consistency, and amount of drainage (for each wound); the presence and location of drains
● additional procedures, such as irrigation, packing, or application of a topical medication
● type and amount of new dressing or pouch applied
● patient's tolerance of the procedure.

Expected outcomes
The patient will:
● express pain relief
● exhibit wound healing.

Complications
A complication of a dressing change is an allergic reaction to an antiseptic cleaning agent, a prescribed topical medication, or adhesive tape. This reaction may lead to skin redness, a rash, excoriation, or infection. Other complications for patients with surgical wounds include wound dehiscence and evisceration or infection.

Documentation
Document special or detailed wound care instructions and pain management steps and the patient's response on the care plan. Record the color and amount of drainage on the intake and output sheet. (See *Documenting surgical incision care.*)

Supportive references

Hallett, C. "Infection Control in Wound Care: A Study of Fatalism in Community Nursing," *Journal of Clinical Nursing* 9(1):103-109, January 2000.

Perry, A.G., and Potter, P.A. *Clinical Nursing Skills and Techniques,* 6th ed. St Louis: Mosby–Year Book, Inc., 2005.

Ultraviolet light therapy

Light therapy is a viable alternative for a variety of conditions, such as psoriasis, eczema, vitiligo, mycosis fungoides, and other dermatoses. Typically, patients require anywhere from 20 to 30 treatments to see results, depending on the severity of their condition.

According to the Dermatology Nurses' Association, the staff should gather information for immediate needs and also for future reference for a patient about to be treated with light therapy. Important information needed during the initial interview includes:
- chief complaint
- allergies
- current medications
- medical history. **DNA**

Questions should also be asked about family history. Areas of discussion should include a history of skin cancers and of photodermatoses. A family history of a photodermatoses, such as lupus, may negate the use of phototherapy in treatment. **DNA**

Ultraviolet (UV) light causes profound biological changes, including UV light-induced immune suppression and temporary suppression of epidermal basal cell division followed by a later increase in cell turnover. Emitted by the sun, the UV spectrum is subdivided into three bands — A, B, and C — each of which affects the skin differently. Ultraviolet A (UVA) radiation (with a relatively long wavelength of 320 to 400 nm) rapidly darkens preformed melanin pigment, may augment ultraviolet B (UVB) in causing sunburn and skin aging, and may induce phototoxicity in the presence of some drugs. UVB radiation (with a wavelength of 280 to 320 nm) causes sunburn and erythema. Ultraviolet C (UVC) radiation (with a wavelength of 200 to 280 nm) is usually absorbed by the earth's ozone layer and doesn't reach the ground. However, UVC kills bacteria and is used in operating room germicidal lamps.

The drug methoxsalen, a psoralen agent, creates artificial sensitivity to UVA by binding with the deoxyribonucleic acid in epidermal basal cells. Treating skin with a photosensitizing agent, such as methoxsalen, and UVA is called psoralen plus UVA (PUVA) therapy (or photochemotherapy). Administered before a UV light treatment, methoxsalen photosensitizes the skin to enhance therapeutic effect. Other drugs used in photochemotherapy in combination with PUVA include acitretin (Soriatane), an oral vitamin A derivative, and methotrexate. Topical preparations, such as crude coal tar, may be used in combination with UVB (known as the *Goeckerman treatment*).

Contraindications to PUVA and UVB therapy include a history of photosensitivity diseases, skin cancer, arsenic ingestion, or cataracts or cataract surgery; current use of a photosensitivity-inducing drug; and previous skin irradiation (which can induce skin cancer). UV light therapy is also contraindicated in patients who have undergone previous ionizing chemotherapy and patients who are using a photosensitizing drug or an immunosuppressant. PUVA is contraindicated in pregnant women. **DNA**

UV light therapy requires a team approach to be safe and effective. Implementing the treatment plan requires knowledge, skills, and expertise of the entire health care team.

Equipment

UVA radiation
Fluorescent black-light lamp •high-intensity UVA fluorescent bulbs

UVB radiation
Fluorescent sunlamp or hot quartz lamp •sunlamp bulbs

All UV treatments
Oral or topical phototherapeutic medications, if necessary •body-sized light chamber or smaller light box •dark, polarized goggles •sunscreen, if necessary • hospital gown •towels

Preparation of equipment
The patient can undergo UV light therapy in the hospital, physician's office, or at home. Typically set into a reflective cabinet, the light source consists of a bank of high-intensity fluorescent bulbs. (At home, the patient may use a small fluorescent sunlamp.)

Check the practitioner's orders to confirm the light treatment type and dose. For PUVA, the initial dose is based on the patient's skin type and is increased according to the treatment protocol and as tolerated. (See *Comparing skin types*.) The physician calculates the UVB dose based on skin type estimation or by determining a minimal erythema dose—the smallest amount of UV light needed to produce mild erythema.

Implementation

● Confirm the patient's identity using two patient identifiers according to facility policy. **JCAHO**
● Inform the patient that UV light treatments produce a mild sunburn that helps to reduce or resolve skin lesions. **PCP**
● Review the patient's health history for contraindications to UV light therapy. Ask whether he's taking a photosensitizing drug, such as an anticonvulsant, antihypertensive, phenothiazine, salicylate, sulfonamide, tetracycline, tretinoin, or a drug for cancer. **DNA**
● If the patient is to have PUVA therapy, make sure he takes methoxsalen (with food) $1\frac{1}{2}$ hours before treatment.
● To begin therapy, instruct the patient to disrobe and put on a hospital gown. Have him remove the gown or expose just the treatment area after he's in the phototherapy unit. Make sure he wears goggles *to protect his eyes* and sunscreen, towels, or a hospital gown *to protect vulnerable skin areas.* All male patients receiving PUVA must wear protection over the groin area.
● If the patient is having local UVB treatment, position him at the correct distance from the light source. For example, for facial treatment with a sunlamp, position the patient's face about 12″ (30.5 cm) from the lamp. For body treatment, position the patient's body about 30″ (76 cm) from either the sunlamp or the hot quartz lamp.
● During therapy, make sure the patient wears goggles at all times. If you're observing him through light-chamber windows, you should wear goggles as well. If the patient must stand for the treatment, ask him to report dizziness *to ensure his safety.* **DNA**
● After delivering the prescribed UVB dose, help the patient out of the unit, and instruct him to shield exposed areas of skin from sunlight for 8 hours after therapy.

Comparing skin types

Skin type	Sunburn and tanning history
I	Always burns; never tans; sensitive ("Celtic" skin)
II	Burns easily; tans minimally
III	Burns moderately; tans gradually to light brown (average Caucasian skin)
IV	Burns minimally; always tans well to moderately brown (olive skin)
V	Rarely burns; tans profusely to dark (brown skin)
VI	Never burns; deeply pigmented; not sensitive (black skin)

Special considerations

● Overexposure to UV light (sunburn) can result from prolonged treatment and an inadequate distance between the patient and light sources. It can also result from the use of photosensitizing drugs or from overly sensitive skin.
● Prevent eye damage by using gray or green polarized lenses during UVB therapy or UV-opaque sunglasses during PUVA therapy. The patient undergoing PUVA therapy should wear these glasses for 24 hours after treatment *because methoxsalen can cause photosensitivity.*
● Tell the patient to look for marked erythema, blistering, peeling, or other signs of overexposure 4 to 6 hours after UVB therapy and 24 to 48 hours after UVA therapy. In either case, the erythema should disappear within another 24 hours. Tell him that mild dryness and desquamation will occur in 1 to 2 days. Teach him appropriate skin care measures. (See *Skin care guidelines*, page 548.) Advise him to notify the physician if overexposure occurs. Typically, the physician recommends stopping treatment for a few days and then starting over at a lower exposure level. **DNA**
● Before giving methoxsalen or etretinate, check to ensure that baseline liver function studies have been done. Keep in mind that both drugs are hepatotoxic and are never given together. Liver function and blood lipid studies are required before treatment with

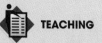

Skin care guidelines

A patient receiving ultraviolet (UV) light treatments must know how to protect his skin from injury. Provide the patient with the following skin care tips:

- Encourage the patient to use emollients and drink plenty of fluids *to combat dry skin and maintain adequate hydration.* Warn him to avoid hot baths or showers and to use soap sparingly. *Heat and soap promote dry skin.*
- Instruct the patient to notify his physician before taking medication, including aspirin, *to prevent heightened photosensitivity.*
- If the patient is receiving psoralen plus UVA therapy, review his methoxsalen dosage schedule. Explain that deviating from it could result in burns or ineffective treatment. Urge him to wear appropriate sunglasses outdoors for at least 24 hours after taking methoxsalen. Recommend yearly eye examinations *to detect cataract formation.*
- If the patient uses a sunlamp at home, advise him to let the lamp warm for 5 minutes before treatment. Stress the importance of exposing his skin to the light for the exact amount of time that the physician has prescribed. Instruct the patient to protect his eyes with goggles and to use a dependable timer or have someone else time his therapy. Above all, urge him never to use the sunlamp when he's tired *to avoid falling asleep under the lamp and sustaining a burn.*
- Teach the patient first aid for localized burning: Tell him to apply cool water soaks for 20 minutes or until skin temperature cools. For more extensive burns, recommend tepid tap water baths after notifying the physician about the burn. After the patient bathes, suggest using an oil-in-water moisturizing lotion (not a petroleum-jelly-based product, which can trap radiant heat).
- Tell the patient to limit natural light exposure, to use a sunscreen when he's outdoors, and to notify his physician immediately if he discovers unusual skin lesions.
- Advise the patient to avoid harsh soaps and chemicals, such as paints and solvents, and to discuss ways to manage physical and psychological stress, which may exacerbate skin disorders.

acitretin and at regular intervals during treatment. Liver function studies and a complete blood count are required before and during methotrexate treatment. **DNA**

- If the physician prescribes tar preparations with UVB treatment, watch for signs of sensitivity, such as erythema, pruritus, and eczematous reactions. If you apply carbonis detergens to the patient's skin before UV light therapy, be sure to remove it completely with mineral oil just before treatment begins *to let the light penetrate the skin.*

Nursing diagnoses

- Deficient knowledge (procedure)

Expected outcomes

The patient will:
- state an understanding of the procedure and postprocedure care.

Complications

Erythema is the major adverse effect of UVB therapy. Minimal erythema without discomfort is acceptable, but treatments are suspended if marked edema, swelling, or blistering occurs.

Erythema, nausea, and pruritus are the three major short-term adverse effects of PUVA therapy. Long-term adverse effects are similar to those caused by excessive exposure to sun — premature aging (xerosis, wrinkles, and mottled skin), lentigines, telangiectasia, increased risk of skin cancer, and ocular damage if eye protection isn't used. The patient can minimize effects by using emollients, sunscreens, and cover-ups.

Documentation

Record the date and time of initial and subsequent treatments, the UV wavelength used, and the name and dose of any oral or topical medications given. Record the exact duration of therapy, the distance between the light source and the skin, and the patient's tolerance. Note safety measures used such as eye protection. Describe the patient's skin condition before and after treatment. Note improvements and adverse reactions, such as increased pruritus, oozing, and scaling.

Supportive references

Lagan, K.M., et al. "Low-intensity Laser Therapy/ Combined Phototherapy in the Management of Chronic Venous Ulceration: A Placebo-controlled Study," *Journal of Clinical Laser Medical Surgery* 20(3):109-16, June 2002.

Venous ulcer care

Venous ulcers may result from trauma or develop after chronic venous insufficiency (CVI). In CVI, venous valves don't close completely, allowing blood to flow back from the deep venous system through the perforator veins into the superficial venous system. Over time, the weight of the backflow of blood causes a build-up of fluid and protein, which leaks into the surrounding tissues, resulting in edema, tissue breakdown, and ulceration. Venous ulcers may be shallow or extend into the deep muscle. The patient at risk for a venous ulcer may have a history of any of these conditions:

- deep vein thrombosis
- venous disease
- edema of the lower extremities.

Assess the intact skin surrounding the wound for pigmentation changes, erythema, induration, and maceration and exudate, and document the type, amount, odor, and color. Auscultate using a Doppler device or palpate for peripheral pulses. Measure and compare calf and ankle circumferences for both legs.

Treatment of venous ulcers is difficult because the damaged vein valves can't be repaired, which means that there's always the potential for new ulcers to form. In addition to providing local wound care, the underlying venous hypertension and edema need to be addressed. Although hospitalization usually isn't necessary, some patients are admitted to the hospital for treatment of cellulitis, which requires an I.V. antibiotic.

Combined with the appropriate dressing, external compression helps heal venous ulcers by compressing superficial veins and enhancing the effects of the calf muscle pump. This increases blood flow velocity in the deep venous system. Studies show that high compression is more effective than low compression. **WOCN**

When choosing a dressing, keep in mind that the goal is to provide a local wound environment that's conducive to healing. A moist environment promotes granulation and epithelial proliferation and migration. Typically, venous ulcers have a large amount of drainage and moisture, which decreases as the ulcer heals. When this occurs, choose a dressing that keeps the wound bed moist. Hydrocolloids, foams, gels, and other moist dressings are easy to apply and don't need to be changed daily. No studies have shown evidence to support one specific type of dressing or frequency of dressing change needed when dressings are used under compression wraps. **WOCN**

Venous ulcers are most commonly found around the ankle. They typically have irregular borders and are more likely to have copious drainage.

Equipment

Bedside table • normal saline solution • sterile and nonsterile 4″ × 4″ gauze pads • foam, gel or hydrocolloid dressing • hypoallergenic tape or elastic netting • piston-type irrigating system • two pairs of gloves • normal saline solution, as ordered • sterile cotton swabs • linen-saver pads • impervious plastic trash bag • disposable wound-measuring device (a square, transparent card with concentric circles arranged in bull's-eye fashion and bordered with a straight-edge ruler)

Preparation of equipment

Assemble equipment at the patient's bedside. Cut tape into strips for securing dressings. Loosen lids on cleaning solutions and medications for easy removal. Loosen existing dressing edges and tapes before putting on gloves. Attach an impervious plastic trash bag to the bedside table to hold used dressings and refuse.

Implementation

- Confirm the patient's identity using two patient identifiers according to facility policy. **JCAHO**
- Premedicate the patient as necessary.
- Wash your hands, and put on clean gloves. **CDC**
- Remove the previous dressing, and place it into the impervious trash bag. If the old dressing is dry, soak it with normal saline solution before removing, so that granulating tissue isn't removed when the dressing is pulled off. **CDC**
- Inspect the wound. Note the color, amount, and odor of drainage and necrotic debris. Measure the wound perimeter with the disposable wound-measuring device. **WOCN**

- Irrigate the wound with the piston-style syringe, using normal saline solution.
- Remove and discard your soiled gloves, and put on a fresh pair. **CDC**
- Insert a cotton-tipped swab into the wound to assess for tunneling depth. **WOCN**
- Use an appropriate supportive topical treatment based on the amount of exudate and as ordered. For example, use an absorbent dressing for ulcers with copious drainage. Maintain a moist healing environment.
- To apply a moist dressing, squeeze out the excess saline solution from the gauze layers. Place the layer of moist gauze into the wound. If there's tunneling, make sure the dressing is tucked loosely into the tunneled areas and that there's a moist dressing next to all the tissue in the wound, filling up all of the wound's dead space. Avoid overpacking the wound.
- Elevate the leg as ordered.
- Use compression therapy (Unna's boot, stockings, or electronic compression devices) and debridement as ordered.
- Provide patient support and education.
- Provide information about other therapies the patient may use including the following:
– Horse chestnut seed extract has been found to control pain and reduce edema of venous disease.
– Ultrasound has been found to aid in healing.
– Recombinant human keratinocyte growth factor-2 (Repifermin) can be used to accelerate wound healing. **WOCN**

Nursing diagnoses

- Acute pain
- Risk for infection

Expected outcomes

The patient will:
- express pain relief
- remain free from infection.

Complications

The common complication of a venous ulcer is infection.

Documentation

Document the ulcer's anatomic location; its length, width, and depth; and any tunneling. Record the appearance of the wound bed and the history of the patient's ulcer, including previous injuries or related surgeries. Record previous and current topical treatments and the date, time, and frequency of dressing changes.

Supportive references

McMullin, G.M. "Improving the Treatment of Leg Ulcers," *Medical Journal of Australia* 175(7):375-78, October 2001.

Wound, Ostomy and Continence Nurses Society (WOCN). *Guideline for Management of Wounds in Patients with Lower-Extremity Venous Disease.* Glenview, Ill.: WOCN; June 2005.

Zafar, A. "Management of Diabetic Foot — Two Years Experience," *Journal of Ayub Medical College, Abbottabad* 13(1):14-16, January-March 2001.

12

Obstetric, neonatal, and postpartum care

More than 4 million infants are born in the United States each year. Many of them are born with considerably less medical intervention than was customary in previous decades, yet many are conceived with considerably more medical intervention. Accompanying changes in maternal care are changes in neonatal care — thanks to the advanced knowledge and techniques for improving fetal monitoring and promoting neonatal survival.

If you're working with a pregnant patient, you'll need to employ all your teaching skills. You'll also need to be aware of what the best practice is for caring for the pregnant patient as recommended by such organizations as the American College of Obstetricians and Gynecologists **ACOG** and the Association of Women's Health, Obstetric, and Neonatal Nurses **AWHONN**. Care of the neonate requires knowledge of new clinical evaluation methods and electronic and biochemical monitoring techniques as well as knowledge of best practices as recommended by the National Association of Neonatal Nurses **NANN** and the American Academy of Pediatrics **AAP**. Organizations, such as the National Institutes of Health **NIH**, the Centers for Disease Control and Prevention **CDC**, the Joint Commission on Accreditation of Health Care Organizations **JCAHO**, and the American Hospital Association **AHospA** also offer guidelines to best practices in obstetric and neonatal care. Additional practices are evidence-based **EB**, grounded in the principles of fundamental science **Science**, or related to the American Hospital Association's Patient Care Partnership **PCP**. In addition, equipment manufacturers **MFR** may have specific guidelines or recommendations for the use of their equipment.

Because of its profound impact on mother and child, maternal-neonatal care requires expertise that goes beyond clinical skills. Such care requires clinical competence, sensitivity, and good judgment. It must consider the patient's sexuality and self-image and recognize changing social attitudes and values — especially those concerning childbirth and alternative methods of conception and childbirth. The information presented in this chapter covers the fundamentals of maternal-child care and presents evidence-based information so that you can provide the best care for both of your patients.

Amnioinfusion

Amnioinfusion is the replacement of amniotic fluid volume through an intrauterine infusion. It involves the infusion of a warmed isotonic solution, such as normal saline or lactated Ringer's solution, via an intrauterine pressure catheter into the amniotic cavity.

Amnioinfusion is indicated when umbilical cord compression is a factor or when repetitive variable decelerations aren't alleviated by maternal position change and oxygen administration. It also helps to relieve umbilical cord compression in such conditions as oligohydramnios associated with postmaturity, intrauterine growth retardation, preterm labor, and premature rupture of membranes. Although this procedure can be done to dilute meconium before aspiration occurs, a recent study suggests that for women in labor who have thick meconium staining of their amniotic fluid, amnioinfusion didn't decrease the risk of perinatal death, severe meconium aspiration syndrome, or other major neonatal or maternal disorders. **EB1**

Contraindications include amnionitis, placental abnormalities, hydramnois, and multiple gestation.

Equipment

Fetal heart rate (FHR) monitor • sterile intrauterine pressure catheter • normal saline solution or lactated Ringer's solution at room temperature • I.V. tubing

Implementation

- Confirm the patient's identity using two patient identifiers according to facility policy. **JCAHO**
- Explain the procedure and rationale for its use.
- Prepare the patient for the procedure, and encourage her to lie in a lateral recumbent position.
- Inform the patient that she'll feel fluid flowing out of her vagina during the procedure. **PCP**
- Be sure that the solution for the infusion is warmed to the patient's body temperature to avoid chilling.
- Institute continuous FHR monitoring if not already in place; obtain a baseline FHR tracing.
- The practitioner ruptures the membranes if they haven't ruptured spontaneously.
- The practitioner inserts a sterile pressure catheter through the cervix into the uterus.
- The catheter is attached via I.V. tubing to warmed isotonic solution.
- The fluid is administered rapidly over 20 to 30 minutes, usually 250 to 500 ml initially, and then the flow rate is adjusted based on FHR patterns. **EB2**
- Assist with infusion, and adjust flow rate as ordered to maintain fetal heart rate pattern demonstrating no variable decelerations.

After the procedure

- Continuously monitor FHR and uterine contractions.
- Assess temperature at least every hour to detect infection.
- Monitor the patient for a continuous flow of fluid via the vagina.
- Provide comfort measures, including frequent bed linen changes.
- Notify the practitioner if the fluid suddenly stops, an indication that the fetal head is engaged and fluid is collecting in the uterus — this could lead to hydramnios and, possibly, uterine rupture.

Nursing diagnoses

- Deficient knowledge (procedure)
- Risk for infection

Expected outcomes

The patient will:
- state an understanding of procedure and reason for doing it
- remain free from infection
- not exhibit an increase in body temperature.

Complications

Amnioinfusion is considered safe and effective, and complications are rare. Possible complications include umbilical cord prolapse, uterine scar disruption, iatrogenic polyhydramnios, elevated intrauterine pressure leading to fetal bradycardia, and amniotic fluid embolism.

Documentation

Document that the patient has signed an informed consent form. Keep accurate intake and output records during the procedure. Document FHR along with the maternal vital signs and response to treatment.

Supportive references

Fraser, W.D. et al. "Amnioinfusion for the Prevention of Meconium Aspiration Syndrome," *New England Journal of Medicine* 353(9):909-17, September 2005. **EB1**

Pillitteri, A. *Maternal & Child Health Nursing: Care of the Childbearing & Childrearing Family,* 5th ed. Philadelphia: Lippincott Williams & Wilkins, 2007. **EB2**

Apgar scoring

The Apgar assessment is a screening tool to assist health care providers in determining which medical and nursing interventions are needed to help the neonate successfully adapt from an intrauterine to an extrauterine environment.

Named after its developer, Virginia Apgar, the Apgar score quantifies the neonatal heart rate, respiratory effort, muscle tone, reflexes, and color. Each category is assessed 1 minute after birth and again 5 minutes later. Scores in each category range from 0 to 2. The highest Apgar score is 10 — the greatest possible sum of the five categories.

CONTROVERSIAL ISSUE *Several controversial issues surround the use of Apgar scores. First, Apgar scores may not be reliable when applied to premature neonates. Several criteria mea-*

Recording the Apgar score

Use this chart to record the neonatal Apgar score — assigning 0, 1, or 2 points for each of five signs — at 1 minute and at 5 minutes after birth. A score of 7 to 10 indicates good condition; 4 to 6, fair condition — the infant may have moderate central nervous system depression, muscle flaccidity, cyanosis, and poor respirations; 0 to 3, danger — the infant needs immediate resuscitation, as ordered.

Sign	Apgar score		
	0	1	2
Heart rate	Absent	Less than 100 beats/minute (slow)	More than 100 beats/minute
Respiratory effort	Absent	Slow, irregular	Good crying
Muscle tone	Flaccid	Some flexion and resistance to extension of extremities	Active motion
Reflex irritability	No response	Grimace or weak cry	Vigorous cry
Color	Pallor, cyanosis	Pink body, blue extremities	Completely pink

sured in the Apgar score are developmentally determined. These include muscle tone, which increases with gestational age; reflex irritability, which is more pronounced in a full-term neonate; and respiratory effort, which is decreased in a preterm neonate because of a decrease in surfactant production. Second, Apgar scores have been used to document birth asphyxia. The American Academy of Physicians (AAP) states that neither Apgar score nor low pH values alone can define the degree of perinatal asphyxia in a neonate. The AAP suggests that the term asphyxia should be reserved to describe a neonate with these conditions:
- profound metabolic or mixed acidemia (pH less than 7.0)
- Apgar score of 0 to 3 for longer than 5 minutes
- neonatal neurologic manifestations (seizures, coma, or hypotonia) **AAP**
- multisystem organ dysfunction.

Finally, the Apgar score should be assigned by health care providers who haven't provided direct nursing or medical care to the mother or fetus during labor. These individuals have direct involvement with birth outcomes, which may bias the scoring.

The evaluation at 1 minute indicates the neonate's initial adaptation to extrauterine life. The evaluation at 5 minutes gives a clearer picture of overall status after medical interventions have been implemented based on the appearance of the neonate at birth. If the neonate doesn't breathe or his heart rate is less than 100 beats/minute, call for help and begin resuscitation at once. Don't wait for a 1-minute Apgar test score.

Equipment

Apgar score sheet or neonatal assessment sheet • stethoscope • a clock with a second hand or Apgar timers • gloves (see *Recording the Apgar score*)

Preparation of equipment

If you use Apgar timers, make sure both timers are on at the instant of birth.

Implementation

- Note the exact time of delivery. Wear gloves for protection from blood and body fluids. Dry the neonate to prevent heat loss. **AWHONN** **CDC**
- Place the neonate in a 15-degree Trendelenburg position to promote mucus drainage. Position his head with the nose slightly tilted upward to straighten the airway. **Science**
- Assess the neonate's respiratory efforts. If necessary, supply stimulation by rubbing his back or gently flicking his foot. **NANN**
- If the neonate exhibits abnormal respiratory responses, begin neonatal resuscitation according to the

Dealing with a stillbirth

If a fetus that's mature enough to survive extrauterine life dies before or during delivery, the event is called a *stillbirth* and the fetus a *stillborn*. Features of maturity include gestational age of 16 weeks or more and length of 6¼" (16 cm) or more. Delivery of a less-mature fetus is called a *spontaneous abortion.*

Nursing interventions

In addition to measuring, weighing, identifying, and preparing the stillborn for the morgue, you'll need to provide emotional support to the parents. Whether the parents expected the stillbirth, they'll need comfort and care.

If the parents expected the stillbirth, help them continue working through their grief — especially if they have delayed grieving while waiting for delivery. If the parents didn't expect the stillbirth, help them to express their anger and relieve grief in positive ways. Refer them to appropriate support groups.

Offer bereaved parents the opportunity to hold the stillborn. If possible, provide a photograph, identification bracelet, or other memento. If they refuse these mementos now, file them with the chart so that they may obtain them later if desired.

guidelines of the American Heart Association (AHA) and the AAP. Use the Apgar score and the neonatal resuscitation AHA guidelines to judge the progress and success of resuscitation efforts. Should resuscitation efforts prove futile, you'll need to implement measures for dealing with stillbirth. (See *Dealing with a stillbirth.*)

● If the neonate exhibits normal responses, proceed to assign the Apgar score at 1 minute after birth.

● Repeat the evaluation and record the score at 5 minutes after birth.

Assessing heart rate

● Using a stethoscope, listen to the heartbeat for 30 seconds, and record the rate. To obtain beats per minute, double the rate. Alternatively, palpate the umbilical cord where it joins the abdomen, monitor pulsations for 6 seconds, and multiply by 10 to obtain beats per minute. Assign a 0 for no heart rate, a 1 for

a rate less than 100 beats/minute, and a 2 for a rate greater than 100 beats/minute. **NANN**

Assessing respiratory effort

● Count unassisted respirations for 60 seconds, noting quality and regularity (a normal rate is 30 to 60 respirations/minute). Assign a 0 for no respirations; a 1 for slow, irregular, shallow, or gasping respirations; and a 2 for regular respirations and vigorous crying.

Assessing muscle tone

● Observe the extremities for flexion and resistance to extension. This can be done by extending the limbs and observing their rapid return to flexion — the neonate's normal state. Assign a 0 for flaccid muscle tone, a 1 for some flexion and resistance to extension, and a 2 for normal flexion of elbows, knees, and hips, with good resistance to extension.

Assessing reflex irritability

● Observe the neonate's response to nasal suctioning or to flicking the sole of his foot. Assign a 0 for no response, a 1 for a grimace or weak cry, and a 2 for a vigorous cry.

Assessing color

● Observe skin color, especially at the extremities. Assign a 0 for complete pallor and cyanosis, a 1 for a pink body with blue extremities (acrocyanosis), and a 2 for a completely pink body. To assess color in a dark-skinned neonate, inspect the oral mucous membranes and conjunctivae, the lips, the palms, and the soles.

Special considerations

● If the patient and her support person don't know about the Apgar score, discuss it with them during early labor, when they're more receptive to new information. *To prevent confusion or misunderstanding at delivery,* explain to them what will occur and why. Explain to the parents that Apgar scores serve as a guide to assess the neonate's initial adaptation to extrauterine life.

● If the neonate requires emergency care, make sure a member of the delivery team provides appropriate support.

● Closely observe the neonate whose mother receives heavy sedation just before delivery. Despite a high Apgar score at birth, he may show secondary effects of sedation in the nursery. Be alert for depression or unresponsiveness.

Nursing diagnoses

- Anticipatory grieving
- Risk for delayed development

Expected outcomes

The patient will:
- express and accept feelings about anticipated death.

The neonate will:
- have an Apgar score between 7 and 10.

Complications

Neonate will have a score of less than 7. If the heart rate is less than 100 beats/minute or the neonate doesn't breath, begin resuscitation efforts.

Documentation

Record the Apgar score on the Apgar score sheet or the neonatal assessment sheet required by your facility. Be sure to indicate the total score and the signs for which points were deducted *to guide postnatal care.*

Supportive references

American Academy of Pediatrics and American College of Obstetricians and Gynecologists. *Guidelines for Perinatal Care,* 5th ed. Elk Grove Village, Ill.: AAP; Washington, D.C.: ACOG, 2002.

Casy, B.M., et al. "The Continuing Value of Apgar Score for the Assessment of Newborn Infants," *New England Journal of Medicine* 344(7):461-71, February 2001.

Olds, S.B., et al. *Clinical Handbook, Maternal-Newborn Nursing. A Family and Community Based Approach,* 6th ed. Upper Saddle River, N.J.: Prentice Hall Health, 2000.

Wong, D.L., et al. *Maternal-Child Nursing Care,* 3rd ed. St. Louis: Mosby–Year Book, Inc., 2006.

Apnea monitoring

Apnea in a neonate is defined as cessation of breathing for 20 seconds or longer, or for a shorter period if accompanied by cyanosis or bradycardia. (See *Categories of apnea.*) Apnea monitors provide an early alert to the caregiver when the breathing rate ceases, allowing for immediate life-saving interventions. These monitors may be used for vulnerable neonates,

Categories of apnea NIH

Apnea has long been recognized as a clinical problem in neonates. Considerable investigative and clinical attention has been directed toward this condition. Although progress has been made and certain categories of apnea have been delineated, the cause remains unclear in many situations.

- *Apnea* is the cessation of respiratory airflow. This pause in respiration can be the result from central or diaphragmatic (no respiratory effort), obstructive (usually due to upper airway obstruction), or mixed causes. Short (15 seconds), central apnea can be normal at all ages.
- *Pathologic apnea* is characterized by cyanosis; abrupt, marked pallor or hypotonia; or bradycardia and a prolonged respiratory pause.
- *Periodic breathing* is a breathing pattern in which there are three or more respiratory pauses of greater than 3 seconds' duration with less than 20 seconds of respiration between pauses. Periodic breathing can be a normal event.
- *Apnea of prematurity* is periodic breathing with pathologic apnea in a premature neonate. Apnea of prematurity usually ceases by 37 weeks' gestation but occasionally persists to several weeks past term.
- *Apparent life-threatening event* is an episode characterized by some combination of apnea (central or occasionally obstructive), color change (usually cyanotic or pallid but occasionally erythematous or plethoric), marked change in muscle tone (usually marked limpness), choking, or gagging.
- *Apnea of infancy* is an unexplained episode of cessation of breathing for 20 seconds or longer, or a shorter respiratory pause associated with bradycardia, cyanosis, pallor, and marked hypotonia.

Source: "Infantile Apnea and Home Monitoring." *NIH Consensus Statement Online* 6(6):1-10, September-October, 1986.

such as those born prematurely, those who have survived a life-threatening medical emergency, and those who have a neurologic disorder, neonatal respiratory distress syndrome, bronchopulmonary dysplasia, congenital heart disease with heart failure, a tracheostomy, a history of sleep-induced apnea, a family history of sudden infant death syndrome, or acute drug with-

Using a home apnea monitor

When a neonate in your care requires the use of a home apnea monitor, you'll need to prepare his parents to operate the equipment safely, correctly, and confidently. First, review the neonate's breathing problem with his parents. Explain that the monitor warns them of breathing or heart rate changes. Then offer the following guidelines:

- Advise the parents to prepare their home and family for the equipment — for example, by providing a sturdy, flat surface for the monitor and by posting emergency telephone numbers (physician, nurse, equipment supplier, and ambulance) accessibly.
- Teach other responsible family members how to use the monitor safely. Suggest that older siblings, grandparents, babysitters, and other caregivers learn cardiopulmonary resuscitation (CPR).
- Instruct the parents to notify local service authorities — police, ambulance, telephone company, and electric company — if their neonate uses an apnea monitor *so that alternative power can be supplied if a failure occurs.*
- Explain to the parents how a monitor with electrodes works. Advise them to make sure the respiration indicator goes on each time the neonate breathes. If it doesn't, describe troubleshooting techniques, such as moving the electrodes slightly. Tell them to try this technique several times.
- Show the parents how to respond to either the apnea or bradycardia alarm. Direct them to check the color of the neonate's oral tissues. If the tissues appear bluish and the neonate isn't breathing, tell them to call loudly and touch him — gently at first, then more urgently as needed. Tell them to stop short of shaking him. If he doesn't respond, urge them to begin CPR.
- Also, advise the parents to keep the operator's manual attached to or beside the monitor and to consult it as needed. Explain that an activated loose-lead alarm, for example, may indicate a dirty electrode, a loose electrode patch, a loose belt, or a disconnected or malfunctioning wire or monitor.

drawal. According to the American Academy of Pediatrics, cardiorespiratory monitoring shouldn't be done at home for neonates to prevent sudden infant death syndrome. Research hasn't proven that monitoring has prevented sudden infant death. **AAP**

Two types of monitors are used most commonly. The thoracic impedance monitor uses chest electrodes to detect conduction changes caused by respirations. The newest models have alarm systems and memories that record cardiorespiratory patterns. The apnea mattress, or underpad monitor, relies on a transducer connected to a pressure-sensitive pad, which detects pressure changes resulting from altered chest movements.

To guard against potentially life-threatening apneic episodes in vulnerable neonates, monitoring begins in the hospital or birthing center and continues at home. Parents need to learn how to operate the monitor, which actions to take when the alarm sounds, and how to revive a neonate with cardiopulmonary resuscitation (CPR). Crucial steps for correctly using a monitor include testing the alarm system, positioning the sensor properly, and setting the controls correctly. (See *Using a home apnea monitor.*)

According to the National Institutes of Health (NIH), the criteria for discontinuing monitoring should be based on the neonate's clinical condition. **NIH** Clinical experience and the literature support monitor discontinuation when neonates with apparent life-threatening events have had 2 to 3 months free from significant alarms or apnea (vigorous stimulation or resuscitation wasn't needed). Additionally, assessing the neonate's ability to tolerate stress (such as immunizations and illnesses) during this time is advisable. Requiring one or more normal pneumograms before discontinuing the monitor may needlessly prolong the monitoring period.

Equipment

Monitor unit • electrodes • lead wires • electrode belt • electrode gel, if needed • pressure transducer pad, if using apnea mattress • stable surface for monitor placement

Prepackaged and pretreated disposable electrodes are available.

Implementation

- Confirm the neonate's identity using two patient identifiers according to facility policy. **JCAHO**
- Explain the procedure to the parents, as appropriate, and wash your hands. **CDC** **PCP**
- Plug the monitor's power cord into a grounded wall outlet. Attach the leadwires to the electrodes, and attach the electrodes to the belt. If appropriate, apply conduction gel to the electrodes. (Or, apply gel to the neonate's chest, place the electrodes atop the gel, and attach the electrodes to the leadwires. Secure the belt.) **MFR**
- To hold the electrodes securely in position, wrap the belt snugly but not restrictively around the neonate's chest at the point of greatest movement — optimally at the right and left midaxillary line about 3/4″ (2 cm) below the axillae. Be sure to position the leadwires according to the manufacturer's instructions.
- Follow the color code to connect the leadwires to the patient cable. Connect the cable to the proper jack at the rear of the monitoring unit.
- Turn the sensitivity controls to maximum to facilitate tuning when adjusting the system.
- Set the alarms according to recommendations so that an apneic period lasting for a specified time activates the signal.
- Turn on the monitor. If the monitor has two alarms — one to signal apnea, one to signal bradycardia — both will sound until you adjust the monitor and reset the alarms according to the manufacturer's instructions.
- Adjust the sensitivity controls until the indicator lights blink with each breath and heartbeat.
- If you use an apnea mattress, assemble the monitor and pressure transducer pad according to the manufacturer's directions.
- Plug the monitor into a grounded wall outlet. Plug the cable of the transducer pad into the monitor.
- Touch the pad to make sure it works. Watch for the monitor's respiration light to blink.
- Follow the manufacturer's instructions for pad placement.
- If you have difficulty obtaining a signal, place a foam rubber pad under the mattress, and sandwich the transducer pad between the foam pad and the mattress.
- If you hear the apnea or bradycardia alarm during monitoring, immediately check the neonate's respira-

tions and color, but don't touch or disturb him until you confirm apnea.
- If he's still breathing and his color is good, readjust the sensitivity controls or reposition the electrodes, if necessary.
- If he isn't breathing but his color looks normal, wait 10 seconds to see if he starts breathing spontaneously. If he isn't breathing and he appears pale, dusky, or blue, immediately try to stimulate breathing in these ways: Sequentially, place your hand on the neonate's back, rub him gently, or flick his soles gently. If he doesn't begin to breathe at once, start CPR. (For detailed instructions, see "Cardiopulmonary resuscitation," page 217.)

Special considerations

- *To ensure accurate operation,* don't put the monitor on top of another electrical device. Make sure that it's on a level surface and that it can't be easily bumped.
- Avoid applying lotions, oils, or powders to the neonate's chest, *where they could cause the electrode belt to slip.* Periodically check the alarm by disconnecting the sensor plug. Listen for the alarm to sound after the preset time delay.
- In addition to apnea monitoring, the neonate will frequently receive a respiratory stimulant, such as theophylline or caffeine. **EB**

🔖 **TEACHING** *Safety must be emphasized during patient teaching because monitors may cause electrical burns. Parental instruction should include the following points:*
- *Remove the electrodes when the neonate isn't attached to the monitor.*
- *Unplug the cord from the electrical outlet when the cord isn't plugged into the monitor.*
- *Use safety covers over electrical outlets to prevent injury to children.*
- *Supervise children when in contact with the neonate on the home apnea monitor.*
- *Teach children that the apnea monitor isn't a toy.*

Nursing diagnoses

- Ineffective breathing pattern

Expected outcomes

The neonate will:
- show no signs of respiratory distress
- exhibit a normal respiratory rate.

Complications

An apneic episode resulting from upper airway obstruction may not trigger the alarm if the neonate continues to make respiratory efforts without gas exchange. However, the monitor's bradycardia alarm may be triggered by the decreased heart rate resulting from the vagal stimulation (which accompanies obstruction).

If you're using a thoracic impedance monitor without a bradycardia alarm, you may interpret bradycardia during apnea as shallow breathing. That's because this type of monitor fails to distinguish between respiratory movement and the large cardiac stroke volume associated with bradycardia. In this case, the alarm won't sound until the heart rate drops below the apnea limit. Use of thoracic impedance apnea monitors would require an additional cardiac respiratory monitor so that bradycardia could be assessed when the heart rate begins to drop at 100 beats/ minute.

Documentation

Record all alarm incidents. Document the time and duration of apnea. Describe the neonate's color, the event that occurred before the apneic episode, the stimulation measures implemented, and other pertinent information. Document any medications given.

Supportive references

American Academy of Pediatrics. "Policy Statement: Apnea, Sudden Infant Death Syndrome, and Home Monitoring," *Pediatrics* 111(4):914-17, April 2003.

Bhatia, J. "Current Options in the Management of Apnea of Prematurity," *Clinical Pediatrics* 39(6):327-36, June 2000. **EB**

Pillitteri, A. *Maternal & Child Health Nursing: Care of the Childbearing & Childrearing Family,* 5th ed. Philadelphia: Lippincott Williams & Wilkins, 2007.

Wong, D.L., et al. *Maternal-Child Nursing Care,* 3rd ed. St. Louis: Mosby–Year Book, Inc., 2006.

Circumcision

Steeped in controversy and history, circumcision (the removal of the penile foreskin) is thought to promote a clean glans and to minimize the risk of phimosis (tightening of the foreskin) in later life.

Current scientific evidence indicates potential medical benefits for the circumcised male neonate. Stud-

ies have shown that circumcision may reduce the risk of penile cancer, decreases the risk of contracting a urinary tract infection, and reduces the risk of contracting a sexually transmitted disease. After reviewing available research, however, the American Academy of Pediatrics (AAP) concluded that there are no absolute medical indications for routine circumcision. They recommend that the parents should be provided with information about the potential benefits and risks and counseled to make a decision that's in the best interest of their child. The AAP also states that if the decision is made for circumcision, procedural analgesia should be provided. **AAP**

In Judaism, circumcision is a religious rite (known as a *bris*) performed by a *mohel* (a specialist trained in both the medical procedure and Jewish law) on the 8th day after birth, when the neonate officially receives his name. Because most neonates are discharged before this time, the bris rarely occurs in the hospital.

There are two methods used in practice for performing circumcision. These include use of the Gomco or Mogen clamp and use of the Plastibell.

Circumcision using a Gomco or Mogen clamp involves using the clamp to stabilize the penis while removing the foreskin. With this device, a cone that fits over the glans provides a cutting surface and protects the glans penis. The other technique uses a plastic circumcision bell (Plastibell) over the glans and a suture tied tightly around the base of the foreskin. This method prevents bleeding. The resultant ischemia causes the foreskin to slough off within 5 to 8 days. This method is thought to be painless because it stretches the foreskin, which inhibits sensory conduction.

Circumcision is contraindicated in neonates who are ill or who have bleeding disorders, ambiguous genitalia, or congenital anomalies of the penis, such as hypospadias or epispadias, because the foreskin may be needed for later reconstructive surgery. **AAP**

Equipment

Circumcision tray (contents vary but usually include circumcision clamps, various-sized cones, scalpel, probe, scissors, forceps, sterile basin, sterile towel, and sterile drapes) • povidone-iodine solution or chlorhexidine solution • restraining board with arm and leg restraints • sterile gloves • petroleum gauze • sterile 4″ × 4″ gauze pads • optional: sutures, plastic circumcision bell, antimicrobial ointment, topical or local anesthetic • sterile marker • sterile labels • overhead warmer

Preparation of equipment

Circumcision using a Gomco clamp: Assemble the sterile tray and other equipment in the procedure area. Open the sterile tray, and pour povidone-iodine solution into the sterile basin. Using sterile technique, place sterile 4″ × 4″ gauze pads and petroleum gauze on the sterile tray. Arrange the restraining board, and direct adequate light on the area.

    Circumcision using a plastic circumcision bell: Assemble sterile gloves, sutures, restraining board, petroleum gauze and, if ordered, antibiotic ointment.

    A *mohel* usually brings his own equipment.

Preparing for analgesia administration **AAP**

Several methods are available to provide analgesia to the neonate during a circumcision.
- Label all medications, medication containers, and other solutions on and off the sterile field. **JCAHO**
- Eutectic mixture of local anesthetics (EMLA) cream consists of the application of a cream containing 2.5% lidocaine and 2.5% prilocaine, administered 60 to 90 minutes before the procedure along with the application of an occlusive dressing. Research indicates that neonates who receive EMLA cream spend less time crying and have less of an increase in heart rate during the procedure.
- Dorsal penile nerve block (DPNB) is administered using a 27G needle to inject 0.4 ml of 1% lidocaine at both the 10 and 2 o'clock positions at the base of the penis. Bruising at the injection site is the most reported complication.
- Subcutaneous ring block (SRB) involves administration of 0.8 ml of 1% lidocaine at the midshaft of the penis. The SRB appears to prevent crying and increases in heart rate more consistently than DPNB or EMLA cream. No complications have been reported to date.
- Neonates should also be given acetaminophen immediately postcircumcision for pain relief.

Implementation
- Confirm the neonate's identity using two patient identifiers according to facility policy. **JCAHO**

- Make sure the parents understand the procedure and have signed the proper consent form. **PCP**
- Withhold feeding for at least 1 hour before the procedure to reduce the possibility of emesis and aspiration. **AAP**
- Place the neonate on a padded restraining board. To decrease distress during the procedure, restrain his arms and legs only while the procedure is in progress. Remain with the neonate to offer comfort and provide a safe environment. **NANN**
- Assist the physician as necessary throughout the procedure, and comfort the neonate as needed.

Using a Gomco clamp
- After putting on sterile gloves, the physician cleans the penis and scrotum with povidone-iodine or chlorhexidine solution and drapes the neonate. **AAP** **AWHONN** **CDC**
- He then applies a Gomco clamp to the penis, loosens the foreskin, inserts the cone under it *to provide a cutting surface and to protect the penis,* and removes the foreskin.
- He covers the wound with sterile petroleum gauze *to prevent infection and control bleeding.*

Using a plastic bell
- The physician slides the plastic bell device between the foreskin and the glans penis.
- He then ties a suture tightly around the foreskin at the coronal edge of the glans. The foreskin distal to the suture becomes ischemic and then atrophic. After 5 to 8 days, the foreskin drops off with the plastic bell attached, leaving a clean, well-healed excision. No special care is required, but watch for swelling that may indicate infection or interfere with urination.

Providing aftercare
- Remove the neonate from the restraining board, and assess for bleeding.
- If povidone-iodine was used before the procedure, wash it off with sterile water. **AWHONN**
- Place him on his back to minimize pressure on the excision area. Leave him diaperless for 1 to 2 hours to observe for bleeding and to reduce possible chafing and irritation.
- Show the neonate to his parents to reassure them that he's all right.
- When you rediaper the neonate, change his diaper as soon as he voids. If the dressing falls off, clean the

wound with warm water *to minimize pain from urine on the circumcised area and prevent irritation.* Don't remove the original dressing until it falls off (usually after the first or second voiding).

● Check for bleeding every 15 minutes for the 1st hour and then every hour for the next 24 hours. If bleeding occurs, apply pressure with sterile gauze pads. Notify the physician if bleeding continues. **NANN**

● Loosely diaper the neonate *to prevent irritation.* At each diaper change, apply ordered antimicrobial ointment, petroleum jelly, or petroleum gauze until the wound appears healed. Avoid leaving the neonate under the radiant warmer after placing petroleum gauze on the penis *because the area might burn.*

● Watch for drainage, redness, or swelling. Don't remove the thin, yellow-white exudate that forms over the healing area within 1 to 2 days. *This normal incrustation protects the wound until it heals in 3 to 4 days.* **NANN**

● Don't discharge the neonate until he has voided.

Special considerations

● Show parents the circumcision before discharge so they can ask questions and you can teach them how to care for the area.

● If the neonate's mother has human immunodeficiency virus (HIV) infection, circumcision is delayed until the physician knows the neonate's HIV status. The neonate whose mother has HIV infection has a higher-than-normal risk of infection.

TEACHING *Inform the mother that the circumcision site will have a yellowish discharge on the glans for several days after the circumcision. Tell her that this signifies healing and isn't a cause for concern.*

Instruct the mother to observe the circumcision site regularly for pus or bloody discharge, which may indicate delayed healing or infection. If these signs occur, she should notify the physician.

Tell the mother that the rim of the Plastibell device used for circumcision may remain in place after discharge from the facility. Reassure her that the rim will fall off harmlessly in 1 week. However, if the rim doesn't fall off after 1 week, tell her to notify the physician. A retained rim may lead to infection.

Instruct the mother to clean the circumcised area with cotton balls moistened with tap water for the

first 3 to 4 days to prevent irritation. **AWHONN** *Don't apply soap to the area until it's well healed.*

Nursing diagnoses

● Risk for infection

Expected outcomes

The neonate will:

● remain free from infection.

Complications

After a Gomco clamp procedure, bleeding, the most frequent complication, is observed in about 0.1% of all circumcisions. Infection is the second most common complication and is usually minor. The skin of the penile shaft can adhere to the glans, resulting in scarring or fibrous bands. The most severe complications are urethral fistulae, penile necrosis, necrotizing fasciitis, sepsis, and meningitis. Incomplete amputation of the foreskin can follow application of the plastic circumcision bell.

Documentation

Note the time, date, and type of circumcision performed. Record the neonate's vital signs, the appearance of the circumcision site, parent teaching, and any excessive bleeding. Most neonates are observed until their first voiding postprocedure and then discharged home.

Supportive references

American Academy of Pediatrics. "Prevention and Management of Pain and Stress in the Neonate," *Pediatrics* 105(2):454-61, February 2000.

Anand, K.J.S., and the International Evidence-Based Group for Neonatal Pain. "Consensus Statement for the Prevention of Pain in the Newborn," *Archives of Pediatric and Adolescent Medicine* 155:1730-780, 2001.

Association of Women's Health, Obstetric and Neonatal Nurses (AWHONN). Neonatal Skin Care. Evidence-based Clinical Practice Guideline. Washington, D.C.: AWHONN, January 2001. *www.guideline.gov.*

Byers, J.F., and Thornley, K. "Cuing into Infant Pain," *The American Journal of Maternal/Child Nursing* 29(2):84-89, March-April 2004.

Kaufman, M.W., et al. "Neonatal Circumcision — Benefits, Risks, and Family Teaching," *The American*

Journal of Maternal Child/Nursing 26(4):197-201, July-August 2001.

Emergency delivery

Emergency delivery, the unplanned birth of a neonate outside of a health care facility, may occur when labor progresses quickly or when circumstances prevent the mother from entering a facility. Whether assisting at an emergency delivery or instructing the person who is, your objectives include establishing a clean, safe, and private birth area; promoting a controlled delivery; preventing injury, infection, and hemorrhage; and maintaining a calm, supportive environment.

Equipment

Unopened newspaper or a large, clean cloth (such as a tablecloth, towel, or curtain) • bath towel, blanket, or coat • gloves • at least two small, clean cloths • clean, sharp object (such as scissors, new razor blade, knife, or nail file) • ligating material (such as string, yarn, ribbon, or new shoelaces) • a clean blanket or towel (to cover the neonate) • boiling water

Preparation of equipment

Boil the ligating and cutting materials for at least 5 minutes, if possible.

Implementation

● Offer support and reassurance *to help relieve the patient's anxiety.* Encourage the patient to pant or blow during contractions *to promote a controlled delivery.* As possible, provide privacy, wash your hands, and put on gloves. **CDC**
● Position the patient comfortably on a bed, a couch, or the ground. Open the newspaper or the large, clean cloth, and place it under the patient's buttocks *to provide a clean delivery area.* Elevate the buttocks slightly with the bath towel, blanket, or coat *to cushion and support the patient's buttocks.*
● The mother should lie on her side until the neonate is nearly ready to be delivered.
● Check for signs of imminent delivery — bulging perineum, an increase in bloody show, urgency to push, and crowning of the presenting part. **ACOG**
● As the fetal head reaches and begins to pass the perineum, instruct the patient to pant or blow through the contractions *because forceful bearing down could cause extensive maternal lacerations.* Place one hand against the area below the vaginal opening, and apply gentle pressure during each contraction. Your other hand should be placed gently against the vaginal opening over the neonate's head, which controls how quickly the neonate's head is delivered. **ACOG**
● Avoid forcibly restraining fetal descent because undue pressure can cause cephalohematoma or scalp lacerations, head trauma, and vagal stimulation. Undue pressure may also occlude the umbilical cord, which may cause fetal bradycardia, circulatory depression, and hypoxia.
● As the fetal head emerges, immediately break the amniotic sac if it's intact. Support the head as it emerges. Instruct the patient to continue blowing and panting. **ACOG**
● Locate the umbilical cord. Insert one or two fingers along the back of the emergent head *to be sure the cord isn't wrapped around the neck.* If the cord is wrapped loosely around the neck, slip it over the head *to prevent prolonged cord compression, tearing of the cord, or interrupted delivery.* If it's wrapped tightly around the neck, ligate the cord in two places using string, yarn, ribbon, or new shoelaces. Carefully cut between the ligatures, using a clean, sharp object or, if possible, a sterile one. **ACOG**

✓ **CLINICAL IMPACT** *If the delivery takes place outside of the health care facility, don't cut the umbilical cord unless you have a cutting instrument (scissors or knife) that has been boiled in water for at least 10 minutes. Instead, continue trying to deliver the rest of the fetus.*

● Carefully support the head with both hands as it rotates to one side (external rotation). Gently wipe mucus and amniotic fluid from the nose and mouth with a clean, small cloth *to prevent aspiration.* **ACOG**
● Instruct the patient to bear down with the next contraction *to aid delivery of the shoulders.* Position your hands on either side of the neonate's head, and support the neck. Exert gentle downward pressure *to deliver the anterior shoulder.* Exert gentle upward pressure *to deliver the posterior shoulder.*
● Remember that amniotic fluid and vernix are slippery, so take care to support the neonate's body securely after freeing the shoulders.
● Keep the neonate in a slightly head-down position *to encourage mucus to drain from the respiratory tract.* Wipe excess mucus from his face. If the neo-

nate doesn't breathe spontaneously, gently pat the soles of his feet or stroke his back. *Never suspend a neonate by his feet.* **ACOG**

● Dry and cover the neonate quickly with the blanket or towel. Ensure that his head is well covered *to minimize exposure and prevent heat loss.*

● Cradle the neonate at the level of the maternal uterus until the umbilical cord stops pulsating. This prevents the neonatal blood from flowing to or from the placenta and leading to hypovolemia or hypervolemia, respectively. Hypovolemia can lead to circulatory collapse and neonatal death; hypervolemia can cause hyperbilirubinemia.

● Place the neonate on the mother's abdomen in a slightly head-down position.

● Ligate the umbilical cord at two points, 1″ to 2″ (2.5 to 5 cm) apart. Place the first ligature 4″ to 6″ (10 to 15 cm) from the neonate. *Ligation prevents autotransfusion, which may cause hemolysis and hyperbilirubinemia.*

✓ CLINICAL IMPACT *In a normal delivery, there's no rush to cut the umbilical cord; it should be cut only with sterilized instruments. Placing one tie around the cord and leaving it alone is better than cutting it with instruments that haven't been sterilized.*

● Use sterile instruments to cut the umbilical cord. *Using unsterile ones may cause infection.*

● Watch for signs of placental separation, such as a slight gush of dark blood from the vagina, cord lengthening, and a firm uterine fundus rising within the abdominal area. Usually, the placenta separates from the uterus within 5 minutes after delivery (although it may take as long as 30 minutes). When you see these signs, encourage the patient to bear down *to expel the placenta.* As she does, apply gentle downward pressure on her abdomen *to aid placental delivery.* Never tug on the umbilical cord at this time *because doing so may invert the uterus or sever the cord from the placenta.* **ACOG**

● Examine the expelled placenta for intactness. Retained placental fragments may cause hemorrhage or lead to intrauterine infection. **ACOG** **AWHONN**

● Place the cord and the placenta inside the towel or blanket covering the neonate to provide extra warmth and also *to ensure that the cord and placenta will be transported to the hospital for closer examination.*

● Palpate the maternal uterus *to make sure it's firm.* Gently massage the atonic uterus *to encourage con-*

traction and prevent hemorrhage. Encourage breastfeeding, if appropriate, *to stimulate uterine contraction.*

● Check the patient for excessive bleeding from perineal lacerations. Apply a perineal pad, if available, and instruct the patient to press her thighs together. Provide comfort and reassurance, and offer fluids, if available. Have someone summon an emergency medical service, or arrange transportation to the hospital for the mother and neonate. Make sure the mother and neonate are warm and dry while they await transport. **AWHONN**

Special considerations

● Never introduce an object into the vagina to facilitate delivery. This increases the risk of intrauterine infection as well as injury to the cervix, uterus, fetus, umbilical cord, and placenta.

● In a breech presentation, make every effort to transport the patient to a nearby hospital. If the patient begins to deliver, carefully support the fetal buttocks with both hands. Gently lift the body to deliver the posterior shoulder. Lower the neonate slightly to deliver the anterior shoulder. Flexion of the head usually follows. Never apply traction to the body to avoid lodging the head in the cervix. Allow the neonate to rotate and emerge spontaneously.

● If the umbilical cord emerges first, elevate the presenting part, using your fingers to move the presenting part off of the umbilical cord to prevent cord compression, which causes fetal hypoxia. Because this obstetric emergency usually necessitates a cesarean delivery, arrange for immediate transport to a nearby hospital.

● If the neonate fails to breathe spontaneously after birth, clear the airway and begin to breathe for him. Place your opened mouth over his nose and mouth. Using air collected in your cheeks, deliver two effective breaths (produce visible chest rise). Next, check the umbilical cord for pulsation. If the neonate's heart rate is less than 60 beats/minute, begin cardiopulmonary resuscitation (CPR). Compressions should be delivered on the lower third of the sternum, with the depth of compressions equaling $1/2$″ to $3/4$″ (1 to 2 cm). There are two techniques for external cardiac massage. One method involves placing two thumbs on the sternum, superimposed or adjacent to each other depending on the neonate's size, with fingers encircling the chest and supporting the back. Administer a breath of air, and then use your thumbs gently but firmly to pump the heart. The second method involves placing the tips of the middle and index fingers of one hand on the lower third of the sternum for compressions. Pump three times for each ventilation. Continue performing CPR until the neonate breathes and his heart rate is 60 beats/minute or higher. **AHA**

Nursing diagnoses
● Risk for injury

Expected outcomes
The patient will:
● establish a good labor pattern
● deliver the neonate without complications.

Complications
Injury to mother or neonate, infection, and hemorrhage are all possible complications.

Documentation
Give the medical care team the following information if possible: the time of delivery; the presentation and position of the fetus; delivery complications, such as the cord wrapped around the neonate's neck; the color, character, and amount of amniotic fluid; and the mother's blood type and Rh factor, if known. Note the time of placental expulsion, the placental appearance and intactness, the amount of postpartum bleeding, the status of uterine firmness (tone) and contractions, and the mother's response.

Document the sex of the neonate, estimate the Apgar score, and define any resuscitative measures used. Record whether the mother began breast-feeding the neonate. Identify and quantify fluids given to the mother.

Supportive references
American Academy of Pediatrics and American College of Obstetricians and Gynecologists. *Guidelines for Perinatal Care,* 5th ed. Elk Grove Village, Ill.: AAP; Washington, D.C.: ACOG, 2002.

Kattwinkel, J., et al. *Maternal and Fetal Evaluation and Immediate Newborn Care.* Charlottesville, Va.: Perinatal Continuing Education Program, 2001. *www.pcep.org/book_1.html.*

Olds, S.B., et al. *Clinical Handbook, Maternal-Newborn Nursing. A Family and Community Based Approach,*

6th ed. Upper Saddle River, N.J.: Prentice Hall Health, 2000.

Wong, D.L., et al. *Maternal-Child Nursing Care,* 3rd ed. St. Louis: Mosby–Year Book, Inc., 2005.

Eye prophylaxis

The instillation of antibiotic ointment into the neonate's eyes prevents blindness and eye damage from conjunctivitis due to *Neisseria gonorrhoeae* and *Chlamydia,* which the neonate may have acquired from the mother as he passed through the birth canal. This treatment is legally required in most states. **CDC** It's recommended to prevent gonococcal ophthalmia, but whether it's effective against chlamydial eye infections is unclear. The best way to prevent gonococcal and chlamydial ophthalmia is to treat pregnant women prenatally, but because many women don't get prenatal care, eye prophylaxis is required. **CDC** **EB**

The Centers for Disease Control and Prevention recommends a single application of erythromycin (0.5%) ointment or tetracycline ophthalmic ointment (1%).

Equipment
Antibiotic ointment or aqueous solution in a single dose ointment tube • sterile gloves • dry gauze pads

Implementation
● Confirm the neonate's identity using two patient identifiers according to facility policy. **JCAHO**
● Explain the procedure to the parents if present, informing them that the neonate will probably cry and that eye irritation may occur. **PCP**
● Wash your hands and put on gloves.
● Wipe the neonate's face with dry gauze.
● To ensure comfort and effectiveness, shield the neonate's eye's from direct light and tilt his head slightly to the side of the intended treatment.
● Using your nondominant hand, gently raise the neonate's upper eyelid with your index finger and pull the lower eyelid down with your thumb.
● Using your dominant hand, instill a 1- to 2-cm ribbon of ointment along the lower conjunctival sac, from the inner canthus to the outer canthus. (See *Instilling eye medication,* page 564.)

Instilling eye medication

Using your nondominant hand, gently raise the neonate's upper eyelid with your index finger and pull down the lower eyelid with your thumb. Using your dominant hand, apply the ordered ophthalmic antibiotic ointment in a line along the lower conjunctival sac (as shown below). Then close the eyes to allow ointment to spread across the conjunctiva. Repeat the procedure for the other eye.

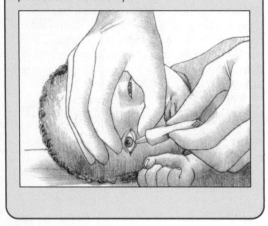

- Close the neonate's eye to allow the ointment to be distributed across the conjunctiva.
- Repeat the steps with the other eye.

Special considerations

- Use a single-dose ointment tube to prevent contamination and the spread of infection.
- Keep in mind that although the procedure may be administered in the birthing room, treatment can be delayed for up to 1 hour to allow initial parent-child bonding.
- Assess the neonate's eyes for chemical conjunctivitis evidenced by redness, swelling, and drainage or discoloration of the skin around the neonate's eyes.
- If chemical conjunctivitis or discoloration occurs, inform the parents that these effects are temporary and will subside within a few days.
- Document the procedure appropriately on the birthing room record or in the progress notes.

Nursing diagnoses

- Risk for infection

Expected outcomes

The neonate will:
- remain free from infection.

Complications

Failure to instill the eye prophylaxis can result in the neonate developing blindness or eye damage from conjunctivitis from *Neisseria gonorrhoeae*.

Documentation

Document the drug, dose, route, site, date, and time of administration.

Supportive references

Department of Health and Human Services, Centers for Disease Control and Prevention. "Sexually Transmitted Diseases Treatment Guidelines 2002." *www.cdc.gov/ STD/treatment/4-2002TG.htm.* **EB**

Fetal heart rate

Fetal heart rate (FHR) is the best way to determine fetal well-being during gestation and labor. It may be assessed by auscultating with a fetoscope or a Doppler ultrasound stethoscope placed on the maternal abdomen. The fetoscope relies on bone conduction to assist with hearing the opening and closing of the fetal ventricular heart valves. The Doppler device uses ultrasound technology to detect heart motion, such as moving heart walls or valves. Both methods have been approved by the American College of Obstetricians and Gynecologists and the Association of Women's Health, Obstetric, and Neonatal Nurses.

Normal FHR ranges from 110 to 160 beats/minute. Auscultation can easily be used to detect fetal tachycardia (heart rate greater than 160 beats/minute) and bradycardia (heart rate less than 110 beats/minute), and it allows the examiner to determine whether the rhythm is regular or irregular.

Auscultation requires the ability to distinguish among the fetal heart sounds generated. FHR must also be distinguished from similar sounds created by the maternal pulse in the uterine vessels. The uterine bruit, or souffle sounds that are simultaneous with the maternal pulse, could be confused with the FHR. Practitioners should check maternal and fetal heart rates because false conclusions about fetal status could be reached if the maternal sounds are considered to be fetal heart sounds. **ACOG** **AWHONN**

Instruments for hearing fetal heart sounds

The fetoscope and the Doppler stethoscope are basic instruments for auscultating fetal heart sounds and assessing fetal heart rate (FHR).

Fetoscope

A fetoscope can detect fetal heartbeats as early as the 20th gestational week. As an assessment tool during labor, the fetoscope is helpful for hearing fetal heart sounds when contractions are mild and infrequent.

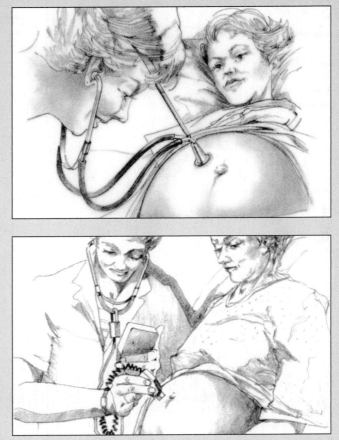

Doppler stethoscope

The Doppler stethoscope can detect fetal heartbeats as early as the 10th gestational week. Useful throughout labor, the Doppler stethoscope is more sensitive than the fetoscope.

With a clear sound that both the mother and the examiner can easily hear, this device provides a digital display of the FHR. Features include a "freeze" button to hold the reading until it's recorded, an optional 10-second manual count mode, and an automatic shutoff to save power.

Baseline rhythm can also be assessed with auscultation. The presence of an irregularity in the baseline rate can best be detected when listening with an auscultation device that allows practitioners to hear the actual heart sounds. **AWHONN**

CLINICAL IMPACT *An irregular rate can also be heard with the Doppler device; however, it's important to keep in mind that the sound that the Doppler generates isn't the actual heart sound but a mechanical representation of the heart rate.*

Because auscultation can detect gross (but in many instances late) fetal distress signs (tachycardia and bradycardia), the technique remains useful in an uncomplicated, low-risk pregnancy. In a high-risk pregnancy, indirect external or direct internal electronic fetal monitoring gives more accurate information on fetal status.

Equipment

Fetoscope or Doppler stethoscope (see *Instruments for hearing fetal heart sounds*) • water-soluble lubri-

Performing Leopold's maneuvers

You can determine fetal position, presentation, engagement, and attitude by performing Leopold's maneuvers. Ask the patient to empty her bladder, assist her to a supine position, and place a small rolled towel under her right hip to prevent supine hypotension syndrome. Expose her abdomen, and then perform the four maneuvers in order.

First maneuver

Face the patient and warm your hands. Place them on her abdomen *to determine fetal presentation in the uterine fundus.* Curl your fingers around the fundus. With the fetus in vertex position, the buttocks feel irregularly shaped and firm. With the fetus in breech presentation, the head feels hard, round, and movable.

Second maneuver

Move your hands down the sides of the abdomen, and apply gentle pressure. If the fetus lies in vertex position, you'll feel a smooth, hard surface on one side — the fetal back. Opposite, you'll feel lumps and knobs — the knees, hands, feet, and elbows. If the fetus lies in breech position, you may not feel the back at all.

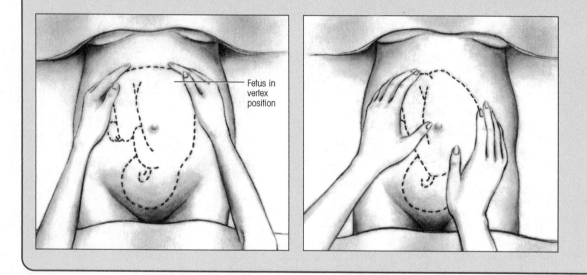

Fetus in vertex position

cant (for ultrasound instrument) • watch with second hand

Implementation

● Confirm the patient's identity using two patient identifiers according to facility policy. **JCAHO**
● Explain the procedure to the patient, wash your hands, and provide privacy. **PCP** Reassure the patient that you may reposition the listening instrument frequently *to hear the loudest fetal heart sounds.*
● Assist the patient to a supine position, placing a wedge under the right hip, and drape her appropri-

ately *to minimize exposure.* If you're using the Doppler stethoscope, apply the water-soluble lubricant to the patient's abdomen or Doppler stethoscope. *This gel or paste creates an airtight seal between the skin and the instrument and promotes optimal ultrasound wave conduction and reception.*

Calculating FHR during gestation

● To assess FHR in a fetus age 20 weeks or older, place the earpieces in your ears and position the bell of the fetoscope or Doppler stethoscope on the abdominal midline above the pubic hairline. After 20

Third maneuver

Spread apart the thumb and fingers of one hand. Place them just above the patient's symphysis pubis. Bring your fingers together. If the fetus lies in vertex presentation (and hasn't descended), you'll feel the head. If the fetus lies in vertex presentation (and has descended), you'll feel a less distinct mass. Apply gentle pressure to the fundus with your other hand to help facilitate the maneuver.

Fourth maneuver

Use this maneuver in late pregnancy. The purpose of the fourth maneuver is to determine flexion or extension of the fetal head and neck. Place your hands on both sides of the lower abdomen. Apply gentle pressure with your fingers as you slide your hands downward, toward the symphysis pubis. If the head presents, one hand's descent will be stopped by the cephalic prominence. The other hand will be unobstructed. If the cephalic prominence is on the side opposite the back, the attitude is flexion; if it's on the same side as the fetal back, then the attitude is extension.

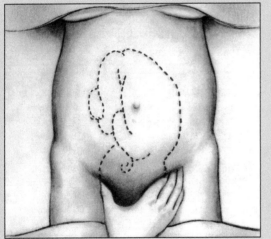

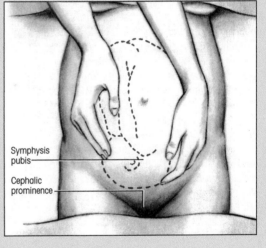

Symphysis pubis

Cephalic prominence

weeks, when you can palpate fetal position, use Leopold's maneuvers *to locate the back of the fetal thorax.* Position the listening instrument over the fetal back. (See *Performing Leopold's maneuvers.*) Because the presentation and position of the fetus may change, most clinicians don't perform Leopold's maneuvers until 32 to 34 weeks' gestation. **AWHONN**

● Using a Doppler stethoscope, place the earpieces in your ears, and press the bell gently on the patient's abdomen. Start listening at the midline, midway between the umbilicus and the symphysis pubis. Or, using a fetoscope, place the earpieces in your ears with the fetoscope positioned centrally on your forehead. Gently press the bell about 1/2″ (1 cm) into the patient's abdomen. Remove your hands from the fetoscope *to avoid extraneous noise.* **AWHONN**

● Move the bell of either instrument slightly from side to side, as necessary, *to locate the loudest heart sounds.* After locating these tones, palpate the maternal pulse.

● While monitoring the maternal pulse rate (*to avoid confusing maternal heart sounds with fetal heart sounds*), count the fetal heartbeats for at least 15 seconds. If the maternal radial pulse and the FHR are the same, try to locate the fetal thorax by using Leopold's maneuvers; then reassess FHR. Usually, the fetal heart beats faster than the maternal heart does. Record the FHR.

Counting FHR during labor

● Allow the mother and her support person to listen to the fetal heart if they wish. *This helps to make the fetus a greater reality for them.* Record their participation. **AWHONN**

● Position the fetoscope or Doppler stethoscope on the abdomen — midway between the umbilicus and symphysis pubis *for cephalic presentation,* or at the umbilicus or above *for breech presentation.* Locate the loudest heartbeats, and simultaneously palpate the maternal pulse *to ensure that you're monitoring the fetal pulse rate rather than the maternal one.* **AWHONN**

● Monitor maternal pulse rate, and count fetal heartbeats for 60 seconds during the relaxation period between contractions *to determine baseline FHR.* In a low-risk labor, assess FHR every 60 minutes during the latent phase, every 30 minutes during the active phase, and every 15 minutes during the second stage of labor. In a high-risk labor, assess FHR every 30 minutes during the latent phase, every 15 minutes during the active phase, and every 5 minutes during the second stage of labor. **AWHONN** **EB**

● Auscultate FHR during a contraction and for 30 seconds after the contraction *to identify the response to the contraction.*

● Notify the physician or nurse-midwife immediately if you observe marked changes in FHR from baseline values (especially during or immediately after a contraction when signs of fetal distress typically occur). If fetal distress develops, begin indirect or direct electronic fetal monitoring. **AWHONN**

● Repeat the procedure as ordered.

● Auscultate before administration of medications, before ambulation, and before artificial rupture of membranes.

● Auscultate after rupture of membranes, after changes in the characteristics of the contractions, after ambulation, after vaginal examinations, and after administration of medications. **AWHONN**

Special considerations

● If you're auscultating FHR with a Doppler stethoscope, be aware that obesity and hydramnios can interfere with sound-wave transmission, making accurate results more difficult to obtain. If the physician orders continuous FHR monitoring, apply the ultrasound transducer to the patient's abdomen. The monitor will provide a printed record of the FHR.

● The tocotransducer may also be applied to monitor the contractile pattern at this time.

Nursing diagnoses

● Deficient knowledge (procedure)

Expected outcomes

The patient will:

● recognize the need for monitoring.

Complications

None

Documentation

Record FHR and the maternal pulse rate on the flowchart. Record each auscultation, and note tolerance to activity or treatment.

Supportive references

ACOG, Practice Bulletin, Clinical Management Guidelines for Obstetrician-Gynecologists No. 62. "Intrapartum Fetal Heart Rate Monitoring," *Obstetrics and Gynecology* 105(5 Pt 1):1161-169, May 2005. **EB**

Chez, B.F., et al. "Intrapartum Fetal Monitoring: Past, Present, and Future," *Journal of Perinatal Neonatal Nursing* 14(3):1-18, December 2000.

Feinstein, N.F., et al. "Fetal Heart Rate Auscultation: Comparing Auscultation to Electronic Fetal Monitoring," *AWHONN Lifelines* 4(3):35-44, June-July 2000.

Goodwin, L. "Intermittent Auscultation of the Fetal Heart Rate: A Review of General Principles," *Journal of Perinatal Neonatal Nursing* 14(3):53-61, December 2000.

Fetal monitoring, external

External monitoring is an indirect, noninvasive procedure that uses two devices strapped to the mother's abdomen to evaluate fetal well-being during labor. One device, an ultrasound transducer, transmits high-frequency sound waves through soft body tissues to the fetal heart. The waves rebound from the heart, and the transducer relays them to a monitor. The other, a pressure-sensitive tocotransducer, responds to the pressure exerted by uterine contractions and si-

Applying an external electronic fetal monitor

Fetal heart rate monitor

Palpate the uterus to locate the fetus's back. If possible, place the ultrasound transducer over this site where the fetal heartbeat sounds the loudest. Then tighten the belt. Use the fetal heart tracing on the monitor strip to confirm the transducer's position.

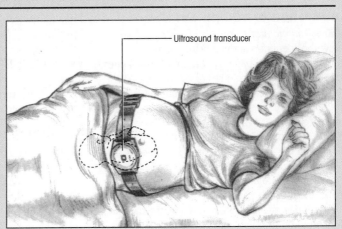

Ultrasound transducer

Labor monitor

A tocotransducer records uterine motion during contractions. Place the tocotransducer over the uterine fundus where it contracts, either midline or slightly to one side. Place your hand on the fundus, and palpate a contraction to verify proper placement. Secure the tocotransducer's belt, and then adjust the pen set so that the baseline values read between 5 and 15 mm Hg on the monitor strip.

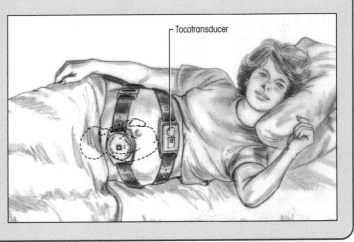

Tocotransducer

multaneously records their duration and frequency. (See *Applying an external electronic fetal monitor*.) The monitoring apparatus traces fetal heart rate (FHR) and uterine contraction data onto the same paper.

Indications for external fetal monitoring include high-risk pregnancy, oxytocin-induced labor, maternal medical illness (such as gestational diabetes, hypertension, or asthma) and antepartal nonstress, contraction stress tests, and psychosocial factors, such as tobacco, alcohol, drug use, and lack of prenatal care. Many labor and delivery units use external fetal monitoring for all patients. The procedure has no contraindications, but it may be difficult to perform on patients with hydramnios, on obese patients, or on hyperactive or premature fetuses. **AAP**

Equipment

Electronic fetal monitor • ultrasound transducer • tocotransducer • conduction gel • transducer straps • damp cloth • printout paper

Monitoring devices, such as phonotransducers and abdominal electrocardiogram transducers, are commercially available. However, facilities use these devices less frequently than they use the ultrasound transducer.

Preparation of equipment

Because fetal monitor features and complexity vary, review the operator's manual before proceeding. If the monitor has two paper speeds, select the higher speed (typically 3 cm/minute) *to ensure an easy-to-read tracing.* At slower speeds (for example, 1 cm/minute), the printed tracings are difficult to decipher and interpret accurately.

Plug the tocotransducer cable into the uterine activity jack and the ultrasound transducer cable into the phono-ultrasound jack. Attach the straps to the tocotransducer and the ultrasound transducer. **MFR**

Label the printout paper with the patient's identification number or birth date and name, the date, maternal vital signs and position, the paper speed, and the number of the strip paper *to maintain accurate, consecutive monitoring records.*

If your facility has central monitoring capabilities, enter the patient data into the central computer *to ensure accurate labeling of monitor strips.*

Implementation

● Explain the procedure to the patient, and provide emotional support. Inform her that the monitor may make noise if the pen set tracer moves above or below the printed paper. Reassure her that this doesn't indicate fetal distress. As appropriate, explain other aspects of the monitor *to help reduce maternal anxiety about fetal well-being.* **PCP**
● Make sure the patient has signed a consent form, if required.
● Wash your hands, and provide privacy. **CDC**
● Confirm the patient's identity using two patient identifiers according to facility policy. **JCAHO**

Beginning the procedure

● Assist the patient to the semi-Fowler or a left-lateral position with her abdomen exposed. Don't let her lie in a supine position *because pressure from the gravid uterus on the maternal inferior vena cava may cause maternal hypotension and decreased uterine perfusion and may induce fetal hypoxia.* **Science**
● Palpate the patient's abdomen to locate the fundus — the area of greatest muscle density in the uterus. Using transducer straps, secure the tocotransducer over the fundus. **AWHONN**

● Adjust the pen set tracer controls so that the baseline values read between 5 and 15 mm Hg on the monitor strip. This prevents triggering of the alarm that indicates that the tracer has dropped below the paper's margins. The proper setting varies among tocotransducers.
● Apply conduction gel to the ultrasound transducer crystals to promote an airtight seal and optimal sound-wave transmission.
● Use Leopold's maneuvers to palpate the fetal back, through which fetal heart sounds resound most audibly. **AWHONN**
● Start the monitor. Apply the ultrasound transducer directly over the site having the strongest heart sounds. **AWHONN**
● Activate the control that begins the printout. On the printout paper, note coughing, position changes, drug administration, vaginal examinations, and blood pressure readings that may affect interpretation of the tracings.
● Explain to the patient and her support person how to time and anticipate contractions with the monitor. Inform them that the distance from one dark vertical line to the next on the printout grid represents 1 minute. The support person can use this information to prepare the patient for the onset of a contraction and to guide and slow her breathing as the contraction subsides. **PCP**

Monitoring the patient

● Observe the tracings *to identify the frequency and duration of uterine contractions,* but palpate the uterus to determine intensity of contractions.
● Mentally note the baseline FHR — the rate between contractions — *to compare with suspicious-looking deviations.* FHR normally ranges from 110 to 160 beats/minute. **AWHONN**
● Assess periodic accelerations or decelerations from the baseline FHR. Compare FHR patterns with those of the uterine contractions. Note the time relationship between the onset of an FHR deceleration and the onset of a uterine contraction, the time relationship of the lowest level of an FHR deceleration to the peak of a uterine contraction, and the range of FHR deceleration. *These data help distinguish fetal distress from benign head compression.* **AWHONN**
● Move the tocotransducer and the ultrasound transducer to accommodate changes in maternal or fetal position. Readjust both transducers every hour, and

assess the patient's skin for reddened areas caused by the strap pressure. Document skin condition.

● Clean the ultrasound transducer periodically with a damp cloth *to remove dried conduction gel,* which can interfere with ultrasound transmission. Apply fresh gel as necessary. After using the ultrasound transducer, replace the cover over it.

Special considerations

● If the monitor fails to record uterine activity, palpate for contractions. Check for equipment problems according to the manufacturer's instructions and readjust the tocotransducer.
● If the patient reports discomfort in the position that provides the clearest signal, try to obtain a satisfactory 5- to 10-minute tracing with the patient in this position before assisting her to a more comfortable position. As the patient progresses through labor and abdominal pressure increases, the pen set tracer may exceed the alarm boundaries.

Nursing diagnoses

● Deficient knowledge (procedure)

Expected outcomes

The patient will:
● state an understanding of and the reason for the procedure.

Complications

None

Documentation

Make sure you numbered each monitor strip in sequence and labeled each printout sheet with the patient's identification number or birth date and name, the date, the time, and the paper speed. Record the time of vaginal examinations, membrane rupture, drug administration, and maternal or fetal movements. Record maternal vital signs and the intensity of uterine contractions. Document each time that you moved or readjusted the tocotransducer and ultrasound transducer, and summarize this information in your notes.

Supportive references

ACOG Practice Bulletin. Clinical Management Guidelines for Obstetrician-Gynecologists. No. 62. "Intrapartum Fetal Heart Rate Monitoring," *Obstetrics and Gynecology* 105(5 Pt 1):1161-169, May 2005.

Chez, B.F., et al. "Intrapartum Fetal Monitoring: Past, Present, and Future," *Journal of Perinatal Neonatal Nursing* 14(3):1-18, July 2000.

Mahlmeister, L. "Legal Implications of Fetal Heart Assessment," *Journal of Obstetric, Gynecologic, and Neonatal Nurses* 29(5):517-26, September-October 2000.

Pillitteri, A. *Maternal & Child Health Nursing: Care of the Childbearing & Childrearing Family,* 5th ed. Philadelphia: Lippincott Williams & Wilkins, 2007.

Wong, D.L., et al. *Maternal-Child Nursing Care,* 3rd ed. St. Louis: Mosby–Year Book, Inc., 2005.

Fetal monitoring, internal

Also called *direct fetal monitoring,* internal fetal monitoring is a sterile, invasive procedure that uses a spiral electrode and an intrauterine catheter to evaluate fetal status during labor. By providing an electrocardiogram (ECG) of the fetal heart rate (FHR), internal electronic fetal monitoring assesses fetal response to uterine contractions more accurately than external fetal monitoring. Internal FHR monitoring allows evaluation of short- and long-term FHR variability. The intrauterine catheter measures uterine pressure during contraction and relaxation.

Internal fetal monitoring is indicated whenever direct, beat-to-beat FHR monitoring is required. Specific indications include maternal diabetes or hypertension, fetal postmaturity, suspected intrauterine growth retardation, and meconium-stained fluid. However, internal monitoring is performed only if the amniotic sac has ruptured, the cervix is dilated at least 2 cm, and the presenting part of the fetus is at least at the –1 station. **ACOG** **AWHONN**

Contraindications for internal fetal monitoring include maternal blood dyscrasias, suspected fetal immune deficiency, placenta previa, face presentation or uncertainty about the presenting part, maternal human immunodeficiency virus-positive status, and cervical or vaginal herpetic lesions. **ACOG**

A spiral electrode is the most commonly used device for internal fetal monitoring. Shaped like a corkscrew, the electrode is attached to the presenting fetal part (usually the scalp). It detects the fetal heartbeat and then transmits it to the monitor, which converts the signals to a fetal ECG waveform.

A pressure-sensitive catheter, though not as widely used as the tocotransducer, is the most accurate method of determining the true intensity of contractions. Although it's especially helpful in dysfunctional labor and in preventing or rapidly determining the need for a cesarean section, the risk of infection or uterine perforation associated with this device is high.

Equipment

Electronic fetal monitor • spiral electrode and a drive tube • disposable leg plate pad or reusable leg plate with Velcro belt • conduction gel • antiseptic solution • hypoallergenic tape • two pairs of sterile gloves • intrauterine catheter connection cable and pressure-sensitive catheter • graph paper • operator's manual

Preparation of equipment

Be sure to review the operator's manual before using the equipment. **MFR** If the monitor has two paper speeds, set the speed at 3 cm/minute *to ensure a readable tracing.* A tracing at 1 cm/minute is more condensed and harder to interpret accurately. **AWHONN**

Connect the intrauterine cable to the uterine activity outlet on the monitor. Wash your hands and open the sterile equipment, maintaining sterile technique.

Implementation

● Describe the procedure to the patient and her partner, if present, and explain how the equipment works. Tell the patient that a physician or specially trained nurse will perform a vaginal examination *to identify the position of the fetus.* **PCP**
● Make sure the patient is fully informed about the procedure and that a signed consent form has been obtained.
● Confirm the patient's identity using two patient identifiers according to facility policy. **JCAHO** Then label the printout paper with the patient's identification number or name and birth date, the date, the paper speed, and the number on the monitor strip.

Monitoring contractions

● Assist the patient into the lithotomy position *for a vaginal examination.* The physician puts on sterile gloves.
● Attach the connection cable to the appropriate outlet on the monitor marked UA (uterine activity). Con-

nect the cable to the intrauterine catheter. Next, zero the catheter with a gauge provided on the distal end of the catheter. *This helps to determine the resting tone of the uterus, usually 5 to 15 mm Hg.*
● Cover the patient's perineum with a sterile drape, if facility policy dictates. Clean the perineum with antiseptic solution, according to facility policy. Using sterile technique, the physician inserts the catheter into the uterine cavity while performing a vaginal examination. The catheter is advanced to the black line on the catheter and secured with hypoallergenic tape along the inner thigh. **AWHONN**
● Observe the monitoring strip *to verify proper placement of the catheter guide and to ensure a clear tracing.* Periodically evaluate the monitoring strip to determine the exact amount of pressure exerted with each contraction. Note all such data on the monitoring strip and on the patient's medical record. **AWHONN**
● The intrauterine catheter is usually removed during the second stage of labor or at the physician's discretion. Dispose of the catheter, and clean and store the cable according to facility policy. (See *Applying an internal electronic fetal monitor.*)

Monitoring FHR

● Apply conduction gel to the leg plate. Secure the leg plate to the patient's inner thigh with Velcro straps or 2″ tape. Connect the leg plate cable to the ECG outlet on the monitor.
● Inform the patient that she'll undergo a vaginal examination to identify the fetal presenting part (which is usually the scalp or buttocks), to determine the level of fetal descent, and to apply the electrode. Explain that this examination is done to ensure that the electrode isn't attached to the suture lines, fontanels, face, or genitalia of the fetus. The spiral electrode will be placed in a drive tube and advanced through the vagina to the fetal presenting part. *To secure the electrode,* mild pressure will be applied and the drive tube will be turned clockwise 360 degrees. **PCP**
● After the electrode is in place and the drive tube has been removed, connect the color-coded electrode wires to the corresponding color-coded leg plate posts.
● Turn on the recorder and note the time on the printout paper.

Applying an internal electronic fetal monitor

During internal electronic fetal monitoring, a spiral electrode monitors the fetal heart rate (FHR), and an internal catheter monitors uterine contractions.

Monitoring FHR

The spiral electrode is inserted after a vaginal examination that determines the position of the fetus. As shown at right, the electrode is attached to the presenting fetal part, usually the scalp or buttocks.

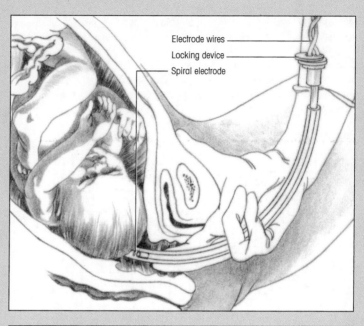

Electrode wires

Locking device

Spiral electrode

Monitoring uterine contractions

The intrauterine catheter is inserted up to a premarked level on the tubing and then connected to a monitor that interprets uterine contraction pressure.

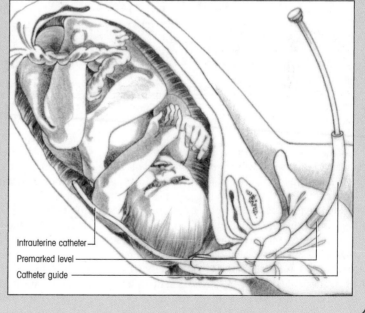

Intrauterine catheter

Premarked level

Catheter guide

Reading a fetal monitor strip

Presented in two parallel recordings, the fetal monitor strip records the fetal heart rate (FHR) in beats per minute in the top recording and uterine activity (UA) in mm Hg in the bottom recording. You can obtain information on fetal status and labor progress by reading the strips horizontally and vertically.

Reading horizontally on the FHR or the UA strip, each small block represents 10 seconds. Six consecutive small blocks, separated by a dark vertical line, represent 1 minute.

Reading vertically on the FHR strip, each block represents an amplitude of 10 beats/minute. Reading vertically on the UA strip, each block represents 5 mm Hg of pressure.

Assess the baseline FHR—the "resting" heart rate—between uterine contractions when fetal movement diminishes. This baseline FHR (normal range, 110 to 160 beats/minute) pattern serves as a reference for subsequent FHR tracings produced during contractions.

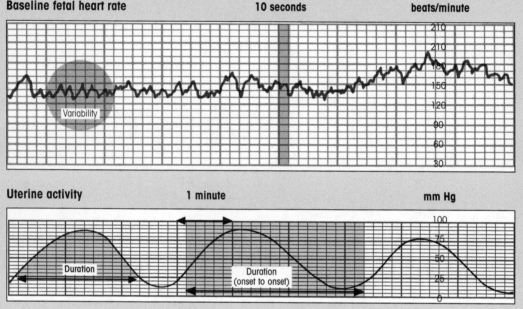

● Assist the patient to a comfortable position, and evaluate the strip *to verify proper placement and a clear FHR tracing.*

Monitoring the patient
● Begin by noting the frequency, duration, and intensity of uterine contractions. Normal intrauterine pressure ranges from 8 to 12 mm Hg. (See *Reading a fetal monitor strip.*) **AWHONN**
● Next, check the baseline FHR. Assess periodic accelerations or decelerations from the baseline FHR.

● Compare the FHR pattern with the uterine contraction pattern. Note the interval between the onset of an FHR deceleration and the onset of a uterine contraction, the interval between the lowest level of an FHR deceleration and the peak of a uterine contraction, and the range of FHR deceleration. **AWHONN**
● Check for FHR variability, which is a measure of fetal oxygen reserve and neurologic integrity and stability.
● When removing the spinal electrode, perform a vaginal examination and turn the electrode counter-

clockwise or until it releases from the fetal presenting part. Don't pull on the electrode. If it won't disconnect easily from the presenting part, it may be removed after delivery under direct visualization. The electrode should be removed just before a cesarean delivery. It should be brought through the uterine incision. If unable to detach, cut the wire at the perineum and notify the physician.

Special considerations

● Interpret the FHR and uterine contractions at regular intervals. Guidelines of the Association of Women's Health, Obstetric, and Neonatal Nurses specify that high-risk patients need continuous FHR monitoring, whereas low-risk patients should have the FHR auscultated every 30 minutes after a contraction during the first stage of labor and every 15 minutes after a contraction during the second stage of labor. **AWHONN**

● First, determine the baseline FHR within 10 beats/minute, and then assess the degree of baseline variability. Note the presence or absence of short- or long-term variability. Identify periodic FHR changes, such as decelerations (early, late, variable, or mixed), or nonperiodic changes, such as a sinusoidal pattern.

● Keep in mind that acute fetal distress can result from any change in the baseline FHR that causes fetal compromise. If necessary, take steps to counteract FHR changes. (See *Identifying baseline fetal heart rate irregularities,* pages 576 and 577.)

● If vaginal delivery isn't imminent (within 30 minutes) and fetal distress patterns don't improve, cesarean delivery is necessary.

CLINICAL IMPACT *Scalp electrode monitoring of the fetus provides the most accurate information used to assess fetal status. As with any electronic device, problems may occur that require immediate intervention. One critical inaccuracy that may occur is the recording of the maternal pulse when the fetus has expired in utero or is stillborn. With the loss of the fetal heartbeat, the monitor with a spiral electrode will pick up, conduct, and record the maternal heart rate. To verify that the heart rate being monitored is fetal, assess and document the maternal radial pulse with a Doppler ultrasound device. Ultrasound imaging can be used to document fetal heart motion and can verify the accuracy of the FHR.*

Nursing diagnoses

● Risk for infection

Expected outcomes

The mother and fetus will:
● remain free from infection.

Complications

Maternal complications of internal electronic fetal monitoring (EFM) may include uterine perforation and intrauterine infection. Fetal complications may include abscess, hematoma, and infection.

Documentation

Document all activity related to monitoring. (A fetal monitoring strip becomes part of the patient's permanent record, so it's considered a legal document.) Be sure to record the type of monitoring your patient received as well as all interventions. Identify the monitoring strip with the patient's name, her physician's name, your name, and the date and time. Document the paper speed and electrode placement.

Record the patient's vital signs according to standard practice. Note her pushing efforts, and record changes in her position. Document I.V. line insertion and changes in the I.V. solution or infusion rate. Note the use of oxytocin, regional anesthetics, or other medications.

After a vaginal examination, document cervical dilation and effacement as well as fetal station, presentation, and position. Document membrane rupture, including the time it occurred and whether it was spontaneous or artificial. Note the amount, color, and odor of the fluid. If internal EFM was used, document electrode placement.

Supportive references

ACOG Practice Bulletin. Clinical Management Guidelines for Obstetrician-Gynecologists. No. 62. "Intrapartum Fetal Heart Rate Monitoring," *Obstetrics and Gynecology* 105(5 Pt 1):1161-169, May 2005.

Chez, B.F., et al. "Intrapartum Fetal Monitoring: Past, Present, and Future," *Journal of Perinatal Neonatal Nursing* 14(3):1-18, December 2000.

Pillitteri, A. *Maternal & Child Health Nursing: Care of the Childbearing & Childrearing Family,* 5th ed. Philadelphia: Lippincott Williams & Wilkins, 2007.

(Text continues on page 578.)

Identifying baseline fetal heart rate irregularities

Irregularity	Possible causes	Clinical significance	Nursing interventions
Baseline tachycardia Beats/minute *[FHR tracing graph, scale 30–240]*	• Early fetal hypoxia • Maternal fever • Parasympathetic agents, such as atropine and scopolamine • Beta-adrenergics, such as ritodrine and terbutaline • Amnionitis (inflammation of inner layer of fetal membrane, or amnion) • Maternal hyperthyroidism • Fetal anemia • Fetal heart failure • Fetal arrhythmias	Persistent tachycardia without periodic changes usually doesn't adversely affect fetal well-being — especially when associated with maternal fever. However, tachycardia is an ominous sign when associated with late decelerations, severe variable decelerations, or lack of variability.	• Intervene to alleviate the cause of fetal distress and provide supplemental oxygen, as ordered. Also, administer I.V. fluids, as prescribed. • Discontinue oxytocin infusion *to reduce uterine activity.* • Turn the patient onto her left side and elevate her legs. • Continue to observe the fetal heart rate (FHR). • Document interventions and outcomes. • Notify the physician; further medical intervention may be necessary.
Baseline bradycardia Beats/minute *[FHR tracing graph, scale 30–240]*	• Late fetal hypoxia • Beta-adrenergic blockers, such as propranolol, and anesthetics • Maternal hypotension • Prolonged umbilical cord compression • Fetal congenital heart block	Bradycardia with good variability and no periodic changes doesn't signal fetal distress if FHR remains above 80 beats/minute. But bradycardia caused by hypoxia and acidosis is an ominous sign when associated with loss of variability and late decelerations.	• Intervene to correct the cause of fetal distress. Administer supplemental oxygen, as ordered. • Start an I.V. line and administer fluids, as prescribed. • Discontinue oxytocin infusion *to reduce uterine activity.* • Turn the patient onto her left side and elevate her legs. • Continue observing the FHR. • Document interventions and outcomes. • Notify the physician; further medical intervention may be necessary.
Early decelerations Beats/minute *[FHR tracing graph, scale 30–240]* mm Hg *[pressure tracing graph, scale 0–100]*	• Fetal head compression	Early decelerations are benign, indicating fetal head compression at dilation of 4 to 7 cm.	• Reassure the patient that the fetus isn't at risk. • Observe the FHR. • Document the frequency of decelerations.

Identifying baseline fetal heart rate irregularities *(continued)*

Irregularity	Possible causes	Clinical significance	Nursing interventions

Late decelerations

Beats/minute

mm Hg

- Uteroplacental circulatory insufficiency (placental hypoperfusion) caused by decreased intervillous blood flow during contractions or a structural placental defect such as abruptio placentae
- Uterine hyperactivity caused by excessive oxytocin infusion
- Maternal hypotension
- Maternal supine hypotension

Late decelerations indicate uteroplacental circulatory insufficiency and may lead to fetal hypoxia and acidosis if the underlying cause isn't corrected.

- Turn the patient onto her left side to increase placental perfusion and decrease contraction frequency.
- Increase the I.V. fluid rate to boost intravascular volume and placental perfusion, as prescribed.
- Administer oxygen by mask to increase fetal oxygenation, as ordered.
- Assess for signs of the underlying cause, such as hypotension or uterine tachysystole.
- Take other appropriate measures, such as discontinuing oxytocin, as prescribed.
- Document interventions and outcomes.
- Notify the physician; further medical intervention may be necessary.

Variable decelerations

Beats/minute

mm Hg

- Umbilical cord compression causing decreased fetal oxygen perfusion

Variable decelerations are the most common deceleration pattern in labor because fetal movement during contractions compresses the umbilical cord.

- Help the patient change position to relieve pressure on the cord. No other intervention is necessary unless you detect fetal distress.
- Assure the patient that the fetus tolerates cord compression well. Explain that cord compression affects the fetus the same way that breath-holding affects her.
- Assess the deceleration pattern for reassuring signs: a baseline FHR that isn't increasing, short-term variability that isn't decreasing, abruptly beginning and ending decelerations, and decelerations lasting less than 50 seconds. If assessment doesn't reveal reassuring signs, notify the physician.
- Start I.V. fluids and administer oxygen by mask at 10 to 12 L/minute, as prescribed.
- Document interventions and outcomes.
- Discontinue oxytocin infusion to decrease uterine activity.

Wong, D.L., et al. *Maternal-Child Nursing Care*, 2nd ed. St. Louis: Mosby–Year Book, Inc., 2002.

Fundal assessment, postpartum

After delivery, the uterus gradually shrinks and descends into its prepregnancy position in the pelvis — a process known as involution. To evaluate the involution process, the nurse will palpate the uterus to determine its size, firmness, and descent. Fundal massage is performed only when the uterus is boggy and soft. (See *Hand placement for fundal palpation and massage.*)

Hand placement for fundal palpation and massage

A full-term pregnancy stretches the ligaments supporting the uterus, placing the uterus at risk for inversion during palpation and massage. To guard against this, use your hands to support and fix the uterus in a safe position. Here's how:
● Place one hand against the patient's abdomen at the symphysis pubis level. This stabilizes the uterus and prevents downward displacement.
● Place the other hand at the top of the fundus, cupping it. Press firmly into the abdomen.

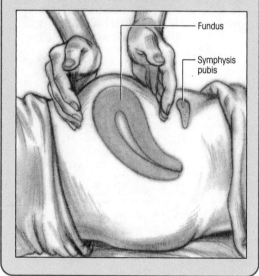

Fundus

Symphysis pubis

CLINICAL IMPACT *The first hour after delivery is potentially the most dangerous time for uterine atony leading to postpartum hemorrhage. Frequent fundal assessments — at least every 15 minutes — should be done so that interventions can be implemented immediately.*
AWHONN

Involution normally begins immediately after delivery, when the firmly contracted uterus lies midway between the umbilicus and the symphysis pubis. By the first postpartum day, the uterus rises to the umbilicus and begins returning to the pelvis. The average descent rate is 1 cm or fingerbreadth daily — slightly slower if the patient had a cesarean delivery. By the 10th postpartum day, the now unpalpable uterus lies deep in the pelvis, at or below the symphysis pubis.

When the uterus fails to connect or remain firm during involution, uterine bleeding or hemorrhage can result. This happens because placental separation after delivery exposes large uterine vessels, which uterine contractions compress. A firmly contracted uterus allows thrombi to form within the uterine sinuses, providing a permanent seal at the placental attachment site. Fundal massage, synthetic oxytocin delivery, or natural oxytocin substances released during breast-feeding help to maintain or stimulate contractions.

Typical nursing procedures that coincide with fundal palpation and massage include care for the perineum and evaluating healing. (See *Postpartum perineal care.*)

Equipment

Gloves ● perineal pad ● optional: urinary catheter

Implementation

● Confirm the patient's identity using two patient identifiers according to facility policy. **JCAHO**
● Explain the procedure to the patient, and provide privacy. Wash your hands, and put on gloves. **CDC** **PCP**

● Unless the physician orders otherwise, schedule fundal assessment every 15 minutes for the 1st hour after delivery, every 30 minutes for the next 2 to 3 hours, every hour for the next 4 hours, every 4 hours for the rest of the postpartum day, and then every 8 hours until the patient's discharge. **AWHONN**

Postpartum perineal care

Vaginal birth (which stretches and sometimes tears the perineal tissues) and episiotomy (which may minimize tissue injury) usually leave the patient with perineal edema and tenderness. Postpartum perineal care aims to relieve this discomfort, promote healing, and prevent infection.

Performed after the patient eliminates, perineal hygiene involves cleaning and drying the perineum and assessing the wound area and the lochia (blood and debris sloughed from the placental site and the decidua). Red immediately after delivery, the lochia turns pinkish brown in 4 to 7 days and appears white during the second and third weeks after delivery. This discharge decreases gradually but may continue for up to 6 weeks.

Cleaning the perineum
Typically, you'll use a water-jet irrigation system or a peribottle to clean the perineum. Assist the patient to the bathroom, wash your hands, and put on gloves.
- If you're using a water-jet irrigation system, insert the prefilled cartridge containing antiseptic or medicated solution into the handle, and push the disposable nozzle into the handle until you hear it click into place. Instruct the patient to sit on the commode. Next, place the nozzle parallel to the perineum, and turn on the unit. Rinse the perineum for at least 2 minutes from front to back. Then turn off the unit, remove the nozzle, and discard the cartridge. Dry the nozzle, and store it appropriately labeled with the patient's name for later use.
- If you're using a peri bottle, fill it with cleaning solution, and instruct the patient to pour it over the perineal area.
- Help the patient to stand up before you flush the commode *to avoid spraying the perineum with contaminated water.*
- Also assist her in applying a new perineal pad before returning to bed. Instruct her to apply the pad front to back *to avoid infection.* Provide her with a belt to keep the pad in place. However, if she had a cesarean delivery, offer safety pins to secure the pad to her underwear *because a belt may irritate the incision site.*

Assessing the healing process
- Inspect the perineum regularly. To do so, first put on gloves.
- Ensure adequate lighting, and place the patient in the lateral Sims' position *to best expose the perineum and anal area.*
- When inspecting the wound area, be alert for signs of infection, such as unusual swelling, redness, and foul-smelling drainage.

- For the patient who has had a cesarean delivery, plan the fundal assessment during a time when she has received an analgesic and is comfortable.
- Encourage the patient's efforts to urinate before fundal palpation *because bladder distention impairs uterine contraction by pushing the uterus up and aside.* You may need to catheterize the patient if she can't urinate or if the uterus becomes displaced with increased bleeding. **Science**
- Lower the head of the bed until the patient lies in a supine position. If this position causes discomfort — especially if she has had a cesarean delivery — keep the head of the bed slightly elevated or ask the patient to bend her knees.
- Expose the abdomen for palpation and the perineum for observation. Watch for bleeding, clots, and tissue expulsion while palpating the fundus.

- Gently compress the uterus between both hands to evaluate uterine firmness. Note the level of the fundus above or below the umbilicus in fingerbreadths or centimeters.
- If the uterus seems soft and boggy, gently massage the fundus with a circular motion until it becomes firm. Simply cupping the uterus between your hands may also stimulate contraction. Alternatively, massage the fundus with the side of the hand above the fundus. Without digging into the abdomen, gently compress and release, always supporting the lower uterine segment with the other hand. Observe for lochia flow during massage. **AWHONN**
- Massage long enough to produce firmness. The sensitive fundus needs only gentle pressure. This should produce the desired results without causing excessive discomfort. **AWHONN**

• Notify the physician or nurse-midwife immediately should the uterus fail to contract and should heavy bleeding occur. If the fundus becomes firm after massage, keep one hand on the lower uterus and press gently toward the pubis *to expel clots.* **AWHONN**

• Clean the perineum and apply a clean perineal pad. Help the patient into a comfortable position.

Special considerations

• If the patient has had a vertical abdominal incision for cesarean delivery, palpate the uterus from the sides to determine tone.

⚠ ALERT *The absence of lochia may signal a clot blocking the cervical os. Subsequent heavy bleeding may result if a position change dislodges the clot. Take vital signs to assess for hypovolemic shock.*

Nursing diagnoses

• Risk for injury

Expected outcomes

The patient will:

• experience fundal assessment and massage without pain or complications.

Complications

Because the uterus and its supporting ligaments are usually tender after delivery, pain is the most common complication of fundal palpation and massage. Excessive massage causes myometrium relaxation, causing undue muscle fatigue and leading to uterine atony or inversion.

Documentation

Record vital signs, fundal height in centimeters or fingerbreadths, and also record position (midline or off-center) and tone (firm, or soft and boggy). Document massage, and note the passage of clots. Record excessive bleeding.

Supportive references

American Academy of Pediatrics and American College of Obstetricians and Gynecologists. *Guidelines for Perinatal Care,* 5th ed. Elk Grove Village, Ill.: AAP, 1997; Washington, D.C.: ACOG, 2002.

Pillitteri, A. *Maternal & Child Health Nursing: Care of the Childbearing & Childrearing Family,* 5th ed. Philadelphia: Lippincott Williams & Wilkins, 2007.

Oxytocin administration

The hormone oxytocin stimulates the uterus to contract, thereby facilitating cervical dilation. The physician may order synthetic oxytocin (Pitocin, Syntocinon) to induce or augment labor or to control bleeding and enhance uterine contraction after the placenta is delivered. Usually, the nurse administers oxytocin I.V. *To regulate dosage and to help prevent uterine hyperstimulation*, an infusion pump is always used. Additional nursing responsibilities include managing the infusion and monitoring maternal and fetal responses. Indications for oxytocin administration include the following maternal and fetal conditions:

• Maternal conditions: gestational hypertension, premature rupture of membranes, preeclampsia or eclampsia, diabetes, renal disease, chronic hypertension, and chronic obstructive cardiopulmonary disease. Other maternal situations in which induction may be considered include risk of rapid labor and delivery and being far from the health care facility. If induction is scheduled in these situations, term gestation and fetal lung maturity should be confirmed.

• Fetal conditions: postterm gestation, macrosomia, fetal demise, fetal anomaly, blood group sensitization, nonreassuring fetal testing, fetal hydrops, and intrauterine growth restriction.

⬢ CONTROVERSIAL ISSUE *A review of the literature indicates that routine induction after 40 weeks' gestation isn't mandatory. Antenatal testing is a safe and effective monitoring tool that allows the woman to progress to 42 weeks' gestation — which is a true postterm — without increasing the mother's or the fetus's risk of death. However, induction at 40 to 41 weeks is the latest that many physicians will allow, most likely related to their own comfort level and medical-legal concerns. Current clinical practices related to timing of induction when considering a postdate pregnancy need to be modified and based on current research findings.*

Assessment of the pregnant client scheduled for an induction should include a determination of labor readiness. One way to determine the woman's readiness for delivery is by using the Bishop scoring method. (See *Bishop score.*) This assessment includes determination of the woman's cervical dilation, effacement, station, and consistency of the position of

Bishop score

This scoring system was created to determine whether the cervix is "ripe" — that is, ready for cervical dilation. If a woman's total score is eight or more, the cervix is considered to be ready for birth and should respond to induction.

Scoring factor	Score			
	0	**1**	**2**	**3**
Dilation (cm)	0	1 to 2	3 to 4	5 to 6
Effacement (%)	0 to 30	40 to 50	60 to 70	80
Station	−3	−2	−1 to 0	+1 to +2
Consistency	Firm	Medium	Soft	
Position	Posterior	Midposition	Anterior	

Adapted with permission from Searing, K.A. "Induction vs. Post-date Pregnancies: Exploring the Controversy of Who's Really at Risk," *AWHONN Lifelines* 5(2):44-48, April-May 2001. Originally published by Bishop, E.H. "Pelvic Scoring for Elective Induction," *Obstetrics and Gynecology* 24:266, 1964.

the cervix. A score of 4 or less indicates that the cervix isn't ready for labor and delivery. **AWHONN**

Contraindications include placenta previa or vasa previa, diagnosed cephalopelvic disproportion, fetal distress, previous classic uterine incision or uterine surgery, transverse fetal lie, prolapsed umbilical cord, or active genital herpes. Oxytocin should be administered cautiously and requires special attention in a patient who has an overdistended uterus or a history of cervical surgery, uterine surgery, or grand multiparity, breech presentation, maternal heart disease, polyhydramnios, presenting part above the pelvic inlet, severe hypertension, or abnormal fetal heart rate (FHR) patterns not necessitating emergency delivery. **ACOG** **AWHONN**

Equipment

Administration set for primary I.V. line • infusion pump and tubing • I.V. solution, as ordered • external or internal fetal monitoring equipment • oxytocin • 20G 1″ needle • label • venipuncture equipment with an 18G through-the-needle catheter • optional: autosyringe

Preparation of equipment

Prepare the oxytocin solution as ordered. Rotate the I.V. bag *to disperse the drug throughout the solution.* Label the I.V. container with the name of the medication. Attach the infusion pump tubing to the I.V. container, and connect the tubing to the pump.

Because infusion pump features vary, review the operator's manual before proceeding. Attach the 20G 1″ needle or a needleless system adapter to the tubing to piggyback it to the primary I.V. line. Or, if using a needleless system, attach the infusion pump tubing to a needleless adapter and then connect the adapter to the primary I.V. line, or use an autosyringe connected to the primary I.V. line. Set up the equipment for internal or external fetal monitoring.

Implementation

● Confirm the patient's identity using two patient identifiers according to facility policy. **JCAHO**
● Explain the procedure to the patient and provide privacy. Wash your hands. Describe the equipment, and forewarn the patient that she may feel a pinch from the venipuncture. **CDC** **PCP**

Administering oxytocin during labor and delivery

● Help the patient to a lateral-tilt position, and support her hip with a pillow. Don't let her lie in a supine position. In the supine position, the gravid uterus presses on the maternal great vessels, producing maternal hypotension and reduced uterine perfusion. **Science**

● Identify and record the FHR, and assess uterine contractions occurring in a 20-minute span to establish baseline fetal status and evaluate spontaneous maternal uterine activity. **AWHONN**

● Start the primary I.V. line using an 18G through-the-needle catheter. Use this line to deliver oxytocin and fluids, blood, or other medications as needed.

● Piggyback the oxytocin solution (metered by the infusion pump) to the primary I.V. line at the Y injection site closest to the patient. Piggybacking maintains I.V. line patency (which you'll need to preserve should you discontinue the oxytocin infusion). Using the Y injection site nearest the venipuncture ensures that the primary line holds the lowest concentration of oxytocin if you must stop the infusion. **ACOG**

● Begin the oxytocin infusion as ordered (either high- or low-dose regimen). If starting the patient on a low-dose regimen, begin the infusion at 0.5 to 1.0 mU/minute with incremental increases for the desired results at 30- to 40-minute intervals in increments of 1 mU/minute, or begin the oxytocin administration at 1 to 2 mU/minute and increase the dose by 2 mU/minute every 15 minutes. **ACOG**

● If starting the patient on high-dose oxytocin, begin the infusion at 6 mU/minute, increasing the dose by 6 mU every 15 minutes, or begin the infusion at 6 mU/minute and increase the dose by 1, 3, or 6 mU every 20 to 40 minutes. The maximum dose is usually 20 mU/minute. **ACOG**

● Because oxytocin begins acting immediately, be prepared to start monitoring uterine contractions.

● Increase the oxytocin dosage as ordered, and based on your assessment of the contraction pattern and fetal response. When induced labor stimulates normal labor (when contractions occur every 2 to 3 minutes and last 40 to 60 seconds) and cervical dilation progresses at least 1 cm/hour in first-stage, active-phase labor, you can stop increasing the dosage. However, continue the infusion at the dosage and rate that maintain activity closest to normal labor.

● Before each increase, be sure to time the frequency and duration of contractions, palpate the uterus to identify contraction intensity, and assess maternal vital signs and fetal heart rhythm and rate *to ensure safety and to anticipate possible complications.* If you're using an external fetal monitor, the uterine activity strip or grid should show contractions occurring every 2 to 3 minutes. The contractions should last for about 60 seconds and be followed by uterine relaxation. If you're using an internal fetal monitor, look for an optimal baseline value ranging from 5 to 15 mm Hg. Your aim is to verify uterine relaxation between contractions. **AWHONN**

● Assist with comfort measures, such as repositioning the patient on her other side, as needed.

● Continue assessing maternal and fetal responses to the oxytocin. For example, every 10 to 15 minutes, evaluate FHR, maternal response to increased contraction activity and subsequent discomfort, and maternal pulse rate and pattern, blood pressure, respiration rate and quality, and uterine contractions. Review the infusion rate to prevent uterine hyperstimulation. Signs and symptoms of hyperstimulation include contractions less than 2 minutes apart and lasting 90 seconds or longer (tetanic contraction), uterine pressure that doesn't return to baseline between contractions, and intrauterine pressure that rises over 75 mm Hg. **AWHONN**

● *To reduce uterine irritability,* try to increase uterine blood flow. Do this by changing the patient's position and increasing the infusion rate of the primary I.V. line. Avoid exceeding the maximum total infusion of 20 mU/minute. **AWHONN**

● *To manage hyperstimulation,* discontinue the infusion, administer oxygen, and notify the physician.

● After hyperstimulation resolves, resume the oxytocin infusion. Depending on maternal and fetal conditions, select one of the following methods: Resume the infusion beginning with oxytocin 0.5 mU/minute, increase the dosage to 1 mU/minute every 15 minutes, and increase the rate, as before; resume the infusion at one-half of the last dose given and increase the rate, as before; or resume the infusion at the dosage given before hyperstimulation signs occurred. Check your facility's policy for the appropriate method.

● Monitor and record intake and output. Output should be at least 30 ml/hour. Oxytocin has an antidiuretic effect at rates of 16 mU/minute and more, so you may need to administer an electrolyte-containing I.V. solution to maintain electrolyte balance. **ACOG**

Administering oxytocin after delivery
● As ordered after delivery, administer 10 to 40 units of oxytocin added to 1,000 ml of physiologic electrolyte solution. Infuse at a rate titrated to decrease postpartum bleeding or uterine atony after placental delivery. As an alternative, administer 10 units of oxytocin I.M. until you can establish the I.V. line.

Special considerations
● Most facilities require the use of an infusion pump to ensure accurate dosage and titration. (See *Conversion formulas for oxytocin administration.*)
● Without an infusion pump, administer oxytocin through a minidrop system (60 drops/ml) or an autosyringe, and observe the patient closely. Without an electronic fetal monitor, frequently palpate and assess contractions. Auscultate FHR every 5 to 15 minutes. (See "Fetal heart rate," page 564.)

Nursing diagnoses
● Acute pain
● Risk for injury

Expected outcomes
The patient will:
● identify characteristics of pain and describe factors that intensify and relieve it
● establish a good labor pattern, delivering the neonate without complications.

Complications
Oxytocin can cause uterine hyperstimulation. Other complications include fetal distress, abruptio placentae, uterine rupture, precipitate delivery, hemorrhage, amniotic fluid embolism, maternal hypotension, and water intoxication.

Watch for signs of oxytocin hypersensitivity, such as elevated blood pressure. Rarely, oxytocin leads to maternal seizures or coma from water intoxication.

Documentation
Monitor uterine activity response to oxytocin infusion rate. Document the baseline FHR, variability, accelerations, decelerations, and changes in FHR response to uterine contraction pattern. Document interventions related to assessment of contractile pattern and fetal response, and record maternal response to contractions, blood pressure, pulse rate and pattern, and respiratory rate and quality on the labor progression chart. Record oxytocin infusion rate and intake and output amounts.

Conversion formulas for oxytocin administration

To ensure that all members of the health care team are referring to the same amounts when administering oxytocin, use the following formulas, as needed, to convert milliliters (ml) per minute or drops (gtt) per minute to milliunits (mU) per minute. Conversion to mU per minute gives the actual drug dosage instead of the fluid dosage. The conversion formula used depends on the infusion pump being used. Synthetic oxytocin for I.V. administration comes in a concentration of 10 U/ml in 10-ml vials, in 0.5- and 1-ml ampules, and in 1-ml disposable syringes.

To calculate oxytocin dilution (in mU/ml):

$$\frac{\text{\# of units oxytocin}}{\text{ml of fluid}} \times 1,000 = \text{mU/ml}$$

To convert ml/minute to mU/minute:

$$\frac{mU}{ml} \times \frac{ml}{minute} = \frac{mU}{minute}$$

To convert gtt/minute to mU/minute:

$$\frac{gtt}{minute} \times \frac{mU}{ml} \times \frac{ml}{gtt} = \frac{mU}{minute}$$

Supportive references
Pillitteri, A. *Maternal & Child Health Nursing: Care of the Childbearing & Childrearing Family,* 5th ed. Philadelphia: Lippincott Williams & Wilkins, 2007.
Searing, K.A. "Induction vs. Post-date Pregnancies: Exploring the Controversy of Who's Really at Risk," *AWOHNN Lifelines* 5(2):44-48, April-May 2001.
Tucker, S.M. *Fetal Monitoring and Assessment,* 5th ed. St. Louis: Mosby–Year Book, Inc., 2004.
Wong, D.L., et al. *Maternal-Child Nursing Care,* 3rd ed. St. Louis: Mosby–Year Book, Inc., 2006.

AAP phototherapy guidelines (AAP)

The American Academy of Pediatrics (AAP) has recommendations on when to initiate phototherapy for treating hyperbilirubinemia in neonates. Term neonates who are clinically jaundiced before 24 hours aren't considered healthy and require further evaluation.

Age (hours)	Total serum bilirubin (TSB) level Consider phototherapy (based on clinical judgment)	TSB Level Treat with phototherapy
25 to 48	≥ 12	≥ 15
49 to 72	≥ 15	≥ 18
> 72	≥ 17	≥ 20

Adapted from American Academy of Pediatrics. "Practice Guideline: Management of Hyperbilirubinemia in the Healthy Term Newborn," *Pediatrics* 94(4):1-18, October 1994.

Phototherapy

In utero, the fetus's liver processes little bilirubin (a pigment of red blood cells [RBCs]) because the mother's circulation does it for the fetus. Exposure to light at birth usually triggers the liver to assume this function. When the liver doesn't begin to process bilirubin effectively, phototherapy treatment is ordered to help the liver speed up its conversion potential. Each year about 60% of the 4 million neonates in the United States become clinically jaundiced.

Phototherapy involves exposing the neonate to high-intensity fluorescent light that breaks down bilirubin for transport to the GI system and excretion. The treatment is commonly given to neonates with hyperbilirubinemia — a symptom of physiologic jaundice, breast-milk jaundice, or hemolytic disease. Phototherapy continues until bilirubin drops to a normal level because unchecked hyperbilirubinemia can lead to kernicterus (deposits of unconjugated bilirubin in the brain cells), permanent brain damage, and even death.

Physiologic jaundice — resulting from the neonate's high RBC count and short RBC life span — may develop in 2 to 3 days after delivery in about 50% of full-term neonates and in 3 to 5 days in about 80% of premature neonates. Breast-milk jaundice typically develops 3 to 4 days after delivery in about 25% of breast-feeding neonates and 4 to 5 days after delivery in less than 5%.

Experts think that this hyperbilirubinemia results from reduced calorie and fluid intake (before the mother develops an adequate milk supply) or from constituents in breast milk that reduce bilirubin de-

composition. They encourage frequent breast-feeding (at least 8 to 10 times every 24 hours) to increase fluid and calorie intake until the bilirubin level reaches about 15 mg/dl. Breast-feeding may be discontinued for 48 hours with formula supplementation while the bilirubin level decreases. (AAP)

Treatment for hemolytic disease, a much more serious condition, includes phototherapy and exchange transfusions. In pathologic jaundice, which occurs within 24 hours of birth and raises serum bilirubin levels about 13 mg/dl, phototherapy may be used with appropriate treatment for the underlying cause.

There's continuing controversy over the management of jaundice in the healthy neonate. Several key issues include determining when to initiate phototherapy using total serum bilirubin (TSB) level as an indicator, adverse effects of phototherapy versus adverse effects of hyperbilirubinemia, and whether phototherapy should be continuous or intermittent. The American Academy of Pediatrics (AAP) has guidelines regarding initiating phototherapy treatment in the neonate. (See *AAP phototherapy guidelines.*)

CLINICAL IMPACT *Controversy continues when comparing intermittent and continuous phototherapy for the treatment of neonatal hyperbilirubinemia. Clinical studies have yielded conflicting results. The AAP recommends that intensive phototherapy should be administered for a neonate with a TSB level of 25 mg/dl or more until a satisfactory decline occurs. Intensive phototherapy should produce a decline in the TSB level of 1 to 2 mg/dl within 4 to 6 hours. In many cases these neonates can be removed from therapy during feedings and for brief parental visits.*

Equipment

Phototherapy unit • photometer • opaque eye mask • thermometer • urinometer • surgical face mask or small diaper • optional: thermistor (if the phototherapy unit is combined with a temperature-controlled radiant heat warmer) or incubator (if the neonate is small for his gestational age), bilimeter

Prepackaged eye coverings are available.

Preparation of equipment

Set up the phototherapy unit about 18" (45.5 cm) above the neonate's crib. Verify placement of the light-bulb shield *because this device filters ultraviolet rays and protects the neonate from broken bulbs.* If the neonate is in an incubator, place the phototherapy unit at least 3" (7.5 cm) above the incubator *to promote sufficient airflow and prevent overheating.* (See *Understanding the phototherapy unit.*)

Turn on the lights. Place a photometer probe in the middle of the crib *to measure the energy emitted by the lights.* The energy should range between 6 and 8 $\mu w/cm^2/nanometer$.

Implementation

● Confirm the neonate's identity using two patient identifiers according to facility policy. **JCAHO**
● Verify the physician's or the neonatal nurse practitioner's orders to initiate therapy.
● Explain the procedure to the parents to reduce their anxiety and guilt and to ensure cooperation. **PCP**
● Record the neonate's initial bilirubin level and his axillary temperature to establish baseline measurements. **NANN**
● Place the opaque eye mask over the neonate's closed eyes. Fasten the mask securely enough to stay in place and to prevent the neonate from opening his eyes, but loosely enough to ensure circulation and avoid pressure on the eyeballs. This protects the eyes and prevents reflex bradycardia and head molding. **AAP**
● Clean the eyes daily and as needed *to remove drainage and check circulation.*
● Remove eye patches for 5 to 10 minutes every 4 hours to observe for irritation or drainage, and also remove them for short periods during parental visits to encourage bonding. **NANN**
● Undress the neonate to expose the most skin to the most light. Remember to place a diaper under the neonate and to cover genitalia with a surgical mask

> ### Understanding the phototherapy unit
>
> Whether you use fluorescent or daylight bulbs, blue lights, or high-intensity quartz lamps in your neonatal phototherapy unit, you'll prepare the neonate in much the same way. You'll position the unit at a correct distance according to whether the neonate is in a crib, radiant warmer, or incubator. You'll also take care to expose as much skin surface as possible to as much light as possible. That's because the light decomposes harmful, excess bilirubin in the skin and subcutaneous tissues to a more water-soluble form that's easily excreted from the body.

or a small diaper to catch urine and to prevent possible testicular damage from the heat and light waves.
● Take the neonate's axillary temperature every 2 to 4 hours to make sure the neonate maintains a normal and stable body temperature. **NANN**
● If the neonate uses a servo-controlled incubator or a radiant warmer, place the thermistor on the neonate's side and cover it with opaque or reflective tape. This prevents frequent sensor changes and protects the sensor from direct energy.
● Provide additional warmth, if necessary, by adjusting the warming unit's thermostat.
● Monitor elimination. Note urine and stool amounts and frequency. Weigh the neonate once or twice daily as ordered by the physician, and watch for signs of dehydration (such as dry skin, poor turgor, and depressed fontanels) because phototherapy increases fluid loss through stools and evaporation. **AAP NANN**
● Clean the neonate carefully after each bowel movement because the loose green stools that result from phototherapy can excoriate the skin. Don't apply ointment because this can cause burns under phototherapy lights.
● Check urine specific gravity with a urinometer, as ordered, *to gauge the neonate's hydration status.*
● Feed the formula-fed neonate every 3 to 4 hours; water may be offered between feedings to ensure adequate hydration and to boost gastric motility. Make sure water intake doesn't replace formula. The breast-fed neonate should be encouraged to eat every 2 to 3 hours (8 to 10 times in 24 hours). Don't give the breast-feeding neonate supplements with water or

dextrose. Take the neonate out of the crib, turn off the phototherapy lights, and unmask his eyes at least every 3 to 4 hours with feedings, if possible, to provide visual stimulation and human contact. **NANN**

● Reposition the neonate every 2 hours to expose all body surfaces to the light and to prevent head molding and skin breakdown from pressure. **NANN**

● Assess jaundice by blanching the skin with digital pressure over a bony prominence and determine the underlying color of the skin in the blanched area.

✓ CLINICAL IMPACT *Assessment of jaundice must be done in natural light or a well-lit room. Note the progression of jaundice, which may assist in quantifying the degree of jaundice.*

● Check the bilirubin level at least once every 24 hours — more often if levels rise significantly. If you don't use a bilimeter, turn off the phototherapy unit before drawing venous blood for testing because the lights may degrade bilirubin in the blood sample and thereby produce inaccurate test results. **AAP**

● When bilirubin is being drawn, turn the phototherapy unit off. **NANN**

● Notify the physician if the bilirubin level nears 20 mg/dl in full-term neonates or 15 mg/dl in premature neonates, *because such levels may lead to kernicterus.* **AAP**

● Review the neonatal and maternal histories for clues to possible hyperbilirubinemia causes. Watch for signs of infection and metabolic disorders, and check the neonate's hematocrit for polycythemia. Inspect the neonate for hematoma, bruising, petechiae, and cyanosis. If the phototherapy unit has blue lights, turn them off for the examination *because these lights can mask cyanosis.* **AAP**

Special considerations

● If the neonate cries excessively during phototherapy, place a blanket roll at each side *to give him a feeling of security.*

● If the physician diagnoses breast-feeding jaundice (suspending breast-feeding temporarily), teach the mother to express milk manually or with a pump. Encourage continued breast-feeding when indicated. Reassure the parents by explaining that jaundice is transitory. If possible, give phototherapy treatment in the mother's room *to facilitate bonding and to decrease parental anxiety and guilt feelings.*

● For neonates discharged less than 48 hours after birth, arrange for follow-up by a health care profes-

sional in an office, clinic, or at home within 2 to 3 days after discharge.

📋 TEACHING *Home phototherapy programs are safe and effective alternatives for treating uncomplicated neonatal jaundice. Teach families how to perform the procedure, and encourage their compliance. Explain that testing continues until results show serum bilirubin at an acceptable level. Provide written instructions at discharge.*

For fiber-optic phototherapy, teaching should focus on the application of the BiliBlanket. Be sure to inform the parents that the neonate's back or chest should be placed on the white side of the blanket, to make sure the neonate's skin is in direct contact with the blanket; that if the neonate is positioned on his back his eyes should be covered with eyepatches; and that the brightness selector switch should be set on high or as ordered by the physician.

Nursing diagnoses
● Interrupted breast-feeding
● Risk for injury

Expected outcomes
The mother will:
● express an understanding of the factors that necessitate the interruption of breast-feeding
● express and store breast milk appropriately
● resume breast-feeding when interfering factors cease.
   The neonate will:
● not develop complications related to phototherapy.

Complications
Phototherapy may cause complications, such as dehydration due to increases in insensible water loss, hypothermia or hyperthermia as a result of total skin surface exposure, diarrhea, and bronze baby syndrome (an idiopathic darkening of the skin, serum, and urine). Changes in feeding and activity patterns and hormonal secretions may follow prolonged therapy.

Documentation
Document when phototherapy was initiated. At least once every 2 hours, note the progress of phototherapy and ensure that the neonate's eyes remain protected. Record the time of all bilirubin testing, and plot results. Document eye covering changes and eye care

given. Keep records of measured radiant energy — initially and then every 8 hours. Document neonatal time away from lights — for example, for feeding or other procedures. Note fluid intake and the amount of urine and stool eliminated. Describe changes in skin appearance and character, in feeding patterns, and in activity level.

Supportive references

American Academy of Pediatrics. Subcommittee on Hyperbilirubinemia. "Management of Hyperbilirubinemia in the Newborn Infant 35 or More Weeks of Gestation: Practice Guideline," *Pediatrics* 114(1):297-316, July 2004.

National Association of Neonatal Nurses. Position Statement 3040 Prevention of Bilirubin Encephalopathy and Kernicterus in Newborns. August 2003.

Pillitteri, A. *Maternal & Child Health Nursing: Care of the Childbearing & Childrearing Family,* 5th ed. Philadelphia: Lippincott Williams &Wilkins, 2007.

Wong, D.L., et al. *Maternal-Child Nursing Care,* 3rd ed. St. Louis: Mosby–Year Book, Inc., 2006.

RhoGAM administration

Theoretically, there's no direct connection between fetal and maternal circulation. In reality, however, especially during the third trimester of pregnancy, placental villi can tear and a drop or two of fetal blood can enter the maternal circulation. *To prevent the maternal immune system from responding to the "foreign" material with the production of anti-Rho antibodies,* the mother receives an intramuscular injection of RhoGAM — a concentrated solution of immune globulin containing $Rh_o(D)$ antibodies.

RhoGAM prevents the Rh-negative mother from producing active antibody responses and forming anti-$Rh_o(D)$ antibodies to Rh-positive fetal blood cells and endangering future Rh-positive neonates. Maternal sensitization to the Rh antigen commonly results from transplacental hemorrhage during gestation or delivery. If unchecked during gestation, incompatible fetal and maternal blood can lead to hemolytic disease in the neonate.

It's indicated for the Rh-negative mother after abortion, ectopic pregnancy, or delivery of a neonate having $Rh_o(D)$-positive or Du-positive blood and Coombs'-negative cord blood, accidental transfusion of Rh-positive blood, amniocentesis, abruptio placentae, or abdominal trauma. After the above situations, a RhoGAM injection should be given within 72 hours to prevent future maternal sensitization.

Subsequent pregnancies of the Rh-negative mother require screening to detect previous inadequate RhoGAM administration or low Rh-positive antibody titers.

When RhoGAM is administered at about 28 weeks' gestation, it can also protect the fetus of the Rh-negative mother. The dose is determined according to the fetal packed red blood cell (RBC) volume that enters the mother's blood. A volume under 15 ml usually calls for one vial of RhoGAM; a significant feto-maternal hemorrhage calls for more than one vial if the fetal packed RBC volume is greater than 15 ml.

CLINICAL IMPACT *Mothers who are Rh-negative and who deliver Rh-positive neonates are given a second shot of RhoGAM 72 hours after delivery.*

Equipment

3-ml syringe • 22G 1½″ needle • RhoGAM vial • alcohol pads • gloves • triplicate form and patient identification (from the blood bank or laboratory)

Implementation

● Confirm the patient's identity using two patient identifiers according to facility policy. **JCAHO**
● Explain RhoGAM administration to the patient, and answer her questions. If the patient refuses the injection, notify the practitioner. **PCP**
● Obtain a history of allergies and reaction to immunizations.
● Two nurses must check the vial's identification numbers and sign the triplicate form that comes with the RhoGAM. Complete the form as indicated. Attach the top copy to the patient's chart. Send the remaining two copies, along with the empty RhoGAM vial, to the laboratory or blood bank.
● Provide privacy, wash your hands, and put on gloves. **CDC**
● Withdraw the RhoGAM from the vial with the needle and syringe. Clean the gluteal injection site, and administer the RhoGAM I.M.
● Give the patient a card that identifies her Rh-negative status, and instruct her to carry it with her or keep it in a convenient location.

Special considerations

● After the procedure, watch for redness and soreness at the injection site.
● Provide an opportunity for the patient to voice any guilt or anxiety she may feel if she perceives her body is acting against the fetus.

Nursing diagnoses

● Deficient knowledge (procedure)

Expected outcomes

The patient will:
● state an understanding of the need for RhoGAM administration.

Complications

Complications rarely occur after a single RhoGAM injection; when they do, they're mild and confined to the injection site. After multiple injections (given after Rh mismatch), complications may include fever, myalgia, lethargy, discomfort, splenomegaly, or hyperbilirubinemia.

Documentation

Record the date, the time, and the site of the RhoGAM injection. If applicable, note the patient's refusal to accept a RhoGAM injection. Document patient teaching about RhoGAM. Note whether the patient received a card identifying her Rh-negative status.

Supportive references

Olds, S.E., et al. *Clinical Handbook, Maternal-Newborn Nursing: A Family and Community-Based Approach,* 6th ed. Upper Saddle River, N.J.: Prentice Hall Health, 2000.
Pillitteri, A. *Maternal & Child Health Nursing: Care of the Childbearing & Childrearing Family,* 5th ed. Philadelphia: Lippincott Williams & Wilkins, 2007.

Thermoregulation

A large body surface-to-mass ratio, reduced metabolism per unit area, limited amounts of insulating subcutaneous fat, vasomotor instability, and limited metabolic capacity make all neonates susceptible to hypothermia. To stay warm when he's cold, the neonate metabolizes brown fat. Unique to neonates,

brown fat has energy-producing mitochondria in its cells, which enhance its capacity for heat production.

Brown-fat metabolism effectively warms the body, but only within a narrow temperature range. Without careful external thermoregulation, the neonate may become chilled. Hypoxia, acidosis, hypoglycemia, pulmonary vasoconstriction, and even death may result.

Thermoregulation provides a neutral thermal environment that helps the neonate maintain a normal core temperature with minimal oxygen consumption and caloric expenditure. Although it varies with the neonate, the average core temperature is 97.7° F (36.5° C).

Two kinds of thermoregulators are common in a hospital nursery: radiant warmers and incubators. The radiant warmer, through use of a servocontrol probe attached to the neonate's skin over soft tissue, maintains the skin temperature at a preselected temperature. When the neonate arrives in the nursery, another radiant warmer may be used until his temperature stabilizes and he can occupy a bassinet, or open crib. If the temperature doesn't stabilize or if the neonate has a condition that affects thermoregulation, a temperature-controlled incubator will house him. (See *Understanding thermoregulators.*)

Equipment

Radiant warmer or incubator (if necessary) ● blankets ● washcloths or towels ● skin probe ● adhesive pad ● water-soluble lubricant ● thermometer ● clothing (including a cap) ● optional: stockinette gauze

Preparation of equipment

Turn on the radiant warmer in the delivery room, and set the desired temperature. Warm the blankets, washcloths, or towels under a heat source.

Implementation

● Continue nursing measures to conserve neonatal body warmth until the neonate is transferred to the nursery.

In the delivery room

● Place the neonate under the radiant warmer, and dry him with the warm washcloths or towels *to prevent heat loss by evaporation.*
● Pay special attention to drying his scalp and hair. If you take him off the warmer, make sure you cover his

Understanding thermoregulators

Thermoregulators preserve neonatal body warmth in various ways. A radiant warmer maintains the neonate's temperature by *radiation.* Neonates placed in a radiant warmer have increased convective and evaporative heat losses.

Α *Stretching* plastic wrap over the neonate from the side panels of the warmer will decrease insensible water loss while allowing the radiant heat to warm the neonate. An incubator maintains the neonate's temperature by *conduction* and *convection. Use of a double-walled incubator will decrease radiant heat loss.*

Temperature settings

Radiant warmers and incubators have two operating modes: *nonservo* and *servo.* The nurse manually sets temperature controls on nonservo equipment; a probe on the neonate's skin controls temperature settings on servo models. The nonservo mode is used to prewarm the radiant warmer bed but shouldn't be used after placing the neonate in the warmer because the neonate may experience overheating.

Other features

Most thermoregulators come with alarms. Incubators have the added advantage of providing a stable, enclosed environment, which protects the neonate from evaporative heat loss.

Radiant warmer

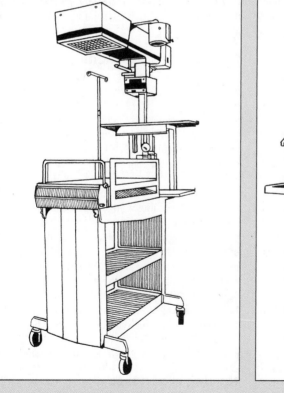

Incubator

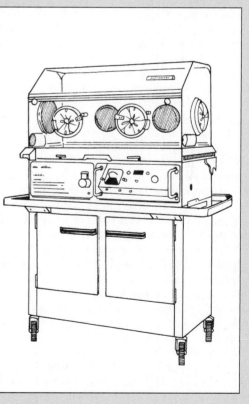

head (which makes up about 25% of neonatal body surface) with a ready-made cap *to prevent heat loss.* **NANN**

● Perform required procedures quickly to reduce the neonate's exposure to cool, delivery-room air.
● Wrap him in the warmed blankets. If his condition permits, give him to his parents *to promote bonding.* **NANN**
● Transport the neonate to the nursery in the transport incubator *to prevent convective heat loss.*

In the nursery

● Remove the blankets and cap, and place the neonate under the radiant warmer.
● Use the adhesive pad to attach the temperature control probe to his skin in the right upper abdominal quadrant. *This lets the servo control maintain neonatal skin temperature between 96.8° and 97.7° F (36° and 36.5° C).* If the neonate will lie in a prone position, put the skin probe on his back *to ensure accurate temperature control and avoid false-high readings from the neonate lying on the probe.* Don't cover the device with anything *because this could interfere with the servo control.* Be sure to raise the warmer's side panels *to prevent accidents.* **NANN**
● Lubricate the thermometer, and take the neonate's rectal temperature on admission *to identify core temperature and to establish anal patency.* The rectal thermometer shouldn't be inserted more than 1¼″ (3 cm) because the sigmoid colon turns at an angle 1¼″ from the rectum. Take axillary temperatures thereafter *to avoid injuring delicate rectal mucosa.* Usually, axillary temperature readings are lower than the core temperature. Take axillary temperatures every 15 to 30 minutes until the temperature stabilizes and then every 4 hours *to ensure stability.* **NANN**
● Sponge-bathe the neonate under the warmer only after his temperature stabilizes and his glucose level is normal, and leave him under the warmer until his temperature remains stable for at least 1 minute.
● Take appropriate action if the temperature doesn't stabilize. The neonate should be warmed slowly, because rapid warming may cause heat-induced apnea, hypotension, and shock. If the neonate is in a double-walled incubator, begin by setting the air temperature at 96.8° F (36° C). Increase humidity to decrease heat loss. Retake the neonate's temperature in 15 to 30 minutes. If the temperature continues to fall, increase the incubator air temperature to 98.6° F (37° C) and evaluate the environment for missed

sources of heat loss. If the neonate's temperature continues to fall after 15 minutes, increase the air temperature to 99.5° F (37.5° C) and consider adding a radiant warmer over the incubator to increase external wall temperatures. Check for signs of infection, which can cause hypothermia. **NANN**
● Apply a skin probe to the neonate in an incubator as you would for a neonate in a radiant warmer. Move the incubator away from cold walls or objects.
● Perform all required procedures quickly *to maintain a neutral thermal environment and to minimize heat loss.* Close portholes in the hood immediately after completing any procedure, *also to reduce heat loss.* If procedures must be performed outside the incubator, do them under a radiant warmer. **NANN**
● To leave the hospital or to move to a bassinet or open crib, a neonate must be weaned from the incubator. Slowly reduce the incubator's temperature to that of the nursery. Check periodically for hypothermia. *To ensure temperature stability,* never discharge the neonate to home directly from an incubator.
● When the normal neonate's temperature stabilizes, dress him, put him in a bassinet, and cover him with a blanket.

Special considerations

● Always warm oxygen before administering it to a neonate *to avoid initiating heat loss from his head and face.*
● *To prevent conductive heat loss,* preheat the radiant warmer bed and linen, warm stethoscopes and other instruments before use, and pad the scale with paper or a preweighed, warmed sheet before weighing the neonate.
● *To avoid convective heat loss,* place the neonate's bed out of direct line with an open window, a fan, or an air-conditioning vent.
● *To control evaporative heat loss,* dry the neonate immediately after delivery. When bathing the neonate, expose only one body part at a time, wash each part thoroughly, and then dry it immediately.
● Review the reasons for regulating body temperature with the neonate's family. Instruct them to keep him wrapped in a blanket and out of drafts when he isn't in the bassinet, in the facility and at home. In a warm place, guard against overheating the neonate.

Nursing diagnoses

● Ineffective thermoregulation

Expected outcomes

The neonate will:
- maintain body temperature within normal limits
- have warm, dry skin
- maintain heart rate, respiratory rate, and blood pressure within normal limits.

Complications

Hypothermia from ineffective natural or external thermoregulation can inhibit weight gain because the neonate must use caloric energy to maintain his temperature. Hyperthermia can cause increased oxygen consumption and apnea. Both conditions can result from equipment failure or insufficient monitoring.

Documentation

Name the heat source, and record its temperature and the neonate's temperature, whenever taken. Document complications that result from using thermoregulatory equipment.

Supportive references

Deacon, J., and O'Neill, P. *Core Curriculum for Neonatal Intensive Care Nursing,* 3rd ed. Philadelphia: W.B. Saunders Co., 2004.

Merenstein, G., and Gardner, S. *Handbook of Neonatal Intensive Care,* 6th ed. St. Louis: Mosby–Year Book, Inc., 2006.

National Association of Neonatal Nurses. Guidelines for Practice: Neonatal Thermoregulation. CA, 1999.

Pillitteri, A. *Maternal & Child Health Nursing: Care of the Childbearing & Childrearing Family,* 5th ed. Philadelphia: Lippincott Williams &Wilkins, 2007.

Tocolytic therapy

Tocolytic therapy involves the use of medications to suppress uterine activity — that is, to stop preterm labor contractions or prevent preterm labor. They may prolong pregnancy for 2 to 7 days and therefore allow the patient to receive a steroid to improve fetal lung maturity before birth. Several drugs may be used including magnesium sulfate, terbutaline, nifedipine, or indomethacin. (See *Tocolytic drugs,* page 592.)

Tocolytic therapy is contraindicated if the gestation is less than 20 weeks, cervical dilation is greater than 4 cm, or if cervical effacement is greater than 50%.

Equipment

I.V. line •medication as ordered by the physician

Implementation

- Assess baseline uterine contractions and fetal heart rate patterns.
- Confirm the patient's identity using two patient identifiers according to facility policy. **JCAHO**
- Explain the drug therapy ordered, including the route used and possible adverse effects. **PCP**
- Start an I.V. line for the woman who's to receive magnesium sulfate or terbutaline I.V.
- Obtain baseline maternal vital signs.
- Obtain laboratory studies, such as complete blood count, hematocrit, and hemoglobin and serum electrolyte levels.
- Obtain baseline electrocardiogram and urinary, vaginal, and cervical cultures as ordered.
- Closely observe the patient in preterm labor for signs of fetal or maternal distress, and provide comprehensive supportive care.
- Provide guidance about the hospital stay, potential for delivery of a preterm neonate, and the possible need for neonatal intensive care.
- Encourage the patient to assume the side-lying position to maximize placental blood flow and relieve pressure on the cervix.
- During attempts to suppress preterm labor, make sure the patient maintains bed rest; provide appropriate diversionary activities.
- Administer a tocolytic agent as ordered. Give nifedipine and indomethacin orally, magnesium sulfate I.V. piggybacked into a primary line and terbutaline subcutaneously or I.V. piggybacked into a primary line.

After the procedure

- Continue administration of tocolytic therapy as ordered.
- Monitor blood pressure, pulse rate, respirations, fetal heart rate (FHR), and uterine contraction pattern when administering a beta-adrenergic stimulant. (See *Administering terbutaline,* page 593.)
- Minimize adverse reactions by keeping the patient in a side-lying position as much as possible *to ensure adequate placental perfusion*
- Monitor the status of contractions, notifying the practitioner if the patient experiences more than four contractions per hour. If the mother's pulse rises

Tocolytic drugs

This chart highlights the major drugs used to halt uterine contractions.

Drug	Indications	Effects on the mother	Effects on the fetus	Antidote
Terbutaline (Brethine)	Beta$_2$ receptor stimulator that causes smooth-muscle relaxation	Tachycardia, diarrhea, nervousness and tremors, nausea and vomiting, headache, hyperglycemia or hypoglycemia, hypokalemia, and pulmonary edema	Tachycardia, hypoxia, hypoglycemia, and hypocalcemia	Propranolol (Inderal)
Magnesium sulfate	Central nervous system (CNS) depressant that prevents reflux of calcium into the myometrial cells, thereby keeping the uterus relaxed Prostaglandin synthesis inhibitor; typically not used after 32 weeks' gestation, *to avoid premature closure of the ductus arteriosus*	Drowsiness, flushing, warmth, nausea, headache, slurred speech, and blurred vision (toxicity is manifested by CNS depression, respirations less than 12 breaths/minute, hyporeflexia, oliguria, cardiac arrhythmias, and cardiac arrest)	Hypotonia and bradycardia	Calcium gluconate
Indomethacin (Indocin)	Nonsteroidal anti-inflammatory that decreases production of prostaglandins, which are lipid compounds associated with the initiation of labor	Nausea, vomiting, and dyspepsia; additive CNS effects if given with magnesium sulfate	Premature closure of ductus arteriosus	None; discontinuation of drug necessary
Nifedipine (Procardia)	Calcium channel blocker that decreases the production of calcium, a substance associated with the initiation of labor	Headache, flushing; additive CNS effects if given with magnesium sulfate	Minimal	None; discontinuation of drug necessary

above 120 beats/minute or her systolic blood pressure drops below 90 mm Hg, or if the fetus's heart rate rises above 180 beats/minute or drops below 110 beats/minute, notify the practitioner.
● Assess the patient's level of consciousness.
● Administer fluids, as ordered, *to ensure adequate hydration.* Monitor intake and output *to prevent fluid overload.* Output less than 30 ml/hour may promote magnesium sulfate toxicity.
● Frequently assess deep tendon reflexes when administering magnesium sulfate. (See *Safety with magnesium,* page 594.)
● Monitor serum magnesium sulfate levels *to assess for toxicity.*
● Prepare patient for possible delivery if therapy is unsuccessful; if preterm labor continues, expect to administer a corticosteroid *to promote lung maturity in the fetus.*

● Keep calcium gluconate at the patient's bedside *to counteract magnesium sulfate toxicity.*
● If labor isn't stopped and preterm neonate is delivered, monitor the neonate for signs of magnesium toxicity, including neuromuscular and respiratory depression.
● If labor is suppressed, begin discharge teaching with the patient and her support person about tocolytic therapy at home; anticipate referral for home care follow-up.

TEACHING *Instruct the patient in drug dosage, frequency, route, and possible adverse effects. Teach the patient how to monitor contraction pattern, pulse rate, and fetal movement. Teach her the signs and symptoms of true labor. Review with the patient any activity restrictions as well as danger signs about which she should to notify physician.*

Administering terbutaline

I.V. terbutaline may be ordered for a woman in premature labor. When administering this drug, follow these steps:
- Obtain baseline maternal vital signs, fetal heart rate (FHR), and laboratory studies, including serum glucose and electrolyte levels and hematocrit.
- Institute external monitoring of uterine contractions and FHR.
- Prepare the drug with lactated Ringer's solution instead of dextrose and water to prevent additional glucose load and possible hyperglycemia.
- Administer the drug as an I.V. piggyback infusion into a main I.V. solution so that the drug can be discontinued immediately if the patient experiences adverse reactions.
- Use microdrip tubing and infusion pump *to ensure an accurate flow rate.*
- Expect to adjust infusion flow rate every 10 minutes until contractions cease or adverse reactions become problematic.
- Monitor maternal vital signs every 15 minutes while infusion rate is being increased and then every 30 minutes thereafter until contractions cease; monitor FHR every 15 to 30 minutes.
- Auscultate breath sounds for evidence of crackles or changes; monitor the patient for complaints of dyspnea and chest pain.
- Be alert for maternal pulse rate greater than 120 beats/minute, blood pressure less than 90/60 mm Hg, or per-

sistent tachycardia or tachypnea, chest pain, dyspnea, or abnormal breath sounds because these could indicate developing pulmonary edema. Notify the physician immediately.
- Watch for fetal tachycardia or late or variable decelerations in FHR pattern because these could indicate uterine bleeding or fetal distress necessitating an emergency birth.
- Monitor intake and output closely, every hour during the infusion and then every 4 hours thereafter.
- Expect to continue the infusion for 12 to 24 hours after contractions have ceased and then switch to oral therapy.
- Administer the first dose of oral therapy 30 minutes before discontinuing the I.V. infusion.
- Instruct the patient on how to take the oral therapy, continuing therapy until 37 weeks' gestation or until fetal lung maturity has been confirmed by amniocentesis; alternatively, if the patient is prescribed subcutaneous terbutaline therapy via a continuous pump, teach the patient how to use the pump.
- Teach the patient how to measure her pulse rate before each dose of oral terbutaline, or at the recommended times with subcutaneous therapy; instruct the patient to call the physician if her pulse rate exceeds 120 beats/minute or she experiences palpitations or severe nervousness.

Nursing diagnoses
- Anxiety
- Deficient knowledge (procedure)

Expected outcomes
The patient will:
- express feelings of anxiety
- make use of available emotional support
- express an understanding of the procedure.

Complications
Complications include fetal and/or maternal distress and adverse effects of specific drug used in tocolytic therapy.

Documentation
Document the drug, dosage, route, site, and date and time of drug administration as well as adverse effects and nursing interventions. Also document status of contractions, mother's vital signs, FHR, and intake and output according to facility policy.

Supportive references
ACOG. "Management of Preterm Labor," ACOG Practice Bulletin No. 43, Washington (D.C.): May 2003. Available at: *www.guideline.gov.*

Berkman, N.D. et al. "Tocolytic Treatment for the Management of Preterm Labor: A Review of the Evidence," *American Journal of Obstetrics and Gynecology* 188(6):1648-659, June 2003.

Safety with magnesium

Use caution when administering I.V. magnesium therapy by following these guidelines.

● Always administer the drug as a piggyback infusion so that if the patient develops signs and symptoms of toxicity, the drug can be discontinued immediately.
● Obtain a baseline serum magnesium level before initiating therapy, and monitor frequently thereafter.
● Keep in mind that to be effective as an anticonvulsant, the serum magnesium level should be between 5 and 8 mg/dl. A level above 8 mg/dl indicates toxicity and places the patient at risk for respiratory depression, cardiac arrhythmias, and cardiac arrest.
● Assess the patient's deep tendon reflexes. Ideally, this should be the patellar reflex. However, if the patient has received epidural anesthesia, test the biceps or triceps reflex. Diminished or hypoactive reflexes suggest magnesium toxicity.
● Assess for ankle clonus by rapidly dorsiflexing the patient's ankle three times in succession and then remove your hand, observing foot movement. If no further motion is noted, ankle clonus is absent; if the foot continues to move voluntarily, clonus is present. Moderate (three to five) or severe (six or more) movements may suggest magnesium toxicity.
● Have calcium gluconate readily available at the patient's bedside. Anticipate administering this antidote for magnesium toxicity.

Pillitteri, A. *Maternal & Child Health Nursing: Care of the Childbearing & Childrearing Family,* 5th ed. Philadelphia: Lippincott Williams & Wilkins, 2007.

Uterine contraction palpation

Periodic, involuntary uterine contractions characterize normal labor and cause progressive cervical effacement and dilation, impelling the fetus to descend. Uterine palpation can tell you the frequency, duration, and intensity of contractions and the relaxation time between them. The character of contractions varies with the stage of labor and the body's response to labor-inducing drugs, if administered.

Uterine palpation isn't typically used as the sole method of monitoring contractions in the United States, but it's a major assessment tool in countries that don't have fetal monitoring technology. The American College of Obstetricians and Gynecologists and the Association of Women's Health, Obstetric, and Neonatal Nurses recommend the standards of practice and guidelines regarding fetal assessment (including palpation). As labor advances, contractions become more intense, occur more often, and last longer. (See *Four stages of labor.*) **ACOG** **AWHONN**

Equipment

Watch with a second hand ● sheet (for draping)

Implementation

● Review the patient's admission history *to determine the onset, frequency, duration, and intensity of contractions.* Note where contractions feel strongest or exert the most pressure. **AWHONN**
● Wash your hands, and follow standard precautions, as appropriate. Provide privacy. **CDC** **PCP**
● Confirm the patient's identity using two patient identifiers according to facility policy. **JCAHO**
● Describe the palpation procedure to the patient. *Because she may be ticklish or sensitive to touch,* forewarn her that you'll palpate her abdominal area over the uterus. **PCP**
● Assist the patient to a comfortable side-lying position to relieve pressure on the inferior vena cava and promote uteroplacental circulation. This position also relieves direct pressure on the sacral area from the fetal head and eases backache. **Science**
● Drape the patient with a sheet.
● Plant the palmar surface of your fingers on the uterine fundus and palpate lightly *to assess contractions.* Note the uterine tightening and abdominal lifting that occur with contractions. Each contraction has three phases: increment (rising), acme (peak), and decrement (letting down or ebbing). **ACOG** **AWHONN**
● Palpate several contractions. Simultaneously use the second hand on your watch to assess and measure such contraction qualities as frequency, duration, and intensity. **ACOG** **AWHONN**
● *To assess frequency,* time the interval from the beginning of one contraction to the beginning of the

Four stages of labor

Normal labor advances through the four stages summarized below. Offer your patient encouragement and progress reports throughout the stages.

First stage
Regular contractions, which repeat at 15- to 20-minute intervals and last between 10 and 30 seconds, signal the onset of labor's first stage. This stage has three phases: latent, active, and transitional. In primiparous patients, the first stage of labor may range from 3.3 to 19.7 hours; in multiparous patients, from 0.1 to 14.3 hours.

In the *latent phase* (characterized by irregular, brief, and mild contractions), the cervix dilates to 3 to 4 cm. Other signs and symptoms include abdominal cramping and backache. The patient may expel the mucus plug during this phase. This phase averages 8.6 hours in primiparous patients and 5.3 hours in multiparous patients.

During the *active phase,* cervical dilation increases to between 5 and 7 cm. Contractions occur every 3 to 5 minutes, last 30 to 45 seconds, and become moderately intense. In primiparous patients, this phase averages 5.8 hours; in multiparous patients, 2.5 hours.

In the *transitional phase,* the cervix dilates completely (8 to 10 cm). Uterine contractions grow intense, last between 45 and 60 seconds, and repeat at least every 2 minutes. The patient may thrash about, lose control of breathing techniques, and experience nausea and vomiting. This phase typically lasts less than 3 hours in primiparous patients and less than 1 hour in multiparous patients. The first stage of labor concludes when complete dilation occurs.

Second stage
In the second stage of labor, contractions occur often (every 1¼ to 2 minutes) and last up to 90 seconds. This stage commonly ends within 1 hour for a primiparous patient and possibly 15 minutes for a multiparous patient.

Signs and symptoms signaling onset of the second stage include increased bloody show, rupture of membranes (if they're still intact), severe rectal pressure and flaring, and reflexive bearing down with each contraction. The fetal head approaches the perineal floor and emerges at the vaginal opening. The second labor stage concludes with birth.

Third stage
In the third stage, strong but less painful contractions expel the placenta, which normally emerges within 30 minutes after the neonate emerges. Signs indicating normal separation of the placenta from the uterine wall include lengthening of the umbilical cord, a sudden gush of dark blood from the vagina, and a palpable change in uterine shape from disclike to globular.

Fourth stage
The fourth stage begins with placental expulsion and extends through the next 4 hours, while the patient's body rests and begins adjusting to the postpartum state.

next. In normal labor, contractions begin slowly and gradually occur more frequently with briefer relaxation intervals. **ACOG** **AWHONN**

● *To assess duration,* time the period from when the uterus begins tightening until it relaxes. As labor progresses, contractions usually last longer. **ACOG** **AWHONN**

● *To assess intensity,* press your fingertips into the uterine fundus when the uterus tightens. During mild contractions, the fundus indents easily and feels like a chin; during moderate contractions, the fundus indents less easily and feels like a nose; during strong contractions, the fundus resists indenting and feels like a forehead. **ACOG** **AWHONN**

● Determine how the patient copes with discomfort by assessing her breathing and relaxation techniques, if any. *This assessment may help guide your intervention choices.* Naturally, you'll provide ongoing emotional support in any event.

● Observe the patient's response to contractions to evaluate whether she needs an analgesic, an anesthetic, or another appropriate measure, such as repositioning and back massage.

● For a patient at low risk for complications, assess contractions at least every 30 to 60 minutes during the latent phase of first-stage labor and every 30 minutes throughout the active phase. During second-stage labor, assess contractions every 15 minutes. For a patient at high risk for complications, assess contractions and fetal well-being every 30 minutes during the latent phase, every 15 minutes during the active phase, and every 5 minutes during the second stage. **ACOG AWHONN**

Special considerations

● Because the patient may become irritable or anxious during the transitional phase of first-stage labor — when the cervix dilates fully — and because abdominal palpation may aggravate her distress, assess contractions only as necessary. If appropriate, teach her support person to palpate and record contractions.

● If a contraction lasts longer than 90 seconds and isn't followed by uterine muscle relaxation, notify the physician immediately so that he can evaluate maternal and fetal well-being. Report a brief relaxation (less than 60 seconds) period between contractions because inadequate relaxation intervals increase the risk of fetal hypoxia and exhaust the mother.

● Be aware that false labor (or Braxton Hicks) contractions occur at irregular intervals and vary in intensity. They're felt over the abdomen and are usually relieved by walking. Membranes remain intact, and there's no show of blood or progressive cervical dilation or effacement.

Nursing diagnoses

● Deficient knowledge (procedure)

Expected outcomes

The patient will:

● state an understanding of uterine contraction palpation.

Complications

None

Documentation

Record the frequency, duration, and intensity of contractions. Keep track of the relaxation time between contractions, and describe the patient's response to contractions.

Supportive references

Association of Women's Health, Obstetric, and Neonatal Nurses. *Fetal Heart Monitoring Principles and Practices,* 3rd ed. Dubuque, Iowa: Kendall-Hunt, 2003.

Pillitteri, A. *Maternal & Child Health Nursing: Care of the Childbearing & Childrearing Family,* 5th ed. Philadelphia: Lippincott Williams & Wilkins, 2007.

Tucker, S.M. *Pocket Guide to Fetal Monitoring and Assessment,* 5th ed. St. Louis: Mosby–Year Book, Inc., 2004.

Vacuum extraction

Vacuum extraction, also called *vacuum-assisted birth,* is an alternative to forceps delivery. It may be used when the second stage of labor is prolonged or if fetal heart tones are nonreassuring. It's associated with a lower incidence of vaginal, cervical, and third and fourth-degree lacerations; less maternal discomfort, because the cup doesn't occupy additional space in the birth canal; and less anesthesia (as compared with that required for forceps delivery). Vacuum extraction is also associated with a marked caput succedaneum of the neonate's head, lasting as long as 7 days after birth.

Tentorial tears are possible from extreme pressure, and renewed bleeding from the scalp can occur if used for a fetus that has undergone fetal blood sampling. Its use in preterm neonates is problematic because of the extreme softness of their skulls. **EB**

The use of vacuum extraction is contraindicated in the event of cephalopelvic disproportion, non-vertex presentation, coagulation disorders, and hydrocephalus.

Equipment

Vacuum extractor ● pressure regulator ● suction source

Implementation

● Explain the procedure to the patient and her partner. **PCP**

● Frequently monitor uterine contractions and fetal heart rate.

● Inform the patient that pressure and traction will be applied during contractions; encourage her to push when directed. **PCP**

● Assess the woman for possible contraindications to the procedure, including true cephalopelvic disproportion, nonvertex presentation, maternal or suspected fetal coagulation problems, hydrocephalus (known or suspected), or trauma to the fetal scalp.

● Inform the woman and her partner that the neonate may have a misshaped head resulting from the suction. **PCP**

● Encourage the patient to participate in the labor process as much as possible.

● A plastic vacuum cup connected to a suction source via tubing is applied to the fetal head over the posterior fontanel. (See *Understanding vacuum extraction.*)

● Negative pressure of 50 to 60 mm Hg is exerted, causing air beneath the cup to be removed.

● The cup adheres tightly to the fetal head.

● In conjunction with contractions, the physician applies traction.

● With each contraction, traction is applied until the head is delivered.

● Once the head is delivered, the vacuum cup is removed.

● After delivery of the neonate, provide postpartum care as usual.

● Inspect the neonate's head for evidence of caput succedaneum, which is common due to vacuum cup.

● Assess the neonate for possible complications, such as cephalhematoma and for signs of trauma and infection.

● Monitor the neonate for signs of listlessness or poor sucking, which may indicate cerebral irritation.

● Offer support to the parents about the neonate's misshapen head; advise them that the swelling will resolve with time.

● Inform neonatal caregivers and personnel that vacuum extraction was used.

Nursing diagnoses

● Risk for injury

Expected outcomes

The neonate will:

● remain free from injury or complications.

Complications

Cephalohematomas and subgleal hemorrhages (rare) may occur. Scalp bruising and lacerations may also occur. Maternal perineal and vaginal lacerations may occur.

Understanding vacuum extraction

With vacuum extraction, a suction cup is applied to the fetal head at the posterior fontanel. Negative pressure via suction is used, and traction is applied to achieve delivery.

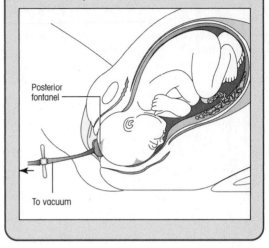

Posterior fontanel

To vacuum

Documentation

Document that the delivery was performed with vacuum extraction assistance. Document the amount of pressure used and the condition of the neonate at delivery.

Supportive references

Caughey, A.B., et al. "Forceps Compared with Vacuum: Rates of Neonatal and Maternal Morbidity," *Obstetrics and Gynecology* 106(5 Pt 1):908-12, November 2005.

Groom, K., et al. "A Prospective Randomised Controlled Trial of the Kiwi Omnicup Versus Conventional Ventouse Cups for Vacuum-assisted Vaginal Delivery," *British Journal of Obstetrics and Gynecology* 113(2):183-89, February 2006.

Mollberg, M., et al. "Risk Factors for Obstetric Brachial Plexus Palsy Among Neonates Delivered by Vacuum Extraction," *Obstetrics and Gynecology* 106(5 Pt 1):913-18, November 2005.

O'Grady, J.P. "Instrumental Delivery: A Critique of Current Practice," In Nichols D, ed. *Gynecologic, Obstetric, and Related Surgery.* St. Louis: Mosby–Year Book, Inc., 2000.

Pillitteri, A. *Maternal & Child Health Nursing: Care of the Childbearing & Childrearing Family*, 5th ed. Philadelphia: Lippincott Williams & Wilkins, 2007. **EB**

Vaginal examination

Vaginal examination is necessary to determine the extent of cervical effacement and dilation and confirm the fetal presentation, position, and engagement. The examination may be performed either between or during contractions. More of the fetal skull can be palpated during a contraction because the cervix retracts more at that time; however, performing a vaginal examination during a contraction is more painful to the mother and rarely results in additional information.

Important considerations during the examination include respecting the patient's privacy, providing simple explanations for her and her support person, maintaining eye contact when possible, and using aseptic technique. With experience, the typical examiner develops a well-honed routine for collecting the necessary information. This enables the examination to proceed precisely and efficiently.

Contraindications to a vaginal examination include excessive vaginal bleeding, which may signal placenta previa. Performing a vaginal examination in this instance might tear the placenta and cause hemorrhage, resulting in danger to the mother and fetus. **ACOG**

Equipment

Sterile gloves and clean disposable gloves • sterile, water-soluble lubricant or sterile water • mild soap and water, or cleaning solution • linen-saver pads • antiseptic solution • sterile gauze

Implementation

● Confirm the patient's identity using two patient identifiers according to facility policy. **JCAHO**
● Explain the procedure to the patient, and give her an opportunity to empty her bladder. **PCP** A distended bladder may interfere with accurate examination findings.
● Assess the patient for latex allergies. If latex allergies exist, use nonlatex sterile gloves and place an allergy band on the patient's wrist.
● Use Leopold's maneuvers to identify the fetal presenting part and position. Help the patient into a lithotomy position for the vaginal examination. **ACOG**

CLINICAL IMPACT *For an alternative position for vaginal examination, have the patient flex and abduct her thighs and put the heels of her feet together. This position allows her thighs to rest on the bed and provides easy access for a vaginal examination.*

● Place a linen-saver pad under the patient's buttocks.
● Inform the patient when you're about to touch her *to avoid startling her.*
● Clean the perineum with mild soap and water or cleaning solution, using clean disposable gloves.
● Put on sterile gloves. **CDC**
● Lubricate the index and middle fingers of your examining hand with sterile water or sterile water-soluble lubricant to facilitate insertion. If the membranes are ruptured, use an antiseptic solution. **ACOG**
● Spread the labia gently apart with your nondominant hand *to avoid contaminating your examining hand.*
● Ask the patient to relax by taking several deep breaths and slowly releasing the air. Insert your lubricated fingers (palmar surface down) into the vagina. Keep your uninserted fingers flexed *to avoid the rectum.* (See *Step-by-step vaginal examination.*) **ACOG**
● Palpate the cervix, keeping in mind that it may assume a posterior position in early labor and may be difficult to locate. When you find the cervix, note its consistency. The cervix gradually softens throughout pregnancy, reaching a buttery consistency before labor begins. (See *Cervical effacement and dilation,* page 600.)
● After identifying the presenting fetal part and position, evaluating dilation and effacement, assessing fetal engagement and station, and verifying membrane status, gently withdraw your fingers. Let the patient clean her perineum herself with sterile gauze if she can walk to the bathroom. If she's confined to bed, you can clean her perineum and change the linen-saver pad.
● *To encourage the patient and help reduce her anxiety,* describe how labor is progressing, and define her stage and phase if appropriate.

Special considerations

● In early labor, perform the vaginal examination between contractions, focusing primarily on the extent of cervical dilation and effacement. At the end of first-stage labor, perform the examination during a

Step-by-step vaginal examination EB

Begin the vaginal examination — usually in early labor — by inserting your gloved index and middle fingers palm side down into the vagina. Use your nondominant hand to gently but firmly press on the uterus *to steady the fetal presenting part against the cervix for examination.*

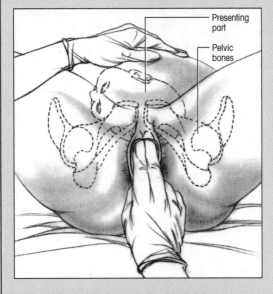

Presenting part

Pelvic bones

Confirm the presenting part and position

Rotate your fingers to palpate and confirm the fetal presenting part (a fetal head feels firm, the buttocks soft) and position (left, right, anterior, posterior, or transverse) identified by using Leopold's maneuvers.

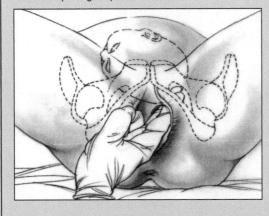

Assess cervical effacement and dilation

Estimate cervical dilation by palpating the internal os. Each fingerbreadth of dilation averages 1.5 to 2 cm, depending on the width of the examiner's finger.

Next, determine the percentage of effacement by palpating the ridge of tissue around the cervix. Assign a low percentage of effacement to defined and thick cervical tissue. Indistinct, wafer-thin cervical tissue scores 100%.

Assess fetal engagement and station

Estimate the extent of fetal engagement (descent of the fetal presenting part into the pelvis).

Palpate the presenting part and grade the fetal station (where the presenting part lies in relation to the ischial spines of the maternal pelvis). A zero grade indicates that the presenting part lies level with the ischial spine.

Station grades range from −3 (3 cm above the maternal ischial spines) to +4 (4 cm below the maternal ischial spines, causing the perineum to bulge).

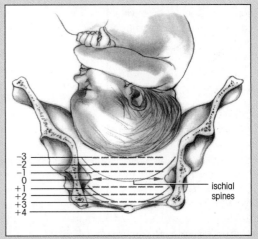

−3
−2
−1
0
+1
+2
+3
+4

ischial spines

Evaluate membrane status

If appropriate, also check amniotic membrane status. If you feel a bulging, slick surface over the presenting fetal part, you know the membranes are intact.

To test for amniotic fluid leakage, use Nitrazine test tape before applying lubricant for performing a vaginal examination. If amniotic fluid is present, the Nitrazine test tape changes color to deep blue.

Cervical effacement and dilation

As labor advances, so do cervical effacement and dilation, thereby facilitating birth. During effacement, the cervix shortens and its walls become thin, progressing from 0% effacement (palpable and thick) to 100% effacement (fully indistinct — or effaced — and paper thin). Full effacement obliterates the constrictive uterine neck to create a smooth, unobstructed passage for the fetus.

At the same time, dilation occurs. This progressive widening of the cervical canal — from the upper internal cervical os to the lower external cervical os — advances from 0 to 10 cm. As the cervical canal opens, resistance decreases. This further eases fetal descent.

No effacement or dilation

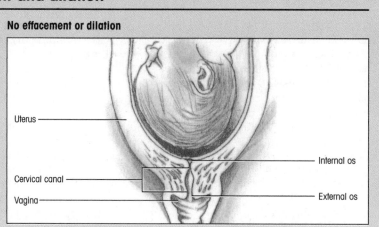

Uterus

Internal os

Cervical canal

External os

Vagina

Early effacement and dilation

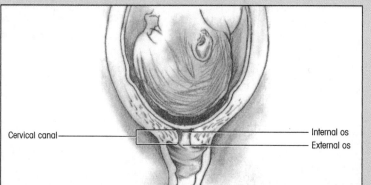

Cervical canal

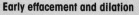

Internal os
External os

Full effacement and dilation

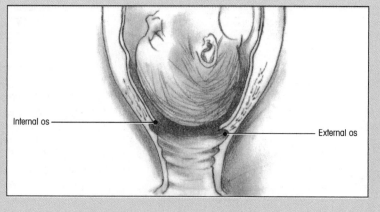

Internal os

External os

contraction, when the uterine muscle pushes the fetus downward. This examination will focus on assessing fetal descent.

● If the amniotic membrane ruptures during the examination, record the fetal heart rate (FHR). Note the time, and describe the color, odor, and approximate amount of fluid. If the FHR becomes unstable, determine fetal station, check for umbilical cord prolapse, and notify the physician. After the membranes rupture, perform the vaginal examination only when labor changes significantly *to minimize the risk of introducing intrauterine infection.*

Nursing diagnoses
● Anxiety

Expected outcomes
The patient will:
● express feelings of anxiety
● identify positive aspects of her ability to cope during childbirth.

Complications
Placental tears and hemorrhage may occur if procedure is performed during excessive vaginal bleeding.

Documentation
After each examination, record the percentage of effacement, dilation, the station of the presenting fetal part, amniotic membrane status, and the patient's tolerance of the procedure.

Supportive references
McKinney, E.S., et al. *Maternal-Child Nursing,* 2nd ed. Philadelphia: W.B. Saunders Co., 2004.

Olds, S.B., et al. *Clinical Handbook, Maternal-Newborn Nursing: A Family and Community-Based Approach,* 6th ed. Upper Saddle River, N.J.: Prentice Hall Health, 2000.

Pillitteri, A. *Maternal & Child Health Nursing: Care of the Childbearing & Childrearing Family,* 5th ed. Philadelphia: Lippincott Williams & Wilkins, 2007. **EB**

Wong, D.L., et al. *Maternal-Child Nursing Care,* 3rd ed. St. Louis: Mosby–Year Book, Inc., 2006.

Appendices
Index

Evaluating a research article

Research is a major force in nursing. The knowledge generated from research can influence and change nursing practice, education, and health policy. The use of research to provide a foundation for nursing practice and policy is called *evidence-based practice.* Evaluating or critiquing research is vital for developing and refining nursing knowledge. Often, the word *critique* has been made synonymous with the word *criticize,* which is commonly viewed as negative. In reality, a critique should be associated with critical thinking and appraisal and requires carefully developed intellectual skills.

Evaluating a research study involves careful examination of all aspects of the study to judge the strengths, weaknesses, meaning, and significance of the research.

Quality research should focus on a significant problem, demonstrate sound methodology, produce credible findings, and have the capacity to be replicated by others.

Evaluation of a research article should focus on the major components of the study, including problem statement, review of the literature, conceptual framework, hypothesis, method, results, and the conclusion derived from those results. When evaluating a research article, ask these questions.

Problem statement

- What is studied?
- What are the dependent variables (the response or behavior predicted in the research) and the independent variables (the treatment implemented by the researcher to create a response or behavior)?
- Why is the problem important?

The problem statement should be clear and concise and needs to focus on significant practice problems, if a sound knowledge base is to be identified.

Review of the literature

- Does the literature review relate to the study? How?
- Is the review current?
- Is previous research on the topic included in the review?

The literature review should also include a range of opinions and varying points of view about the problem.

Conceptual framework

- Does the study relate to the previous research conducted on the problem? How?
- Does the study fit with current knowledge about the problem?

The relationship identified in the conceptual framework should be clear; if not, the research may not be cohesive.

Hypothesis

- What relationship is tested?
- Can the question be answered by the data collected?

The hypothesis or research question is directly derived from the problem statement. If the question can't be answered by the research, then the research has little value.

Method

Evaluation of the method used determines if the research can be generalized. The method of a research study includes the sample, treatment, instruments used, and data analysis.

● Sample — How are the subjects chosen? What's the size of the sample and is it appropriate for the research study? How does the sample relate to the population (demographic) data?

● Treatment — How is the treatment assigned to the subjects? How and where is the treatment carried out (in a clinical or nonclinical setting)?

● Instruments — What are the instruments used? Are the instruments appropriate for the study? Are the instruments valid? Are they reliable? If the instruments are developed for the study, how are they developed? What's the procedure to develop the instruments?

● Data analysis — How's the data analyzed? Is the analytical method appropriate for the research? If graphics (tables, charts, and graphs) are used, are they presented clearly? Are they clearly presented in the text?

Results

● What are the results of the study?

● Are the results discussed in relation to the theoretical or conceptual framework?

● Are all the questions answered?

The results section of a research article deserves special attention because this is the outcome of the research.

Conclusions

● What conclusion (or meaning) does the researcher draw from the results?

● Do the results make sense?

● What are the limitations in using the results? (This may identify the strengths and weaknesses of the study.)

● What recommendations does the researcher make for the current practice and for further research?

Implications for practice should consider limitations of the study that would affect the generalizability of the results to similar populations. Only well structured comprehensive studies should be considered when being used for evidence-based practice.

All studies have their strengths and weaknesses. Recognizing these strengths is imperative for generating scientific knowledge and using the findings in practice.

Supportive references

Burns, N., and Grove, S. *The Practice of Nursing Research, Conduct, Critique, & Utilization,* 5th ed. Philadelphia: W.B. Saunders Co., 2005.

DiCenso, A., et al. *Evidence-Based Nursing — A Guide to Clinical Practice,* St. Louis: Mosby–Year Book, Inc., 2005.

Drevdahl, D., et al. "Uncontested Categories: The Use of Race and Ethnicity Variables in Nursing Research," *Nursing Inquiry* (1):52-63, March 2006.

Klardie, K., et al. "Integrating the Principles of Evidence-Based Practice into Clinical Practice," *Journal of American Academy of Nurse Practitioners* 16(3):98-105, March 2004.

LoBiondo-Wood, G., and Haber, J. *Nursing Research: Methods and Critical Appraisal for Evidence-Based Practice,* 6th ed. St. Louis: Mosby–Year Book, Inc., 2006.

Olsen, D. "HIPAA Privacy Regulations and Nursing Research," *Nursing Research* 52(5):344-48, September-October 2003.

Polit, D., and Fineout-Overholt, E. *Essentials of Nursing Research: Methods, Appraisal, and Utilization,* 6th ed. Philadelphia: Lippincott Williams & Wilkins, 2006.

Whittemore, R. "Combining Evidence in Nursing Research: Methods and Implications," *Nursing Research* 54(1):56-62, January-February 2005.

Resources

This list of national organizations can provide information on health care services and treatment.

American Academy of Dermatology
1350 I St. N.W., Suite 870
Washington, DC 20005-4355
www.aad.org

American Academy of Orthopaedic Surgeons
6300 North River Rd.
Rosemont, IL 60018-4262
www.aaos.org

American Academy of Pain Management
13947 Mono Way #A
Sonora, CA 95370
www.aapainmanage.org

American Academy of Pediatrics
141 Northwest Point Blvd.
Elk Grove Village, IL 60007
www.aap.org

American Association for Respiratory Care
9425 N. MacArthur Blvd., Suite 100
Irving, TX 75063-4706
www.aarc.org

American Association of Critical-Care Nurses
101 Columbia
Aliso Viejo, CA 92656-4109
www.aacn.org

American Cancer Society
1599 Clifton Rd. N.E.
Atlanta, GA 30329
www.cancer.org

American Chronic Pain Association
P.O. Box 850
Rocklin, CA 95677
www.theacpa.org

American College of Cardiology
Heart House
9111 Old Georgetown Rd.
Bethesda, MD 20814-1699
www.acc.org

American College of Obstetricians and Gynecologists
409 12th St. S.W.
P.O. Box 96920
Washington, DC 20090-6920
www.acog.com

American Gastroenterological Association
4930 Del Ray Ave.
Bethesda, MD 20814
www.gastro.org

American Heart Association
National Center
7272 Greenville Ave.
Dallas, TX 75231
www.americanheart.org

American Hospital Association
One North Franklin
Chicago IL 60606-3421
www.aha.org

American Kidney Fund
6110 Executive Blvd., Suite 1010
Rockville, MD 20852
www.kidneyfund.org

American Liver Foundation
75 Maiden Lane, Suite 603
New York, NY 10038
www.liverfoundation.org

American Lung Association
61 Broadway, 6th Floor
New York, NY 10006
www.lungusa.org

American Nephrology Nurses' Association
East Holly Ave.
P.O. Box 56
Pitman, NJ 08071-0056
www.anna.inurse.com

American Nurses Association
8515 Georgia Ave., Suite 400
Silver Spring, MD 20910
www.ana.org

American Pain Society
4700 W. Lake Ave.
Glenview, IL 60025
www.ampainsoc.org

American Physical Therapy Association
1111 N. Fairfax St.
Alexandria, VA 22314-1488
www.apta.org

American Society for Parenteral and Enteral Nutrition
8630 Fenton St., Suite 412
Silver Spring, MD 20910
www.clinnutr.org

Arthritis Foundation
P.O. Box 7669
Atlanta, GA 30357-0669
www.arthritis.org

Association of Women's Health, Obstetric and Neonatal Nurses
2000 L St. N.W., Suite 740
Washington, DC 20036
www.awhonn.org

Best Practice Network (American Association of Critical Care Nurses)
101 Columbia
Aliso Viejo, CA 92656-4109
www.aacn.org/aacn/aacnsite.nsf/htmlmedia/
best_practice_network.html

Centers for Disease Control and Prevention
1600 Clifton Rd.
Atlanta, GA 30333
www.cdc.gov

Centers for Medicare & Medicaid Services
7500 Security Blvd.
Baltimore, MD 21244
www.cms.hhs.gov

Dermatology Nurses' Association
East Holly Ave.
P.O. Box 56
Pitman, NJ 08071-0056
www.dna.inurse.com

Emergency Nurses Association
915 Lee St.
Des Plaines, IL 60016-6569
www.ena.org

Hospice Patients Alliance
4541 Gemini St.
P.O. Box 744
Rockford, MI 49341-0744
www.hospicepatients.org

Infusion Nurses Society
220 Norwood Park South
Norwood, MA 02062
www.ins1.org

Institute for Safe Medication Practices
1800 Byberry Rd., Suite 810
Huntingdon Valley, PA 19006
www.ismp.org

Institute of Medicine of the National Academies
500 Fifth St. N.W.
Washington, DC 20001
www.iom.edu

International Foundation for Functional Gastrointestinal Disorders
P.O. Box 170864
Milwaukee, WI 53217-8076
www.iffgd.org

Joint Commission on Accreditation of Healthcare Organizations
One Renaissance Blvd.
Oakbrook Terrace, IL 60181
www.jcaho.org

National Association for Continence
P.O. Box 1019
Charleston, SC 29402-1019
www.nafc.org

National Association of Orthopaedic Nurses
401 North Michigan Ave., Suite 200
Chicago, IL 60611
www.orthonurse.com

National Cancer Institute
9000 Rockville Pike
Bethesda, MD 20314
www.cancer.gov

National Heart, Lung, and Blood Institute
P.O. Box 30105
Bethesda, MD 20824-0105
www.nhlbi.nih.gov/

National Hospice and Palliative Care Organization
1700 Diagonal Rd., Suite 625
Alexandria, VA 22314
www.nhpco.org

National Institute for Occupational Safety and Health
1600 Clifton Rd. N.E.
Atlanta, GA 30333
www.cdc.gov/niosh

National Institute of Diabetes, Digestive & Kidney Diseases
Bldg. 31, Rm. 9A04 Center Dr., MSC 2560
Bethesda, MD 20892-2560
www.niddk.nih.gov

National Institute of Neurological Disorders and Stroke
P.O. Box 5801
Bethesda, MD 20824
www.ninds.nih.gov

National Institutes of Health
9000 Rockville Pike
Bethesda, MD 20892
www.nih.gov

National Kidney Foundation
30 E. 33rd St.
New York, NY 10016
www.kidney.org

National Osteoporosis Foundation
1232 22nd St. N.W.
Washington, DC 20037-1292
www.nof.org

National Stroke Association
9707 E. Easter Lane
Englewood, CO 80112
www.stroke.org

Occupational Safety & Health Administration
U.S. Department of Labor
200 Constitution Ave.
Washington, DC 20210
www.osha.gov

Oncology Nursing Society
125 Enterprise Dr.
Pittsburgh, PA 15275
www.ons.org

Planned Parenthood Federation of America, Inc.
434 West 33rd St.
New York, NY 10001
www.plannedparenthood.org

U.S. Department of Health and Human Services
200 Independence Ave. S.W.
Washington, DC 20201
www.hhs.gov

Wound, Ostomy & Continence Nurses Society
15000 Commerce Parkway, Suite C
Mt. Laurel, NJ 08054
www.wocn.org

Index

i refers to an illustration; t refers to a table.

i refers to an illustration; t refers to a table.

i refers to an illustration; t refers to a table.

---

i refers to an illustration; t refers to a table.

---

i refers to an illustration; t refers to a table.

---

i refers to an illustration; t refers to a table.

i refers to an illustration; t refers to a table.

i refers to an illustration; t refers to a table.

i refers to an illustration; t refers to a table.

---

i refers to an illustration; t refers to a table.

i refers to an illustration; t refers to a table.

---

i refers to an illustration; t refers to a table.

i refers to an illustration; t refers to a table.

i refers to an illustration; t refers to a table.

i refers to an illustration; t refers to a table.

i refers to an illustration; t refers to a table.

i refers to an illustration; t refers to a table.